CALCULATION OF DRUG DOSAGES

A Work Text

CALCULATION OF DRUG DOSAGES

A Work Text

ELEVENTH EDITION

Sheila J. Ogden, MSN, RN
President and CEO
SJOgden Consulting, Inc.
Indianapolis, Indiana

Linda K. Fluharty, MSN, RN
Professor
School of Nursing
Ivy Tech Community College
Indianapolis, Indiana

ELSEVIER

ELSEVIER

3251 Riverport Lane
St. Louis, Missouri 63043

CALCULATION OF DRUG DOSAGES:
A WORK TEXT, ELEVENTH EDITION

ISBN: 978-0-323-55128-1

Notices

Knowledge and best practice in this field are constantly changing. As new research and experience broaden our understanding, changes in research methods, professional practices, or medical treatment may become necessary.

Practitioners and researchers must always rely on their own experience and knowledge in evaluating and using any information, methods, compounds, or experiments described herein. In using such information or methods they should be mindful of their own safety and the safety of others, including parties for whom they have a professional responsibility.

With respect to any drug or pharmaceutical products identified, readers are advised to check the most current information provided (i) on procedures featured or (ii) by the manufacturer of each product to be administered, to verify the recommended dose or formula, the method and duration of administration, and contraindications. It is the responsibility of practitioners, relying on their own experience and knowledge of their patients, to make diagnoses, to determine dosages and the best treatment for each individual patient, and to take all appropriate safety precautions.

To the fullest extent of the law, neither the Publisher nor the authors, contributors, or editors, assume any liability for any injury and/or damage to persons or property as a matter of products liability, negligence or otherwise, or from any use or operation of any methods, products, instructions, or ideas contained in the material herein.

Library of Congress Control Number: 2018944862

Senior Content Strategist: Yvonne Alexopoulos
Content Development Manager: Lisa Newton
Senior Content Development Specialist: Danielle M. Frazier
Publishing Services Manager: Catherine A. Jackson
Senior Project Manager: Carrie Stetz
Design Direction: Margaret Reid

Printed in Canada

Last digit is the print number: 9 8 7 6 5 4

To David, my husband and best friend, for your patience, support, and love;
and to our wonderful family, John, Shannon, Kate, Claire,
Amy, Ryan, Connor, Carter, Justin, and Celeste.
Love, Sheila, Mom, and Nana.

S.J.O.

To my parents, Richard and Arlene Duke,
for their love and support when I said I wanted to be a nurse.
Love, Linda.

L.K.F.

CONTENT AND MATH REVIEWERS

Emily R. Berkowitz, RN, MSN, CEN, CCRN, CNE, ANP-C, PhD
Nursing Faculty and Coordinator
Nursing Department
El Centro College
Dallas, Texas

Lou Ann Boose, MSN, RN
Senior Professor
Harrisburg Area Community College
Harrisburg, Pennsylvania

Jessica Gonzales, ARNP
Advanced Registered Nurse Practitioner
Private Practice
Redmond, Washington

Stephanie Holmes-Thomas, MSN, BSN, RN, CDP
DNP Student
Health & Legal Studies, Nursing Faculty
El Centro College
Dallas, Texas

Quanza Elise Mooring, PhD, RN
Assistant Professor
Hunt School of Nursing
Gardner-Webb University
Boiling Springs, North Carolina

Paula D. Silver, BS, PharmD
Medical Instructor
Medical Careers School of Health Sciences and Technology
ECPI University
Newport News, Virginia

ACKNOWLEDGMENTS

We are grateful to the students and instructors who have chosen to use this book; we continue to learn so much from each of you. You have helped us understand the problems that students have with basic mathematics and with the calculation of drug dosages. We appreciate the physicians, nurses, pharmacists, and representatives of various health care agencies who took the time to discuss topics with us. We hope this book will provide readers with a feeling of confidence when working with a variety of mathematical problems.

We want to give special thanks to the reviewers of this text. Your sincere evaluation and critique played an integral part in the revision of this edition, and your attention to detail was most helpful.

We would also like to acknowledge Carrie Stetz, Danielle Frazier, and Yvonne Alexopoulos for their help and support during the writing of this eleventh edition. Danielle supplied answers to many questions, pushed to meet deadlines, and offered her services as needed. She also remained calm and offered guidance during the entire revision process. Yvonne has been diligent in providing clarity on the needs of students, faculty, and hospitals as the scope and use of the book continue to grow.

Thank you all so much!

Sheila J. Ogden

Linda K. Fluharty

This work text is designed for students in professional and vocational schools of nursing and for nurses returning to practice after being away from the clinical setting. It can be used in the classroom or for individual study. The work text contains an extensive review of basic mathematics to assist students who have not mastered the subject in previous educational experiences. It can also be used by those who have not attended school for a number of years and feel a lack of confidence in the area of mathematics computations.

ORGANIZATION OF MATERIAL

A pretest precedes each chapter in Parts One and Two and may be used for evaluating present skills. For those students who are comfortable with basic mathematics, a quick assessment of each area will confirm their competency in the subject matter.

Part Two begins with the use of the metric system, which is predominant in the medical field. The apothecary system continues to decline in use to the point of being almost extinct. However, in remembering that differences in practice exist throughout the United States and the world, it was felt that some of that content should remain in the book. Therefore it has been placed in the Appendix for reference. Chapter 7 emphasizes calculations used in patient assessments.

Part Three helps students prepare for the actual calculation of drug dosages. Chapter 8 combines material from all previous chapters and discusses various points concerning patient safety as it relates to medication administration. This chapter also includes safety issues for the nurse in the dispensing of medication. The case scenarios emphasize the importance of delivering the correct medication to the patient as ordered. Chapter 9 emphasizes the interpretation of the licensed prescribers' orders, and Chapter 10 explains how to read medication labels.

Part Four is named the Calculation of Drug Dosages. As students begin their clinical experiences, they start with basic medical-surgical patients. Therefore the content moves from oral to parenteral, units, reconstitution, and, finally, intravenous flow rates. Part Four includes substantial content on dimensional analysis as a method for solving problems of drug calculations. This method has become the preferred method of use by numerous schools of nursing.

However, many schools have remained with the ratio/proportion or formula methods. Examples of each type of calculation are shown first with dimensional analysis followed by the proportion and formula methods. The division of the three methods will allow instructors to target the area of study they prefer for their students and/or schools.

The actual drug labels have been updated and increased in number in all chapters that discuss the calculation of drug dosages. Also in Part Four, the content has been separated and expanded for dosages measured in units (Chapter 13) and the reconstitution of medications (Chapter 14). These are two separate concepts and are sometimes difficult for students to understand. This separation allows for extended practice and attention to each chapter's content.

More medications are being delivered to patients via the intravenous route, not only in intensive care units, but also in progressive care and medical-surgical areas as well. Chapter 15, Intravenous Flow Rates, and Chapter 16, Intravenous Flow Rates for Dosages Measured in Units, address this reality. Chapter 17 remains focused on Critical Care Intravenous Flow Rates. Chapter 18, Pediatric Dosages, continues to include oral, parenteral, and intravenous flow rate problems. Chapter 19, Obstetric Dosages, remains to address calculation in regards to obstetric patients.

The majority of the calculation problems relating to drug dosages continue to represent actual licensed prescribers' orders in various health care settings.

FEATURES IN THE ELEVENTH EDITION

- **Learning objectives** are listed at the beginning of each chapter so students will know the goals that must be achieved.
- Chapter **work sheets** provide the opportunity to practice solving realistic problems.
- Almost every chapter contains two **posttests** designed to evaluate the student's learning.
- A **comprehensive posttest** at the end of the book will help students assess their total understanding of the process of calculation of drug dosages.
- A **glossary** is included to define important terms.
- Numerous **full-color drug labels** continue to provide a more realistic representation of medication administration.

ANCILLARIES

Evolve resources for instructors and students can be found online at http://evolve.elsevier.com/Ogden/calculation/

The instructor resources are designed to help instructors present the material in this text and include the following:

- Drug Label Glossary
- TEACH Lesson Plan
- TEACH Lecture Outlines
- TEACH PowerPoint Slides
- Test Bank
- Chapter Teaching Strategies
- Suggested Class Schedules
- Image Collection

Student Resources provide students with additional tools for learning and include the following:

- Student Practice Problems and Learning Activities
- Flash Cards

NEW! Elsevier's Interactive Drug Calculation Application, Version 1. This interactive drug calculations application provides hands on, interactive practice for the user to master drug calculations. Users can select the mode (Study, Exam, or Comprehensive Exam) and then the category for study and exam modes. Eight categories cover the main drug calculation topics. Users are able to select the number of problems they want to complete and their preferred drug calculation method. A calculator is available for easy access within any mode, and the application also provides history of the work done by the user.

DESCRIPTION AND FEATURES

Calculation of Drug Dosages is an innovative drug calculation work text designed to provide you with a systematic review of mathematics and a simplified method of calculating drug dosages. It affords you the opportunity to move at a comfortable pace to ensure success. It includes information on the dimensional analysis, ratio and proportion, and formula methods of drug calculation, as well as numerous practice problems. Take a look at the following features so that you may familiarize yourself with this text and maximize its value.

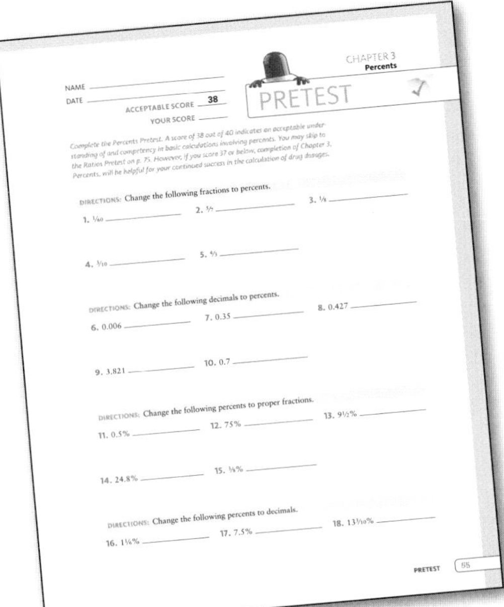

CHAPTER 3
Percents

PRETEST

NAME ________
DATE ________
ACCEPTABLE SCORE **38**
YOUR SCORE ________

Complete the Percents Pretest. A score of 38 out of 40 indicates an acceptable understanding of and competency in basic calculations involving percents. You may skip to the Ratios Pretest on p. 75. However, if you score 37 or below, completion of Chapter 3, Percents, will be helpful for your continued success in the calculation of drug dosages.

DIRECTIONS: Change the following fractions to percents.

1. 1/60 ________ 2. 5/7 ________ 3. 1/8 ________
4. 3/10 ________ 5. 4/3 ________

DIRECTIONS: Change the following decimals to percents.

6. 0.006 ________ 7. 0.35 ________ 8. 0.427 ________
9. 3.821 ________ 10. 0.7 ________

DIRECTIONS: Change the following percents to proper fractions.

11. 0.5% ________ 12. 75% ________ 13. 9½% ________
14. 24.8% ________ 15. 1/8% ________

DIRECTIONS: Change the following percents to decimals.

16. 1⅙% ________ 17. 7.5% ________ 18. 13 3/10% ________

PRETEST 65

Pretests evaluate your present skills in utilizing mathematics, units, and measurements.

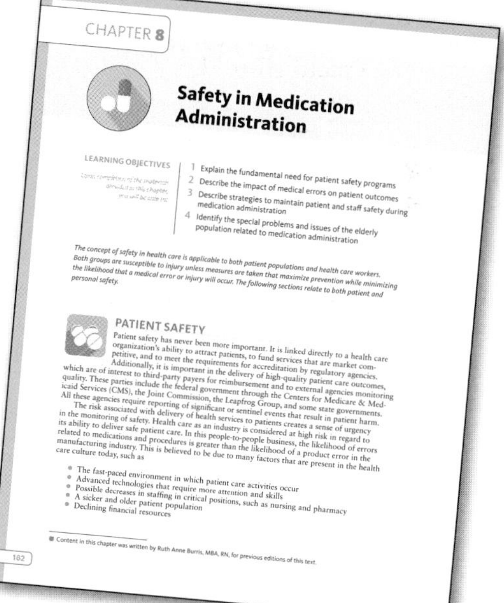

CHAPTER 8

Safety in Medication Administration

LEARNING OBJECTIVES

1 Explain the fundamental need for patient safety programs
2 Describe the impact of medical errors on patient outcomes
3 Describe strategies to maintain patient and staff safety during medication administration
4 Identify the special problems and issues of the elderly population related to medication administration

The concept of safety in health care is applicable to both patient populations and health care workers. Both groups are susceptible to injury unless measures are taken that maximize prevention while minimizing the likelihood that a medical error or injury will occur. The following sections relate to both patient and personal safety.

PATIENT SAFETY

Patient safety has never been more important. It is linked directly to a health care organization's ability to attract patients, to fund services that are market competitive, and to meet the requirements for accreditation by regulatory agencies.

Additionally, it is important in the delivery of high-quality patient care outcomes, which are of interest to third-party payers for reimbursement and to external agencies monitoring quality. These parties include the federal government through the Centers for Medicare & Medicaid Services (CMS), the Joint Commission, the Leapfrog Group, and some state governments. All these agencies require reporting of significant or sentinel events that result in patient harm.

The risk associated with delivery of health services to patients creates a sense of urgency in the monitoring of safety. Health care as an industry is considered at high risk in regard to its ability to deliver safe patient care. In this people-to-people business, the likelihood of errors related to medications and procedures is greater than the likelihood of a product error in the manufacturing industry. This is believed to be due to many factors that are present in the health care culture today, such as

- The fast-paced environment in which patient care activities occur
- Advanced technologies that require more attention and skills
- Possible decreases in staffing in critical positions, such as nursing and pharmacy
- A sicker and older patient population
- Declining financial resources

Content in this chapter was written by Ruth Anne Burris, MBA, RN, for previous editions of this text.

182

Learning Objectives highlight key content and goals that must be achieved.

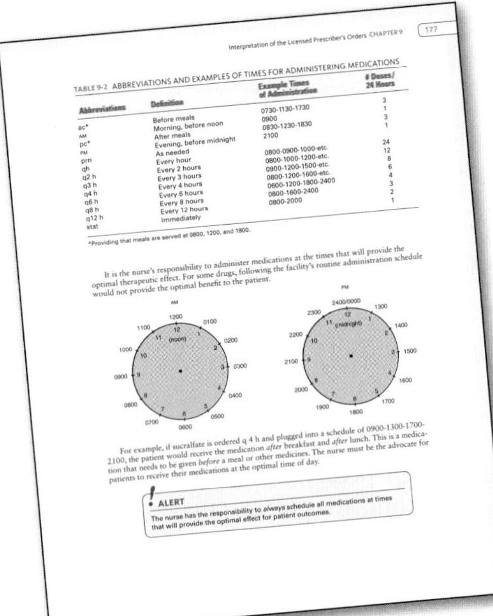

Interpretation of the Licensed Prescriber's Orders CHAPTER 9 177

TABLE 9-2 ABBREVIATIONS AND EXAMPLES OF TIMES FOR ADMINISTERING MEDICATIONS

Abbreviations	Definition	Example Times of Administration	# Doses/24 Hours
ac*	Before meals	0730-1130-1730	3
AM	Morning, before noon	0900	1
pc*	After meals	0830-1230-1830	3
PM	Evening, before midnight	2100	1
prn	As needed		
qh	Every hour	0800-0900-1000-etc.	24
q2 h	Every 2 hours	0800-1000-1200-etc.	12
q3 h	Every 3 hours	0900-1200-1500-etc.	8
q4 h	Every 4 hours	0800-1200-1600-etc.	6
q6 h	Every 6 hours	0600-1200-1800-2400	4
q8 h	Every 8 hours	0800-1600-2400	3
q12 h	Every 12 hours	0800-2000	2
stat	Immediately		1

*Providing that meals are served at 0800, 1200, and 1800.

It is the nurse's responsibility to administer medications at the times that will provide the optimal therapeutic effect. For some drugs, following the facility's routine administration schedule would not provide the optimal benefit to the patient.

For example, if sucralfate is ordered q 4 h and plugged into a schedule of 0900-1300-1700-2100, the patient would receive the medication *after* breakfast and *after* lunch. This is a medication that needs to be given *before* a meal or other medicines. The nurse must be the advocate for patients to receive their medications at the optimal time of day.

ALERT

The nurse has the responsibility to always schedule all medications at times that will provide the optimal effect for patient outcomes.

Alerts highlight potential and common drug calculation errors.

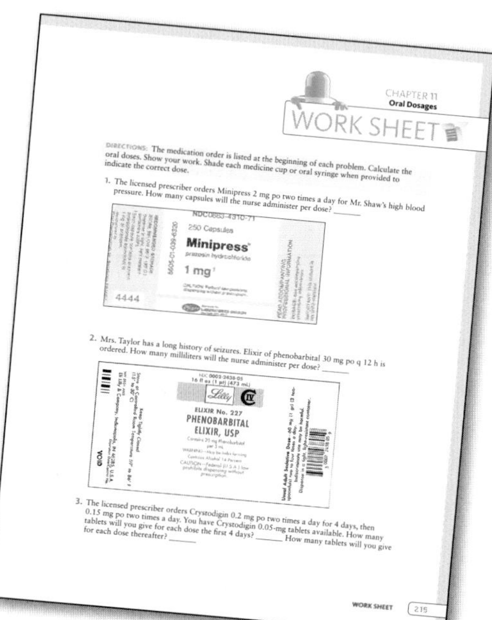

CHAPTER 11 Oral Dosages

WORK SHEET

DIRECTIONS: The medication order is listed at the beginning of each problem. Calculate the oral doses. Show your work. Shade each medicine cup or oral syringe when provided to indicate the correct dose.

1. The licensed prescriber orders Minipress 2 mg po two times a day for Mr. Shaw's high blood pressure. How many capsules will the nurse administer per dose? _____

2. Mrs. Taylor has a long history of seizures. Elixir of phenobarbital 30 mg po q 12 h is ordered. How many milliliters will the nurse administer per dose? _____

3. The licensed prescriber orders Crystodigin 0.2 mg po two times a day for 4 days, then 0.15 mg po two times a day. You have Crystodigin 0.05-mg tablets available. How many tablets will you give for each dose the first 4 days? _____ How many tablets will you give for each dose thereafter? _____

WORK SHEET 215

Work Sheets provide you with the opportunity to practice solving realistic problems.

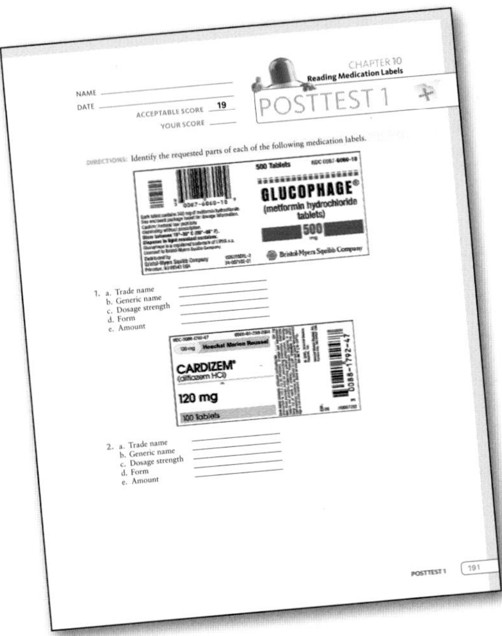

CHAPTER 10 Reading Medication Labels

POSTTEST 1

NAME _____
DATE _____
ACCEPTABLE SCORE 19
YOUR SCORE _____

DIRECTIONS: Identify the requested parts of each of the following medication labels.

1. a. Trade name
   b. Generic name
   c. Dosage strength
   d. Form
   e. Amount

2. a. Trade name
   b. Generic name
   c. Dosage strength
   d. Form
   e. Amount

POSTTEST 1 191

Posttests are designed to assess your learning and identify your strengths and weaknesses.

NEW! Elsevier's Interactive Drug Calculation Application, Version 1. This interactive drug calculations application provides hands on, interactive practice for the user to master drug calculations. Users can select the mode (Study, Exam, or Comprehensive Exam) and then the category for study and exam modes. Eight categories cover the main drug calculation topics. Users are also able to select the number of problems they want to complete and their preferred drug calculation method. A calculator is available for easy access within any mode, and the application also provides history of the work done by the user.

evolve Look for this icon at the end of the chapters. It will refer to *Elsevier's Interactive Drug Calculation Application, Version 1* for additional practice problems and content information.

USING THIS WORK TEXT

A pretest precedes each chapter in Parts One and Two to assess previous learning. If your grade on the pretest is acceptable (an acceptable score is noted at the top of the test), you may continue to the next pretest. If your score on the pretest indicates a need for further study, read the introduction to the chapter, study the method of solving the problems, and complete the work sheet. If you have difficulty with a problem, refer to the examples in the introduction.

On completion of the work sheet, refer to the answer key at the end of each chapter to verify that your answers are correct. Rework all the incorrect problems to find your errors. It may be necessary to refer again to the examples in each chapter. Then proceed to the first posttest and grade the test. if your grade is acceptable, as indicated at the top of the test, continue to the next chapter. If your grade is less than acceptable, rework all incorrect problems to find your errors. Review as necessary before completing the second posttest. Again, verify that your answers are correct. At this point, if you have followed the system of study, your grade on the second posttest should be more than acceptable. Follow the same system of study in each of the chapters.

When all the chapters in the work text are completed with acceptable scores (between 95% and 100%), you should be proficient in solving problems relating to drug dosages; more important, you will have completed the first step toward becoming a safe practitioner of medication administration.

On completion of the material provided in this work text, you will have mastered the following mathematical concepts for use in the accurate performance of computations:

1. Solving problems using fractions, decimals, percents, ratios, proportions, and dimensional analysis
2. Solving problems involving the apothecary, metric, and household systems of measurements
3. Solving problems measured in units and milliequivalents
4. Solving problems related to oral and parenteral dosages
5. Solving problems involving intravenous flow rates and critical care intravenous flow rates
6. Solving problems confirming the correct dosage of pediatric medications
7. Solving problems confirming the correct dosages of obstetric medications
8. Solving problems by using dimensional analysis, ratio and proportion, and formula methods.

You are now ready to begin Chapter 1!

CONTENTS

REVIEW of MATHEMATICS

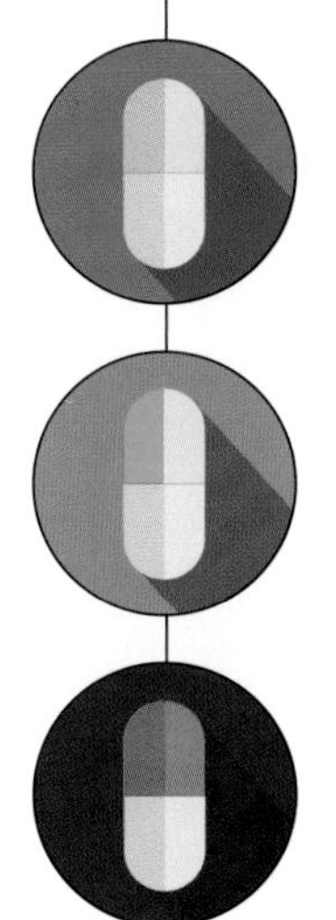

A solid knowledge base of general mathematics is necessary before you will be able to use these concepts in the more complicated calculations of drug dosages. It is this knowledge that allows for the safe administration of medications to your patients and prevents medication errors.

For students who have been away from basic mathematics awhile, please take the time and effort to review the multiplication tables of one through twelve. These tables must be memorized to allow ease in the computation of all problems found in this textbook.

As you prepare to learn how to calculate drug dosages, an assessment of your current basic mathematics understanding and competency is essential. A general mathematics pretest is provided. Allow 1 to 2 hours in a quiet study area to complete the pretest. This is your opportunity to assess your true capability of performing basic math problems. Calculators are very useful tools. In most areas of health care, the use of a calculator is actually required to ensure accuracy in the delivery of medications. Follow the direction of your instructor as to the acceptable use of calculators while using this text on your path to safe administration of medications.

The pretest allows you to assess your need for a more extensive review. After completion of the test, check your answers with the key provided. A score of 95%, or 48 out of 50 problems correct, indicates a firm foundation in basic mathematics. You may then skip to Part 2, Units and Measurements for the Calculation of Drug Dosages. However, a score of 47 or below indicates a need to review fraction, decimal, percent, ratio, and/or proportion calculations. Chapters 1 through 5 allow you to work on these basic mathematical skills at your leisure.

The pretest and review chapters are provided to ensure your success in the calculation and administration of your future patients' medications. Begin now, and good luck!

NAME ____________________

DATE ____________________

ACCEPTABLE SCORE 48

YOUR SCORE ______

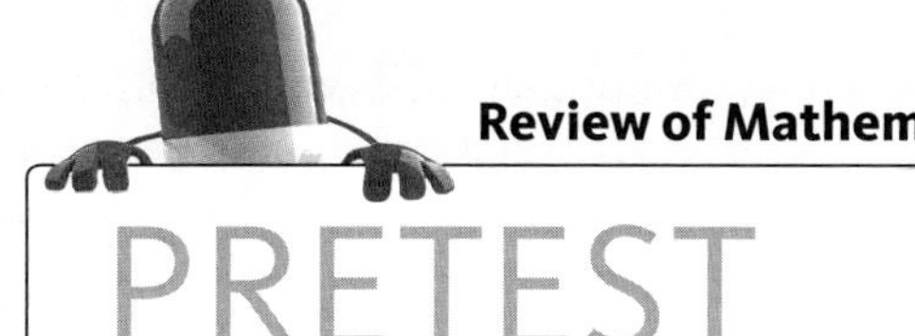

Review of Mathematics

PRETEST

DIRECTIONS: Perform the indicated computations. Reduce fractions to lowest terms.

1. $\frac{3}{8} + \frac{1}{3} =$ ______

2. $2\frac{3}{7} + 1\frac{2}{3} =$ ______

3. $1\frac{3}{5} + \frac{7}{8}/\frac{1}{3} =$ ______

4. $1.03 + 2.2 + 1.134 =$ ______

5. $1.479 + 28.68 + 4.5 =$ ______

6. $\frac{14}{15} - \frac{1}{6} =$ ______

7. $2\frac{1}{3} - \frac{1}{2} =$ ______

8. $2.04 - 0.987 =$ ______

9. $8.53 - 7.945 =$ ______

10. $3 \times \frac{4}{7} =$ ______

11. $2\frac{1}{2} \times 3\frac{3}{5} =$ ______

12. $0.315 \times 5.8 =$ ______

13. $4.884 \times 6.51 =$ ______

14. $\frac{3}{5} \div \frac{5}{6} =$ ______

15. $\frac{1}{150} \div \frac{1}{20} =$ ______

16. $2\frac{3}{4} \div 6\frac{2}{3} =$ ______

17. $241.73 \div 3.6 =$ ______

18. $22.68 \div 4.2 =$ ______

DIRECTIONS: Circle the decimal fraction that has the *least* value.

19. 0.3, 0.03, 0.003

20. 0.9, 0.45, 0.66

21. 0.72, 0.721, 0.0072

DIRECTIONS: Circle the decimal fraction that has the *greatest* value.

22. 0.1, 0.15, 0.155

23. 0.249, 0.1587, 0.00633

24. 2.913, 2.99, 2.9

DIRECTIONS: Change the following fractions to decimals.

25. $5/8$ = ________________ **26.** $17/25$ = ________________

DIRECTIONS: Change the following decimals to fractions reduced to lowest terms.

27. 0.375 = ________________ **28.** 0.05 = ________________

DIRECTIONS: Perform the indicated computations.

29. Express 0.432 as a percent.

30. Express 65% as a proper fraction and reduce to the lowest terms.

31. Express 0.3% as a ratio.

32. What percent of 2.5 is 0.5?

33. What is $1/4$% of 60?

34. What is 65% of 450?

DIRECTIONS: Change the following fractions and decimals to ratios reduced to lowest terms.

35. $9/42$ = ________________ **36.** $1\frac{1}{2}/2\frac{2}{3}$ = ________________ **37.** 0.34 = ________________

DIRECTIONS: Find the value of x.

38. $7 : 7/100 :: x : 4$

39. $x : 40 :: 7 : 56$

40. $2.5 : 6 :: 10 : x$

41. $x : 1/4\% :: 9.6 : 1/300$

42. $1/150 : 1/100 :: x : 30$

43. $0.10 : 0.20 :: x : 200$

44. $\frac{1}{200} : \frac{1}{40} :: 100 : x$

45. $x : 85 :: 6 : 10$

46. $\frac{1}{20}/\frac{1}{5} : 5 :: x : 50$

47. $100 : 5 :: x : 3.4$

48. $75 : x :: 36 : 6$

49. $\frac{1}{3} : \frac{2}{5} :: x : 30$

50. $x : 9 :: 98 : 7$

ANSWERS ON P. 6.

ANSWERS

REVIEW OF MATHEMATICS PRETEST, pp. 3–5

1. $\frac{17}{24}$
2. $4\frac{2}{21}$
3. $4\frac{9}{40}$
4. 4.364
5. 34.659
6. $\frac{23}{30}$
7. $1\frac{5}{6}$
8. 1.053
9. 0.585
10. $1\frac{5}{7}$
11. 9
12. 1.827
13. 31.79484
14. $\frac{18}{25}$
15. $\frac{2}{15}$
16. $\frac{33}{80}$
17. 67.14722
18. 5.4
19. 0.003
20. 0.45
21. 0.0072
22. 0.155
23. 0.249
24. 2.99
25. 0.625
26. 0.68
27. $\frac{3}{8}$
28. $\frac{1}{20}$
29. 43.2%
30. $\frac{13}{20}$
31. 3:1000
32. 20%
33. 0.15
34. 292.5
35. 3:14
36. 9:16
37. 17:50
38. 400
39. 5
40. 24
41. $7\frac{1}{5}$ or 7.2
42. 20
43. 100
44. 500
45. 51
46. $2\frac{1}{2}$ or 2.5
47. 68
48. 12.5
49. 25
50. 126

NAME ______________________

DATE ______________________

ACCEPTABLE SCORE **29**

YOUR SCORE ______

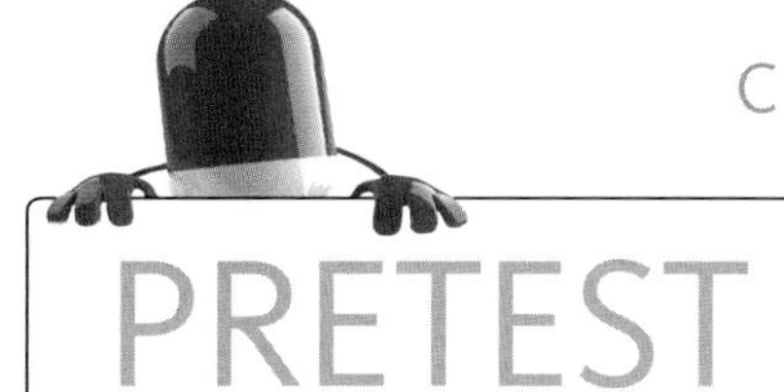

PRETEST

Complete the Fractions Pretest. A score of 29 out of 30 indicates an acceptable understanding of and competency in basic calculations involving fractions. You may skip to the Decimals Pretest on p. 31. However, if you scored 28 or below, completion of Chapter 1, Fractions, will be helpful for your continued success in the calculation of drug dosages.

DIRECTIONS: Perform the indicated calculations and reduce fractions to lowest terms.

1. $\frac{5}{7} + \frac{4}{9} =$ ______ **2.** $2\frac{1}{2} + 8\frac{1}{6} =$ ______ **3.** $3\frac{13}{20} + 1\frac{3}{10} + 4\frac{4}{5} =$ ______

4. $2\frac{5}{16} + 3\frac{1}{4} =$ ______ **5.** $5\frac{6}{11} + 3\frac{1}{2} =$ ______ **6.** $3\frac{2}{3} + 4\frac{2}{9} =$ ______

7. $1\frac{3}{4} + 2\frac{3}{8} + 1\frac{5}{6} =$ ______ **8.** $\frac{9}{10} - \frac{3}{5} =$ ______ **9.** $2\frac{1}{4} - 1\frac{3}{8} =$ ______

10. $6\frac{1}{8} - 3\frac{1}{2} =$ ______ **11.** $4\frac{5}{6} - 2\frac{1}{8} =$ ______ **12.** $3\frac{3}{4} - 1\frac{11}{12} =$ ______

13. $7\frac{1}{2} - 5\frac{7}{10} =$ ______ **14.** $6\frac{1}{2} - 4\frac{2}{3} =$ ______ **15.** $\frac{4}{5} \times \frac{1}{12} =$ ______

16. $1\frac{1}{3} \times 3\frac{3}{4} =$ ______ **17.** $3\frac{2}{7} \times 2\frac{2}{9} =$ ______ **18.** $\frac{5}{8} \times 1\frac{5}{7} =$ ______

19. $\frac{1}{1000} \times \frac{1}{10} =$ ______ **20.** $2\frac{4}{9} \times 1\frac{3}{4} =$ ______ **21.** $4\frac{1}{6} \times 2\frac{9}{10} =$ ______

22. $1\frac{1}{8} \times 2\frac{4}{7} =$ ______ **23.** $\frac{1}{4} \div \frac{4}{5} =$ ______ **24.** $2\frac{1}{6} \div 1\frac{5}{8} =$ ______

25. $\frac{1}{3} \div \frac{1}{100} =$ ___________ **26.** $1\frac{3}{4} \div 2 =$ ___________ **27.** $\frac{4}{5}/\frac{3}{5} =$ ___________

28. $\frac{1}{3}/\frac{3}{5} =$ ___________ **29.** $2\frac{5}{6}/1\frac{2}{3} =$ ___________ **30.** $4\frac{1}{2}/2\frac{1}{4} =$ ___________

ANSWERS ON P. 29.

CHAPTER 1

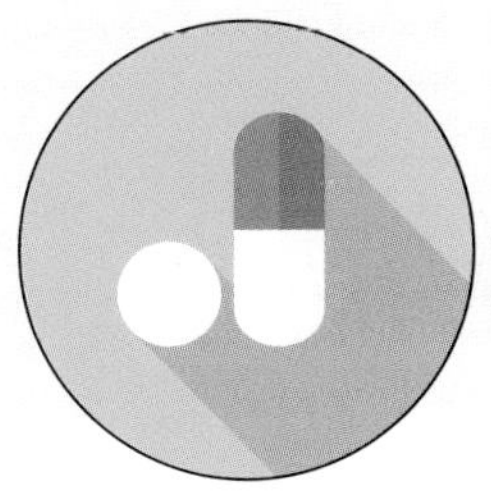

Fractions

LEARNING OBJECTIVES

Upon completion of the materials provided in this chapter, you will be able to perform computations accurately by mastering the following mathematical concepts:

1. Changing an improper fraction to a mixed number
2. Changing a mixed number to an improper fraction
3. Changing a fraction to an equivalent fraction with the lowest common denominator
4. Changing a mixed number to an equivalent fraction with the lowest common denominator
5. Adding fractions having the same denominator, having unlike denominators, or involving whole numbers and unlike denominators
6. Subtracting fractions having the same denominator, having unlike denominators, or involving whole numbers and unlike denominators
7. Multiplying fractions and mixed numbers
8. Dividing fractions and mixed numbers
9. Reducing a complex fraction
10. Reducing a complex fraction involving mixed numbers

Study the introductory material for fractions. The processes for the calculation of fraction problems are listed in steps. Memorize the steps for each type of calculation before beginning the work sheet. Complete the work sheet at the end of this chapter, which provides extensive practice in the manipulation of fractions. Check your answers. If you have difficulties, go back and review the steps for that type of calculation. When you feel ready to evaluate your learning, take the first posttest. Check your answers. An acceptable score (number of answers correct) as indicated on the posttest signifies that you are ready for the next chapter. An unacceptable score signifies a need for further study before you take the second posttest.

A **fraction** indicates the number of equal parts of a whole. For example, $3/4$ means three of four equal parts.

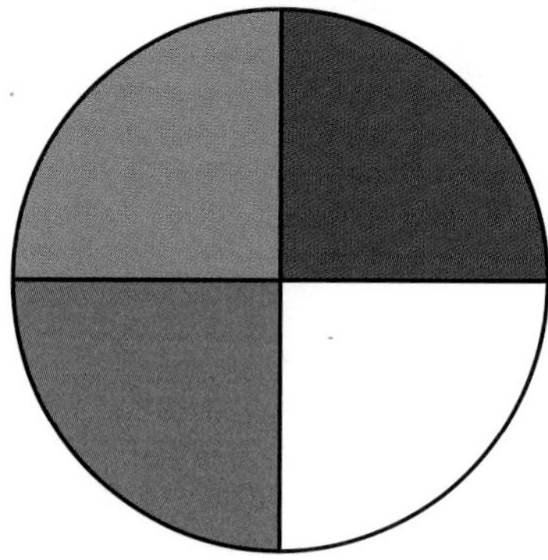

The **denominator** indicates the number of parts into which a whole has been divided. The denominator is the number *below* the fraction line. The **numerator** designates the number of parts that you have of a divided whole. It is the number *above* the fraction line. The line also indicates division to be performed and can be read as "divided by." The example $3/4$, or three fourths, can therefore be read as "three divided by four." In other words the numerator is "divided by" the denominator. The numerator is the **dividend,** and the denominator is the **divisor.** When numbers are multiplied, the answer is the **product.** When numbers are divided, the answer is the **quotient.**

A fraction can often be expressed in smaller numbers without any change in its real value. This is what is meant by the direction "Reduce to lowest terms." The reduction is accomplished by dividing both numerator and denominator by the same number.

EXAMPLE 1: $6/8$

Step 1. $6 \div 2 = 3$

Step 2. $8 \div 2 = 4$

Step 3. $\frac{6}{8} = \frac{3}{4}$

EXAMPLE 2: $3/9$

Step 1. $3 \div 3 = 1$

Step 2. $9 \div 3 = 3$

Step 3. $\frac{3}{9} = \frac{1}{3}$

EXAMPLE 3: $4/10$

Step 1. $4 \div 2 = 2$

Step 2. $10 \div 2 = 5$

Step 3. $\frac{4}{10} = \frac{2}{5}$

There are several different types of fractions. A **proper fraction** is one in which the numerator is smaller than the denominator. A proper fraction is sometimes called a *common* or *simple fraction.*

EXAMPLES: $2/3$, $1/8$, $5/12$

An **improper fraction** is a fraction in which the numerator is larger than or equal to the denominator.

EXAMPLES: $8/7$, $6/6$, $4/2$

A **complex fraction** is one that contains a fraction in its numerator, its denominator, or both.

EXAMPLES: $2\frac{1}{3}/3$, $2/\frac{1}{2}$, $\frac{3}{4}/\frac{3}{8}$

Sometimes a fraction is seen in conjunction with a whole number. This combination is called a **mixed number.**

EXAMPLES: $2\frac{3}{8}$, $4\frac{1}{3}$, $6\frac{1}{2}$

IMPROPER FRACTIONS

Changing an Improper Fraction to a Mixed Number

1. Divide the numerator by the denominator.
2. Place any remainder over the denominator and write this proper fraction beside the whole number found in step 1.

EXAMPLE 1: $\frac{5}{3}$

$$3\overline{)5} = 1 \text{ remainder } 2 = 1\frac{2}{3}$$
$$\begin{array}{r} 3 \\ \hline 2 \end{array}$$

EXAMPLE 2: $\frac{7}{2}$

$$2\overline{)7} = 3 \text{ remainder } 1 = 3\frac{1}{2}$$
$$\begin{array}{r} 6 \\ \hline 1 \end{array}$$

When an improper fraction is reduced, it will *always* result in a mixed number or a whole number.

Changing a Mixed Number to an Improper Fraction

1. Multiply the denominator of the fraction by the whole number.
2. Add the product to the numerator of the fraction.
3. Place the sum over the denominator.

EXAMPLE 1: $3\frac{1}{4}$

Step 1. $4 \times 3 = 12$

Step 2. $12 + 1 = 13$

Step 3. $3\frac{1}{4} = \frac{13}{4}$

EXAMPLE 2: $1\frac{3}{8}$

Step 1. $8 \times 1 = 8$

Step 2. $8 + 3 = 11$

Step 3. $1\frac{3}{8} = \frac{11}{8}$

EXAMPLE 3: $2\frac{7}{10}$

Step 1. $10 \times 2 = 20$

Step 2. $20 + 7 = 27$

Step 3. $2\frac{7}{10} = \frac{27}{10}$

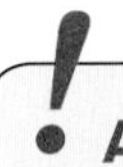

ALERT

If fractions are to be added or subtracted, it is necessary for their *denominators to be the same.*

LOWEST COMMON DENOMINATOR

Computations are facilitated when the lowest common denominator is used. The term **lowest common denominator** is defined as the smallest whole number that can be divided evenly by all denominators within the problem.

When trying to determine the lowest common denominator, first observe whether one of the denominators in the problem is evenly divisible by each of the other denominators. If so, this will be the lowest common denominator for the problem.

EXAMPLE 1: $\frac{2}{3}$ and $\frac{5}{12}$
You find that 12 is evenly divisible by 3; therefore 12 is the lowest common denominator.

EXAMPLE 2: $\frac{1}{2}$ and $\frac{3}{8}$
You find that 8 is evenly divisible by 2; therefore 8 is the lowest common denominator.

EXAMPLE 3: $\frac{2}{7}$ and $\frac{5}{14}$ and $\frac{1}{28}$
You find that 28 is evenly divisible by 7 and 14; therefore 28 is the lowest common denominator.

Changing a Fraction to an Equivalent Fraction with the Lowest Common Denominator

1. Divide the lowest common denominator by the denominator of the fraction to be changed.
2. Multiply the quotient by the numerator of the fraction to be changed.
3. Place the product over the lowest common denominator.

EXAMPLE 1: $2/3 = ?/12$

Step 1. $12 \div 3 = 4$

Step 2. $4 \times 2 = 8$

Step 3. $\frac{2}{3} = \frac{8}{12}$

EXAMPLE 2: $1/2 = ?/8$

Step 1. $8 \div 2 = 4$

Step 2. $4 \times 1 = 4$

Step 3. $\frac{1}{2} = \frac{4}{8}$

EXAMPLE 3: $2/7 = ?/14$

Step 1. $14 \div 7 = 2$

Step 2. $2 \times 2 = 4$

Step 3. $\frac{2}{7} = \frac{4}{14}$

Changing a Mixed Number to an Equivalent Fraction with the Lowest Common Denominator

1. Change the mixed number to an improper fraction.
2. Divide the lowest common denominator by the denominator of the fraction.
3. Multiply the quotient by the numerator of the improper fraction.
4. Place the product over the lowest common denominator.

EXAMPLE 1: $1\frac{3}{4}$ and $5/12$

Step 1. $1\frac{3}{4} = \frac{?}{12}$

$4 \times 1 = 4$

$4 + 3 = 7$

Step 2. $\frac{7}{4} = \frac{?}{12}$

$12 \div 4 = 3$

Step 3. $3 \times 7 = 21$

Step 4. $1\frac{3}{4} = \frac{21}{12}$

EXAMPLE 2: $3\frac{2}{3}$ and $4/9$

Step 1. $3\frac{2}{3} = \frac{?}{9}$

$3 \times 3 = 9$

$9 + 2 = 11$

Step 2. $\frac{11}{3} = \frac{?}{9}$

$9 \div 3 = 3$

Step 3. $3 \times 11 = 33$

Step 4. $3\frac{2}{3} = \frac{33}{9}$

If one of the denominators in the problem is not the lowest common denominator for all, you must look further. One suggestion is to multiply two of the denominators together and if possible use that number as the lowest common denominator.

EXAMPLE: $3\frac{1}{2}$ and $2/3$

Multiply the two denominators: $2 \times 3 = 6$

Step 1. $3\frac{1}{2} = \frac{?}{6}$

$2 \times 3 = 6$

$6 + 1 = 7$

Step 2. $\frac{7}{2} = \frac{?}{6}$

Step 3. $6 \div 2 = 3$

Step 4. $3 \times 7 = 21$

Step 5. $3\frac{1}{2} = \frac{21}{6}$

Step 1. $\frac{2}{3} = \frac{?}{6}$

Step 2. $6 \div 3 = 2$

Step 3. $2 \times 2 = 4$

Step 4. $\frac{2}{3} = \frac{4}{6}$

Another method is to multiply one of the denominators by 2, 3, or 4. Determine whether the resulting number can be used as a common denominator.

EXAMPLE: $\frac{3}{4}$ and $\frac{1}{8}$ and $\frac{5}{12}$

Multiply the denominator 8 by 3: $8 \times 3 = 24$

Step 1. $\frac{3}{4} = \frac{?}{24}$

Step 2. $24 \div 4 = 6$

Step 3. $6 \times 3 = 18$

Step 4. $\frac{3}{4} = \frac{18}{24}$

Step 1. $\frac{1}{8} = \frac{?}{24}$

Step 2. $24 \div 8 = 3$

Step 3. $3 \times 1 = 3$

Step 4. $\frac{1}{8} = \frac{3}{24}$

Step 1. $\frac{5}{12} = \frac{?}{24}$

Step 2. $24 \div 12 = 2$

Step 3. $2 \times 5 = 10$

Step 4. $\frac{5}{12} = \frac{10}{24}$

ADDITION OF FRACTIONS

Addition of Fractions with the Same Denominator

1. Add the numerators.
2. Place the sum over the common denominator.
3. Reduce to lowest terms.

EXAMPLE 1: $\frac{1}{7} + \frac{2}{7} =$ ______

Step 1. $\frac{1}{7} + \frac{2}{7} =$

Step 2. $\frac{1+2}{7} =$

Step 3. $\frac{3}{7}$

EXAMPLE 2: $\frac{1}{8} + \frac{3}{8} =$ ______

Step 1. $\frac{1}{8} + \frac{3}{8} =$

Step 2. $\frac{1+3}{8} =$

Step 3. $\frac{4}{8} = \frac{1}{2}$

Addition of Fractions with Unlike Denominators

1. Change the fractions to equivalent fractions with the lowest common denominator.
2. Add the numerators.
3. Place the sum over the lowest common denominator.
4. Reduce to lowest terms.

EXAMPLE 1: $\frac{2}{3} + \frac{1}{5} =$ ______

To find the lowest common denominator, multiply the two denominators together.

$3 \times 5 = 15$

Change each fraction to an equivalent fraction with 15 as the denominator.

Step 1. $\frac{2}{3} = \frac{?}{15}$

$15 \div 3 = 5$

$5 \times 2 = 10$

$\frac{2}{3} = \frac{10}{15}$

Step 1. $\frac{1}{5} = \frac{?}{15}$

$15 \div 5 = 3$

$3 \times 1 = 3$

$\frac{1}{5} = \frac{3}{15}$

Step 2. $\frac{10}{15} + \frac{3}{15} =$

Step 3. $\frac{10+3}{15} = \frac{13}{15}$

EXAMPLE 2: $\frac{1}{6} + \frac{1}{4} + \frac{1}{3} =$ ______

To find a common denominator, try multiplying two of the denominators together and check to see whether that number is divisible by the other denominator.

$4 \times 3 = 12$

Is 12 divisible by the other denominator, 6? The answer is YES.

Step 1. $\frac{1}{6} = \frac{?}{12}$

$12 \div 6 = 2$

$2 \times 1 = 2$

$\frac{1}{6} = \frac{2}{12}$

Step 1. $\frac{1}{4} = \frac{?}{12}$

$12 \div 4 = 3$

$3 \times 1 = 3$

$\frac{1}{4} = \frac{3}{12}$

Step 1. $\frac{1}{3} = \frac{?}{12}$

$12 \div 3 = 4$

$4 \times 1 = 4$

$\frac{1}{3} = \frac{4}{12}$

Step 2. $\frac{2}{12} + \frac{3}{12} + \frac{4}{12} =$

Step 3. $\frac{2+3+4}{12} = \frac{9}{12}$

Step 4. $\frac{9}{12} = \frac{3}{4}$ (reduced to lowest terms)

Addition of Fractions Involving Whole Numbers and Unlike Denominators

1. Change the fractions to equivalent fractions with the lowest common denominator.
2. Add the numerators.
3. Place the sum over the lowest common denominator.
4. Reduce to lowest terms.
5. Write the reduced fraction next to the sum of the whole numbers.

EXAMPLE 1: $1\frac{1}{3} + 2\frac{3}{8} =$ ______

To find the lowest common denominator, multiply the two denominators together.

$3 \times 8 = 24$

Change the fractions $\frac{1}{3}$ and $\frac{3}{8}$ to equivalent fractions with 24 as their denominators.

Step 1. $\frac{1}{3} = \frac{?}{24}$

$24 \div 3 = 8$

$8 \times 1 = 8$

$\frac{1}{3} = \frac{8}{24}$

Step 1. $\frac{3}{8} = \frac{?}{24}$

$24 \div 8 = 3$

$3 \times 3 = 9$

$\frac{3}{8} = \frac{9}{24}$

Step 2. $1\frac{8}{24} + 2\frac{9}{24} =$

Step 3.

$$\begin{array}{r} 1\frac{8}{24} \\ +2\frac{9}{24} \\ \hline \end{array}$$

Step 4. $3\frac{17}{24}$

EXAMPLE 2: $5\frac{1}{2} + 3\frac{3}{10} =$ ______

Because 10 is evenly divisible by 2, 10 is the lowest common denominator. Therefore ½ needs to be changed to an equivalent fraction with 10 as the denominator.

Step 1. $\frac{1}{2} = \frac{?}{10}$

$10 \div 2 = 5$

$5 \times 1 = 5$

$\frac{1}{2} = \frac{5}{10}$

Step 2. $5\frac{5}{10} + 3\frac{3}{10} =$

Step 3.

$$\begin{array}{r} 5\frac{5}{10} \\ +3\frac{3}{10} \\ \hline 8\frac{8}{10} \end{array}$$

$8\frac{8}{10} = 8\frac{4}{5}$ (reduced to lowest terms)

SUBTRACTION OF FRACTIONS

Subtraction of Fractions with the Same Denominator

1. Subtract the numerator of the **subtrahend** (the number being subtracted) from the numerator of the **minuend** (the number from which another number is subtracted).
2. Place the difference over the common denominator.
3. Reduce to lowest terms.

EXAMPLE 1: $\frac{6}{8} - \frac{4}{8} =$ ______

Step 1. $\frac{6}{8} - \frac{4}{8} =$

Step 2. $\frac{6-4}{8} =$

Step 3. $\frac{2}{8} = \frac{1}{4}$ (reduced to lowest terms)

EXAMPLE 2: $\frac{7}{12} - \frac{1}{12} =$ ______

Step 1. $\frac{7}{12} - \frac{1}{12} =$

Step 2. $\frac{7-1}{12} =$

Step 3. $\frac{6}{12} = \frac{1}{2}$ (reduced to lowest terms)

Subtraction of Fractions with Unlike Denominators

1. Change the fractions to equivalent fractions with the lowest common denominator.
2. Subtract the numerator of the subtrahend from that of the minuend.
3. Place the difference over the lowest common denominator.
4. Reduce to lowest terms.

EXAMPLE 1: $\frac{2}{3} - \frac{1}{6} =$ ______

The lowest common denominator is 6, because 6 is evenly divisible by 3. Therefore the fraction ⅔ needs to be changed to an equivalent fraction with 6 as the denominator.

Step 1. $\frac{2}{3} = \frac{?}{6}$

$6 \div 3 = 2$

$2 \times 2 = 4$

$\frac{2}{3} = \frac{4}{6}$

Step 2. $\frac{4}{6} - \frac{1}{6} =$

Step 3. $\frac{4-1}{6} =$

Step 4. $\frac{3}{6} = \frac{1}{2}$ (reduced to lowest terms)

EXAMPLE 2: $\frac{7}{10} - \frac{3}{5} =$ ______

The lowest common denominator is 10, because 10 is evenly divisible by 5. Therefore the fraction $\frac{3}{5}$ needs to be changed to an equivalent fraction with 10 as the denominator.

Step 1. $\frac{3}{5} = \frac{?}{10}$

$10 \div 5 = 2$

$2 \times 3 = 6$

$\frac{3}{5} = \frac{6}{10}$

Step 2. $\frac{7}{10} - \frac{6}{10} =$

Step 3. $\frac{7-6}{10} = \frac{1}{10}$

Subtraction of Fractions Involving Whole Numbers and Unlike Denominators

1. Change the fractions to equivalent fractions with the lowest common denominator.
2. Subtract the numerator of the subtrahend from that of the minuend, borrowing 1 from the whole number if necessary.
3. Place the difference over the lowest common denominator.
4. Reduce to lowest terms.
5. Write the reduced fraction next to the difference of the whole numbers.

EXAMPLE 1: $3\frac{2}{3} - 1\frac{1}{4} =$ ______

The lowest common denominator is 12 (determined by multiplying 3×4). Each fraction needs to be changed to an equivalent fraction with 12 as the common denominator.

Step 1. $\frac{2}{3} = \frac{?}{12}$

$12 \div 3 = 4$

$4 \times 2 = 8$

$\frac{2}{3} = \frac{8}{12}$

Step 1. $\frac{1}{4} = \frac{?}{12}$

$12 \div 4 = 3$

$3 \times 1 = 3$

$\frac{1}{4} = \frac{3}{12}$

Step 2. $3\frac{8}{12} - 1\frac{3}{12} =$

Step 3.

$$\begin{array}{r} 3\frac{8}{12} \\ -1\frac{3}{12} \\ \hline 2\frac{5}{12} \end{array}$$

EXAMPLE 2: $8\frac{1}{2} - 3\frac{4}{7} =$ ______

The lowest common denominator is 14 (determined by multiplying 2×7). Each fraction needs to be changed to an equivalent fraction with 14 as the common denominator.

Step 1. $\frac{1}{2} = \frac{?}{14}$

$14 \div 2 = 7$

$7 \times 1 = 7$

$\frac{1}{2} = \frac{7}{14}$

Step 1. $\frac{4}{7} = \frac{?}{14}$

$14 \div 7 = 2$

$2 \times 4 = 8$

$\frac{4}{7} = \frac{8}{14}$

Step 2. $8\frac{7}{14} - 3\frac{8}{14} =$

To perform the subtraction, it is necessary to borrow 1 from the whole number. "One" for this problem can be expressed as $\frac{14}{14}$. Therefore $8\frac{7}{14} = 7\frac{21}{14}$. Now the mathematics may be completed.

Step 3. $\begin{array}{r} 8\frac{7}{14} \\ -3\frac{8}{14} \\ \hline \end{array}$ = **Step 4.** $\begin{array}{r} 7\frac{21}{14} \\ -3\frac{8}{14} \\ \hline 4\frac{13}{14} \end{array}$

MULTIPLICATION OF FRACTIONS

1. Multiply the numerators.
2. Multiply the denominators.
3. Place the product of the numerators over the product of the denominators.
4. Reduce to lowest terms.

EXAMPLE 1: $\frac{2}{3} \times \frac{3}{5} =$ ______

$\frac{2}{3} \times \frac{3}{5} =$

Step 1. $\frac{2 \times 3}{3 \times 5} = \frac{6}{15}$

Step 2. $\frac{6}{15} = \frac{2}{5}$ (reduced to lowest terms)

EXAMPLE 2: $\frac{4}{9} \times \frac{4}{5} =$ ______

$\frac{4}{9} \times \frac{4}{5} =$

Step 1. **Step 2.** $\frac{4 \times 4}{9 \times 5} = \frac{16}{45}$ (reduced to lowest terms)

The process of multiplying fractions may be shortened by **canceling.** In other words, numbers common to the numerators and denominators may be divided or canceled out.

EXAMPLE 1: $\frac{2}{3} \times \frac{3}{5} =$ ______

$\frac{2}{\overset{}{\cancel{3}}_{1}} \times \frac{\overset{1}{\cancel{3}}}{5} = \frac{2 \times 1}{1 \times 5} = \frac{2}{5}$

EXAMPLE 2: $\frac{7}{20} \times \frac{2}{5} \times \frac{3}{14} =$ ______

$\frac{\overset{1}{\cancel{7}}}{\underset{10}{\cancel{20}}} \times \frac{\overset{1}{\cancel{2}}}{5} \times \frac{3}{\underset{2}{\cancel{14}}} =$

$\frac{1 \times 1 \times 3}{10 \times 5 \times 2} = \frac{3}{100}$

EXAMPLE 3: $\frac{2}{6} \times \frac{3}{4} =$ ______

$$\frac{\overset{1}{\cancel{2}}}{\underset{2}{\cancel{6}}} \times \frac{\overset{1}{\cancel{3}}}{\underset{2}{\cancel{4}}} = \frac{1 \times 1}{2 \times 2} = \frac{1}{4}$$

Multiplication of Mixed Numbers

1. Change each mixed number to an improper fraction.
2. Multiply the numerators.
3. Multiply the denominators.
4. Place the product of the numerators over the product of the denominators.
5. Reduce to lowest terms.

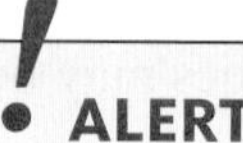

ALERT

*Remember the denominator of a whole number is *always* 1.

$$6 = \frac{6}{1}$$

$$12 = \frac{12}{1}$$

EXAMPLE 1: $1\frac{1}{2} \times 2\frac{1}{4} =$ ______

Step 1. $\frac{3}{2} \times \frac{9}{4} =$

Step 2. $\frac{3 \times 9}{2 \times 4} = \frac{27}{8} = 3\frac{3}{8}$ (reduced to lowest terms)

EXAMPLE 2: $2 \times 3\frac{5}{6} =$ ______

Step 1. $\frac{2}{1} \times \frac{23}{6} =$

Step 2. $\frac{\overset{1}{\cancel{2}}}{1} \times \frac{23}{\underset{3}{\cancel{6}}} =$

Step 3. $\frac{1 \times 23}{1 \times 3} = \frac{23}{3} = 7\frac{2}{3}$ (reduced to lowest terms)

DIVISION OF FRACTIONS

1. Invert (or turn upside down) the divisor.
2. Multiply the two fractions.
3. Reduce to lowest terms.

EXAMPLE 1: $\frac{2}{3} \div \frac{6}{8} =$ ______

$$\frac{2}{3} \div \frac{6}{8} =$$

Step 1. $\frac{2}{3} \times \frac{8}{6} =$

Step 2.
Step 3. $\frac{\overset{1}{\cancel{2}}}{3} \times \frac{8}{\underset{3}{\cancel{6}}} = \frac{1 \times 8}{3 \times 3} = \frac{8}{9}$

EXAMPLE 2: $\frac{3}{4} \div \frac{8}{9} =$ ______

$$\frac{3}{4} \div \frac{8}{9} =$$

Step 1. $\frac{3}{4} \times \frac{9}{8} =$

Step 2.
Step 3. $\frac{3 \times 9}{4 \times 8} = \frac{27}{32}$

Division of Mixed Numbers

1. Change each mixed number to an improper fraction.
2. Invert (or turn upside down) the divisor.
3. Multiply the two fractions.
4. Reduce to lowest terms.

EXAMPLE 1: $1\frac{3}{4} \div 2\frac{1}{8} =$ ______

Step 1. $\frac{7}{4} \div \frac{17}{8} =$

Step 2.
Step 3. $\frac{7}{\cancel{4}_{1}} \times \frac{\cancel{8}^{2}}{17} = \frac{7 \times 2}{1 \times 17} = \frac{14}{17}$

EXAMPLE 2: $\frac{1}{7} \div 7 =$ ______

Step 1. $\frac{1}{7} \div \frac{7}{1} =$

Step 2.
Step 3. $\frac{1}{7} \times \frac{1}{7} = \frac{1 \times 1}{7 \times 7} = \frac{1}{49}$

REDUCTION OF A COMPLEX FRACTION

1. Rewrite the complex fraction as a division problem.
2. Invert (or turn upside down) the divisor.
3. Multiply the two fractions.
4. Reduce to lowest terms.

EXAMPLE 1: $\frac{3}{8}/\frac{1}{4} =$ ______

Step 1. $\frac{3}{8} \div \frac{1}{4} =$

Step 2. $\frac{3}{8} \times \frac{4}{1} =$

Step 3. $\frac{3}{\cancel{8}_{2}} \times \frac{\cancel{4}^{1}}{1} = \frac{3 \times 1}{2 \times 1} = \frac{3}{2} = 1\frac{1}{2}$ (reduced to lowest terms)

EXAMPLE 2: $\frac{1}{2}/\frac{2}{7} =$ ______

Step 1. $\frac{1}{2} \div \frac{2}{7} =$

Step 2. $\frac{1}{2} \times \frac{7}{2} =$

Step 3. $\frac{1 \times 7}{2 \times 2} = \frac{7}{4} = 1\frac{3}{4}$ (reduced to lowest terms)

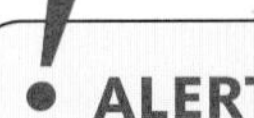

ALERT

- Remember the / in a complex fraction means the same as the sign for division ÷.

$3/6/1/4 \qquad 2\frac{1}{2}/1\frac{1}{3}$

Reduction of a Complex Fraction with Mixed Numbers

1. Rewrite the complex fraction as a division problem.
2. Change the mixed numbers to improper fractions.
3. Invert (or turn upside down) the divisor.
4. Multiply the two fractions.
5. Reduce to lowest terms.

EXAMPLE 1: $2\frac{1}{2}/1\frac{1}{3}$ = ______

Step 1. $2\frac{1}{2} \div 1\frac{1}{3} =$

Step 2. $\frac{5}{2} \div \frac{4}{3} =$

Step 3. $\frac{5}{2} \times \frac{3}{4} =$

Step 4. $\frac{5 \times 3}{2 \times 4} = \frac{15}{8} = 1\frac{7}{8}$ (reduced to lowest terms)

EXAMPLE 2: $3\frac{3}{4}/2\frac{1}{6}$ = ______

Step 1. $3\frac{3}{4} \div 2\frac{1}{6} =$

Step 2. $\frac{15}{4} \div \frac{13}{6} =$

Step 3. $\frac{15}{4} \times \frac{6}{13} =$

Step 4. $\frac{15 \times \overset{3}{\cancel{6}}}{\underset{2}{\cancel{4}} \times 13} = \frac{45}{26} = 1\frac{19}{26}$ (reduced to lowest terms)

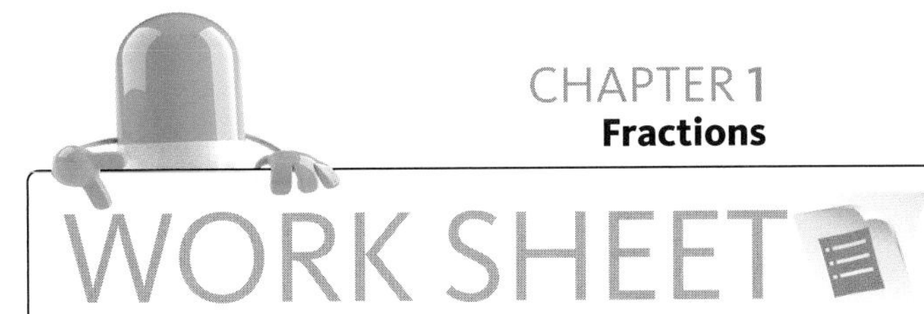

DIRECTIONS: Change the following improper fractions to mixed numbers.

1. $4/3$ = ________ **2.** $6/2$ = ________ **3.** $16/5$ = ________ **4.** $13/4$ = ________

5. $15/10$ = ________ **6.** $9/8$ = ________ **7.** $10/6$ = ________ **8.** $26/12$ = ________

9. $21/6$ = ________ **10.** $11/8$ = ________ **11.** $7/2$ = ________ **12.** $112/100$ = ________

DIRECTIONS: Change the following mixed numbers to improper fractions.

1. $1\,1/2$ = ________ **2.** $3\,3/4$ = ________ **3.** $2\,2/3$ = ________ **4.** $2\,5/6$ = ________

5. $1\,3/5$ = ________ **6.** $3\,4/7$ = ________ **7.** $4\,7/8$ = ________ **8.** $3\,7/100$ = ________

9. $2\,7/10$ = ________ **10.** $6\,5/8$ = ________ **11.** $1\,3/25$ = ________ **12.** $4\,1/4$ = ________

DIRECTIONS: Add and reduce fractions to lowest terms.

1. $2/3 + 5/6$ = ________ **2.** $2/5 + 3/7$ = ________ **3.** $3\,1/8 + 2/3$ = ________

4. $2\,1/2 + 3/4$ = ________ **5.** $2\,1/4 + 3\,2/5$ = ________ **6.** $1\,6/13 + 1\,2/3$ = ________

7. $1\frac{1}{2} + 3\frac{3}{4} + 2\frac{3}{8} =$ ____ 8. $4\frac{3}{11} + 2\frac{1}{2} =$ ____ 9. $2\frac{2}{3} + 3\frac{7}{9} =$ ____

10. $1\frac{3}{10} + 4\frac{2}{5} + \frac{2}{3} =$ ____ 11. $3\frac{1}{2} + 2\frac{5}{6} + 2\frac{2}{3} =$ ____ 12. $5\frac{5}{6} + 2\frac{2}{5} =$ ____

DIRECTIONS: Subtract and reduce fractions to lowest terms.

1. $\frac{2}{3} - \frac{3}{7} =$ ____ 2. $\frac{7}{8} - \frac{5}{16} =$ ____ 3. $\frac{9}{16} - \frac{5}{12} =$ ____

4. $1\frac{1}{3} - \frac{5}{6} =$ ____ 5. $2\frac{17}{20} - 1\frac{3}{4} =$ ____ 6. $5\frac{1}{4} - 3\frac{5}{16} =$ ____

7. $5\frac{3}{8} - 4\frac{3}{4} =$ ____ 8. $3\frac{1}{4} - 1\frac{11}{12} =$ ____ 9. $6\frac{1}{2} - 3\frac{7}{8} =$ ____

10. $4\frac{1}{6} - 2\frac{3}{4} =$ ____ 11. $5\frac{2}{3} - 3\frac{7}{8} =$ ____ 12. $2\frac{5}{16} - 1\frac{3}{8} =$ ____

DIRECTIONS: Multiply and reduce fractions to lowest terms.

1. $\frac{1}{3} \times \frac{4}{5} =$ ____ 2. $\frac{7}{8} \times \frac{2}{3} =$ ____ 3. $6 \times \frac{2}{3} =$ ____

4. $\frac{3}{8} \times 4 =$ ____ 5. $2\frac{1}{3} \times 3\frac{3}{4} =$ ____ 6. $4\frac{3}{8} \times 2\frac{5}{7} =$ ____

7. $2\frac{5}{12} \times 5\frac{1}{4} =$ ____ 8. $\frac{3}{4} \times 2\frac{3}{8} =$ ____ 9. $\frac{3}{8} \times \frac{4}{5} \times \frac{2}{3} =$ ____

10. $\frac{1}{10} \times \frac{3}{100} =$ ____ 11. $3\frac{1}{2} \times 1\frac{5}{6} =$ ____ 12. $2\frac{4}{9} \times 1\frac{3}{11} =$ ____

DIRECTIONS: Divide and reduce fractions to lowest terms.

1. $1\frac{2}{3} \div 3\frac{1}{2} =$ ________

2. $5\frac{1}{2} \div 2\frac{1}{2} =$ ________

3. $3\frac{1}{2} \div 2\frac{1}{4} =$ ________

4. $4\frac{3}{8} \div 1\frac{3}{4} =$ ________

5. $3\frac{1}{2} \div 1\frac{6}{7} =$ ________

6. $\frac{9}{10} \div \frac{2}{3} =$ ________

7. $3 \div 1\frac{5}{6} =$ ________

8. $6\frac{2}{3} \div 1\frac{7}{10} =$ ________

9. $\frac{7}{8}/\frac{1}{4} =$ ________

10. $6\frac{1}{2}/2\frac{5}{6} =$ ________

11. $5\frac{1}{2}/2\frac{2}{3} =$ ________

12. $2\frac{2}{3}/1\frac{7}{9} =$ ________

ANSWERS ON P. 29.

NAME ____________________

DATE ____________________

ACCEPTABLE SCORE **29**

YOUR SCORE ______

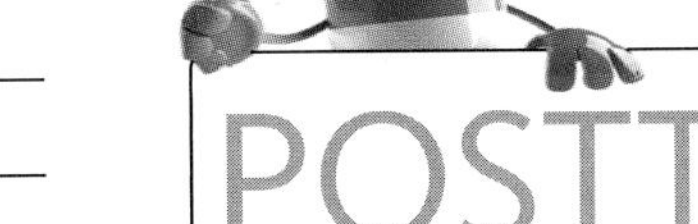

CHAPTER 1
Fractions

POSTTEST 1

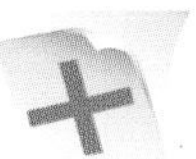

DIRECTIONS: Perform the indicated calculations and reduce fractions to lowest terms.

1. $\frac{2}{3} + \frac{4}{9} =$ ______
2. $\frac{3}{8} + \frac{1}{3} =$ ______
3. $2\frac{3}{4} + 2\frac{1}{3} =$ ______
4. $2\frac{2}{3} + \frac{3}{7} =$ ______
5. $\frac{3}{4} + \frac{3}{100} =$ ______
6. $4\frac{2}{5} + 3\frac{3}{4} =$ ______
7. $4\frac{1}{6} + \frac{2}{3} + 2\frac{3}{4} =$ ______
8. $1\frac{3}{10} - \frac{2}{5} =$ ______
9. $2\frac{1}{2} - 1\frac{2}{3} =$ ______
10. $\frac{5}{7} - \frac{1}{2} =$ ______
11. $3\frac{1}{2} - 1\frac{9}{16} =$ ______
12. $2\frac{5}{7} - 1\frac{2}{9} =$ ______
13. $9\frac{1}{5} - 3\frac{1}{2} =$ ______
14. $2\frac{1}{4} - \frac{7}{9}/\frac{2}{3} =$ ______
15. $\frac{3}{4} \times \frac{6}{7} =$ ______
16. $3 \times \frac{4}{5} =$ ______
17. $\frac{2}{9} \times 9 =$ ______
18. $2\frac{3}{4} \times 1\frac{1}{6} =$ ______
19. $1\frac{1}{4} \times 2\frac{2}{3} =$ ______
20. $10\frac{1}{2} \times 1\frac{2}{5} =$ ______
21. $5\frac{6}{7} \times \frac{3}{5} =$ ______
22. $\frac{1}{4} \times 3\frac{1}{2} =$ ______
23. $\frac{2}{3} \div \frac{5}{8} =$ ______
24. $\frac{1}{5} \div \frac{1}{50} =$ ______

25. $\frac{1}{3} \div \frac{1}{2} =$ ______ 26. $\frac{5}{6} \div \frac{2}{3} =$ ______ 27. $\frac{1}{5}/\frac{1}{3} =$ ______

28. $1\frac{1}{5}/\frac{8}{9} =$ ______ 29. $\frac{3}{4}/\frac{1}{6} =$ ______ 30. $3\frac{1}{8}/2\frac{3}{4} =$ ______

ANSWERS ON P. 29.

NAME ____________________

DATE ____________________

ACCEPTABLE SCORE **29**

YOUR SCORE ______

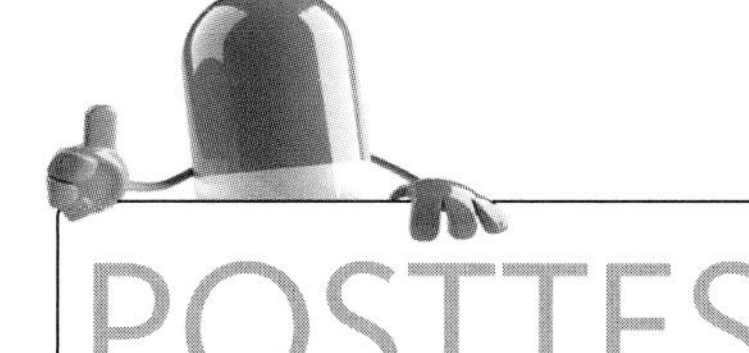

CHAPTER 1
Fractions

POSTTEST 2

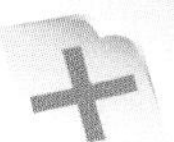

DIRECTIONS: Perform the indicated calculations and reduce fractions to lowest terms.

1. $\frac{1}{4} + \frac{5}{6} =$ ______ **2.** $2\frac{3}{5} + 1\frac{1}{2} =$ ______ **3.** $\frac{2}{3} + 2\frac{3}{7} =$ ______

4. $1\frac{7}{8} + 3\frac{2}{5} =$ ______ **5.** $1\frac{3}{4} + \frac{5}{8} + 2\frac{5}{12} =$ ______ **6.** $10\frac{1}{2} + 1\frac{3}{10} =$ ______

7. $1\frac{5}{14} + 2\frac{3}{21} =$ ______ **8.** $\frac{4}{9} - \frac{1}{3} =$ ______ **9.** $2\frac{3}{4} - \frac{7}{8} =$ ______

10. $3\frac{1}{2} - 1\frac{2}{3} =$ ______ **11.** $3\frac{5}{8} - 1\frac{5}{16} =$ ______ **12.** $7\frac{1}{3} - 5\frac{5}{6} =$ ______

13. $7\frac{7}{10} - 3\frac{4}{5} =$ ______ **14.** $3\frac{4}{15} - 2\frac{2}{3} =$ ______ **15.** $\frac{2}{7} \times \frac{2}{3} =$ ______

16. $3\frac{4}{9} \times 1\frac{4}{5} =$ ______ **17.** $2 \times \frac{2}{3} =$ ______ **18.** $\frac{5}{6} \times 2\frac{1}{3} =$ ______

19. $\frac{1}{100} \times \frac{1}{10} =$ ______ **20.** $6\frac{3}{4} \times 5\frac{1}{3} =$ ______ **21.** $2\frac{5}{8} \times 1\frac{1}{3} =$ ______

22. $3\frac{1}{2} \times 3\frac{3}{14} =$ ______ **23.** $\frac{3}{4} \div \frac{8}{9} =$ ______ **24.** $1\frac{1}{2} \div 1\frac{6}{7} =$ ______

25. $2\frac{1}{3} \div \frac{3}{8} =$ ______ **26.** $\frac{1}{7} \div 7 =$ ______ **27.** $\frac{5}{6}/1\frac{1}{3} =$ ______

28. $1\frac{1}{2}/2\frac{2}{7}$ = ____________ **29.** $2\frac{1}{4}/1\frac{1}{3}$ = ____________ **30.** $\frac{3}{8}/\frac{3}{9}$ = ____________

ANSWERS ON P. 29.

ANSWERS

CHAPTER 1 Fractions—Pretest, pp. 7–8

1. $1\frac{10}{63}$
2. $10\frac{2}{3}$
3. $9\frac{3}{4}$
4. $5\frac{9}{16}$
5. $9\frac{1}{22}$
6. $7\frac{8}{9}$
7. $5\frac{23}{24}$
8. $\frac{3}{10}$
9. $\frac{7}{8}$
10. $2\frac{5}{8}$
11. $2\frac{17}{24}$
12. $1\frac{5}{6}$
13. $1\frac{4}{5}$
14. $1\frac{5}{6}$
15. $\frac{1}{15}$
16. 5
17. $7\frac{19}{63}$
18. $1\frac{1}{14}$
19. $\frac{1}{10{,}000}$, 0.0001
20. $4\frac{5}{18}$
21. $12\frac{1}{12}$
22. $2\frac{25}{28}$
23. $\frac{5}{16}$
24. $1\frac{1}{3}$
25. $33\frac{1}{3}$
26. $\frac{7}{8}$
27. $1\frac{1}{3}$
28. $\frac{5}{9}$
29. $1\frac{7}{10}$
30. 2

CHAPTER 1 Fractions—Work Sheet, pp. 21–23

Improper Fractions to Mixed Numbers, *p. 21*

1. $1\frac{1}{3}$
2. 3
3. $3\frac{1}{5}$
4. $3\frac{1}{4}$
5. $1\frac{1}{2}$
6. $1\frac{1}{8}$
7. $1\frac{2}{3}$
8. $2\frac{1}{6}$
9. $3\frac{1}{2}$
10. $1\frac{3}{8}$
11. $3\frac{1}{2}$
12. $1\frac{3}{25}$

Mixed Numbers to Improper Fractions, *p. 21*

1. $\frac{3}{2}$
2. $\frac{15}{4}$
3. $\frac{8}{3}$
4. $\frac{17}{6}$
5. $\frac{8}{5}$
6. $\frac{25}{7}$
7. $\frac{39}{8}$
8. $\frac{307}{100}$
9. $\frac{27}{10}$
10. $\frac{53}{8}$
11. $\frac{28}{25}$
12. $\frac{17}{4}$

Addition, *pp. 21–22*

1. $1\frac{1}{2}$
2. $\frac{29}{35}$
3. $3\frac{19}{24}$
4. $3\frac{1}{4}$
5. $5\frac{13}{20}$
6. $3\frac{5}{39}$
7. $7\frac{5}{8}$
8. $6\frac{17}{22}$
9. $6\frac{4}{9}$
10. $6\frac{11}{30}$
11. 9
12. $8\frac{7}{30}$

Subtraction, *p. 22*

1. $\frac{5}{21}$
2. $\frac{9}{16}$
3. $\frac{7}{48}$
4. $\frac{1}{2}$
5. $1\frac{1}{10}$
6. $1\frac{15}{16}$
7. $\frac{5}{8}$
8. $1\frac{1}{3}$
9. $2\frac{5}{8}$
10. $1\frac{5}{12}$
11. $1\frac{19}{24}$
12. $\frac{15}{16}$

Multiplication, *p. 22*

1. $\frac{4}{15}$
2. $\frac{7}{12}$
3. 4
4. $1\frac{1}{2}$
5. $8\frac{3}{4}$
6. $11\frac{7}{8}$
7. $12\frac{11}{16}$
8. $1\frac{25}{32}$
9. $\frac{1}{5}$
10. $\frac{3}{1000}$
11. $6\frac{5}{12}$
12. $3\frac{1}{9}$

Division, *p. 23*

1. $\frac{10}{21}$
2. $2\frac{1}{5}$
3. $1\frac{5}{9}$
4. $2\frac{1}{2}$
5. $1\frac{23}{26}$
6. $1\frac{7}{20}$
7. $1\frac{7}{11}$
8. $3\frac{47}{51}$
9. $3\frac{1}{2}$
10. $2\frac{5}{17}$
11. $2\frac{1}{16}$
12. $1\frac{1}{2}$

CHAPTER 1 Fractions—Posttest 1, pp. 25–26

1. $1\frac{1}{9}$
2. $\frac{17}{24}$
3. $5\frac{1}{12}$
4. $3\frac{2}{21}$
5. $\frac{39}{50}$
6. $8\frac{3}{20}$
7. $7\frac{7}{12}$
8. $\frac{9}{10}$
9. $\frac{5}{6}$
10. $\frac{3}{14}$
11. $1\frac{15}{16}$
12. $1\frac{31}{63}$
13. $5\frac{7}{10}$
14. $1\frac{1}{12}$
15. $\frac{9}{14}$
16. $2\frac{2}{5}$
17. 2
18. $3\frac{5}{24}$
19. $3\frac{1}{3}$
20. $14\frac{7}{10}$
21. $3\frac{18}{35}$
22. $\frac{7}{8}$
23. $1\frac{1}{15}$
24. 10
25. $\frac{2}{3}$
26. $1\frac{1}{4}$
27. $\frac{3}{5}$
28. $1\frac{7}{20}$
29. $4\frac{1}{2}$
30. $1\frac{3}{22}$

CHAPTER 1 Fractions—Posttest 2, pp. 27–28

1. $1\frac{1}{12}$
2. $4\frac{1}{10}$
3. $3\frac{2}{21}$
4. $5\frac{11}{40}$
5. $4\frac{19}{24}$
6. $11\frac{4}{5}$
7. $3\frac{1}{2}$
8. $\frac{1}{9}$
9. $1\frac{7}{8}$
10. $1\frac{5}{6}$
11. $2\frac{5}{16}$
12. $1\frac{1}{2}$
13. $3\frac{9}{10}$
14. $\frac{3}{5}$
15. $\frac{4}{21}$
16. $6\frac{1}{5}$
17. $1\frac{1}{3}$
18. $1\frac{17}{18}$
19. $\frac{1}{1000}$
20. 36
21. $3\frac{1}{2}$
22. $11\frac{1}{4}$
23. $\frac{27}{32}$
24. $\frac{21}{26}$
25. $6\frac{2}{9}$
26. $\frac{1}{49}$
27. $\frac{5}{8}$
28. $\frac{21}{32}$
29. $1\frac{11}{16}$
30. $1\frac{1}{8}$

NAME ____________________

DATE ____________________

ACCEPTABLE SCORE **36**

YOUR SCORE ______

PRETEST

Complete the Decimals Pretest. A score of 36 out of 38 indicates an acceptable understanding of and competency in basic calculations involving decimals. You may skip to the Percents Pretest on p. 55. However, if you score 35 or below, completion of Chapter 2, Decimals, will be helpful for your continued success in the calculation of drug dosages.

DIRECTIONS: Write the following numbers in words.

1. 0.04 ____________________

2. 1.6 ____________________

3. 16.06734 ____________________

____

4. 1.015 ____________________

5. 0.009 ____________________

DIRECTIONS: Circle the decimal with the *least value.*

6. 0.2, 0.25, 0.025, 0.02

7. 0.4, 0.48, 0.04, 0.004

8. 1.6, 1.64, 1.682, 1.69

9. 2.8, 2.82, 2.082, 2.822

10. 0.3, 0.33, 0.003, 0.033

DIRECTIONS: Perform the indicated calculations.

11. 6.8 + 2.986 + 14.7 + 0.89 = ______

12. 141.71 + 84.98 + 9.98 + 87.63 = ______

13. 1006.48 + 0.008 + 6.2 + 0.179 = ______

14. 47.21 + 48.496 + 0.2976 + 54.67 = ______

15. 5.971 + 63.1 + 8.264 + 7.23 = ______

16. 2.176 − 1.098 = ______

17. 2.006 − 0.998 = ______

18. 836.2 − 76.8 = ______

19. 100.3 − 98.6 = ______

20. 12.6 − 1.654 = ________ **21.** 0.63 × 0.09 = ________ **22.** 41.545 × 0.16 = ________

23. 5.25 × 0.37 = ________ **24.** 44.08 × 0.67 = ________ **25.** 56.7 × 3.29 = ________

26. 0.89 ÷ 4.32 = ________ **27.** 1.436 ÷ 0.08 = ________ **28.** 0.689 ÷ 62.8 = ________

29. 12.54 ÷ 0.02 = ________ **30.** 23 ÷ 1236 = ________

DIRECTIONS: Change the following decimal fractions to proper fractions.

31. 0.008 = ________ **32.** 0.25 = ________ **33.** 0.322 = ________ **34.** 0.004 = ________

DIRECTIONS: Change the following proper fractions to decimal fractions.

35. $\frac{3}{5}$ = ________ **36.** $\frac{2}{3}$ = ________ **37.** $\frac{3}{500}$ = ________ **38.** $\frac{7}{20}$ = ________

ANSWERS ON P. 51.

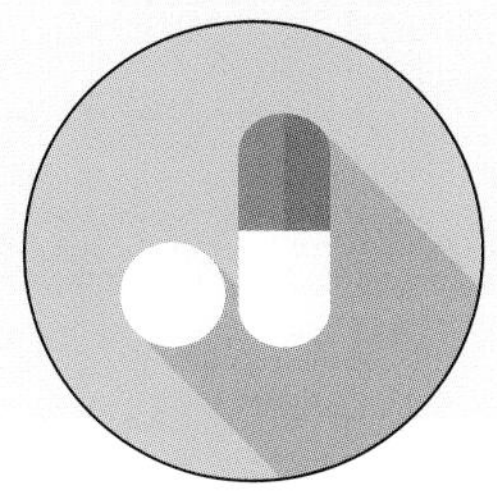

Decimals

LEARNING OBJECTIVES

Upon completion of the materials provided in this chapter, you will be able to perform computations accurately by mastering the following mathematical concepts:

1. Reading and writing decimal numbers
2. Determining the value of decimal fractions
3. Adding, subtracting, multiplying, and dividing decimals
4. Rounding decimal fractions to an indicated place value
5. Multiplying and dividing decimals by 10 or a power of 10
6. Multiplying and dividing decimals by 0.1 or a multiple of 0.1
7. Converting a decimal fraction to a proper fraction
8. Converting a proper fraction to a decimal fraction

Study the introductory material for decimals. The processes for the calculation of decimal problems are listed in steps. Memorize the steps for each calculation before beginning the work sheet. Complete the work sheet at the end of this chapter, which provides for extensive practice in the manipulation of decimals. Check your answers. If you have difficulties, go back and review the steps for that type of calculation. When you feel ready to evaluate your learning, take the first posttest. Check your answers. An acceptable score as indicated on the posttest signifies that you are ready for the next chapter. An unacceptable score signifies a need for further study before you take the second posttest.

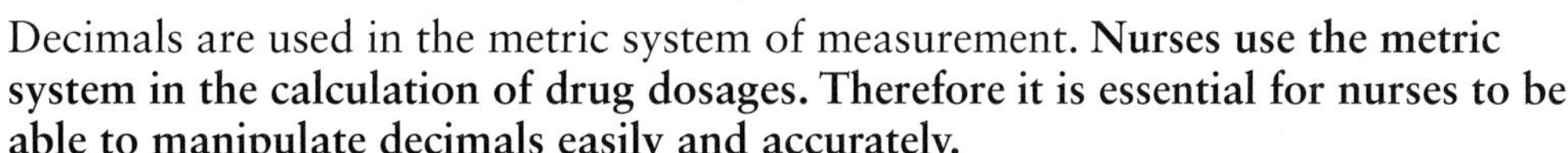

Decimals are used in the metric system of measurement. **Nurses use the metric system in the calculation of drug dosages. Therefore it is essential for nurses to be able to manipulate decimals easily and accurately.**

Each **decimal fraction** consists of a numerator that is expressed in numerals; a decimal point placed to designate the value of the denominator; and the denominator, which is understood to be 10 or some power of 10. **In writing a decimal fraction, always place a zero to the left of the decimal point so that the decimal point can readily be seen. The omission of the zero may result in a critical medication error.** Some examples are as follows:

Fraction	Decimal fraction
$\frac{7}{10}$	0.7
$\frac{13}{100}$	0.13
$\frac{227}{1000}$	0.227

Decimal numbers include an integer (or whole number), a decimal point, and a decimal fraction. The value of the combined integer and decimal fraction is determined by the placement of the decimal point. Whole numbers are written to the *left* of the decimal point, and decimal fractions to the *right*. Figure 2-1 illustrates the place occupied by the numeral that has the value indicated.

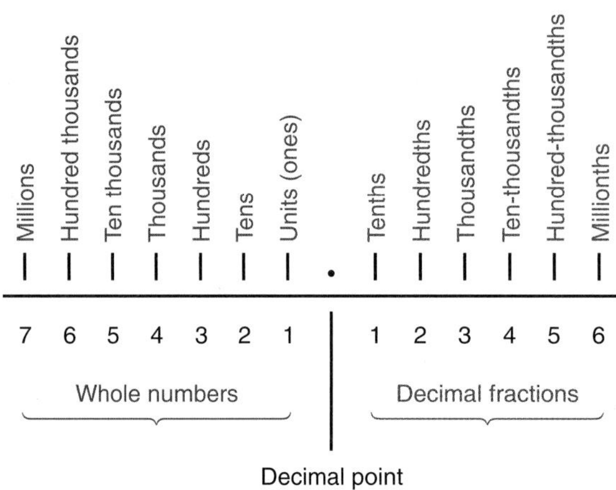

FIGURE 2-1 Decimal place values.

READING DECIMAL NUMBERS

The reading of a decimal number is determined by the place value of the integers and decimal fractions.

1. Read the whole number.
2. Read the decimal point as "and" or "point."
3. Read the decimal fraction.

EXAMPLES:	
0.4	four tenths
0.86	eighty-six hundredths
3.659	three and six hundred fifty-nine thousandths
182.0012	one hundred eighty-two and twelve ten-thousandths
9.47735	nine and forty-seven thousand seven hundred thirty-five hundred-thousandths

! ALERT

- Remember when reading a decimal number the decimal point is read as "and" or "point."

DETERMINING THE VALUES OF DECIMAL FRACTIONS

1. Place the numbers in a vertical column with the decimal points in a vertical line.
2. Add zeros on the right in the decimal fractions to make columns even.
3. The largest number in the first column to the right of the decimal point has the *greatest* value.
4. If two numbers in a column are of equal value, examine the next column to the right, and so on.
5. The smallest number in the first column to the right of the decimal point has the *least* value. If two numbers in the first column are of equal value, examine the second column to the right, and so on.

EXAMPLE 1: Of the following fractions (0.623, 0.841, 0.0096, 0.432), which has the greatest value? the least value?

0.6320
0.8410
0.0096
0.4320

0.841 has the greatest value; 0.0096 has the least value.

EXAMPLE 2: Which decimal number (0.4, 0.25, 1.2, 1.002) has the greatest value? the least value?

0.400
0.250
1.200
1.002

1.2 has the greatest value; 0.25 has the least value.

NOTE: In mixed numbers the values of both the integer and the fraction are considered.

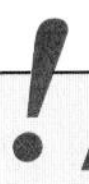

ALERT

- Remember both the integer and the decimal fraction are considered in determining which number has the greatest or least value.

ADDITION AND SUBTRACTION OF DECIMALS

1. Write the numerals in a vertical column with the decimal points in a straight line.
2. Add zeros as needed to complete the columns.
3. Add or subtract each column as indicated by the symbol.
4. Place the decimal point in the sum or difference directly below the decimal points in the column.
5. Place a zero to the left of the decimal point in a decimal fraction.

EXAMPLE 1: Add: 14.8 + 6.29 + 3.028

$$\begin{array}{r} 14.800 \\ 6.290 \\ +\ 3.028 \\ \hline 24.118 \end{array}$$

EXAMPLE 2: Subtract: 5.163 − 4.98

$$\begin{array}{r} 5.163 \\ -\ 4.980 \\ \hline 0.183 \end{array}$$

MULTIPLICATION OF DECIMALS

1. Place the shorter group of numbers under the longer group of numbers.
2. Multiply.
3. Add the number of places to the right of the decimal point in the **multiplicand** and the **multiplier** (i.e., the numbers being multiplied). The sum determines the placement of the decimal point within the product.
4. Count from right to left of the value of the sum and place the decimal point.

EXAMPLE 1: 0.19×0.2

$$
\begin{array}{rl}
0.19 & \text{two place values} \\
\times\ 0.2 & \text{one place value} \\
\hline
038 & \\
000\ \ & \\
\hline
0.038 & \text{three place values}
\end{array}
$$

EXAMPLE 2: 0.459×0.52

$$
\begin{array}{rl}
0.459 & \text{three place values} \\
\times\ \ 0.52 & \text{two place values} \\
\hline
0918 & \\
2295\ \ & \\
0000\ \ \ \ & \\
\hline
0.23868 & \text{five place values}
\end{array}
$$

EXAMPLE 3: 8.265×4.36

$$
\begin{array}{rl}
8.265 & \text{three place values} \\
\times\ \ \ 4.36 & \text{two place values} \\
\hline
49590 & \\
24795\ \ & \\
33060\ \ \ \ & \\
\hline
36.03540 & \text{five place values}
\end{array}
$$

EXAMPLE 4: 160.41×3.527

$$
\begin{array}{rl}
160.41 & \text{two place values} \\
\times\ \ \ 3.527 & \text{three place values} \\
\hline
112287 & \\
32082\ \ & \\
80205\ \ \ \ & \\
48123\ \ \ \ \ \ & \\
\hline
565.76607 & \text{five place values}
\end{array}
$$

Multiplying a Decimal by 10 or a Power of 10 (100, 1000, 10,000, 100,000)

1. Move the decimal point to the right the *same number of places as there are zeros in the multiplier.*
2. Zeros may be added as indicated.

EXAMPLE 1: $0.132 \times 10 = 1.32$

EXAMPLE 2: $0.053 \times 100 = 5.3$

EXAMPLE 3: $2.64 \times 1000 = 2640$

EXAMPLE 4: $49.6 \times 10{,}000 = 496{,}000$

Multiplying a Whole Number or Decimal by 0.1 or a Multiple of 0.1 (0.01, 0.001, 0.0001, 0.00001)

1. Move the decimal point to the left the *same number of spaces as there are numbers to the right of the decimal point in the multiplier.*
2. Zeros may be added as indicated.

EXAMPLE 1: $354.86 \times 0.0001 = 0.035486$

EXAMPLE 2: $0.729 \times 0.1 = 0.0729$

EXAMPLE 3: $12.73 \times 0.01 = 0.1273$

EXAMPLE 4: $5.752 \times 0.001 = 0.005752$

ROUNDING A DECIMAL FRACTION

1. Find the number to the right of the place value desired.
2. If the number is 5, 6, 7, 8, or 9, add 1 to the number in the place value desired and drop the rest of the numbers.
3. If the number is 0, 1, 2, 3, or 4, remove all numbers to the right of the desired place value.

EXAMPLE 1: Round the following decimal fractions to the nearest tenth.

Step 1. 0.268

0.2)68 — 6 is the number to the right of the tenths place. Therefore 1 should be added to the number 2 and the 68 dropped.

0.3 — correct answer

Step 2. 4.374

4.3)74 — 7 is the number to the right of the tenths place. Therefore 1 should be added to the number 3 and the 74 dropped.

4.4 — correct answer

Step 3. 5.723

5.7)23 — 2 is the number to the right of the tenths place. Therefore all numbers to the right of the tenths place should be removed.

5.7 — correct answer

EXAMPLE 2: Round the following decimal fractions to the nearest hundredth.

Step 1. 0.876

0.87)6 — 6 is the number to the right of the hundredths place. Therefore 1 should be added to the number 7 and the 6 dropped.

0.88 — correct answer

Step 2. 2.3249

2.32)49 — 4 is the number to the right of the hundredths place. Therefore all numbers to the right of the hundredths place should be removed.

2.32 — correct answer

EXAMPLE 3: Round the following decimal fractions to the nearest thousandth.

Step 1. 3.1325

3.132)5 — 5 is the number to the right of the thousandths place. Therefore 1 should be added to the number 2 and the 5 dropped.

3.133 — correct answer

Step 2. 0.4674

0.467)4 — 4 is the number to the right of the thousandths place. Therefore all numbers to the right of the thousandths place should be removed.

0.467 — correct answer

Rounding numbers helps to estimate values, compare values, have more realistic and workable numbers, and spot errors. Decimal fractions may be rounded to any designated place value.

DIVISION OF DECIMALS

1. Place a caret (/\) to the right of the last number in the divisor, signifying the movement of the decimal point that will make the divisor a whole number.
2. Count the number of spaces that the decimal point is moved in the divisor.
3. Count to the right an equal number of spaces in the dividend and place a caret to signify the movement of the decimal.
4. Place a decimal point on the quotient line directly above the caret.
5. Divide, extending the decimal fraction three places to the right of the decimal point.
6. Zeros may be added as indicated to extend the decimal fraction dividend.
7. Round the quotient to the nearest hundredth.

EXAMPLE 1: 8.326 ÷ 1.062

```
            7 . 839  or 7.84
1.062 ^)8.326 ^ 000
        7 434
        892 0
        849 6
          42 40
          31 86
          10 540
           9 558
```

EXAMPLE 2: 386 ÷ 719

```
      0.536 or 0.54
719)386.000
     359 5
      26 50
      21 57
       4 930
       4 314
```

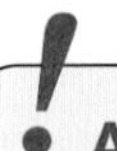

ALERT

- The decimal fraction is emphasized by the placement of a zero to the left of the decimal point.

Dividing a Decimal by 10 or a Multiple of 10 (100, 1000, 10,000, 100,000)

1. Move the decimal point to the left the same number of places as there are zeros in the divisor.
2. Zeros may be added as indicated.

EXAMPLE 1: 6.41 ÷ 10 = 0.641

EXAMPLE 2: 358.0 ÷ 100 = 3.58

Dividing a Whole Number or a Decimal Fraction by 0.1 or a Multiple of 0.1 (0.01, 0.001, 0.0001, 0.00001)

1. Move the decimal point to the right as many places as there are numbers in the divisor.
2. Zeros may be added as indicated.

EXAMPLE 1: 5.897 ÷ 0.01 = 589.7

EXAMPLE 2: 46.31 ÷ 0.001 = 46,310

CONVERSION

Converting a Decimal Fraction to a Proper Fraction

1. Remove the decimal point and the zero preceding it.
2. The numerals are the numerator.
3. The placement of the decimal point indicates what the denominator will be.
4. Reduce to lowest terms.

EXAMPLE 1: 0.3

$$\frac{3}{10}$$

EXAMPLE 2: 0.86

$$\frac{86}{100} = \frac{43}{50}$$

EXAMPLE 3: 0.375

$$\frac{375}{1000} = \frac{3}{8}$$

Converting a Proper Fraction to a Decimal Fraction

1. Divide the numerator by the denominator.
2. Extend the decimal the desired number of places (often three).
3. Place a zero to the left of the decimal point in a decimal fraction.

EXAMPLE 1: $4/5$

$$\begin{array}{r} 0.8 \\ 5\overline{)4.0} \\ \underline{4\,0} \end{array}$$

$4/5 = 0.8$

EXAMPLE 2: $7/8$

$$\begin{array}{r} 0.875 \\ 8\overline{)7.000} \\ \underline{6\,4} \\ 60 \\ \underline{56} \\ 40 \\ \underline{40} \end{array}$$

$7/8 = 0.875$

WORK SHEET

DIRECTIONS: Write the following numbers in words.

1. 0.2 ______

2. 9.68 ______

3. 0.0003 ______

4. 1968.342 ______

______

5. 0.02 ______

DIRECTIONS: Circle the decimal numbers with the *greatest value*.

1. 0.2, 0.15, 0.1, 0.25
2. 0.4, 0.45, 0.04, 0.042
3. 0.9, 0.09, 0.95, 0.98
4. 0.5, 0.065, 0.58, 0.68
5. 1.8, 1.08, 1.18, 1.468
6. 7.4, 7.42, 7.423, 7.44

DIRECTIONS: Circle the decimal numbers with the *least value*.

1. 0.6, 0.66, 0.666, 0.6666
2. 0.3, 0.03, 0.003, 0.0003
3. 1.2, 1.22, 1.022, 1.0022
4. 0.8, 0.08, 0.868, 0.859
5. 0.75, 0.07, 0.007, 0.0075
6. 3.015, 3.1, 3.006, 3.02

DIRECTIONS: Add the following decimal problems.

1. 1.080 + 31.2 + 0.065 + 9.41 = ______
2. 2.2 + 355.6 + 8.125 + 6.75 = ______
3. 24.684 + 5.3697 + 8.025 + 2.9 = ______
4. 18.95 + 1.903 + 8.82 + 9.4 = ______
5. 56.93 + 765.7 + 64.882 + 7.33 = ______
6. 0.3 + 0.874 + 2.763 + 63.2 = ______
7. 13.5 + 1.023 + 8.83 + 3.267 = ______
8. 3.6 + 8.25 + 2.05 + 24 = ______
9. 0.6 + 0.985 + 1.432 + 52.1 = ______

DIRECTIONS: Subtract the following decimal problems.

1. 1321.52 − 63.65 = ____ 2. 4.745 − 2.896 = ______ 3. 1.8 − 1.09 = _________

4. 250.7 − 75.896 = _____ 5. 24.186 − 16.768 = ____ 6. 6.33 − 2.186 = _______

7. 0.486 − 0.025 = ______ 8. 1 − 0.012 = _________ 9. 63 − 0.978 = ________

DIRECTIONS: Multiply the following decimal problems.

1. 1.3 × 12.5 = _______ 2. 127 × 4.8 = _______ 3. 1.69 × 30.8 = _______

4. 9.08 × 6.18 = _______ 5. 52.4 × 0.8 = _______ 6. 420 × 0.08 = _______

7. 2.3 × 45.21 = _______ 8. 7.46 × 54.83 = _______ 9. 1.19 × 0.127 = _______

DIRECTIONS: Multiply the following numbers by 10 by moving the decimal point.

1. 0.09 _________________ 2. 0.2 _________________ 3. 0.18 _________________

4. 0.3 _________________ 5. 0.625 _________________ 6. 2.33 _________________

DIRECTIONS: Multiply the following numbers by 100 by moving the decimal point.

1. 0.023 ________ **2.** 1.5 ________ **3.** 0.004 ________

4. 0.125 ________ **5.** 8.65 ________ **6.** 76.4 ________

DIRECTIONS: Multiply the following numbers by 1000 by moving the decimal point.

1. 0.2 ________ **2.** 0.005 ________ **3.** 0.187 ________

4. 9.65 ________ **5.** 0.46 ________ **6.** 0.489 ________

DIRECTIONS: Multiply the following numbers by 0.1 by moving the decimal point.

1. 30.0 ________ **2.** 0.69 ________ **3.** 1.7 ________

4. 0.95 ________ **5.** 0.138 ________ **6.** 5.67 ________

DIRECTIONS: Multiply the following numbers by 0.01 by moving the decimal point.

1. 0.26 ________ **2.** 90.8 ________ **3.** 5.5 ________

4. 11.2 ________ **5.** 0.875 ________ **6.** 63.3 ________

DIRECTIONS: Multiply the following numbers by 0.001 by moving the decimal point.

1. 56.0 ________ **2.** 12.55 ________ **3.** 126.5 ________

4. 33.3 ________ **5.** 9.684 ________ **6.** 241 ________

DIRECTIONS: Round the following decimal fractions to the nearest tenth.

1. 0.33 ________ **2.** 0.913 ________ **3.** 2.359 ________

4. 0.66 ________ **5.** 58.36 ________ **6.** 8.092 ________

DIRECTIONS: Round the following decimal fractions to the nearest hundredth.

1. 2.555 ________ **2.** 4.275 ________ **3.** 0.284 ________

4. 3.923 ________ **5.** 6.534 ________ **6.** 2.988 ________

DIRECTIONS: Round the following decimal fractions to the nearest thousandth.

1. 27.86314 ________ **2.** 5.9246 ________ **3.** 2.1574 ________

4. 0.8493 ________ **5.** 321.0869 ________ **6.** 455.7682 ________

DIRECTIONS: Divide. Round the quotient to the nearest hundredth.

1. 7.02 ÷ 6 = ________ 2. 124.2 ÷ 0.03 = ______ 3. 5.46 ÷ 0.7 = ________

4. 24 ÷ 0.06 = ________ 5. 24 ÷ 1500 = ________ 6. 4.6 ÷ 35.362 = ______

7. 4.13 ÷ 0.05 = _______ 8. 9.08 ÷ 2.006 = ______ 9. 63 ÷ 132.3 = ________

DIRECTIONS: Divide the following numbers by 10 by moving the decimal point.

1. 6.0 ________________ 2. 0.2 ________________ 3. 9.8 ________________

4. 0.05 ________________ 5. 0.375 ________________ 6. 0.99 ________________

DIRECTIONS: Divide the following numbers by 100 by moving the decimal point.

1. 0.7 ________________ 2. 8.11 ________________ 3. 700.0 ________________

4. 0.19 ________________ 5. 12.0 ________________ 6. 30.2 ________________

DIRECTIONS: Divide the following numbers by 1000 by moving the decimal point.

1. 1.8 ________________ 2. 360.0 ________________ 3. 0.25 ________________

4. 54.6 ________________ 5. 7.5 ________________ 6. 7140 ________________

DIRECTIONS: Divide the following numbers by 0.1 by moving the decimal point.

1. 2.8 ________________ 2. 0.1 ________________ 3. 0.65 ________________

4. 0.987 ________________ 5. 15.0 ________________ 6. 8.25 ________________

DIRECTIONS: Divide the following numbers by 0.01 by moving the decimal point.

1. 36.0 ________________ 2. 0.16 ________________ 3. 0.48 ________________

4. 9.59 ________________ 5. 0.8 ________________ 6. 0.097 ________________

DIRECTIONS: Divide the following numbers by 0.001 by moving the decimal point.

1. 6.2 ________________ 2. 839.0 ________________ 3. 5.0 ________________

4. 0.86 ________________ 5. 13.8 ________________ 6. 0.0156 ________________

DIRECTIONS: Change the following decimal fractions to proper fractions.

1. 0.06 ________ **2.** 0.8 ________ **3.** 0.68 ________ **4.** 0.0025 ________

5. 0.625 ________ **6.** 0.25 ________ **7.** 0.64 ________ **8.** 0.005 ________

DIRECTIONS: Change the following proper fractions to decimal fractions.

1. $\frac{1}{8}$ ________ **2.** $\frac{2}{3}$ ________ **3.** $\frac{16}{25}$ ________ **4.** $\frac{3}{5}$ ________

5. $\frac{8}{200}$ ________ **6.** $\frac{1}{3}$ ________ **7.** $\frac{4}{5}$ ________ **8.** $\frac{7}{8}$ ________

ANSWERS ON PP. 51–53.

NAME ______________________

DATE ______________________

ACCEPTABLE SCORE **31**

YOUR SCORE ______

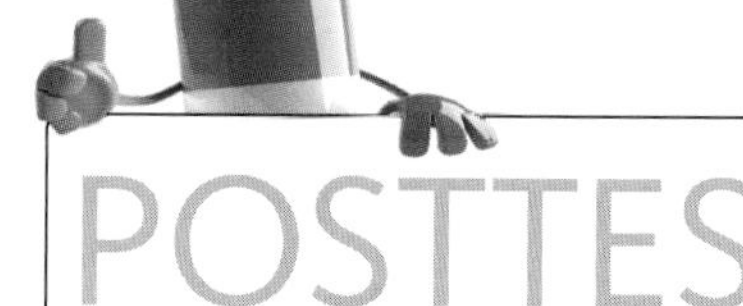

CHAPTER **2**
Decimals

POSTTEST 1

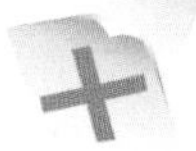

DIRECTIONS: Write the following numbers in words.

1. 634.18 ______________________

2. 0.9 ______________________

3. 64.231 ______________________

DIRECTIONS: Circle the decimal fractions with the *greatest value.*

4. 0.1, 0.01, 0.15, 0.015

5. 0.666, 0.068, 0.006, 0.66

DIRECTIONS: Perform the indicated calculations.

6. 1.342 + 0.987 + 8.062 + 44.269 = ______

7. 0.6 + 0.45 + 2.9 + 4.94 = ______

8. 3.004 + 0.848 + 0.9 + 1.6 = ______

9. 2.875 + 0.75 + 0.094 + 2.385 = ______

10. 1981.62 + 4.876 + 146.35 + 19.78 = ______

11. 1 − 0.661 = ______

12. 2.46 − 1.0068 = ______

13. 844.6 − 521.52 = ______

14. 43.69 − 0.0823 = ______

15. 0.9 − 0.689 = ______

16. 72.8 × 9.649 = ______

17. 1.58 × 0.088 = ______

18. 360 × 0.45 = ________ **19.** 26.2 × 1.69 = ________ **20.** 1.5 × 0.39 = ________

21. 268.8 ÷ 16 = ________ **22.** 8.89 ÷ 0.006 = ________ **23.** 12.54 ÷ 0.02 = ________

24. 56.4 ÷ 40 = ________ **25.** 165.9 ÷ 3.006 = ______

DIRECTIONS: Change the following decimal fractions to proper fractions.

26. 0.09 __________ **27.** 0.0025 ________ **28.** 0.375 ________ **29.** 0.4 __________

DIRECTIONS: Change the following proper fractions to decimal fractions.

30. $\frac{5}{7}$ __________ **31.** $\frac{1}{100}$ __________ **32.** $\frac{1}{250}$ __________ **33.** $\frac{1}{8}$ __________

ANSWERS ON P. 53.

NAME ______________________

DATE ______________________

ACCEPTABLE SCORE **31**

YOUR SCORE ______

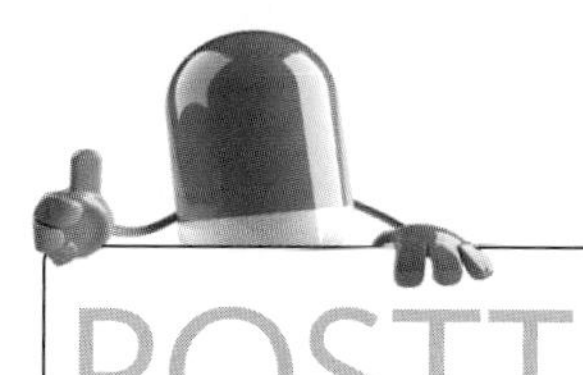

CHAPTER 2
Decimals

POSTTEST 2

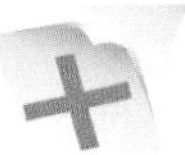

DIRECTIONS: Write the following numbers in words.

1. 0.516 ______________________

2. 4.0002 ______________________

3. 123.69 ______________________

DIRECTIONS: Circle the decimal with the *greatest value.*

4. 0.04, 0.45, 0.8, 0.86

5. 1.202, 1.22, 1.2, 1.222

DIRECTIONS: Perform the indicated calculations.

6. 1.2791 + 327.8 + 123.07 + 4.67 = ______

7. 6.95 + 0.8 + 0.625 + 7.68 = ______

8. 19.29 + 3.5 + 5.869 + 4.55 = ______

9. 1.5 + 6.3 + 10.46 + 29.465 = ______

10. 322 + 0.95 + 6.45 + 9.6 = ______

11. 632.838 − 19.869 = ______

12. 1.572 − 0.985 = ______

13. 6.4 − 3.634 = ______

14. 2.6 − 0.087 = ______

15. 4.819 − 3.734 = ______

16. 57.6 × 2.9 = ______

17. 149.36 × 700 = ______

18. 56.43 × 0.018 = ______

19. 12.8 × 6.5 = ______

20. 27.5 × 5.89 = ______

21. 5.9 ÷ 5.3 = ________ **22.** 0.295 ÷ 0.059 = ______ **23.** 124 ÷ 0.008 = ________

24. 0.7 ÷ 2.3 = ________ **25.** 5.928 ÷ 2.4 = ________

DIRECTIONS: Change the following decimal fractions to proper fractions.

26. 0.005 ________ **27.** 0.35 ________ **28.** 0.125 ________ **29.** 0.85 ________

DIRECTIONS: Change the following proper fractions to decimal fractions.

30. $\frac{1}{6}$ ________ **31.** $\frac{1}{400}$ ________ **32.** $\frac{7}{8}$ ________ **33.** $\frac{1}{150}$ ________

ANSWERS ON P. 54.

ANSWERS

CHAPTER 2 Decimals—Pretest, pp. 31–32

1. Four hundredths
2. One and six tenths
3. Sixteen and six thousand seven hundred thirty-four hundred thousandths
4. One and fifteen thousandths
5. Nine thousandths
6. 0.02
7. 0.004
8. 1.6
9. 2.082
10. 0.003
11. 25.376
12. 324.3
13. 1012.867
14. 150.6736
15. 84.565
16. 1.078
17. 1.008
18. 759.4
19. 1.7
20. 10.946
21. 0.0567
22. 6.6472
23. 1.9425
24. 29.5336
25. 186.543
26. 0.206
27. 17.95
28. 0.01097
29. 627
30. 0.0186
31. 1⁄125
32. 1⁄4
33. 161⁄500
34. 1⁄250
35. 0.6
36. 0.67
37. 0.006
38. 0.35

CHAPTER 2 Decimals—Work Sheet, pp. 41–45

Writing Numbers in Words, *p. 41*

1. Two tenths
2. Nine and sixty-eight hundredths
3. Three ten thousandths
4. One thousand nine hundred sixty-eight and three hundred forty-two thousandths
5. Two hundredths

Decimal Numbers with the Greatest Value, *p. 41*

1. 0.25
2. 0.45
3. 0.98
4. 0.68
5. 1.8
6. 7.44

Decimal Numbers with the Least Value, *p. 41*

1. 0.6
2. 0.0003
3. 1.0022
4. 0.08
5. 0.007
6. 3.006

Addition, *p. 41*

1. 41.755
2. 372.675
3. 40.9787
4. 39.073
5. 894.842
6. 67.137
7. 26.62
8. 37.9
9. 55.117

Subtraction, *p. 42*

1. 1257.87
2. 1.849
3. 0.71
4. 174.804
5. 7.418
6. 4.144
7. 0.461
8. 0.988
9. 62.022

Multiplication, *p. 42*

1. 16.25
2. 609.6
3. 52.052
4. 56.1144
5. 41.92
6. 33.6
7. 103.983
8. 409.0318
9. 0.15113

Multiply by 10, *p. 42*

1. 0.9
2. 2
3. 1.8
4. 3
5. 6.25
6. 23.3

Multiply by 100, *p. 43*

1. 2.3
2. 150
3. 0.4
4. 12.5
5. 865
6. 7640

Multiply by 1000, *p. 43*

1. 200
2. 5
3. 187
4. 9650
5. 460
6. 489

Multiply by 0.1, *p. 43*

1. 3
2. 0.069
3. 0.17
4. 0.095
5. 0.0138
6. 0.567

Multiply by 0.01, *p. 43*

1. 0.0026
2. 0.908
3. 0.055
4. 0.112
5. 0.00875
6. 0.633

Multiply by 0.001, *p. 43*

1. 0.056
2. 0.01255
3. 0.1265
4. 0.0333
5. 0.009684
6. 0.241

Round to the Nearest Tenth, *p. 43*

1. 0.3
2. 0.9
3. 2.4
4. 0.7
5. 58.4
6. 8.1

Round to the Nearest Hundredth, *p. 43*

1. 2.56
2. 4.28
3. 0.28
4. 3.92
5. 6.53
6. 2.99

Round to the Nearest Thousandth, *p. 43*

1. 27.863
2. 5.925
3. 2.157
4. 0.849
5. 321.087
6. 455.768

Division, *p. 44*

1. 1.17
2. 4140
3. 7.8
4. 400
5. 0.016
6. 0.13
7. 82.6
8. 4.53
9. 0.48

Divide by 10, *p. 44*

1. 0.6
2. 0.02
3. 0.98
4. 0.005
5. 0.0375
6. 0.099

Divide by 100, *p. 44*

1. 0.007
2. 0.0811
3. 7
4. 0.0019
5. 0.12
6. 0.302

Divide by 1000, *p. 44*

1. 0.0018
2. 0.36
3. 0.00025
4. 0.0546
5. 0.0075
6. 7.14

Divide by 0.1, *p. 44*

1. 28
2. 1
3. 6.5
4. 9.87
5. 150
6. 82.5

Divide by 0.01, *p. 44*

1. 3600
2. 16
3. 48
4. 959
5. 80
6. 9.7

Divide by 0.001, *p. 44*

1. 6200
2. 839,000
3. 5000
4. 860
5. 13,800
6. 15.6

Decimal Fractions to Proper Fractions, *p. 45*

1. $\frac{3}{50}$
2. $\frac{4}{5}$
3. $\frac{17}{25}$
4. $\frac{1}{400}$
5. $\frac{5}{8}$
6. $\frac{1}{4}$
7. $\frac{16}{25}$
8. $\frac{1}{200}$

Proper Fractions to Decimal Fractions, *p. 45*

1. 0.125
2. 0.67
3. 0.64
4. 0.6
5. 0.04
6. 0.33
7. 0.8
8. 0.875

CHAPTER 2 Decimals—Posttest 1, pp. 47–48

1. Six hundred thirty-four and eighteen hundredths
2. Nine tenths
3. Sixty-four and two hundred thirty-one thousandths
4. 0.15
5. 0.666
6. 54.66
7. 8.89
8. 6.352
9. 6.104
10. 2152.626
11. 0.339
12. 1.4532
13. 323.08
14. 43.6077
15. 0.211
16. 702.4472
17. 0.13904
18. 162
19. 44.278
20. 0.585
21. 16.8
22. 1481.67
23. 627
24. 1.41
25. 55.19
26. $\frac{9}{100}$
27. $\frac{1}{400}$
28. $\frac{3}{8}$
29. $\frac{2}{5}$
30. 0.71
31. 0.01
32. 0.004
33. 0.125

CHAPTER 2 Decimals—Posttest 2, pp. 49–50

1. Five hundred sixteen thousandths
2. Four and two ten thousandths
3. One hundred twenty-three and sixty-nine hundredths
4. 0.86
5. 1.222
6. 456.8191
7. 16.055
8. 33.209
9. 47.725
10. 339
11. 612.969
12. 0.587
13. 2.766
14. 2.513
15. 1.085
16. 167.04
17. 104,552
18. 1.01574
19. 83.2
20. 161.975
21. 1.11
22. 5
23. 15,500
24. 0.30
25. 2.47
26. $1/200$
27. $7/20$
28. $1/8$
29. $17/20$
30. 0.17
31. 0.003
32. 0.875
33. 0.007

NAME ______________________

DATE ______________________

ACCEPTABLE SCORE 38

YOUR SCORE ______

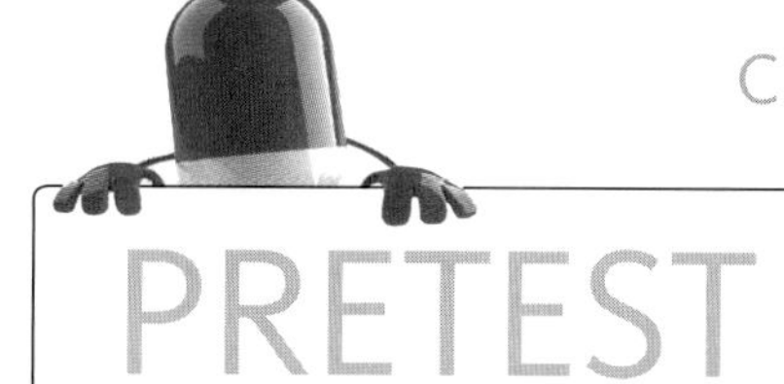

PRETEST

Complete the Percents Pretest. A score of 38 out of 40 indicates an acceptable understanding of and competency in basic calculations involving percents. You may skip to the Ratios Pretest on p. 75. However, if you score 37 or below, completion of Chapter 3, Percents, will be helpful for your continued success in the calculation of drug dosages.

DIRECTIONS: Change the following fractions to percents.

1. $\frac{1}{60}$ ______ **2.** $\frac{5}{7}$ ______ **3.** $\frac{1}{8}$ ______

4. $\frac{3}{10}$ ______ **5.** $\frac{4}{3}$ ______

DIRECTIONS: Change the following decimals to percents.

6. 0.006 ______ **7.** 0.35 ______ **8.** 0.427 ______

9. 3.821 ______ **10.** 0.7 ______

DIRECTIONS: Change the following percents to proper fractions.

11. 0.5% ______ **12.** 75% ______ **13.** $9\frac{1}{2}$% ______

14. 24.8% ______ **15.** $\frac{3}{8}$% ______

DIRECTIONS: Change the following percents to decimals.

16. $1\frac{1}{6}$% ______ **17.** 7.5% ______ **18.** $13\frac{3}{10}$% ______

19. 8/9% ______ 20. 63% ______

DIRECTIONS: What percent of

21. 1.60 is 6 ______ 22. 3/4 is 1/8 ______ 23. 100 is 65 ______

24. 500 is 1 ______ 25. 4.5 is 1.5 ______ 26. 37.8 is 4.6 ______

27. 1 4/9 is 5/8 ______ 28. 1000 is 100 ______ 29. 3 1/2 is 1/4 ______

30. 9.7 is 1/6 ______

DIRECTIONS: What is

31. 3% of 60 ______ 32. 1/4% of 60 ______ 33. 4.5% of 57 ______

34. 2 1/8% of 32 ______ 35. 4% of 77 ______ 36. 9.3% of 46 ______

37. 3/7% of 14 ______ 38. 22% of 88 ______ 39. 7.6% of 156 ______

40. 5% of 300 ______

ANSWERS ON P. 71.

CHAPTER **3**

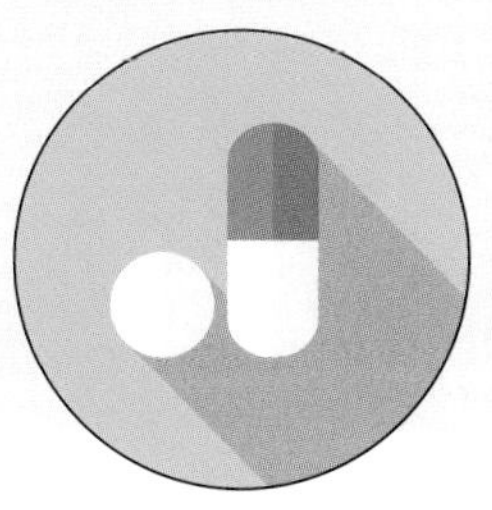

Percents

LEARNING OBJECTIVES

Upon completion of the materials provided in this chapter, you will be able to perform computations accurately by mastering the following mathematical concepts:

1. Changing a fraction or decimal to a percent
2. Changing a percent to a fraction or decimal
3. Changing a percent containing a fraction to a decimal
4. Finding what percent one number is of another
5. Finding the given percent of a number

Study the introductory material on percents. The processes for the calculation of percent problems are listed in steps. Memorize the steps for each calculation before beginning the work sheet. Complete the work sheet at the end of this chapter, which provides for extensive practice in the manipulation of percents. Check your answers. If you have any difficulty, go back and review the steps for that type of calculation. When you feel ready to evaluate your learning, take the first posttest. Check your answers. An acceptable score as indicated on the posttest signifies that you are ready for the next chapter. An unacceptable score signifies a need for further study before taking the second posttest.

A **percent** is a third way of showing a fractional relationship. Fractions, decimals, and percents can all be converted from one form to the others. Conversions of fractions and decimals are discussed in Chapter 2. A percent indicates a value equal to the number of hundredths. Therefore when a percent is written as a fraction, the denominator is *always* 100. The number beside the percent sign (%) becomes the numerator.

! ALERT

- When a percent is written as a fraction, the denominator is ALWAYS 100.
- The number beside the percent sign (%) is the numerator.

Example: $59\% = \frac{59}{100}$

CHANGING A FRACTION TO A PERCENT

1. Multiply by 100.
2. Add the percent sign (%).

EXAMPLE 1: $\frac{2}{5}$

Step 1. $\frac{2}{\cancel{5}_1} \times \frac{\cancel{100}^{20}}{1} =$

Step 2. $\frac{2 \times 20}{1 \times 1} = 40$

Step 3. 40%

EXAMPLE 2: $\frac{3}{10}$

Step 1. $\frac{3}{\cancel{10}_1} \times \frac{\cancel{100}^{10}}{1} =$

Step 2. $\frac{3 \times 10}{1 \times 1} = 30$

Step 3. 30%

CHANGING A MIXED NUMBER TO A PERCENT

1. Change the mixed number to an improper fraction.
2. Multiply by 100.
3. Add the percent sign (%).

EXAMPLE 3: $1\frac{1}{4}$

Step 1. $1\frac{1}{4} = \frac{5}{4}$

Step 2. $\frac{5}{\cancel{4}_1} \times \frac{\cancel{100}^{25}}{1} =$

Step 3. $\frac{5 \times 25}{1 \times 1} = 125$

Step 4. 125%

EXAMPLE 4: $2\frac{1}{3}$

Step 1. $2\frac{1}{3} = \frac{7}{3}$

Step 2. $\frac{7}{3} \times \frac{100}{1} =$

Step 3. $\frac{7 \times 100}{3 \times 1} = \frac{700}{3} = 233\frac{1}{3}$

Step 4. $33\frac{1}{3}\%$

CHANGING A DECIMAL TO A PERCENT

1. Multiply by 100 (by moving the decimal point two places to the right).
2. Add the percent sign (%).

EXAMPLE 1: 0.421

Step 1. $0.421 \times 100 = 42.1$

Step 2. 42.1%

EXAMPLE 2: 0.98

Step 1. $0.98 \times 100 = 98$

Step 2. 98%

EXAMPLE 3: 0.2

Step 1. $0.2 \times 100 = 20$

Step 2. 20%

EXAMPLE 4: 1.1212

Step 1. $1.1212 \times 100 = 112.12$

Step 2. 112.12%

CHANGING A PERCENT TO A FRACTION

1. Drop the % sign.
2. Write the remaining number as the fraction's numerator.
3. Write 100 as the denominator. (The denominator will *always* be 100.)
4. Reduce to lowest terms.

EXAMPLE 1: 45%

Step 1. $\frac{45}{100} = \frac{9}{20}$ (reduced to lowest terms)

EXAMPLE 2: 0.3%

Step 1. $\frac{0.3}{100} =$

Step 2. $\frac{\frac{3}{10}}{100}$

Step 3. $\frac{3}{10} \div \frac{100}{1} =$

Step 4. $\frac{3}{10} \times \frac{1}{100} = \frac{3}{1000}$

EXAMPLE 3: 3½%

Step 1. $\frac{3\frac{1}{2}}{100} = \frac{7/2}{100}$

Step 2. $\frac{7}{2} \div \frac{100}{1} =$

Step 3. $\frac{7}{2} \times \frac{1}{100} = \frac{7}{200}$

CHANGING A PERCENT TO A DECIMAL

1. Drop the % sign.
2. Divide the remaining number by 100 (by moving the decimal point two places to the left).
3. Express the quotient as a decimal. Place a zero before the decimal if there are no whole numbers.

EXAMPLE 1: 32%

0.32

EXAMPLE 2: 125%

1.25

CHANGING A PERCENT CONTAINING A FRACTION TO A DECIMAL

1. Drop the % sign.
2. Change the mixed number to an improper fraction.
3. Divide by 100. Remember, the denominator of all whole numbers is 1.
4. Reduce to lowest terms.
5. Divide the numerator by the denominator, expressing the quotient as a decimal.

EXAMPLE 1: 12½%

Step 1. $\frac{25}{2} \div \frac{100}{1} =$

Step 2. $\frac{\overset{1}{\cancel{25}}}{2} \times \frac{1}{\underset{4}{\cancel{100}}} = \frac{1}{8}$

Step 3.

$$\begin{array}{r} 0.125 \\ 8\overline{)1.000} \\ \underline{8} \\ 20 \\ \underline{16} \\ 40 \\ \underline{40} \end{array}$$

Step 4. 12½% = 0.125

EXAMPLE 2: 3¾%

Step 1. $\frac{15}{4} \div \frac{100}{1} =$

Step 2. $\frac{\overset{3}{\cancel{15}}}{4} \times \frac{1}{\underset{20}{\cancel{100}}} = \frac{3}{80}$

Step 3.

$$\begin{array}{r} 0.0375 \\ 80\overline{)3.0000} \\ \underline{2\,40} \\ 600 \\ \underline{560} \\ 400 \\ \underline{400} \end{array}$$

Step 4. 3¾% = 0.0375

FINDING WHAT PERCENT ONE NUMBER IS OF ANOTHER

1. Write the number following the word *of* as the denominator of a fraction.
2. Write the other number as the numerator of the fraction.
3. Divide the numerator by the denominator, extending the decimal fraction four places to the right of the decimal point.
4. Multiply by 100.
5. Add the % sign.

EXAMPLE 1: What percent of 24 is 9?

Step 1. $\frac{9}{24} = \frac{3}{8}$

Step 2. $8\overline{)3.000} = 0.375$

$$\begin{array}{r} 0.375 \\ 8\overline{)3.000} \\ \underline{2\,4} \\ 60 \\ \underline{56} \\ 40 \\ \underline{40} \end{array}$$

Step 3. $0.375 \times 100 = 37.5$

Step 4. 37.5%

EXAMPLE 2: What percent of 5.4 is 1.2?

Step 1. $\frac{1.2}{5.4} = 5.4\overline{)1.2\ 0000}$

$$\begin{array}{r} 0.2222 \\ 5.4\overline{)1.2\,0000} \\ \underline{1\,0\,8} \\ 1\,20 \\ \underline{1\,08} \\ 120 \\ \underline{108} \\ 120 \\ \underline{108} \end{array}$$

Step 2. $0.2222 \times 100 = 22.22$

Step 3. 22.22%

EXAMPLE 3: What percent of 2 is ¼?

Step 1. ¼/2

Step 2. $\frac{1}{4} \div 2 =$

Step 3. $\frac{1}{4} \div \frac{2}{1} =$

Step 4. $\frac{1}{4} \times \frac{1}{2} = \frac{1}{8}$

Step 5. $\frac{1}{\cancel{8}_{2}} \times \frac{\cancel{100}^{25}}{1} = \frac{25}{2} = 12.5$

Step 6. 12.5%

EXAMPLE 4: What percent of 8.7 is 3½?

Step 1. $\frac{3\frac{1}{2}}{8.7} = \frac{3.5}{8.7}$

Step 2.

$$\begin{array}{r} 0.402 \\ 8.7\overline{)3.5\,000} \\ \underline{3\,4\,8} \\ 20 \\ \underline{00} \\ 200 \\ \underline{174} \end{array}$$

Step 3. $0.402 \times 100 = 40.2$

Step 4. 40.2%

FINDING THE GIVEN PERCENT OF A NUMBER

1. Write the percent as a decimal number.
2. Multiply by the other number.

EXAMPLE 1: What is 40% of 180?

Step 1. $\frac{40}{100} = 100\overline{)40.0}$ = 0.4 (40 0)

Step 2. $180 \times 0.4 = 72.0$

Step 3. 40% of 180 = 72

EXAMPLE 2: What is 3⁄10% of 52?

Step 1. $\frac{\frac{3}{10}}{100} = \frac{3}{10} \div \frac{100}{1} =$

Step 2. $\frac{3}{10} \times \frac{1}{100} = \frac{3}{1000}$

Step 3. $\frac{3}{1000} = 0.003$

Step 4. 0.003×52: 0 006, 00 15, 00.156

Step 5. 3⁄10% of 52 = 0.156

CHAPTER 3
Percents

WORK SHEET

DIRECTIONS: Change each of the following proper fractions to a percent.

1. $3/4$ ____________
2. $3/8$ ____________
3. $4/5$ ____________
4. $8/25$ ____________
5. $3/1000$ ____________
6. $7/200$ ____________
7. $9/400$ ____________
8. $3/20$ ____________
9. $9/150$ ____________
10. $11/16$ ____________
11. $5/6$ ____________
12. $75/10{,}000$ ____________

DIRECTIONS: Change each of the following decimals to a percent.

1. 0.402 ____________
2. 0.0367 ____________
3. 0.163 ____________
4. 0.98 ____________
5. 0.3 ____________
6. 0.145 ____________
7. 0.7 ____________
8. 0.42 ____________
9. 0.159 ____________
10. 0.673 ____________
11. 0.3712 ____________
12. 2.2 ____________

DIRECTIONS: Change each of the following percents to a mixed number or a proper fraction.

1. 3.5% ______ 2. $\frac{3}{4}$% ______ 3. 0.125% ______ 4. 10% ______

5. $\frac{2}{3}$% ______ 6. 20.2% ______ 7. 12% ______ 8. 0.25% ______

9. $2\frac{3}{8}$% ______ 10. $6\frac{1}{4}$% ______ 11. 2.1% ______ 12. $66\frac{2}{3}$% ______

DIRECTIONS: Change each of the following percents to a decimal.

1. 37.5% ______ 2. 3% ______ 3. $6\frac{3}{4}$% ______ 4. 0.42% ______

5. $\frac{1}{4}$% ______ 6. $2\frac{1}{2}$% ______ 7. 0.23% ______ 8. 72.6% ______

9. 16% ______ 10. $\frac{5}{16}$% ______ 11. $\frac{1}{2}$% ______ 12. $\frac{7}{12}$% ______

DIRECTIONS: What percent of

1. 40 is 22 ______ 2. 80 is 6.3 ______ 3. 200 is 4 ______ 4. 500 is 60 ______

5. 20 is 1 ______ 6. 24 is 3.6 ______ 7. 275 is 55 ______ 8. 1000 is 100 ______

9. 800 is 360 ______ 10. 25 is $\frac{1}{4}$ ______ 11. 250 is 5.2 ______ 12. 35 is 7 ______

DIRECTIONS: What is

1. 25% of 478 ____________ **2.** 10% of 34 ____________ **3.** 2.8% of 510 ____________

4. ½% of 28 ____________ **5.** 33⅓% of 3000 ____________ **6.** ⅕% of 65 ____________

7. 2¼% of 26 ____________ **8.** ⅜% of 32 ____________ **9.** 62% of 871 ____________

10. ¼% of 68 ____________ **11.** 41% of 27 ____________ **12.** 8.4% of 128 ____________

ANSWERS ON PP. 71–72.

NAME ______________________

DATE ______________________

ACCEPTABLE SCORE 29

YOUR SCORE ______

CHAPTER 3
Percents

POSTTEST 1

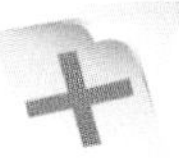

DIRECTIONS: Change the following fractions to percents.

1. $\frac{7}{8}$ ______ **2.** $\frac{11}{20}$ ______ **3.** $\frac{3}{1000}$ ______

DIRECTIONS: Change the following decimals to percents.

4. 0.256 ______ **5.** 0.004 ______ **6.** 0.9 ______

DIRECTIONS: Change the following percents to proper fractions.

7. 85% ______ **8.** 0.3% ______ **9.** $3\frac{1}{2}$% ______

DIRECTIONS: Change the following percents to decimals.

10. 86.3% ______ **11.** $4\frac{5}{8}$% ______ **12.** 0.36% ______

DIRECTIONS: What percent of

13. 70 is 7 ______ **14.** 24 is 1.2 ______ **15.** 300 is 1 ______

16. $66\frac{2}{3}$ is 8 ______ **17.** 3.5 is 1.5 ______ **18.** 2.5 is 0.5 ______

19. $\frac{3}{4}$ is $\frac{3}{8}$ ______ **20.** 160 is 12 ______ **21.** 250 is 20 ______

DIRECTIONS: What is

22. 65% of 800 ________ **23.** 90% of 40 ________ **24.** $\frac{1}{8}$% of 72 ________

25. 8.5% of 2000 ________ **26.** $4\frac{1}{2}$% of 940 ________ **27.** 65% of 450 ________

28. $\frac{1}{4}$% of 60 ________ **29.** 4.3% of 56 ________ **30.** 0.52% of 88 ________

ANSWERS ON P. 72.

NAME ______________________

DATE ______________________

ACCEPTABLE SCORE **29**

YOUR SCORE ______

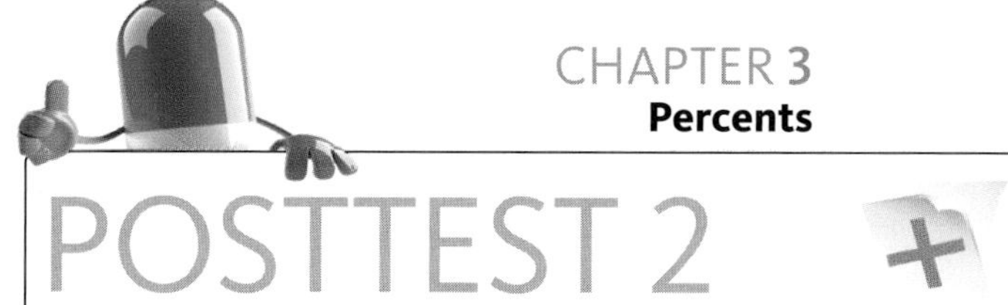

DIRECTIONS: Change the following fractions to percents.

1. $\frac{1}{8}$ ______ **2.** $\frac{2}{5}$ ______ **3.** $\frac{1}{6}$ ______

DIRECTIONS: Change the following decimals to percents.

4. 0.065 ______ **5.** 0.005 ______ **6.** 0.2 ______

DIRECTIONS: Change the following percents to proper fractions.

7. 0.3% ______ **8.** $16\frac{1}{2}$% ______ **9.** 0.25% ______

DIRECTIONS: Change the following percents to decimals.

10. $3\frac{3}{4}$% ______ **11.** 7% ______ **12.** 5.55% ______

DIRECTIONS: What percent of

13. 5.4 is 1.2 ______ **14.** $\frac{1}{4}$ is $\frac{1}{8}$ ______ **15.** 250 is 6 ______

16. 40 is 32 ______ **17.** 160 is 12 ______ **18.** 500 is 50 ______

19. $5\frac{3}{4}$ is $2\frac{3}{8}$ ______ **20.** 120 is 15 ______ **21.** $\frac{9}{16}$ is $\frac{5}{7}$ ______

DIRECTIONS: What is

22. 35% of 650 ________ **23.** $\frac{1}{4}$% of 116 ________ **24.** $4\frac{1}{2}$% of 940 ________

25. 11% of 88 ________ **26.** 16% of 90 ________ **27.** 7.5% of 261 ________

28. 45% of 24.27 ________ **29.** $\frac{7}{8}$% of 64 ________ **30.** 82.4% of 118 ________

ANSWERS ON P. 73.

ANSWERS

CHAPTER 3 Percents—Pretest, pp. 55–56

Fractions to Percents, *p. 55*

1. $1\frac{2}{3}$%, 1.6666%
2. $71\frac{3}{7}$%, 71.4285%
3. $12\frac{1}{2}$%, 12.5%
4. 30%
5. $133\frac{1}{3}$%, 133.3333%

Decimals to Percents, *p. 55*

6. 0.6%
7. 35%
8. 42.7%
9. 382.1%
10. 70%

Percents to Proper Fractions, *p. 55*

11. $\frac{1}{200}$
12. $\frac{3}{4}$
13. $\frac{19}{200}$
14. $\frac{31}{125}$
15. $\frac{3}{800}$

Percents to Decimals, *pp. 55–56*

16. 0.0117
17. 0.075
18. 0.133
19. 0.0088
20. 0.63

What Percent of, *p. 56*

21. 375%
22. $16\frac{2}{3}$%, 16.6666%
23. 65%
24. $\frac{1}{5}$%, 0.2%
25. $33\frac{1}{3}$%, 33.333%
26. $12\frac{32}{189}$%, 12.1693%
27. $43\frac{7}{26}$%, 43.2692%
28. 10%
29. $7\frac{1}{7}$%, 7.1428%
30. $1\frac{209}{291}$%, 1.7182%

What Is, *p. 56*

31. 1.8
32. 0.15
33. 2.565
34. 0.36
35. 3.08
36. 4.278
37. 0.06
38. 19.36
39. 11.856
40. 15

CHAPTER 3 Percents—Work Sheet, pp. 63–65

Fractions to Percents, *p. 63*

1. 75%
2. $37\frac{1}{2}$%
3. 80%
4. 32%
5. $\frac{3}{10}$% or 0.3%
6. $3\frac{1}{2}$%
7. $2\frac{1}{4}$% or 2.25%
8. 15%
9. 6%
10. $68\frac{3}{4}$% or 68.75%
11. $83\frac{1}{3}$% or 83.3%
12. $\frac{3}{4}$% or 0.75%

Decimals to Percents, *p. 63*

1. 40.2%
2. 3.67%
3. 16.3%
4. 98%
5. 30%
6. 14.5%
7. 70%
8. 42%
9. 15.9%
10. 67.3%
11. 37.12%
12. 220%

Percents to Mixed Numbers or Proper Fractions, *p. 64*

1. 7⁄200
2. 3⁄400
3. 1⁄800
4. 1⁄10
5. 1⁄150
6. 101⁄500
7. 3⁄25
8. 1⁄400
9. 19⁄800
10. 1⁄16
11. 21⁄1000
12. 2⁄3

Percents to Decimals, *p. 64*

1. 0.375
2. 0.03
3. 0.0675
4. 0.0042
5. 0.0025
6. 0.025
7. 0.0023
8. 0.726
9. 0.16
10. 0.003125
11. 0.005
12. 0.0058

What Percent of, *p. 64*

1. 55%
2. 7 7⁄8%, 7.875%
3. 2%
4. 12%
5. 5%
6. 15%
7. 20%
8. 10%
9. 45%
10. 1%
11. 2 2⁄25%, 2.08%
12. 20%

What Is, *p. 65*

1. 119.5
2. 3.4
3. 14.28
4. 0.14
5. 999.9 or 1000
6. 0.13
7. 0.585
8. 0.12
9. 540.02
10. 0.17
11. 11.07
12. 10.752

CHAPTER 3 Percents—Posttest 1, pp. 67–68

Fractions to Percents, *p. 67*

1. 87½%, 87.5%
2. 55%
3. 3⁄10%, 0.3%

Decimals to Percents, *p. 67*

4. 25.6%
5. 0.4%
6. 90%

Percents to Proper Fractions, *p. 67*

7. 17⁄20
8. 3⁄1000
9. 7⁄200

Percents to Decimals, *p. 67*

10. 0.863
11. 0.04625
12. 0.0036

What Percent of, *p. 67*

13. 10%
14. 5%
15. 1⁄3%, 0.33%
16. 12%
17. 42 6⁄7%, 42.8571%
18. 20%
19. 50%
20. 7½%, 7.5%
21. 8%

What Is, *p. 68*

22. 520
23. 36
24. 0.09
25. 170
26. 42.3
27. 292.5
28. 0.15
29. 2.408
30. 0.4576

CHAPTER 3 Percents—Posttest 2, pp. 69–70

Fractions to Percents, *p. 69*

1. $12\frac{1}{2}$%, 12.5%	2. 40%	3. $16\frac{2}{3}$%, 16.6666%

Decimals to Percents, *p. 69*

4. 6.5%	5. 0.5%	6. 20%

Percents to Proper Fractions, *p. 69*

7. $\frac{3}{1000}$	8. $\frac{33}{200}$	9. $\frac{1}{400}$

Percents to Decimals, *p. 69*

10. 0.0375	11. 0.07	12. 0.0555

What Percent of, *p. 69*

13. $22\frac{2}{9}$%, 22.2222%	16. 80%	19. $41\frac{7}{23}$%, 41.3043%
14. 50%	17. $7\frac{1}{2}$%, 7.5%	20. $12\frac{1}{2}$%, 12.5%
15. $2\frac{2}{5}$%, 2.4%	18. 10%	21. $126\frac{62}{63}$%, 126.9841%

What Is, *p. 70*

22. 227.5	25. 9.68	28. 10.9215
23. 0.29	26. 14.4	29. 0.56
24. 42.3	27. 19.575	30. 97.232

NAME ______________________

DATE ______________________

ACCEPTABLE SCORE 29

YOUR SCORE ______

PRETEST

Complete the Ratios Pretest. A score of 29 out of 30 indicates an acceptable understanding of and competency in basic calculations involving ratios. You may skip to the Proportions Pretest on p. 91. However, if you score 28 or below, completion of Chapter 4, Ratios, will be helpful for your continued success in the calculation of drug dosages.

DIRECTIONS: Convert to equivalents.

	Ratio	Fraction	Decimal	Percent
1.	17 : 51			
2.			0.715	
3.		8/20		
4.				12½%
5.	21 : 420			
6.		5/32		
7.			0.286	
8.				71 3/7%
9.				16¼%
10.			0.462	

ANSWERS ON P. 88.

CHAPTER **4**

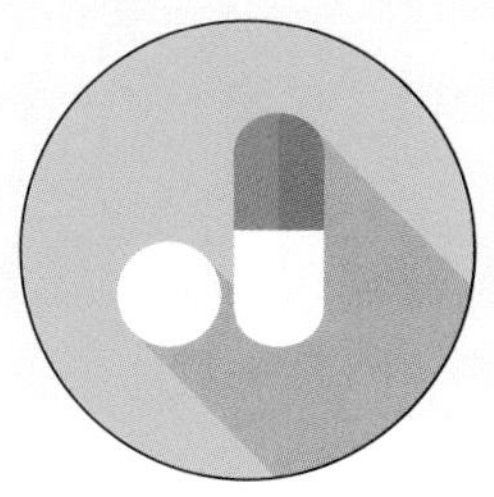

Ratios

LEARNING OBJECTIVES

Upon completion of the materials provided in this chapter, you will be able to perform computations accurately by mastering the following mathematical concepts:

1. Changing a proper fraction, decimal fraction, and percent to a ratio reduced to lowest terms
2. Changing a ratio to a proper fraction, a decimal fraction, and a percent

Study the introductory material on ratios. The processes for the calculation of ratio problems are listed in steps. Memorize the steps for each calculation before beginning the work sheet. Review previous chapters on fractions, decimals, and percents as necessary. Complete the work sheet at the end of this chapter, which provides for extensive practice in the manipulation of ratios. Check your answers. If you have difficulties, go back and review the steps for that type of calculation. When you feel ready to evaluate your learning, take the first posttest. Check your answers. An acceptable score as indicated on the posttest signifies that you are ready for the next chapter. An unacceptable score signifies a need for further study before taking the second posttest.

A **ratio** is another way of indicating a relationship between two numbers. In other words, it is another way to express a fraction. A ratio indicates *division.* The numerator is the first number listed.

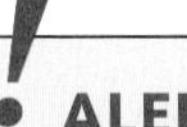

ALERT

- A ratio is another way to represent a fraction.
- A ratio indicates DIVISION.
- The numerator is the first number listed.

EXAMPLE 1: $\frac{3}{4}$ written as a ratio is 3 : 4
In reading a ratio, one reads the colon as "is to." The example would then be read as "three is to four."

EXAMPLE 2: 7 written as a ratio is 7 : 1
To express any whole number as a ratio, the number following the colon is *always* 1. The example would be read as "seven is to one."

CHANGING A PROPER FRACTION TO A RATIO REDUCED TO LOWEST TERMS

1. Reduce the fraction to lowest terms.
2. Write the numerator of the fraction as the first number of the ratio.

3. Place a colon after the first number.
4. Write the denominator of the fraction as the second number of the ratio.

EXAMPLE 1: $\frac{4}{12}$

Step 1. $\frac{4}{12}$ reduced to lowest terms equals $\frac{1}{3}$

Step 2. $\frac{1}{3}$ written as a ratio is 1 : 3

EXAMPLE 2: $\frac{1}{1000}/\frac{1}{10}$

Step 1. $\frac{1}{1000} \div \frac{1}{10} =$

Step 2. $\frac{1}{\cancel{1000}_{100}} \times \frac{\cancel{10}^{1}}{1} = \frac{1}{100}$

Step 3. $\frac{1}{1000}/\frac{1}{10}$ reduced to lowest terms equals $\frac{1}{100}$

Step 4. $\frac{1}{100}$ written as a ratio is 1 : 100

CHANGING A DECIMAL FRACTION TO A RATIO REDUCED TO LOWEST TERMS

1. Express the decimal fraction as a proper fraction reduced to lowest terms.
2. Write the numerator of the fraction as the first number of the ratio.
3. Place a colon after the first number.
4. Write the denominator of the fraction as the second number of the ratio.

EXAMPLE 1: 0.85

Step 1. $\frac{85}{100} = \frac{17}{20}$ (reduced to lowest terms)

Step 2. $\frac{17}{20}$ written as a ratio is 17 : 20

EXAMPLE 2: 0.125

Step 1. $\frac{125}{1000} = \frac{1}{8}$ (reduced to lowest terms)

Step 2. $\frac{1}{8}$ written as a ratio is 1 : 8

CHANGING A PERCENT TO A RATIO REDUCED TO LOWEST TERMS

1. Express the percent as a proper fraction reduced to lowest terms.
2. Write the numerator of the fraction as the first number of the ratio.
3. Place a colon after the first number.
4. Write the denominator of the fraction as the second number of the ratio.

EXAMPLE 1: 30%

Step 1. $\frac{30}{100} = \frac{3}{10}$ (reduced to lowest terms)

Step 2. $\frac{3}{10}$ written as a ratio is 3 : 10

EXAMPLE 2: ½%

Step 1. $\frac{\frac{1}{2}}{100} =$

Step 2. $\frac{1}{2} \div \frac{100}{1} =$

Step 3. $\frac{1}{2} \times \frac{1}{100} = \frac{1}{200}$

Step 4. $\frac{1}{200}$ written as a ratio is 1 : 200

EXAMPLE 3: 3⁹⁄₁₀%

Step 1. $\frac{3\frac{9}{10}}{100} =$

Step 2. $\frac{39}{10} \div \frac{100}{1} =$

Step 3. $\frac{39}{10} \times \frac{1}{100} = \frac{39}{1000}$

Step 4. $\frac{39}{1000}$ written as a ratio is 39 : 1000

CHANGING A RATIO TO A PROPER FRACTION REDUCED TO LOWEST TERMS

1. Write the first number of the ratio as the numerator.
2. Write the second number of the ratio as the denominator.
3. Reduce to lowest terms.

EXAMPLE 1: 9 : 15

$\frac{9}{15} = \frac{3}{5}$ (reduced to lowest terms)

EXAMPLE 2: 11 : 22

$\frac{11}{22} = \frac{1}{2}$ (reduced to lowest terms)

CHANGING A RATIO TO A DECIMAL FRACTION

Divide the first number of the ratio by the second number of the ratio, using long division.

EXAMPLE 1: 4 : 5

Step 1.

```
   0.8
5)4.0
  4 0
  ---
```

Step 2. 4 : 5 written as a decimal is 0.8

EXAMPLE 2: 3½ : 2¼

Step 1. 3.5 : 2.25

Step 2.

```
            1 .555
2.25 ∧)3.50 ∧000
        2 25
        ----
        1 25  0
        1 12  5
        -------
          12  50
          11  25
          ------
           1  250
           1  125
```

Step 3. 3½ : 2¼ written as a decimal is 1.555

CHANGING A RATIO TO A PERCENT

1. Express the ratio as a proper fraction or a decimal fraction, whichever you prefer to work with.
2. Multiply by 100.
3. Add the percent sign (%).

EXAMPLE 1: 3 : 5

Changing to a proper fraction:

Step 1. $\frac{3}{\cancel{5}_{1}} \times \frac{\cancel{100}^{20}}{1} = \frac{60}{1}$

Step 2. 60%

Changing to a decimal fraction:

Step 1. $5\overline{)3.0}$ = 0.6; 3 0

Step 2. $0.6 \times 100 = 60$

Step 3. 60%

EXAMPLE 2: 60 : 180

Changing to a proper fraction:

Step 1. $\frac{60}{180} = \frac{1}{3}$

Step 2. $\frac{1}{3} \times \frac{100}{1} = \frac{100}{3} = 33\frac{1}{3}$

Step 3. $33\frac{1}{3}$%

Changing to a decimal fraction:

Step 1. $180\overline{)60.000}$ = 0.333

```
      0.333
180)60.000
    54 0
    6 00
    5 40
      600
      540
       600
       540
        60
```

Step 2. $0.333 \times 100 = 33.3$

Step 3. 33.3%

WORK SHEET

DIRECTIONS: Change the following fractions to ratios reduced to lowest terms.

1. $^{9}/_{12}$ ____________
2. $^{4}/_{6}$ ____________
3. $^{11}/_{22}$ ____________
4. $^{56}/_{100}$ ____________
5. $^{20}/_{50}$ ____________
6. $^{310}/_{1000}$ ____________
7. $^{10}/_{16}$ ____________
8. $^{5}/_{6}/3^{1}/_{3}$ ____________
9. $1^{3}/_{5}/2^{7}/_{10}$ ____________
10. $^{1}/_{10}/^{1}/_{100}$ ____________
11. $^{14}/_{30}/2$ ____________
12. $3^{1}/_{3}/3^{1}/_{3}$ ____________

DIRECTIONS: Change the following decimal fractions to ratios reduced to lowest terms.

1. 0.896 ____________
2. 0.96 ____________
3. 0.06 ____________
4. 0.6 ____________
5. 0.4032 ____________
6. 0.74 ____________
7. 0.166 ____________
8. 0.26 ____________
9. 0.492 ____________
10. 0.95 ____________
11. 0.235 ____________
12. 0.172 ____________

DIRECTIONS: Change the following percents to ratios reduced to lowest terms.

1. 10% ______ **2.** 33⅓% ______ **3.** ⅜% ______

4. 2 7/10% ______ **5.** 44% ______ **6.** 15.7% ______

7. 7¾% ______ **8.** 0.44% ______ **9.** 7.8% ______

10. 1% ______ **11.** ⅗% ______ **12.** 3 3/7% ______

DIRECTIONS: Change the following ratios to fractions reduced to lowest terms.

1. 4 : 64 ______ **2.** 4 : 800 ______ **3.** 3 : 150 ______

4. ⅜ : ¼ ______ **5.** 8/12 : ⅔ ______ **6.** 2½ : 7½ ______

7. ⅘ : ¼ ______ **8.** 1/10 : 4/20 ______ **9.** 4/75 : 3/10 ______

10. 0.68 : 0.44 ______ **11.** 1.85 : 3.35 ______ **12.** 1.64 : 2.54 ______

DIRECTIONS: Change the following ratios to decimal numbers.

1. 7 : 14 ________
2. 5 : 20 ________
3. 3 : 8 ________
4. 11 : 33 ________
5. $\frac{5}{8} : \frac{1}{10}$ ________
6. $\frac{1}{1000} : \frac{1}{500}$ ________
7. $\frac{3}{4} : \frac{1}{2}$ ________
8. $\frac{3}{1000} : \frac{3}{100}$ ________
9. 2 : 5 ________
10. $\frac{1}{2} : \frac{5}{9}$ ________
11. 7 : 259 ________
12. $1\frac{2}{5} : \frac{12}{30}$ ________

DIRECTIONS: Change the following ratios to percents.

1. 2 : 4 ________
2. 7 : 231 ________
3. 25 : 250 ________
4. 30 : 150 ________
5. $1\frac{1}{4} : 3\frac{3}{8}$ ________
6. 1 : 1000 ________
7. 0.15 : 0.6 ________
8. $\frac{5}{16} : \frac{3}{5}$ ________
9. 1 : 500 ________
10. $1\frac{8}{12} : 2\frac{3}{6}$ ________
11. 2.5 : 4.5 ________
12. $4 : \frac{3}{16}$ ________

ANSWERS ON P. 88.

NAME ______________________

DATE ______________________

ACCEPTABLE SCORE **29**

YOUR SCORE ______

POSTTEST 1

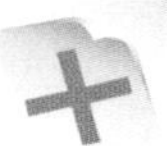

DIRECTIONS: Convert to equivalents.

	Ratio	Fraction	Decimal	Percent
1.	42 : 48			
2.			0.004	
3.		$^{13}/_{20}$		
4.				$2\frac{1}{4}\%$
5.			0.35	
6.		$^{6}/_{25}$		
7.	$^{3}/_{8} : ^{5}/_{9}$			
8.				0.3%
9.			0.205	
10.		$^{4}/_{11}$		

ANSWERS ON P. 88.

NAME ____________________

DATE ____________________

ACCEPTABLE SCORE 29

YOUR SCORE ________

CHAPTER 4
Ratios

POSTTEST 2

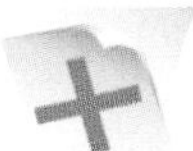

DIRECTIONS: Convert to equivalents.

	Ratio	Fraction	Decimal	Percent
1.	7 : 10			
2.		$\frac{5}{16}$		
3.			0.075	
4.				6%
5.				$\frac{3}{8}$%
6.		$\frac{1}{150}$		
7.			0.007	
8.	6 : 21			
9.			0.322	
10.				18.2%

ANSWERS ON P. 89.

ANSWERS

CHAPTER 4 Ratios—Pretest, p. 75

1. 1/3, 0.3333, 33.33%
2. 143 : 200, 143/200, 71.5%
3. 2 : 5, 0.4, 40%
4. 1 : 8, 1/8, 0.125
5. 1/20, 0.05, 5%
6. 5 : 32, 0.15625, 15.625%
7. 143 : 500, 143/500, 28.6%
8. 5 : 7, 5/7, 0.714
9. 13 : 80, 13/80, 0.1625
10. 231 : 500, 231/500, 46.2%

CHAPTER 4 Ratios—Work Sheet, pp. 81–83

Fractions to Ratios, *p. 81*

1. 3 : 4
2. 2 : 3
3. 1 : 2
4. 14 : 25
5. 2 : 5
6. 31 : 100
7. 5 : 8
8. 1 : 4
9. 16 : 27
10. 10 : 1
11. 7 : 30
12. 1 : 1

Decimals to Ratios, *p. 81*

1. 112 : 125
2. 24 : 25
3. 3 : 50
4. 3 : 5
5. 252 : 625
6. 37 : 50
7. 83 : 500
8. 13 : 50
9. 123 : 250
10. 19 : 20
11. 47 : 200
12. 43 : 250

Percents to Ratios, *p. 82*

1. 1 : 10
2. 1 : 3
3. 3 : 800
4. 27 : 1000
5. 11 : 25
6. 157 : 1000
7. 31 : 400
8. 11 : 2500
9. 39 : 500
10. 1 : 100
11. 3 : 500
12. 6 : 175

Ratios to Fractions, *p. 82*

1. 1/16
2. 1/200
3. 1/50
4. 1 1/2
5. 1
6. 1/3
7. 3 1/5
8. 1/2
9. 8/45
10. 1 6/11
11. 37/67
12. 82/127

Ratios to Decimal Numbers, *p. 83*

1. 0.5
2. 0.25
3. 0.375
4. 0.3333
5. 6.25
6. 0.5
7. 1.5
8. 0.1
9. 0.4
10. 0.9
11. 0.027
12. 3.5

Ratios to Percents, *p. 83*

1. 50%
2. 3 1/33%, 3.0303%
3. 10%
4. 20%
5. 37 1/27%, 37.037%
6. 1/10%, 0.1%
7. 25%
8. 52 1/12%, 52.0833%
9. 1/5%, 0.2%
10. 66 2/3%, 66.6666%
11. 55 5/9%, 55.5555%
12. 2133 1/3%, 2133.3333%

CHAPTER 4 Ratios—Posttest 1, p. 85

1. 7/8, 0.875, 87.5%
2. 1 : 250, 1/250, 0.4%
3. 13 : 20, 0.65, 65%
4. 9 : 400, 9/400, 0.0225
5. 7 : 20, 7/20, 35%
6. 6 : 25, 0.24, 24%
7. 27/40, 0.675, 67.5%
8. 3 : 1000, 3/1000, 0.003
9. 41 : 200, 41/200, 20.5%
10. 4 : 11, 0.3636, 36.36%

CHAPTER 4 Ratios—Posttest 2, p. 87

1. $\frac{7}{10}$, 0.7, 70%
2. 5 : 16, 0.3125, 31.25%
3. 3 : 40, $\frac{3}{40}$, 7.5%
4. 3 : 50, $\frac{3}{50}$, 0.06
5. 3 : 800, $\frac{3}{800}$, 0.00375
6. 1 : 150, 0.0066, 0.66%
7. 7 : 1000, $\frac{7}{1000}$, 0.7%
8. $\frac{2}{7}$, 0.2857, 28.57%
9. 161 : 500, $\frac{161}{500}$, 32.2%
10. 91 : 500, $\frac{91}{500}$, 0.182

NAME ____________________

DATE ____________________

ACCEPTABLE SCORE **19**

YOUR SCORE ______

CHAPTER 5
Proportions

PRETEST

Complete the Proportions Pretest. A score of 19 out of 20 indicates an acceptable understanding of and competency in basic calculations involving proportions. You may skip to the Review of Mathematics Posttest on p. 105. However, if you score 18 or below, completion of Chapter 5, Proportions, will be helpful for your continued success in the calculation of drug dosages.

DIRECTIONS: Find the value of x. Show your work.

1. $25 : 75 :: x : 300$ ______

2. $450 : 15 :: 225 : x$ ______

3. $x : \frac{1}{4}\% :: 8 : 12$ ______

4. $12 : 3 :: x : 0.8$ ______

5. $0.6 : 2.4 :: 32 : x$ ______

6. $150 : x :: 75 : 2$ ______

7. $\frac{1}{8} : \frac{2}{3} :: 75 : x$ ______

8. $\frac{1}{200} : 8 :: x : 800$ ______

9. $x : \frac{1}{2} :: \frac{3}{4} : \frac{7}{8}$ ______

10. $16 : x :: 24 : 12$ ______

11. $\frac{2}{3} : \frac{1}{5} :: x : 24$ ______

12. $x : 9 :: \frac{2}{3} : 36$ ______

13. $\frac{1}{7} : x :: \frac{1}{2} : 49$ ______

14. $0.8 : 4 :: 9.6 : x$ ______

15. $\frac{4}{5} : x :: \frac{2}{3} : \frac{1}{4}$ ______

16. $40 : 80 :: x : 160$ ______

17. $2.5 : x :: 4 : 16$ ______

18. $8 : 72 :: 14 : x$ ______

19. $x : \frac{1}{15} :: 50 : 500$ ______

20. $5 : 100 :: x : 325$ ______

ANSWERS ON P. 104.

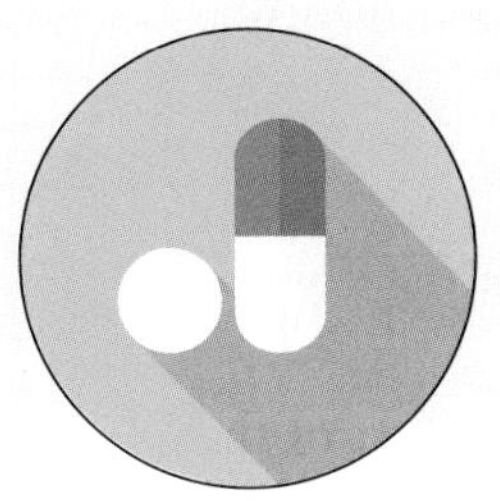

Proportions

LEARNING OBJECTIVES

Upon completion of the materials provided in this chapter, you will be able to perform computations accurately by mastering the following mathematical concepts:

1 Solving simple proportion problems

2 Solving proportion problems involving fractions, decimals, and percents

Most problems concerning drug dosage can be solved by a proportion problem, whether it involves fractions, decimals, or percents. If a proportion problem contains any combination of fractions, decimals, or percents, all forms within the problem must be converted to either fractions or decimals.

Study the introductory material on proportions. The process for the calculation of proportion problems is listed in steps. Memorize the steps before beginning the work sheet. Complete the work sheet at the end of this chapter, which provides for extensive practice in the manipulation of proportions. Check your answers. If you have difficulties, go back and review the necessary steps. When you feel ready to evaluate your learning, take the first posttest. Check your answers. An acceptable score as indicated on the posttest signifies that you are ready for the next chapter. An unacceptable score signifies a need for further study before taking the second posttest.

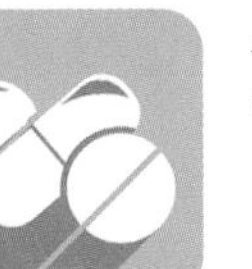

A **proportion** consists of two ratios of equal value. The ratios are connected by a double colon (::), which symbolizes the word *as.*

$$2 : 3 :: 4 : 6$$

Read the above proportion: "Two is to three as four is to six."

The first and fourth terms of the proportion are the **extremes.** The second and third terms are the **means.**

2 and 6 are the extremes

3 and 4 are the means

A helpful way to remember the correct location of the extremes and means is

E = The *end* of the problem

M = The *middle* of the problem

In a proportion the product of the means equals the product of the extremes because the ratios are of equal value. This principle may be used to verify your answer in a proportion problem.

$3 \times 4 = 12$, product of the means

$2 \times 6 = 12$, product of the extremes

If three terms in the proportion are known and one term is unknown, an x is inserted in the space for the unknown term.

$$2 : 3 :: 4 : x$$

SOLVING A SIMPLE PROPORTION PROBLEM

1. Multiply the extremes.
2. Multiply the means.
3. Place the product that includes the x on the *left* of the equal sign and the product of the known terms on the *right* of the equal sign.
4. Divide the product of the known terms by the number next to x. The quotient will be the value of x.

Proportion Problem Involving Whole Numbers

EXAMPLE: $2 : 3 :: 4 : x$

Step 1. $2x = 3 \times 4$

Step 2. $2x = 12$

Step 3. $x = 12 \div 2$

Step 4. $x = \frac{12}{2}$

Step 5. $x = 6$

Proportion Problem Involving Fractions

EXAMPLE: $\frac{1}{150} : \frac{1}{100} :: x : 60$

Step 1. $\frac{1}{100} x = \frac{1}{150} \times 60$

Step 2. $\frac{1}{100} x = \frac{2}{5}$

Step 3. $x = \frac{2}{5} \div \frac{1}{100}$

Step 4. $x = \frac{2}{\cancel{5}_{1}} \times \frac{\cancel{100}^{20}}{1}$

Step 5. $x = 40$

Proportion Problem Involving Decimals

EXAMPLE: $0.4 : 0.8 :: 0.25 : x$

Step 1. $0.4x = 0.8 \times 0.25$

Step 2. $0.4x = 0.2$

Step 3. $x = 0.2 \div 0.4$

Step 4. $x = 0.5$

Proportion Problem Involving Fractions and Percents

EXAMPLE: $x : \frac{1}{4}\% :: 9\frac{3}{5} : \frac{1}{200}$

Convert $\frac{1}{4}\%$ to a proper fraction and $9\frac{3}{5}$ to an improper fraction. Then rewrite the proportion using these fractions.

Step 1. $x : \frac{1}{400} :: \frac{48}{5} : \frac{1}{200}$

Step 2. $\frac{1}{200}x = \frac{1}{400} \times \frac{48}{5}$

Step 3. $\frac{1}{200}x = \frac{1}{\underset{25}{\cancel{400}}} \times \frac{\overset{3}{\cancel{48}}}{5}$

Step 4. $\frac{1}{200}x = \frac{3}{125}$

Step 5. $x = \frac{3}{125} \div \frac{1}{200}$

Step 6. $x = \frac{3}{\underset{5}{\cancel{125}}} \times \frac{\overset{8}{\cancel{200}}}{1}$

Step 7. $x = \frac{24}{5}$

Step 8. $x = 4\frac{4}{5}$

Proportion Problem Involving Decimals and Percents

EXAMPLE: $0.3\% : 1.8 :: x : 14.4$

Convert 0.3% to a decimal.

Step 1. $0.003 : 1.8 = x : 14.4$

Step 2. $1.8x = 0.003 \times 14.4$

Step 3. $1.8x = 0.0432$

Step 4. $x = 0.0432 \div 1.8$

Step 5. $x = 0.024$

Proportion Problem Involving Numerous Zeros

EXAMPLE: $250{,}000 : x :: 500{,}000 : 4$

Step 1. $500{,}000x = 250{,}000 \times 4$

Step 2. $500{,}000x = 1{,}000{,}000$

Step 3. $x = 1{,}000{,}000 \div 500{,}000$

Step 4. $x = \frac{1{,}000{,}000}{500{,}000}$

Step 5. $x = 2$

WORK SHEET

DIRECTIONS: Find the value of x. Show your work.

1. $20 : 400 :: x : 1680$ ____________

2. $0.9 : 2.4 :: x : 75$ ____________

3. $\frac{5}{6} : x :: \frac{5}{9} : \frac{4}{5}$ ____________

4. $3 : 90 :: 1\frac{3}{4} : x$ ____________

5. $75 : x :: 100 : 2$ ____________

6. $\frac{1}{6} : 1 :: \frac{1}{8} : x$ ____________

7. $200{,}000 : x :: 1{,}000{,}000 : 5$ ____________

8. $x : \frac{3}{4}\% :: 3\frac{1}{5} : \frac{1}{200}$ ____________

9. $\frac{1}{150} : 1 :: \frac{1}{100} : x$ ____________

10. $3 : 150 :: 40 : x$ ____________

11. $\frac{1}{8} : x :: 7 : 56$ ____________

12. $\frac{1}{200} : 40 :: \frac{1}{100} : x$ ____________

13. $12\frac{1}{2} : x :: 50 : 2400$ ____________

14. $\frac{1}{2}\% : \frac{1}{100} :: x : 80$ ____________

15. $x : 6.4 :: 0.03 : 6$ ____________

16. $0.25 : 1 :: 0.05 : x$ ____________

17. $\frac{1}{120} : 2 :: 4 : x$ ____________

18. $x : \frac{1}{1000} :: 5 : \frac{1}{5000}$ ____________

19. $6 : 15 :: 8 : x$ ______

20. $x : 3 :: 9 : 54$ ______

21. $1.4 : 0.4 :: 4.2 : x$ ______

22. $x : 0.65 :: 9 : 5$ ______

23. $12\frac{1}{2}\% : 5 :: x : 120$ ______

24. $\frac{1}{300} : 6 :: \frac{1}{120} : x$ ______

25. $25 : 75 :: 16 : x$ ______

26. $0.3 : x :: 7 : 21$ ______

27. $4 : x :: 12 : 48$ ______

28. $x : 12 :: 2 : 4$ ______

29. $\frac{4}{5} : x :: \frac{1}{3} : \frac{5}{9}$ ______

30. $0.6 : x :: 7 : 42$ ______

31. $15 : x :: 20 : 600$ ______

32. $9\% : x :: 11 : 73$ ______

33. $500{,}000 : 1 :: 300{,}000 : x$ ______

34. $\frac{1}{6} : \frac{9}{10} :: \frac{1}{2} : x$ ______

35. $2.8 : 12 :: 40 : x$ ______

36. $8 : \frac{8}{100} :: x : 5$ ______

37. $\frac{1}{8}\% : \frac{1}{200} :: x : 40$ ______

38. $x : 25 :: 18 : 36$ ______

39. $0.15 : 0.25 :: x : 400$ ______

40. $\frac{1}{20} : \frac{1}{15} :: x : 25$ ______

41. 800,000 : 5 :: 960,000 : x ____________

42. 27 : x :: 9 : 60 ____________

43. $\frac{1}{20}$: $\frac{1}{5}$ :: x : 50 ____________

44. $\frac{1}{150}$: $\frac{1}{200}$ :: x : 60 ____________

45. $\frac{1}{2}$% : 4 :: x : 25 ____________

46. 500 : 2.5 :: x : 8.1 ____________

ANSWERS ON P. 104.

NAME ____________________

DATE ____________________

ACCEPTABLE SCORE **19**

YOUR SCORE ______

CHAPTER 5
Proportions

POSTTEST 1

DIRECTIONS: Find the value of x. Show your work.

1. $x : 2.5 :: 4 : 5$ ______ **2.** $\frac{7}{8} : x :: \frac{4}{5} : \frac{2}{3}$ ______ **3.** $30 : 90 :: 2 : x$ ______

4. $x : 3.5 :: 25 : 14$ ______ **5.** $\frac{2}{7} : \frac{1}{2} :: x : 56$ ______ **6.** $\frac{1}{4} : x :: 160 : 320$ ______

7. $x : 7 :: 5 : 14$ ______ **8.** $3 : x :: 18 : 12$ ______ **9.** $\frac{1}{5} : 90 :: x : 250$ ______

10. $1.8 : 4.8 :: x : 96$ ______ **11.** $x : 8 :: 10 : 20$ ______ **12.** $\frac{2}{3} : x :: 4.5 : 27$ ______

13. $\frac{1}{150} : x :: \frac{1}{200} : 6$ ______ **14.** $\frac{2}{3}\% : \frac{1}{5} :: 50 : x$ ______ **15.** $14 : x :: 6 : 18$ ______

16. $x : \frac{2}{3} :: 12 : 18$ ______ **17.** $50 : 250 :: \frac{4}{5} : x$ ______ **18.** $50 : 3 :: x : 6$ ______

19. $\frac{1}{2} : x :: 40 : 80$ ______ **20.** $0.8 : 10 :: x : 40$ ______

ANSWERS ON P. 104.

NAME ____________________

DATE ____________________

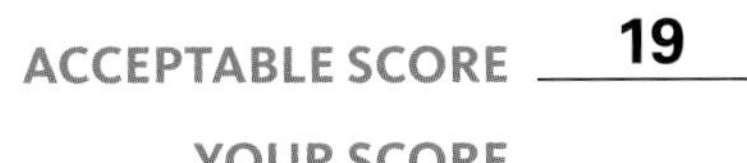

ACCEPTABLE SCORE **19**

YOUR SCORE ______

CHAPTER **5**
Proportions

POSTTEST 2

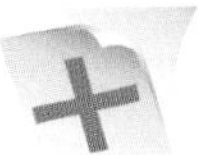

DIRECTIONS: Find the value of x. Show your work.

1. $x : 300 :: 9 : 12$ ______

2. $4 : 32\% :: 16 : x$ ______

3. $18 : x :: 6 : 40$ ______

4. $1.8 : 2.5 :: x : 9.5$ ______

5. $x : 30 :: \frac{1}{3} : \frac{3}{4}$ ______

6. $\frac{7}{8} : x :: \frac{5}{8} : 40$ ______

7. $400 : 500 :: \frac{4}{5} : x$ ______

8. $x : 7.6 :: 3 : 6$ ______

9. $\frac{1}{4} : x :: \frac{2}{3} : \frac{2}{5}$ ______

10. $\frac{1}{150} : \frac{1}{100} :: x : 60$ ______

11. $0.6 : x :: 15 : 90$ ______

12. $3.5 : 12 :: x : 360$ ______

13. $\frac{2}{9} : \frac{4}{5} :: \frac{3}{4} : x$ ______

14. $\frac{1}{8} : x :: \frac{1}{7} : \frac{5}{9}$ ______

15. $x : 2.5 :: 16 : 4$ ______

16. $0.6 : 3 :: 72 : x$ ______

17. $20 : x :: 6 : 4.5$ ______

18. $x : \frac{1}{4} :: 96 : \frac{1}{3}$ ______

19. $300 : 5000 :: x : 18$ ______

20. $\frac{1}{3} : x :: \frac{1}{5} : 90$ ______

ANSWERS ON P. 104.

ANSWERS

CHAPTER 5 Proportions—Pretest, p. 91

1. 100
2. $7\frac{1}{2}$ or 7.5
3. $\frac{1}{600}$
4. 3.2
5. 128
6. 4
7. 400
8. $\frac{1}{2}$
9. $\frac{3}{7}$
10. 8
11. 80
12. $\frac{1}{6}$
13. 14
14. 48
15. $\frac{3}{10}$
16. 80
17. 10
18. 126
19. $\frac{1}{150}$
20. $16\frac{1}{4}$ or 16.25

CHAPTER 5 Proportions—Work Sheet, pp. 97–99

1. 84
2. 28.125
3. $1\frac{1}{5}$
4. $52\frac{1}{2}$
5. $1\frac{1}{2}$ or 1.5
6. $\frac{3}{4}$
7. 1
8. $4\frac{4}{5}$
9. $1\frac{1}{2}$ or 1.5
10. 2000
11. 1
12. 80
13. 600
14. 40
15. 0.032
16. 0.2
17. 960
18. 25
19. 20
20. $\frac{1}{2}$ or 0.5
21. 1.2
22. 1.17
23. 3
24. 15
25. 48
26. 0.9
27. 16
28. 6
29. $1\frac{1}{3}$
30. 3.6
31. 450
32. $\frac{657}{1100}$ or 0.597
33. $\frac{3}{5}$ or 0.6
34. $2\frac{7}{10}$
35. 171.43
36. 500
37. 10
38. $12\frac{1}{2}$ or 12.5
39. 240
40. $18\frac{3}{4}$ or 18.75
41. 6
42. 180
43. $12\frac{1}{2}$ or 12.5
44. 80
45. $\frac{1}{32}$ or 0.03125
46. 1620

CHAPTER 5 Proportions—Posttest 1, p. 101

1. 2
2. $\frac{35}{48}$
3. 6
4. 6.25
5. 32
6. $\frac{1}{2}$
7. $2\frac{1}{2}$ or 2.5
8. 2
9. $\frac{5}{9}$
10. 36
11. 4
12. 4
13. 8
14. 1500
15. 42
16. $\frac{4}{9}$
17. 4
18. 100
19. 1
20. 3.2

CHAPTER 5 Proportions—Posttest 2, p. 103

1. 225
2. $1\frac{7}{25}$ or 1.28
3. 120
4. 6.84
5. $13\frac{1}{3}$
6. 56
7. 1
8. 3.8
9. $\frac{3}{20}$
10. 40
11. 3.6
12. 105
13. $2\frac{7}{10}$
14. $\frac{35}{72}$
15. 10
16. 360
17. 15
18. 72
19. $1\frac{2}{25}$ or 1.08
20. 150

NAME ______________________________

DATE ______________________________

ACCEPTABLE SCORE **95**

YOUR SCORE ______

Review of Mathematics

POSTTEST

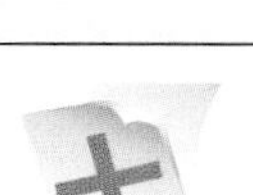

After your successful completion of Chapters 1 through 5, complete the Review of Mathematics Posttest. A score of 95 out of 100 indicates an acceptable understanding of and competency in basic mathematics. You are now ready to begin Part 2, Units and Measurements for the Calculation of Drug Dosages. However, if you score 94 or below, an additional review of previous chapter content may be helpful before beginning Part 2.

DIRECTIONS: Complete the following definitions and exercises.

1. *Improper fractions* can be reduced to a ________ number or a ________ number.

2. In the following fractions, circle only those that are *improper fractions.*

$\frac{4}{12}$ $\frac{7}{6}$ $\frac{6}{3}$ $\frac{4}{7}$ $\frac{9}{9}$ $\frac{14}{21}$

3. A *complex fraction* contains a ________ in its numerator, its denominator, or both.

4. In the following examples, circle only the *complex fractions.*

$1\frac{2}{3}$ $\frac{1}{2}/4$ $\frac{12}{4}$ $\frac{3}{7}/\frac{4}{2}$ $21\frac{9}{6}$ $21/\frac{2}{3}$

5-6. A *ratio* is the ________ between ________ numbers.

Write each of the following numbers as a *ratio.*

7. $\frac{4}{12}$ ______________ **8.** 24% ______________ **9.** 0.03 ______________

10. $\frac{13}{8}$ ______________ **11.** 2.2% ______________ **12.** 1.24 ______________

13. The *divisor* of a fraction is known as the ________.

Division problems can be expressed in different ways. Circle the *divisor* in each of the following examples.

14. $\frac{2}{3}$ **15.** $4 \div 8$ **16.** $10 : 5$ **17.** $4\overline{)12}$

18. $\frac{14}{8}$ **19.** $6 \div 24$ **20.** $42\overline{)7}$ **21.** $7 : 10$

22-24. The number shown in a decimal is the ________ of a fraction. The denominator of this fraction is implied by the number of decimal places shown and is ________ or some power of ________.

Write the fraction values for the following *decimal fraction* numbers.

25. 0.436 ______________ **26.** 0.051 ______________ **27.** 1.0042 ______________

28. 0.9684 ______________ **29.** 0.0019 ______________ **30.** 1.02064 ______________

DIRECTIONS: Add and reduce fractions to lowest terms.

31. $\frac{5}{9} + \frac{2}{5} + \frac{2}{3} =$ ______________________

32. $4\frac{1}{4} + 2\frac{5}{6} =$ ______________________

33. $5\frac{1}{2} + \frac{3}{9} =$ ______________________

34. $\frac{3}{4}/\frac{5}{6} + 4\frac{3}{5} =$ ______________________

DIRECTIONS: Add and round answers to hundredths.

35. $4.02 + 3.4 + 1.099 =$ ______________________

36. $45.009 + 0.076 + 1.2 =$ ______________________

37. $0.0082 + 0.923 + 234 =$ ______________________

38. $456 + 3.56 + 0.0029 =$ ______________________

DIRECTIONS: Subtract and reduce fractions to lowest terms.

39. $\frac{2}{4} - \frac{3}{9} =$ ______________________

40. $\frac{4}{7}/\frac{2}{8} - \frac{2}{3} =$ ______________________

41. $3\frac{4}{5} - 2\frac{8}{9} =$ ______________________

42. $6\frac{1}{2} - \frac{8}{9} =$ ______________________

DIRECTIONS: Subtract and round answers to tenths.

43. $23.98 - 0.0987 =$ ______________________

44. $23.191 - 23.099 =$ ______________________

45. $9.002 - 4.9089 =$ ______________________

46. $2.009 - 0.9834 =$ ______________________

DIRECTIONS: Multiply and reduce fractions to lowest terms.

47. $9 \times \frac{5}{8} =$ ______________________

48. $\frac{3}{4} \times \frac{8}{9} =$ ______________________

49. $4\frac{8}{9} \times 1\frac{5}{6} =$ ______________________

50. $3\frac{4}{5} \times 7 =$ ______________________

DIRECTIONS: Multiply and round answers to hundredths.

51. $3.45 \times 0.56 =$ ______________________

52. $21.4 \times 0.092 =$ ______________________

53. $0.0452 \times 99.1 =$ ______________________

54. $739 \times 0.246 =$ ______________________

DIRECTIONS: Divide and reduce fractions to lowest terms.

55. $\frac{7}{8} \div \frac{4}{9} =$ ______________________

56. $\frac{2}{5} \div \frac{7}{9} =$ ______________________

57. $\frac{1}{300} \div \frac{3}{4} =$ ______________________

58. $4\frac{7}{9} \div 5\frac{9}{11} =$ ______________________

DIRECTIONS: Divide and round answers to thousandths.

59. $52.014 \div 9.2 =$ ______________________

60. $0.0982 \div 75 =$ ______________________

61. $3200 \div 0.04 =$ ______________________

62. $78.09 \div 4.501 =$ ______________________

DIRECTIONS: Number the following decimal numbers in order from *lesser to greater value.*

63. 0.45 ____ 1.46 ____ 0.407 ____ 2.401 ____ 0.048 ____ 0.014 ____

64. 0.15 ____ 0.015 ____ 1.015 ____ 1.15 ____ 0.155 ____ 1.0015 ____

65. 9.09 ____ 0.99 ____ 0.090 ____ 0.90 ____ 90.90 ____ 9.009 ____

66. 0.6 ____ 0.4 ____ 0.7 ____ 0.52 ____ 0.44 ____ 0.24 ____

67. 0.21 ____ 0.191 ____ 0.021 ____ 0.1091 ____ 0.201 ____ 0.2 ____

DIRECTIONS: Change the following fractions to decimals and round the answers to hundredths.

68. $\frac{5}{6}$ ____________ **69.** $\frac{5}{9}$ ____________

70. $\frac{9}{16}$ ____________ **71.** $\frac{1}{150}$ ____________

DIRECTIONS: Change the following decimals to fractions and reduce to lowest terms.

72. 0.225 ____________ **73.** 0.465 ____________

74. 0.06 ____________ **75.** 0.372 ____________

DIRECTIONS: Make the following calculations.

76. Express 0.275 as a percent. ____________ **77.** Express $\frac{3}{8}$ as a percent. ____________

78. Express 42% as a proper fraction and reduce to lowest terms. ____________

79. Express 0.62% as a ratio. ____________ **80.** What percent of 3.2 is 0.4? ____________

81. What percent of $\frac{5}{7}$ is $\frac{5}{28}$? ____________ **82.** What percent of 240 is 36? ____________

83. What is $\frac{1}{2}$% of 48? ____________ **84.** What is $6\frac{1}{2}$% of 840? ____________

85. What is 46% of 325? ____________

DIRECTIONS: Change the following fractions and decimals to ratios reduced to lowest terms.

86. $\frac{10}{45}$ ________ **87.** $1\frac{3}{4}/4\frac{2}{3}$ ________ **88.** 0.584 ________

89. $\frac{250}{375}$ ________ **90.** 0.48 ________

DIRECTIONS: Find the value of x and round decimal answers to hundredths.

91. $8 : \frac{4}{45} :: x : 3$ ________ **92.** $x : 34 :: 4 : 81$ ________ **93.** $4.6 : 3 :: 20 : x$ ________

94. $x : \frac{1}{2}\% :: 4.5 : \frac{1}{50}$ ________ **95.** $\frac{1}{300} : \frac{1}{150} :: x : 300$ ________ **96.** $22 : x :: 4 : 88$ ________

97. $0.35 : 0.75 :: x : 425$ ________ **98.** $400 : x :: \frac{1}{300} : \frac{1}{225}$ ________ **99.** $x : 54 :: 4 : 8$ ________

100. $\frac{1}{2}/\frac{3}{4} : 8 :: x : 45$ ________

ANSWERS ON P. 110.

ANSWERS

REVIEW OF MATHEMATICS POSTTEST, pp. 105–109

1. mixed
   whole
2. $\frac{7}{6}$
   $\frac{6}{3}$
   $\frac{9}{9}$
3. fraction
4. $\frac{1}{2}/4$
   $\frac{3}{7}/\frac{4}{2}$
   $21/\frac{2}{3}$
5. relationship
6. two
7. 4 : 12 or 1 : 3
8. 24 : 100 or 6 : 25
9. 3 : 100
10. 13 : 8
11. 2.2 : 100 or 22 : 1000 (same value)
12. 124 : 100
13. denominator
14. 2 /③
15. 4 ÷ ⑧
16. 10 : ⑤
17. ④$\overline{)12}$
18. 14 /⑧
19. 6 ÷ ㉔
20. ㊷$\overline{)7}$
21. 7 : ⑩
22. numerator
23. 10
24. 10
25. $\frac{436}{1000}$
26. $\frac{51}{1000}$
27. $1\frac{42}{10,000}$
28. $\frac{9684}{10,000}$
29. $\frac{19}{10,000}$
30. $1\frac{2064}{100,000}$
31. $1\frac{28}{45}$
32. $7\frac{1}{12}$
33. $5\frac{5}{6}$
34. $5\frac{1}{2}$
35. 8.52
36. 46.29
37. 234.93
38. 459.56
39. $\frac{1}{6}$
40. $1\frac{13}{21}$
41. $\frac{41}{45}$
42. $5\frac{11}{18}$
43. 23.9
44. 0.1
45. 4.1
46. 1.0
47. $5\frac{5}{8}$
48. $\frac{2}{3}$
49. $8\frac{26}{27}$
50. $26\frac{3}{5}$
51. 1.93
52. 1.97
53. 4.48
54. 181.79
55. $1\frac{31}{32}$
56. $\frac{18}{35}$
57. $\frac{1}{225}$
58. $\frac{473}{576}$
59. 5.654
60. 0.001
61. 80,000
62. 17.349
63. 0.014, 0.048, 0.407, 0.45, 1.46, 2.401
64. 0.015, 0.15, 0.155, 1.0015, 1.015, 1.15
65. 0.090, 0.90, 0.99, 9.009, 9.09, 90.90
66. 0.24, 0.4, 0.44, 0.52, 0.6, 0.7
67. 0.021, 0.1091, 0.191, 0.2, 0.201, 0.21
68. 0.83
69. 0.56
70. 0.56
71. 0.01
72. $\frac{9}{40}$
73. $\frac{93}{200}$
74. $\frac{3}{50}$
75. $\frac{93}{250}$
76. 27.5%
77. 37.5%
78. $\frac{21}{50}$
79. 62 : 10,000 or 31 : 5000
80. 12.5%
81. 25%
82. 15%
83. 0.24
84. 54.6
85. 149.5
86. 2 : 9
87. 3 : 8
88. 73 : 125
89. 2 : 3
90. 12 : 25
91. 270
92. 1.68
93. 13.04
94. 1.13
95. 150
96. 484
97. 198.33
98. $533\frac{1}{3}$ or 533.33
99. 27
100. 3.75

UNITS and MEASUREMENTS for the CALCULATION of DRUG DOSAGES

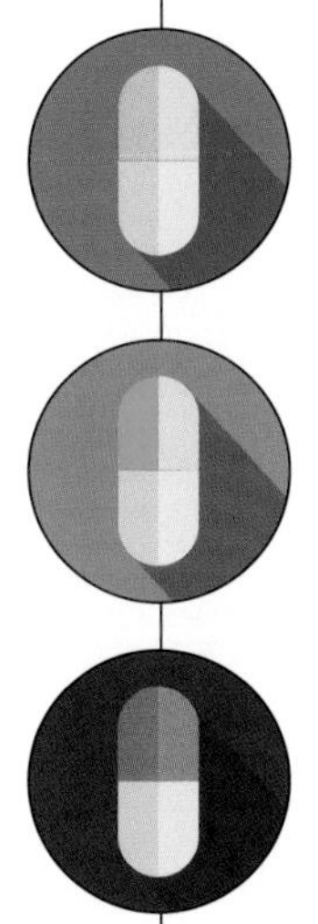

CHAPTERS

Part 2 is designed in the same way as Part 1, Review of Mathematics. After completing Part 1, you have validated that you do have the basic mathematical skills required to progress with Part 2. A pretest precedes each of the two chapters in Part 2. For some of you who have had experience in nursing and the administration of medications (such as a licensed practical nurse, licensed visiting nurse, or registered nurse with an associate's degree), these pretests will allow you to assess your need for a more extensive review of the material. After completion of the test, check your answers with the key provided. A score of 95% correct as indicated on each test indicates a mastery of the material covered in that chapter. You may then skip to the next pretest and follow the same exercises until Part 2 has been completed.

For those of you who have *not* had experience in nursing and the administration of medications, the following chapters of Part 2 should be worked as written *without using the pretests preceding Chapters 6 and 7.*

You are now ready to follow the path that matches your experience to ensure mastery of the following two chapters. Begin now, and good luck!

NAME ______________

DATE ______________

ACCEPTABLE SCORE 29

YOUR SCORE ______

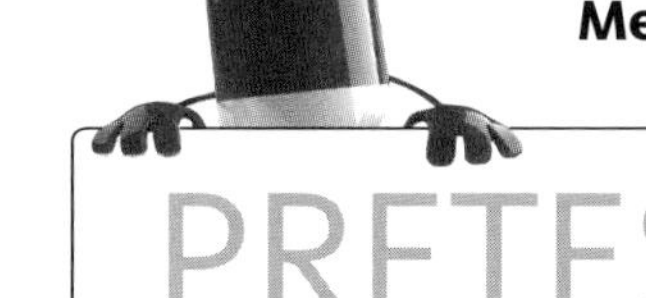

CHAPTER 6

Metric and Household Measurements

PRETEST

DIRECTIONS: Change to equivalent metric or household measurements. Solve each problem and show your work. Convert fractions to decimals before solving the problem.

1. 800,000 mcg = ______ g

2. 3 mg = ______ mcg

3. 255 mg = ______ g

4. 46 mg = ______ mcg

5. 3000 mcg = ______ mg

6. 0.68 g = ______ mg

7. 326 mL = ______ L

8. 33 kg = ______ lb

9. 2.1 g = ______ mg

10. 3000 g = ______ kg

11. 0.1 L = ______ mL

12. 53 kg = ______ lb

13. 0.005 mg = ______ mcg

14. 0.8 kg = ______ g

15. 250 mcg = ______ mg

16. 1¼ cups = ______ mL

17. 22 lb = ______ g

18. 0.63 L = ______ mL

19. 733 g = ______ kg

20. 1.25 g = ______ mcg

21. 60 mg = ______ g

22. 0.25 mg = ______ mcg

23. 0.25 L = ______ mL

24. 45 lb = ______ kg

25. 10,000 mcg = _______ g **26.** 1.2 kg = ___________ g **27.** 1¼ Tbsp = ________ mL

28. 0.71 g = __________ mg **29.** 480 mL = ___________ L **30.** 650 g = ___________ lb

ANSWERS ON P. 131.

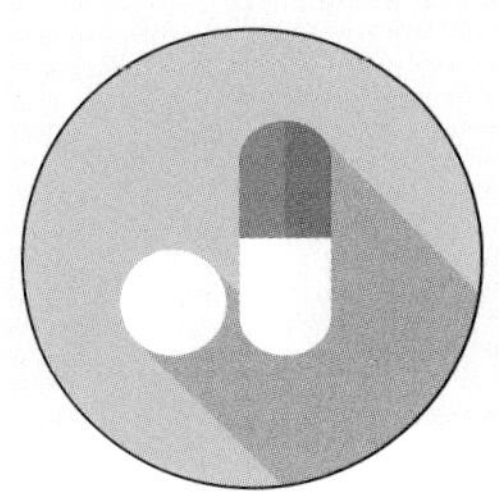

Metric and Household Measurements

LEARNING OBJECTIVES

Upon completion of the materials provided in this chapter, you will be able to perform computations accurately by mastering the following mathematical concepts:

1. Recalling the metric measures of weight, volume, and length
2. Computing equivalents within the metric system by using dimensional analysis or a proportion
3. Recalling approximate equivalents between metric and household measures
4. Computing equivalents between the metric and household systems of measure by using dimensional analysis or a proportion

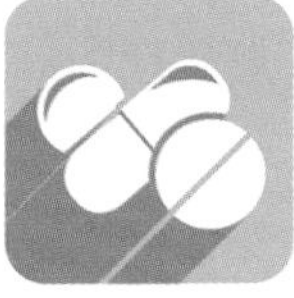

METRIC MEASUREMENTS

The metric system has become the system of choice for dealing with the weights and measures involved in the calculation of drug dosages. This is a result of its accuracy and simplicity because it is based on the decimal system. The use of decimals tends to eliminate errors made when working with fractions. Therefore **all answers within the metric system need to be expressed as decimals, not as fractions.**

EXAMPLES: 0.5, not ½
0.75, not ¾
0.007, not $\frac{7}{1000}$

Certain prefixes identify the multiples of 10 that are being used. The four most commonly used prefixes of the metric system involved with the calculation of drug dosages are the following:

micro = 0.000001 or one millionth
milli = 0.001 or one thousandth
centi = 0.01 or one hundredth
kilo = 1000 or one thousand

These prefixes may be used with any of the base units of weight (gram), volume (liter), or length (meter). The nurse most often uses the following list of metric measures (Box 6-1). Memorize all the entries in the list.

BOX 6-1 COMMON METRIC MEASURES

Metric Measure of Weight

1,000,000 micrograms (mcg) = 1 gram (g)
1000 micrograms (mcg) = 1 milligram (mg)
1000 milligrams (mg) = 1 gram (g)
1000 grams (g) = 1 kilogram (kg)

Metric Measure of Volume

1000 milliliters (mL) = 1 liter (L)
1 cubic centimeter (cc) = 1 milliliter (mL)

Metric Measure of Length

1 meter (m) = 1000 mm or 100 cm
1 centimeter (cm) = 10 mm or 0.01 m
1 millimeter (mm) = 0.1 cm or 0.001 m

Sometimes, to compute drug dosages, the nurse must convert a metric measure to an equivalent measure within the system. This may be done easily by using dimensional analysis or a proportion.

DIMENSIONAL ANALYSIS

Dimensional analysis is one format for setting up problems to calculate equivalents or drug dosages. Dimensional analysis has been around for many years. It was first used in the sciences, such as advanced algebra, chemistry, and physics, to name a few. Recently dimensional analysis has become popular for the calculation of drug dosage problems.

The advantage of dimensional analysis is that only one equation is needed. This format allows a single equation to replace multiple calculations to find the answer.

Three items are required to set up the single equation. These are the desired answer, which goes on the left side of the equation; the equivalent between the two units in the problem; and the given quantity and the unit in which it is supplied.

Let's take a look at some examples that illustrate the dimensional analysis method.

Metric Conversions: Dimensional Analysis Method

EXAMPLE 1: 300 mg equals how many grams?

Step 1. On the left side of the equation, place the name or abbreviation of the drug form of x, or what you are solving for.

$$x \text{ g} =$$

Step 2. On the right side of the equation, place the available information related to the measurement or abbreviation that was placed on the left side. In this example that is *g*. This information is placed in the equation as a common fraction; match the appropriate abbreviation or measurement. Thus the abbreviation that matches the x quantity must be placed in the numerator. We also know there are 1000 mg in 1 g. This information is the denominator of our fraction.

$$x \text{ g} = \frac{1 \text{ g}}{1000 \text{ mg}}$$

Step 3. Next, find the information that matches the measurement or abbreviation used in the denominator of the fraction you created. In this example *mg* is in the denominator and we have 300 mg. Therefore the full equation is

$$x \text{ g} = \frac{1 \text{ g}}{1000 \text{ mg}} \times \frac{300 \text{ mg}}{1}$$

Step 4. Now cancel out the like abbreviations on the right side of the equation. If you have set up the problem correctly, the remaining measurement or abbreviation should match that used on the left side of the equation. You are now ready to solve for x.

$$x \text{ g} = \frac{1 \text{ g}}{\underset{10}{\cancel{1000}}\ \cancel{\text{mg}}} \times \frac{\overset{3}{\cancel{300}}\ \cancel{\text{mg}}}{1}$$

$$x = \frac{1 \times 3}{10 \times 1} = \frac{3}{10}$$

$$x = 0.3 \text{ g}$$

The answer to the problem is 0.3 g.

EXAMPLE 2: 2.5 L equals how many milliliters?

Step 1. On the left side of the equation, place the name or abbreviation of the drug form of x, or what you are solving for.

$$x \text{ mL} =$$

Step 2. On the right side of the equation, place the available information related to the measurement or abbreviation that was placed on the left side. In this example that is *mL*. This information is placed in the equation as a common fraction; match the appropriate abbreviation or measurement. Thus the abbreviation that matches the x quantity must be placed in the numerator. We also know there are 1000 mL in 1 L. This information is the denominator of our fraction.

$$x \text{ mL} = \frac{1000 \text{ mL}}{1 \text{ L}}$$

Step 3. Next, find the information that matches the measurement or abbreviation used in the denominator of the fraction you created. In this example *L* is in the denominator and we have 2.5 L. Therefore the full equation is

$$x \text{ mL} = \frac{1000 \text{ mL}}{1 \text{ L}} \times \frac{2.5 \text{ L}}{1}$$

Step 4. Now cancel out the like abbreviations on the right side of the equation. If you have set up the problem correctly, the remaining measurement or abbreviation should match that used on the left side of the equation. You are now ready to solve for x.

$$x \text{ mL} = \frac{1000 \text{ mL}}{1\ \cancel{\text{L}}} \times \frac{2.5\ \cancel{\text{L}}}{1}$$

$$x = \frac{1000 \times 2.5}{1 \times 1} = \frac{2500}{1}$$

$$x = 2500 \text{ mL}$$

The answer to the problem is 2500 mL.

EXAMPLE 3: 180 mcg equals how many grams?

Step 1. On the left side of the equation, place the name or abbreviation of the drug form of x, or what you are solving for.

$$x \text{ g} =$$

Step 2. On the right side of the equation, place the available information related to the measurement or abbreviation that was placed on the left side. In this example that is *g*. This information is placed in the equation as a common fraction; match the appropriate abbreviation or measurement. Thus the abbreviation that matches the x quantity must be placed in the numerator. We also know there are 1,000,000 mcg in 1 g. This information is the denominator of our fraction.

$$x \text{ g} = \frac{1 \text{ g}}{1{,}000{,}000 \text{ mcg}}$$

Step 3. Next, find the information that matches the measurement or abbreviation used in the denominator of the fraction you created. In this example *mcg* is in the denominator and we have 180 mcg. Therefore the full equation is

$$x \text{ g} = \frac{1 \text{ g}}{1{,}000{,}000 \text{ mcg}} \times \frac{180 \text{ mcg}}{1}$$

Step 4. Now cancel out the like abbreviations on the right side of the equation. If you have set up the problem correctly, the remaining measurement or abbreviation should match that used on the left side of the equation. You are now ready to solve for x.

$$x \text{ g} = \frac{1 \text{ g}}{\underset{50{,}000}{\cancel{1{,}000{,}000}} \cancel{\text{mcg}}} \times \frac{\overset{9}{\cancel{180}} \cancel{\text{mcg}}}{1}$$

$$x = \frac{1 \times 9}{50{,}000} = \frac{9}{50{,}000}$$

$$x = 0.00018 \text{ g}$$

The answer to the problem is 0.00018 g.

EXAMPLE 4: 15 mm equals how many centimeters?

Step 1. On the left side of the equation, place the name or abbreviation of the drug form of x, or what you are solving for.

$$x \text{ cm} =$$

Step 2. On the right side of the equation, place the available information related to the measurement or abbreviation that was placed on the left side. In this example that is *cm*. This information is placed in the equation as a common fraction; match the appropriate abbreviation or measurement. Thus the abbreviation that matches the x quantity must be placed in the numerator. We also know there is 1 cm in 10 mm. This information is the denominator of our fraction.

$$x \text{ cm} = \frac{1 \text{ cm}}{10 \text{ mm}}$$

Step 3. Next, find the information that matches the measurement or abbreviation used in the denominator of the fraction you created. In this example *mm* is in the denominator and the length we are given is 15 mm. Therefore the full equation is

$$x \text{ cm} = \frac{1 \text{ cm}}{10 \text{ mm}} \times \frac{15 \text{ mm}}{1}$$

Step 4. Now cancel out the like abbreviations on the right side of the equation. If you have set up the problem correctly, the remaining measurement or abbreviation should match that used on the left side of the equation. You are now ready to solve for x.

$$x \text{ cm} = \frac{1 \text{ cm}}{\underset{2}{\cancel{10}} \cancel{\text{mm}}} \times \frac{\overset{3}{\cancel{15}} \cancel{\text{mm}}}{1}$$

$$x = \frac{1 \times 3}{2 \times 1} = \frac{3}{2}$$

$$x = 1.5 \text{ cm}$$

The answer to the problem is 1.5 cm.

PROPORTION

Historically, the proportion method was taught as a means of calculating equivalents and also drug dosages. If this is the method you are comfortable with, we have continued to include many examples using this method. If you need a review of the steps in solving proportion problems, see Chapter 5, Proportions, on page 89.

Metric Conversions: Proportion Method

EXAMPLE 1: 300 mg equals how many grams?

Step 1. On the left side of the proportion, place what you know to be an equivalent between milligrams and grams. From Box-1 we know that there are 1000 mg in 1 g. Therefore the left side of the proportion would be

$$1000 \text{ mg} : 1 \text{ g} ::$$

Step 2. The right side of the proportion is determined by the problem and by the abbreviations used on the left side of the proportion. Only *two* different abbreviations may be used in a single proportion. The abbreviations must also be in the same position on the right as they are on the left.

$$1000 \text{ mg} : 1 \text{ g} :: \_\_\_\_ \text{ mg} : \_\_\_\_ \text{ g}$$

From the problem we know we have 300 mg.

$$1000 \text{ mg} : 1 \text{ g} :: 300 \text{ mg} : \_\_\_\_ \text{ g}$$

We need to find the number of grams 300 mg equals, so we use the symbol x to represent the unknown. Therefore the full proportion would be

$$1000 \text{ mg} : 1 \text{ g} :: 300 \text{ mg} : x \text{ g}$$

Step 3. Rewrite the proportion without using the abbreviations.

$$1000 : 1 :: 300 : x$$

Step 4. Solve for x by multiplying the means and extremes. Write the answer as a decimal, because the metric system is based on decimals.

$$1000 : 1 :: 300 : x$$

$$1000x = 300$$

$$x = \frac{300}{1000}$$

$$x = 0.3$$

Step 5. Label your answer, as determined by the abbreviation placed next to x in the original proportion.

$$300 \text{ mg} = 0.3 \text{ g}$$

EXAMPLE 2: 2.5 L equals how many milliliters?

Step 1. 1000 mL : 1 L ::

Step 2. 1000 mL : 1 L ::
_______ mL : _______ L

1000 mL : 1 L :: x mL : 2.5 L

Step 3. 1000 : 1 :: x : 2.5

Step 4. $1x = 2500$

$x = 2500$

Step 5. 2.5 L = 2500 mL

EXAMPLE 3: 180 mcg equals how many grams?

Step 1. 1,000,000 mcg : 1 g ::

Step 2. 1,000,000 mcg : 1 g ::
_______ mcg : _______ g

1,000,000 mcg : 1 g :: 180 mcg : x g

Step 3. 1,000,000 : 1 :: 180 : x

Step 4. $1{,}000{,}000x = 180$

$$x = \frac{180}{1{,}000{,}000}$$

$x = 0.00018$

Step 5. 180 mcg = 0.00018 g

EXAMPLE 4: 15 mm equals how many centimeters?

Step 1. 1 cm : 10 mm

Step 2. 1 cm : 10 mm :: _______ cm : _______ mm

1 cm : 10 mm :: x cm : 15 mm

Step 3. 1 : 10 :: x : 15

Step 4. $10x = 1 \times 15$

$10x = 15$

$$x = \frac{15}{10}$$

$x = 1.5$

Step 5. 15 mm = 1.5 cm

HOUSEHOLD MEASUREMENTS

Household measures are not accurate enough for the nurse to use in the calculation of drug dosages in the hospital. However, their metric equivalents are used in keeping a written record of a patient's "I" and "O," or intake and output. Always use your institution's conversions when documenting intake.

Memorize the following list of approximate equivalents between metric and household measurements (Box 6-2).

BOX 6-2 METRIC HOUSEHOLD EQUIVALENTS

Metric Measure	=	Household Measure
5 milliliters (mL)	=	1 teaspoon (tsp)
15 milliliters (mL)	=	1 tablespoon (Tbsp)
30 milliliters (mL)	=	1 ounce (oz)
240 milliliters (mL)	=	1 standard measuring cup
1 kilogram (kg) or 1000 grams (g)	=	2.2 pounds (lb)
2.5 cm	=	1 inch
		1 foot = 12 inches

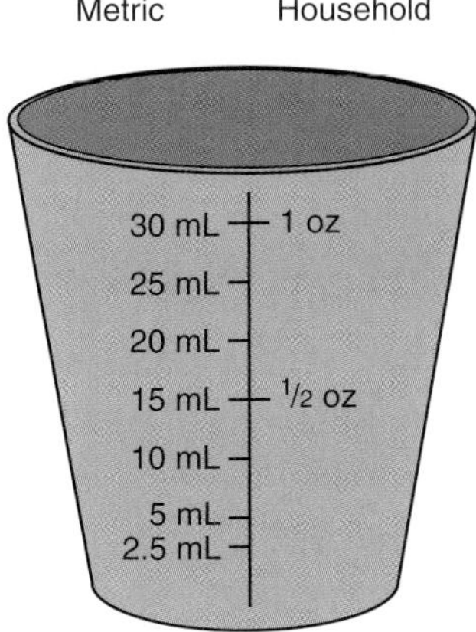

Conversion of measures between the metric and household systems of measure may also be done by using dimensional analysis or a proportion, as has been illustrated.

Household Conversions: Dimensional Analysis Method

EXAMPLE 1: 1½ cups equals how many milliliters?

Step 1. On the left side of the equation, place the name or abbreviation of the drug form of x, or what you are solving for.

$$x \text{ mL} =$$

Step 2. On the right side of the equation, place the available information related to the measurement or abbreviation that was placed on the left side. In this example that is *mL*. This information is placed in the equation as a common fraction; match the appropriate abbreviation or measurement. Thus the abbreviation that matches the x quantity must be placed in the numerator. We also know there are 240 mL in 1 cup. This information is the denominator of our fraction.

$$x \text{ mL} = \frac{240 \text{ mL}}{1 \text{ cup}}$$

Step 3. Next, find the information that matches the measurement or abbreviation used in the denominator of the fraction you created. In this example *cup* is in the denominator and we have 1½ cups. Therefore the full equation is

$$x \text{ mL} = \frac{240 \text{ mL}}{1 \text{ cup}} \times \frac{1.5 \text{ cups}}{1}$$

Step 4. Now cancel out the like abbreviations on the right side of the equation. If you have set up the problem correctly, the remaining measurement or abbreviation should match that used on the left side of the equation. You are now ready to solve for x.

$$x \text{ mL} = \frac{240 \text{ mL}}{1 \cancel{\text{cup}}} \times \frac{1.5 \cancel{\text{cups}}}{1}$$

$$x = \frac{240 \times 1.5}{1 \times 1} = \frac{360}{1}$$

$$x = 360 \text{ mL}$$

The answer to the problem is 360 mL.

EXAMPLE 2: 35 kg equals how many pounds?

Step 1. On the left side of the equation, place the name or abbreviation of the drug form of x, or what you are solving for.

$$x \text{ lb} =$$

Step 2. On the right side of the equation, place the available information related to the measurement or abbreviation that was placed on the left side. In this example that is *lb*. This information is placed in the equation as a common fraction; match the appropriate abbreviation or measurement. Thus the abbreviation that matches the x quantity must be placed in the numerator. We also know there are 2.2 lb in each kilogram. This information is the denominator of our fraction.

$$x \text{ lb} = \frac{2.2 \text{ lb}}{1 \text{ kg}}$$

Step 3. Next, find the information that matches the measurement or abbreviation used in the denominator of the fraction you created. In this example *kg* is in the denominator and the weight we are given is 35 kg. Therefore the full equation is

$$x \text{ lb} = \frac{2.2 \text{ lb}}{1 \text{ kg}} \times \frac{35 \text{ kg}}{1}$$

Step 4. Now cancel out the like abbreviations on the right side of the equation. If you have set up the problem correctly, the remaining measurement or abbreviation should match that used on the left side of the equation. You are now ready to solve for x.

$$x \text{ lb} = \frac{2.2 \text{ lb}}{1 \cancel{\text{kg}}} \times \frac{35 \cancel{\text{kg}}}{1}$$

$$x = \frac{2.2 \times 35}{1 \times 1} = \frac{77}{1}$$

$$x = 77 \text{ lb}$$

The answer to the problem is 77 lb.

EXAMPLE 3: 18 inches equals how many centimeters?

Step 1. On the left side of the equation, place the name or abbreviation of the drug form of x, or what you are solving for.

$$x \text{ cm} =$$

Step 2. On the right side of the equation, place the available information related to the measurement or abbreviation that was placed on the left side. In this example that is *cm*. This information is placed in the equation as a common fraction; match the appropriate abbreviation or measurement. Thus the abbreviation that matches the x quantity must be placed in the numerator. We also know that there are 2.5 cm in each inch. This information is the denominator of our fraction.

$$x \text{ cm} = \frac{2.5 \text{ cm}}{1 \text{ inch}}$$

Step 3. Next, find the information that matches the measurement or abbreviation used in the denominator of the fraction you created. In this example *inch* is in the denominator and the length we are given is 18 inches. Therefore the full equation is

$$x \text{ cm} = \frac{2.5 \text{ cm}}{1 \text{ inch}} \times \frac{18 \text{ inches}}{1}$$

Step 4. Now cancel out the like abbreviations on the right side of the equation. If you have set up the problem correctly, the remaining measurement or abbreviation should match that used on the left side of the equation. You are now ready to solve for x.

$$x \text{ cm} = \frac{2.5 \text{ cm}}{1 \cancel{\text{inch}}} \times \frac{18 \cancel{\text{inches}}}{1}$$

$$x = \frac{2.5 \times 18}{1 \times 1} = \frac{45}{1}$$

$$x = 45 \text{ cm}$$

The answer to the problem is 45 cm.

HOUSEHOLD CONVERSIONS: PROPORTION METHOD

EXAMPLE 1: 1½ cups equals how many milliliters?

Step 1. 1 cup : 240 mL ::

Step 2. 1 cup : 240 mL :: ______ cups : ______ mL

1 cup : 240 mL :: 1½ cups : x mL

Step 3. 1 : 240 :: 1½ : x

Step 4. $x = \frac{240}{1} \times \frac{3}{2}$

$x = \frac{720}{2} = 360$ mL

Step 5. 1½ cups = 360 mL

EXAMPLE 2: 35 kg equals how many pounds?

Step 1. 1 kg : 2.2 lb ::

Step 2. 1 kg : 2.2 lb :: ______ kg : ______ lb

1 kg : 2.2 lb :: 35 kg : x lb

Step 3. 1 : 2.2 :: 35 : x

Step 4. $1x = 2.2 \times 35$

$x = 77$

Step 5. 35 kg = 77 lb

EXAMPLE 3: 18 inches equals how many centimeters?

Step 1. 2.5 cm : 1 inch ::

Step 2. 2.5 cm : 1 inch :: ______ cm : ______ inch

2.5 cm : 1 inch :: x cm : 18 inches

Step 3. 2.5 : 1 :: x : 18

Step 4. $x = 2.5 \times 18$

$x = 45$ cm

Step 5. 18 inches = 45 cm

Memorize the tables of metric and household measurements. Study the material on using dimensional analysis or proportions for the calculation of problems relating to the metric and household systems of measure. Complete the following work sheet, which provides for extensive practice in the manipulation of measurements within the metric and household systems. Check your answers. If you have difficulties, go back and review the necessary material. When you feel ready to evaluate your learning, take the first posttest. Check your answers. An acceptable score as indicated on the posttest signifies that you are ready for the next chapter. An unacceptable score signifies a need for further study before taking the second posttest.

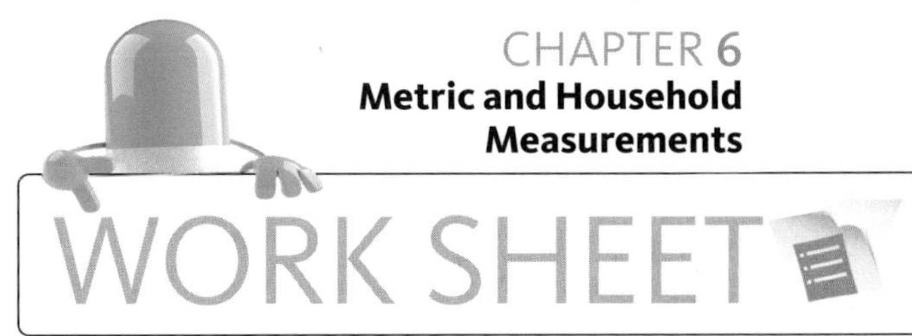

CHAPTER 6
Metric and Household Measurements

WORK SHEET

DIRECTIONS: Change to equivalents within the metric system. Solve the problems and show your work. Convert fractions to decimals before solving the problem.

1. 230 mcg = 0.00023 g **2.** 5 mg = 5000 mcg **3.** 2.5 g = 2,500,000 mcg

4. 4000 mcg = 4 mg **5.** 0.33 g = 330 mg **6.** 6 kg = 6000 g

7. 725 mL = 0.725 L **8.** 2000 mcg = 0.002 g **9.** 3 cm = 30 mm

10. 620 g = 0.62 kg **11.** 0.036 mg = 36 mcg **12.** 460 mL = 0.46 L

13. 0.66 mg = 660 mcg **14.** 0.5 g = 500,000 mcg **15.** 18 inches = 45 cm

16. 350,000 mcg = 0.35 g **17.** 25 mg = 0.025 g **18.** 1.46 L = 1460 mL

19. 2.5 kg = 2500 g **20.** 12 mg = 12,000 mcg **21.** 3.4 kg = 3400 g

22. 920 mcg = 0.00092 g **23.** 25 mm = 2.5 cm **24.** 300 mcg = 0.3 mg

25. 0.16 L = ________ mL **26.** 0.01 g = ________ mg **27.** 500 mcg = ________ mg

28. 360 mg = ________ g **29.** 1.7 L = ________ mL **30.** 0.45 g = ________ mg

31. 240 mL = ________ L **32.** 10 mcg = ________ mg

DIRECTIONS: Change the following measurements into the approximate equivalents within the metric or household system, as indicated. Solve the problems and show your work. Convert fractions to decimals before solving the problem.

33. 3 inches = 7.5 cm **34.** $2\frac{1}{4}$ cups = 540 mL **35.** 2 tsp = 10 mL

36. 3 Tbsp = 45 mL **37.** $1\frac{1}{2}$ cups = 360 mL **38.** 8 kg = 17.6 lb

39. 3825 g = 8.41 lb **40.** 7 inches = 17.5 cm **41.** 3 lb = 1.36 kg

42. 12 kg = 26.4 lb **43.** 1400 g = 3.08 lb **44.** $2\frac{1}{2}$ feet = 30 inches

45. 150 lb = 68.18 kg

ANSWERS ON P. 132.

NAME ______________________

DATE ______________________

ACCEPTABLE SCORE 29

YOUR SCORE ______

POSTTEST 1

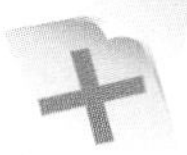

DIRECTIONS: Change to equivalent measurements. Solve each problem and show your work. Convert fractions to decimals before solving the problem.

1. 5000 mcg = ________ g
2. 10 mg = ________ mcg
3. 0.81 L = ________ mL
4. 35 mg = ________ g
5. 2¼ feet = ________ inches
6. 0.12 g = ________ mcg
7. 16 kg = ________ lb
8. 280 mL = ________ L
9. 0.4 kg = ________ g
10. 42 inches = ________ feet
11. 28 lb = ________ g
12. 4 inches = ________ cm
13. 500,000 mcg = ________ g
14. 37 mL = ________ L
15. 20 mL = ________ cc
16. 1⅓ cups = ________ mL
17. 2.5 g = ________ mg
18. 350 mg = ________ g
19. 6700 g = ________ kg
20. 0.3 L = ________ mL
21. 4 mg = ________ mcg
22. 2600 g = ________ lb
23. 1½ tsp = ________ mL
24. 0.2 L = ________ mL

25. 533 mL = __________ L **26.** 1.5 g = __________ mcg **27.** 620 mg = __________ g

28. 2.3 kg = __________ g **29.** 15 inches = ________ feet **30.** 7 lb = __________ kg

ANSWERS ON P. 133.

NAME ____________________

DATE ____________________

ACCEPTABLE SCORE **29**

YOUR SCORE ______

CHAPTER 6
Metric and Household Measurements

POSTTEST 2

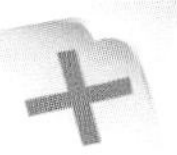

DIRECTIONS: Change to equivalent measurements. Solve each problem and show your work. Convert fractions to decimals before solving the problem.

1. 4000 mcg = ______ mg

2. 150 g = ______ kg

3. 2½ cups = ______ mL

4. 800 g = ______ lb

5. 44 kg = ______ lb

6. 760 mg = ______ g

7. 0.55 L = ______ mL

8. 35 mm = ______ cm

9. 4 Tbsp = ______ mL

10. 2⅛ lb = ______ g

11. 0.1 L = ______ mL

12. 32 mg = ______ mcg

13. 618 mL = ______ L

14. 100,000 mcg = ______ g

15. 28 inches = ______ feet

16. 714 mL = ______ L

17. 350 mg = ______ g

18. 250,000 mcg = ______ g

19. 0.87 g = ______ mg

20. 7 mg = ______ mcg

21. 37 mcg = ______ mg

22. 1.4 L = ______ mL

23. 0.78 g = ______ mg

24. 225 mcg = ______ mg

25. 4500 g = ________ kg **26.** 0.2 L = ________ mL **27.** $3\frac{3}{4}$ feet = ______ inches

28. 420 mg = ________ g **29.** 2.6 g = ________ mcg **30.** 73 lb = ________ kg

ANSWERS ON PP. 134–135.

evolve For additional practice problems, refer to the Conversions and Equivalents section of *Elsevier's Interactive Drug Calculation Application*, version 1.

ANSWERS

CHAPTER 6 Metric and Household Measurements—Pretest, pp. 113–114

1. 0.8 g
2. 3000 mcg
3. 0.255 g
4. 46,000 mcg
5. 3 mg
6. 680 mg
7. 0.326 L
8. 72.6 lb or 72⅗ lb
9. 2100 mg
10. 3 kg
11. 100 mL
12. 116.6 lb or 116⅗ lb
13. 5 mcg
14. 800 g
15. 0.25 mg
16. 300 mL
17. 10,000 g
18. 630 mL
19. 0.733 kg
20. 1,250,000 mcg
21. 0.06 g
22. 250 mcg
23. 250 mL
24. 20.45 kg
25. 0.01 g
26. 1200 g
27. 18.75 mL
28. 710 mg
29. 0.48 L
30. $1\frac{43}{100}$ lb or 1.43 lb

Dimensional Analysis—Pretest, pp. 113–114

1. $x \text{ g} = \frac{1 \text{ g}}{1{,}000{,}000 \text{ mcg}} \times \frac{800{,}000 \text{ mcg}}{1} = 0.8 \text{ g}$
2. $x \text{ mcg} = \frac{1000 \text{ mcg}}{1 \text{ mg}} \times \frac{3 \text{ mg}}{1} = 3000 \text{ mcg}$
3. $x \text{ g} = \frac{1 \text{ g}}{1000 \text{ mg}} \times \frac{255 \text{ mg}}{1} = 0.255 \text{ g}$
4. $x \text{ mcg} = \frac{1000 \text{ mcg}}{1 \text{ mg}} \times \frac{46 \text{ mg}}{1} = 46{,}000 \text{ mcg}$
5. $x \text{ mg} = \frac{1 \text{ mg}}{1000 \text{ mcg}} \times \frac{3000 \text{ mcg}}{1} = 3 \text{ mg}$
6. $x \text{ mg} = \frac{1000 \text{ mg}}{1 \text{ g}} \times \frac{0.68 \text{ g}}{1} = 680 \text{ mg}$
7. $x \text{ L} = \frac{1 \text{ L}}{1000 \text{ mL}} \times \frac{326 \text{ mL}}{1} = 0.326 \text{ L}$
8. $x \text{ lb} = \frac{2.2 \text{ lb}}{1 \text{ kg}} \times \frac{33 \text{ kg}}{1} = 72.6 \text{ lb}$
9. $x \text{ mg} = \frac{1000 \text{ mg}}{1 \text{ g}} \times \frac{2.1 \text{ g}}{1} = 2100 \text{ mg}$
10. $x \text{ kg} = \frac{1 \text{ kg}}{1000 \text{ g}} \times \frac{3000 \text{ g}}{1} = 3 \text{ kg}$
11. $x \text{ mL} = \frac{1000 \text{ mL}}{1 \text{ L}} \times \frac{0.1 \text{ L}}{1} = 100 \text{ mL}$
12. $x \text{ lb} = \frac{2.2 \text{ lb}}{1 \text{ kg}} \times \frac{53 \text{ kg}}{1} = 116.6 \text{ lb}$
13. $x \text{ mcg} = \frac{1000 \text{ mcg}}{1 \text{ mg}} \times \frac{0.005 \text{ mg}}{1} = 5 \text{ mcg}$
14. $x \text{ g} = \frac{1000 \text{ g}}{1 \text{ kg}} \times \frac{0.8 \text{ kg}}{1} = 800 \text{ g}$
15. $x \text{ mg} = \frac{1 \text{ mg}}{1000 \text{ mcg}} \times \frac{250 \text{ mcg}}{1} = 0.25 \text{ mg}$
16. $x \text{ mL} = \frac{240 \text{ mL}}{1 \text{ cup}} \times \frac{1.25 \text{ cups}}{1} = 300 \text{ mL}$
17. $x \text{ g} = \frac{1000 \text{ g}}{2.2 \text{ lb}} \times \frac{22 \text{ lb}}{1} = 10{,}000 \text{ g}$
18. $x \text{ mL} = \frac{1000 \text{ mL}}{1 \text{ L}} \times \frac{0.63 \text{ L}}{1} = 630 \text{ mL}$
19. $x \text{ kg} = \frac{1 \text{ kg}}{1000 \text{ g}} \times \frac{733 \text{ g}}{1} = 0.733 \text{ kg}$
20. $x \text{ mcg} = \frac{1{,}000{,}000 \text{ mcg}}{1 \text{ g}} \times \frac{1.25 \text{ g}}{1} = 1{,}250{,}000 \text{ mcg}$
21. $x \text{ g} = \frac{1 \text{ g}}{1000 \text{ mg}} \times \frac{60 \text{ mg}}{1} = 0.06 \text{ g}$
22. $x \text{ mcg} = \frac{1000 \text{ mcg}}{1 \text{ mg}} \times \frac{0.25 \text{ mg}}{1} = 250 \text{ mcg}$
23. $x \text{ mL} = \frac{1000 \text{ mL}}{1 \text{ L}} \times \frac{0.25 \text{ L}}{1} = 250 \text{ mL}$
24. $x \text{ kg} = \frac{1 \text{ kg}}{2.2 \text{ lb}} \times \frac{45 \text{ lb}}{1} = 20.45 \text{ kg}$
25. $x \text{ g} = \frac{1 \text{ g}}{1{,}000{,}000 \text{ mcg}} \times \frac{10{,}000 \text{ mcg}}{1} = 0.01 \text{ g}$
26. $x \text{ g} = \frac{1000 \text{ g}}{1 \text{ kg}} \times \frac{1.2 \text{ kg}}{1} = 1200 \text{ g}$

27. $x \text{ mL} = \frac{15 \text{ mL}}{1 \text{ Tbsp}} \times \frac{1.25 \text{ Tbsp}}{1} = 18.75 \text{ mL}$

28. $x \text{ mg} = \frac{1000 \text{ mg}}{1 \text{ g}} \times \frac{0.71 \text{ g}}{1} = 710 \text{ mg}$

29. $x \text{ L} = \frac{1 \text{ L}}{1000 \text{ mL}} \times \frac{480 \text{ mL}}{1} = 0.48 \text{ L}$

30. $x \text{ lb} = \frac{2.2 \text{ lb}}{1000 \text{ g}} \times \frac{650 \text{ g}}{1} = 1.43 \text{ lb}$

CHAPTER 6 Metric and Household Measurements—Work Sheet, pp. 125–126

1. 0.00023 g
2. 5000 mcg
3. 2,500,000 mcg
4. 4 mg
5. 330 mg
6. 6000 g
7. 0.725 L
8. 0.002 g
9. 30 mm
10. 0.62 kg
11. 36 mcg
12. 0.46 L
13. 660 mcg
14. 500,000 mcg
15. 45 cm
16. 0.35 g
17. 0.025 g
18. 1460 mL
19. 2500 g
20. 12,000 mcg
21. 3400 g
22. 0.00092 g
23. 2.5 cm
24. 0.3 mg
25. 160 mL
26. 10 mg
27. 0.5 mg
28. 0.36 g
29. 1700 mL
30. 450 mg
31. 0.24 L
32. 0.01 mg
33. 7.5 cm
34. 540 mL
35. 10 mL
36. 45 mL
37. 360 mL
38. $17\frac{3}{5}$ lb or 17.6 lb
39. 8.415 lb, $8\frac{83}{200}$ lb, or 8.41 lb
40. 17.5 cm
41. 1.36 kg
42. $26\frac{2}{5}$ lb or 26.4 lb
43. $3\frac{2}{25}$ lb or 3.08 lb
44. 30 inches
45. 68.18 kg

Dimensional Analysis—Work Sheet, pp. 125–126

1. $x \text{ g} = \frac{1 \text{ g}}{1{,}000{,}000 \text{ mcg}} \times \frac{230 \text{ mcg}}{1}$
$= 0.00023 \text{ g}$

2. $x \text{ mcg} = \frac{1000 \text{ mcg}}{1 \text{ mg}} \times \frac{5 \text{ mg}}{1} = 5000 \text{ mcg}$

3. $x \text{ mcg} = \frac{1{,}000{,}000 \text{ mcg}}{1 \text{ g}} \times \frac{2.5 \text{ g}}{1}$
$= 2{,}500{,}000 \text{ mcg}$

4. $x \text{ mg} = \frac{1 \text{ mg}}{1000 \text{ mcg}} \times \frac{4000 \text{ mcg}}{1} = 4 \text{ mg}$

5. $x \text{ mg} = \frac{1000 \text{ mg}}{1 \text{ g}} \times \frac{0.33 \text{ g}}{1} = 330 \text{ mg}$

6. $x \text{ g} = \frac{1000 \text{ g}}{1 \text{ kg}} \times \frac{6 \text{ kg}}{1} = 6000 \text{ g}$

7. $x \text{ L} = \frac{1 \text{ L}}{1000 \text{ mL}} \times \frac{725 \text{ mL}}{1} = 0.725 \text{ L}$

8. $x \text{ g} = \frac{1 \text{ g}}{1{,}000{,}000 \text{ mcg}} \times \frac{2{,}000 \text{ mcg}}{1}$
$= 0.002 \text{ g}$

9. $x \text{ mm} = \frac{10 \text{ mm}}{1 \text{ cm}} \times \frac{3 \text{ cm}}{1} = 30 \text{ mm}$

10. $x \text{ kg} = \frac{1 \text{ kg}}{1000 \text{ g}} \times \frac{620 \text{ g}}{1} = 0.62 \text{ kg}$

11. $x \text{ mcg} = \frac{1000 \text{ mcg}}{1 \text{ mg}} \times \frac{0.036 \text{ mg}}{1} = 36 \text{ mcg}$

12. $x \text{ L} = \frac{1 \text{ L}}{1000 \text{ mL}} \times \frac{460 \text{ mL}}{1} = 0.46 \text{ L}$

13. $x \text{ mcg} = \frac{1000 \text{ mcg}}{1 \text{ mg}} \times \frac{0.66 \text{ mg}}{1} = 660 \text{ mcg}$

14. $x \text{ mcg} = \frac{1{,}000{,}000 \text{ mcg}}{1 \text{ g}} \times \frac{0.5 \text{ g}}{1}$
$= 500{,}000 \text{ mcg}$

15. $x \text{ cm} = \frac{2.5 \text{ cm}}{1 \text{ in}} \times \frac{18 \text{ in}}{1} = 45 \text{ cm}$

16. $x \text{ g} = \frac{1 \text{ g}}{1{,}000{,}000 \text{ mcg}} \times \frac{350{,}000 \text{ mcg}}{1}$
$= 0.35 \text{ g}$

17. $x \text{ g} = \frac{1 \text{ g}}{1000 \text{ mg}} \times \frac{25 \text{ mg}}{1} = 0.025 \text{ g}$

18. $x \text{ mL} = \frac{1000 \text{ mL}}{1 \text{ L}} \times \frac{1.46 \text{ L}}{1} = 1460 \text{ mL}$

19. $x \text{ g} = \dfrac{1000 \text{ g}}{1 \text{ kg}} \times \dfrac{2.5 \text{ kg}}{1} = 2500 \text{ g}$

20. $x \text{ mcg} = \dfrac{1000 \text{ mcg}}{1 \text{ mg}} \times \dfrac{12 \text{ mg}}{1}$
$= 12{,}000 \text{ mcg}$

21. $x \text{ g} = \dfrac{1000 \text{ g}}{1 \text{ kg}} \times \dfrac{3.4 \text{ kg}}{1} = 3400 \text{ g}$

22. $x \text{ g} = \dfrac{1 \text{ g}}{1{,}000{,}000 \text{ mcg}} \times \dfrac{920 \text{ mcg}}{1}$
$= 0.00092 \text{ g}$

23. $x \text{ cm} = \dfrac{1 \text{ cm}}{10 \text{ mm}} \times \dfrac{25 \text{ mm}}{1} = 2.5 \text{ cm}$

24. $x \text{ mg} = \dfrac{1 \text{ mg}}{1000 \text{ mcg}} \times \dfrac{300 \text{ mcg}}{1} = 0.3 \text{ mg}$

25. $x \text{ mL} = \dfrac{1000 \text{ mL}}{1 \text{ L}} \times \dfrac{0.16 \text{ L}}{1} = 160 \text{ mL}$

26. $x \text{ mg} = \dfrac{1000 \text{ mg}}{1 \text{ g}} \times \dfrac{0.01 \text{ g}}{1} = 10 \text{ mg}$

27. $x \text{ mg} = \dfrac{1 \text{ mg}}{1000 \text{ mcg}} \times \dfrac{500 \text{ mcg}}{1} = 0.5 \text{ mg}$

28. $x \text{ g} = \dfrac{1 \text{ g}}{1000 \text{ mg}} \times \dfrac{360 \text{ mg}}{1} = 0.36 \text{ g}$

29. $x \text{ mL} = \dfrac{1000 \text{ mL}}{1 \text{ L}} \times \dfrac{1.7 \text{ L}}{1} = 1700 \text{ mL}$

30. $x \text{ mg} = \dfrac{1000 \text{ mg}}{1 \text{ g}} \times \dfrac{0.45 \text{ g}}{1} = 450 \text{ mg}$

31. $x \text{ L} = \dfrac{1 \text{ L}}{1000 \text{ mL}} \times \dfrac{240 \text{ mL}}{1} = 0.24 \text{ L}$

32. $x \text{ mg} = \dfrac{1 \text{ mg}}{1000 \text{ mcg}} \times \dfrac{10 \text{ mcg}}{1} = 0.01 \text{ mg}$

33. $x \text{ cm} = \dfrac{2.5 \text{ cm}}{1 \text{ in}} \times \dfrac{3 \text{ in}}{1} = 7.5 \text{ cm}$

34. $x \text{ mL} = \dfrac{240 \text{ mL}}{1 \text{ cup}} \times \dfrac{2.25 \text{ cups}}{1} = 540 \text{ mL}$

35. $x \text{ mL} = \dfrac{5 \text{ mL}}{1 \text{ tsp}} \times \dfrac{2 \text{ tsp}}{1} = 10 \text{ mL}$

36. $x \text{ mL} = \dfrac{15 \text{ mL}}{1 \text{ Tbsp}} \times \dfrac{3 \text{ Tbsp}}{1} = 45 \text{ mL}$

37. $x \text{ mL} = \dfrac{240 \text{ mL}}{1 \text{ cup}} \times \dfrac{1.5 \text{ cups}}{1} = 360 \text{ mL}$

38. $x \text{ lb} = \dfrac{2.2 \text{ lb}}{1 \text{ kg}} \times \dfrac{8 \text{ kg}}{1} = 17.6 \text{ lb}$

39. $x \text{ lb} = \dfrac{2.2 \text{ lb}}{1000 \text{ g}} \times \dfrac{3825 \text{ g}}{1} = 8.415 \text{ lb}$

40. $x \text{ cm} = \dfrac{2.5 \text{ cm}}{1 \text{ in}} \times \dfrac{7 \text{ in}}{1} = 17.5 \text{ cm}$

41. $x \text{ kg} = \dfrac{1 \text{ kg}}{2.2 \text{ lb}} \times \dfrac{3 \text{ lb}}{1} = 1.36 \text{ kg}$

42. $x \text{ lb} = \dfrac{2.2 \text{ lb}}{1 \text{ kg}} \times \dfrac{12 \text{ kg}}{1} = 26.4 \text{ lb}$

43. $x \text{ lb} = \dfrac{2.2 \text{ g}}{1000 \text{ g}} \times \dfrac{1400 \text{ g}}{1} = 3.08 \text{ lb}$

44. $x \text{ inches} = \dfrac{12 \text{ inches}}{1 \text{ foot}} \times \dfrac{2.5 \text{ feet}}{1}$
$= 30 \text{ inches}$

45. $x \text{ kg} = \dfrac{1 \text{ kg}}{2.2 \text{ lb}} \times \dfrac{150 \text{ lb}}{1} = 68.18 \text{ kg}$

CHAPTER 6 Metric and Household Measurements—Posttest 1, pp. 127–128

1. 0.005 g
2. 10,000 mcg
3. 810 mL
4. 0.035 g
5. 27 inches
6. 120,000 mcg
7. $35\frac{1}{5}$ lb or 35.2 lb
8. 0.28 L
9. 400 g
10. $3\frac{1}{2}$ feet
11. 12,727.27 g
12. 10 cm
13. 0.5 g
14. 0.037 L
15. 20 cc
16. 320 mL
17. 2500 mg
18. 0.35 g
19. 6.7 kg
20. 300 mL
21. 4000 mcg
22. $5\frac{18}{25}$ lb or 5.72 lb
23. 7.5 mL
24. 200 mL
25. 0.533 L
26. 1,500,000 mcg
27. 0.62 g
28. 2300 g
29. $1\frac{1}{4}$ fect
30. 3.18 kg

Dimensional Analysis—Posttest 1, pp. 127–128

1. $x \text{ g} = \dfrac{1 \text{ g}}{1{,}000{,}000 \text{ mcg}} \times \dfrac{5000 \text{ mcg}}{1} = 0.005 \text{ g}$
2. $x \text{ mcg} = \dfrac{1000 \text{ mcg}}{1 \text{ mg}} \times \dfrac{10 \text{ mg}}{1} = 10{,}000 \text{ mcg}$
3. $x \text{ mL} = \dfrac{1000 \text{ mL}}{1 \text{ L}} \times \dfrac{0.81 \text{ L}}{1} = 810 \text{ mL}$
4. $x \text{ g} = \dfrac{1 \text{ g}}{1000 \text{ mg}} \times \dfrac{35 \text{ mg}}{1} = 0.035 \text{ g}$
5. $x \text{ inches} = \dfrac{12 \text{ inches}}{1 \text{ foot}} \times \dfrac{2.25 \text{ feet}}{1} = 27 \text{ inches}$
6. $x \text{ mcg} = \dfrac{1{,}000{,}000 \text{ mcg}}{1 \text{ g}} \times \dfrac{0.12 \text{ g}}{1} = 120{,}000 \text{ mcg}$
7. $x \text{ lb} = \dfrac{2.2 \text{ lb}}{1 \text{ kg}} \times \dfrac{16 \text{ kg}}{1} = 35.2 \text{ lb}$
8. $x \text{ L} = \dfrac{1 \text{ L}}{1000 \text{ mL}} \times \dfrac{280 \text{ mL}}{1} = 0.28 \text{ L}$
9. $x \text{ g} = \dfrac{1000 \text{ g}}{1 \text{ kg}} \times \dfrac{0.4 \text{ kg}}{1} = 400 \text{ g}$
10. $x \text{ feet} = \dfrac{1 \text{ foot}}{12 \text{ inches}} \times \dfrac{42 \text{ inches}}{1} = 3.5 \text{ feet}$
11. $x \text{ g} = \dfrac{1000 \text{ g}}{2.2 \text{ lb}} \times \dfrac{28 \text{ lb}}{1} = 12{,}727.27 \text{ g}$
12. $x \text{ cm} = \dfrac{2.5 \text{ cm}}{1 \text{ inch}} \times \dfrac{4 \text{ inches}}{1} = 10 \text{ cm}$
13. $x \text{ g} = \dfrac{1 \text{ g}}{1{,}000{,}000 \text{ mcg}} \times \dfrac{500{,}000 \text{ mcg}}{1} = 0.5 \text{ g}$
14. $x \text{ L} = \dfrac{1 \text{ L}}{1000 \text{ mL}} \times \dfrac{37 \text{ mL}}{1} = 0.037 \text{ L}$
15. $x \text{ cc} = \dfrac{1 \text{ cc}}{1 \text{ mL}} \times \dfrac{20 \text{ mL}}{1} = 20 \text{ cc}$
16. $x \text{ mL} = \dfrac{240 \text{ mL}}{1 \text{ cup}} \times \dfrac{4/3 \text{ cups}}{1} = 320 \text{ mL}$
17. $x \text{ mg} = \dfrac{1000 \text{ mg}}{1 \text{ g}} \times \dfrac{2.5 \text{ g}}{1} = 2500 \text{ mg}$
18. $x \text{ g} = \dfrac{1 \text{ g}}{1000 \text{ mg}} \times \dfrac{350 \text{ mg}}{1} = 0.35 \text{ g}$
19. $x \text{ kg} = \dfrac{1 \text{ kg}}{1000 \text{ g}} \times \dfrac{6700 \text{ g}}{1} = 6.7 \text{ kg}$
20. $x \text{ mL} = \dfrac{1000 \text{ mL}}{1 \text{ L}} \times \dfrac{0.3 \text{ L}}{1} = 300 \text{ mL}$
21. $x \text{ mcg} = \dfrac{1000 \text{ mcg}}{1 \text{ mg}} \times \dfrac{4 \text{ mg}}{1} = 4000 \text{ mcg}$
22. $x \text{ lb} = \dfrac{2.2 \text{ lb}}{1000 \text{ g}} \times \dfrac{2600 \text{ g}}{1} = 5.72 \text{ lb}$
23. $x \text{ mL} = \dfrac{5 \text{ mL}}{1 \text{ tsp}} \times \dfrac{1.5 \text{ tsp}}{1} = 7.5 \text{ mL}$
24. $x \text{ mL} = \dfrac{1000 \text{ mL}}{1 \text{ L}} \times \dfrac{0.2 \text{ L}}{1} = 200 \text{ mL}$
25. $x \text{ L} = \dfrac{1 \text{ L}}{1000 \text{ mL}} \times \dfrac{533 \text{ mL}}{1} = 0.533 \text{ L}$
26. $x \text{ mcg} = \dfrac{1{,}000{,}000 \text{ mcg}}{1 \text{ g}} \times \dfrac{1.5 \text{ g}}{1} = 1{,}500{,}000 \text{ mcg}$
27. $x \text{ g} = \dfrac{1 \text{ g}}{1000 \text{ mg}} \times \dfrac{620 \text{ mg}}{1} = 0.62 \text{ g}$
28. $x \text{ g} = \dfrac{1000 \text{ g}}{1 \text{ kg}} \times \dfrac{2.3 \text{ kg}}{1} = 2300 \text{ g}$
29. $x \text{ feet} = \dfrac{1 \text{ foot}}{12 \text{ inches}} \times \dfrac{15 \text{ inches}}{1} = 1.25 \text{ feet}$
30. $x \text{ kg} = \dfrac{1 \text{ kg}}{2.2 \text{ lb}} \times \dfrac{7 \text{ lb}}{1} = 3.18 \text{ kg}$

CHAPTER 6 Metric and Household Measurements—Posttest 2, pp. 129–130

1. 4 mg
2. 0.15 kg
3. 600 mL
4. $1\frac{19}{25}$ lb or 1.76 lb
5. $96\frac{4}{5}$ lb or 96.8 lb
6. 0.76 g
7. 550 mL
8. 3.5 cm
9. 60 mL
10. 965.909 g
11. 100 mL
12. 32,000 mcg
13. 0.618 L
14. 0.1 g
15. $2\frac{1}{3}$ feet
16. 0.714 L
17. 0.35 g
18. 0.25 g
19. 870 mg
20. 7000 mcg
21. 0.037 mg

22. 1400 mL
23. 780 mg
24. 0.225 mg
25. 4.5 kg
26. 200 mL
27. 45 inches
28. 0.42 g
29. 2,600,000 mcg
30. 33.18 kg

Dimensional Analysis—Posttest 2, pp. 129–130

1. $x \text{ mg} = \dfrac{1 \text{ mg}}{1000 \text{ mcg}} \times \dfrac{4000 \text{ mcg}}{1} = 4 \text{ mg}$
2. $x \text{ kg} = \dfrac{1 \text{ kg}}{1000 \text{ g}} \times \dfrac{150 \text{ g}}{1} = 0.15 \text{ kg}$
3. $x \text{ mL} = \dfrac{240 \text{ mL}}{1 \text{ cup}} \times \dfrac{2.5 \text{ cups}}{1} = 600 \text{ mL}$
4. $x \text{ lb} = \dfrac{2.2 \text{ lb}}{1000 \text{ g}} \times \dfrac{800 \text{ g}}{1} = 1.76 \text{ lb}$
5. $x \text{ lb} = \dfrac{2.2 \text{ lb}}{1 \text{ kg}} \times \dfrac{44 \text{ kg}}{1} = 96.8 \text{ lb}$
6. $x \text{ g} = \dfrac{1 \text{ g}}{1000 \text{ mg}} \times \dfrac{760 \text{ mg}}{1} = 0.76 \text{ g}$
7. $x \text{ mL} = \dfrac{1000 \text{ mL}}{1 \text{ L}} \times \dfrac{0.55 \text{ L}}{1} = 550 \text{ mL}$
8. $x \text{ cm} = \dfrac{1 \text{ cm}}{10 \text{ mm}} \times \dfrac{35 \text{ mm}}{1} = 3.5 \text{ cm}$
9. $x \text{ mL} = \dfrac{15 \text{ mL}}{1 \text{ Tbsp}} \times \dfrac{4 \text{ Tbsp}}{1} = 60 \text{ mL}$
10. $x \text{ g} = \dfrac{1000 \text{ g}}{2.2 \text{ lb}} \times \dfrac{2.125 \text{ lb}}{1} = 965.909 \text{ g}$
11. $x \text{ mL} = \dfrac{1000 \text{ mL}}{1 \text{ L}} \times \dfrac{0.1 \text{ L}}{1} = 100 \text{ mL}$
12. $x \text{ mcg} = \dfrac{1000 \text{ mcg}}{1 \text{ mg}} \times \dfrac{32 \text{ mg}}{1} = 32{,}000 \text{ mcg}$
13. $x \text{ L} = \dfrac{1 \text{ L}}{1000 \text{ mL}} \times \dfrac{618 \text{ mL}}{1} = 0.618 \text{ L}$
14. $x \text{ g} = \dfrac{1 \text{ g}}{1{,}000{,}000 \text{ mcg}} \times \dfrac{100{,}000 \text{ mcg}}{1} = 0.1 \text{ g}$
15. $x \text{ feet} = \dfrac{1 \text{ foot}}{12 \text{ inches}} \times \dfrac{28 \text{ inches}}{1} = 2.33 \text{ feet}$
16. $x \text{ L} = \dfrac{1 \text{ L}}{1000 \text{ mL}} \times \dfrac{714 \text{ mL}}{1} = 0.714 \text{ L}$
17. $x \text{ g} = \dfrac{1 \text{ g}}{1000 \text{ mg}} \times \dfrac{350 \text{ mg}}{1} = 0.35 \text{ g}$
18. $x \text{ g} = \dfrac{1 \text{ g}}{1{,}000{,}000 \text{ mcg}} \times \dfrac{250{,}000 \text{ mcg}}{1} = 0.25 \text{ g}$
19. $x \text{ mg} = \dfrac{1000 \text{ mg}}{1 \text{ g}} \times \dfrac{0.87 \text{ g}}{1} = 870 \text{ mg}$
20. $x \text{ mcg} = \dfrac{1000 \text{ mcg}}{1 \text{ mg}} \times \dfrac{7 \text{ mg}}{1} = 7000 \text{ mcg}$
21. $x \text{ mg} = \dfrac{1 \text{ mg}}{1000 \text{ mcg}} \times \dfrac{37 \text{ mcg}}{1} = 0.037 \text{ mg}$
22. $x \text{ mL} = \dfrac{1000 \text{ mL}}{1 \text{ L}} \times \dfrac{1.4 \text{ L}}{1} = 1400 \text{ mL}$
23. $x \text{ mg} = \dfrac{1000 \text{ mg}}{1 \text{ g}} \times \dfrac{0.78 \text{ g}}{1} = 780 \text{ mg}$
24. $x \text{ mg} = \dfrac{1 \text{ mg}}{1000 \text{ mcg}} \times \dfrac{225 \text{ mcg}}{1} = 0.225 \text{ mg}$
25. $x \text{ kg} = \dfrac{1 \text{ kg}}{1000 \text{ g}} \times \dfrac{4500 \text{ g}}{1} = 4.5 \text{ kg}$
26. $x \text{ mL} = \dfrac{1000 \text{ mL}}{1 \text{ L}} \times \dfrac{0.2 \text{ L}}{1} = 200 \text{ mL}$
27. $x \text{ inches} = \dfrac{12 \text{ inches}}{1 \text{ foot}} \times \dfrac{3.75 \text{ feet}}{1} = 45 \text{ inches}$
28. $x \text{ g} = \dfrac{1 \text{ g}}{1000 \text{ mg}} \times \dfrac{420 \text{ mg}}{1} = 0.42 \text{ g}$
29. $x \text{ mcg} = \dfrac{1{,}000{,}000 \text{ mcg}}{1 \text{ g}} \times \dfrac{2.6 \text{ g}}{1} = 2{,}600{,}000 \text{ mcg}$
30. $x \text{ kg} = \dfrac{1 \text{ kg}}{2.2 \text{ lb}} \times \dfrac{73 \text{ lb}}{1} = 33.18 \text{ kg}$

ANSWERS

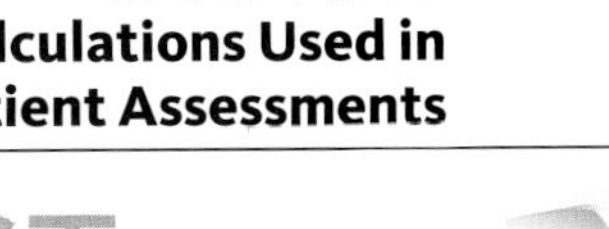

NAME ____________________

DATE ____________________

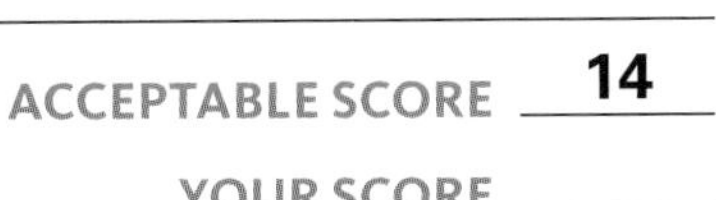

ACCEPTABLE SCORE **14**

YOUR SCORE ______

PRETEST

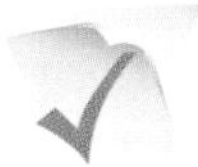

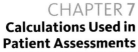

DIRECTIONS: Change to approximate equivalents as indicated. Solve the problems and show your work. (Round weights and temperatures to nearest tenth.) Convert fractions to decimals before solving the problem.

1. 110 lb = ________ kg

2. 480 mL = ________ cups

3. 36 kg = ________ lb

4. 90 mL = ________ fl oz

5. 3 cups = ________ mL

6. 8.2 kg = ________ lb

7. 600 mL = ________ cups

8. 2 cups = ________ mL

9. 7 fl oz = ________ mL

10. 360 mL = ________ fl oz

11. 85 lb = ________ kg

12. 1½ fl oz = ________ mL

13. 98.8° F = ________ ° C

14. 41° C = ________ ° F

15. 97.6° F = ________ ° C

16. 38.5° C = ________ ° F

17. 20 cm = ________ inches

18. 50 inches = ________ cm

ANSWERS ON P. 156.

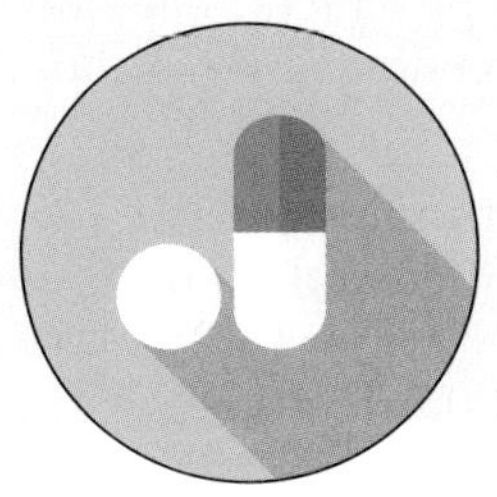

Calculations Used in Patient Assessments

LEARNING OBJECTIVES

Upon completion of the materials provided in this chapter, you will be able to perform computations accurately by mastering the following mathematical concepts:

1. Recalling equivalent apothecary and metric measures
2. Computing equivalents between the apothecary and metric systems by using dimensional analysis to calculate intake and output (I&O), weights, and lengths.
3. Converting from the Fahrenheit scale to the Celsius scale
4. Converting from the Celsius scale to the Fahrenheit scale

In addition to the calculation of drug dosages, nurses calculate aspects of a patient's assessment: intake and output (I&O), weight, lengths, and temperature. The nurse should know the approximate equivalents between the metric and apothecary systems for the calculation of I&O, weight, and lengths. A patient's temperature may require the conversion between the Celsius and Fahrenheit systems. This chapter is devoted to the common calculations that may be used in patient assessments.

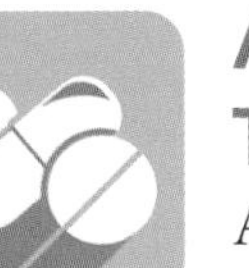

APPROXIMATE EQUIVALENTS BETWEEN THE MEASUREMENT SYSTEMS

A list of the most commonly used equivalents among household, apothecary, and metric systems of measure is provided in Box 7-1. Memorize these equivalents. Sometimes a nurse will have to convert from one system to the other. This can be done by using a proportion or dimensional analysis.

BOX 7-1 HOUSEHOLD/APOTHECARY/METRIC EQUIVALENTS

Household Measure	=	Apothecary Measure	=	Metric Measure
		1 fluid ounce (fl oz)	=	30 milliliters (mL)
		6 fluid ounces (fl oz)	=	180 milliliters (mL)
1 standard measuring cup	=	8 fluid ounces (fl oz)	=	240 milliliters (mL)
		2.2 pounds (lb)	=	1000 grams (g) or 1 kilogram (kg)
		1 inch	=	2.5 cm

CALCULATING INTAKE AND OUTPUT

Intake and output (I&O) is an important assessment performed by health care providers. The unit of measure for I&O calculation is typically milliliters, which may require conversions among the household, apothecary, and metric measurement systems.

EXAMPLE 1: (no conversions): During the 6 AM to 6 PM shift, a patient consumes 240 mL of orange juice and 240 mL of milk for breakfast, 360 mL of coffee and 90 mL of gelatin for lunch, and 120 mL of apple juice and 240 mL of water for dinner. The patient voided four times during the shift for 300 mL, 200 mL, 400 mL, and 300 mL of urine. Calculate the I&O for this shift.

Solution:

Intake	Output
240 mL	300 mL
240 mL	200 mL
360 mL	400 mL
90 mL	300 mL
120 mL	1200 mL
240 mL	
1290 mL	

Therefore 1290 mL would be recorded for the intake and 1200 mL would be recorded for the output during the 6 AM to 6 PM shift.

EXAMPLE 2: (with conversions): During the 6 AM to 6 PM shift, a patient consumes 1 cup of coffee and 6 oz of milk for breakfast, 2 cups of coffee and 2 oz of gelatin for lunch, and ½ cup water and 4 oz of ice cream for dinner. The patient voided four times during the shift for 240 mL, 280 mL, 480 mL, and 360 mL of urine. Calculate the I&O for this shift.

Solution using dimensional analysis method:

1 cup coffee: 1 cup = 240 mL (no conversion needed)

6 oz milk: $x\text{ mL} = \frac{30\text{ mL}}{1\text{ oz}} \times \frac{6\text{ oz}}{1} = 180\text{ mL}$

2 cups coffee: $x\text{ mL} = \frac{240\text{ mL}}{1\text{ cup}} \times \frac{2\text{ cups}}{1} = 480\text{ mL}$

2 oz gelatin: $x\text{ mL} = \frac{30\text{ mL}}{1\text{ oz}} \times \frac{2\text{ oz}}{1} = 60\text{ mL}$

½ cup water: $x\text{ mL} = \frac{240\text{ mL}}{1\text{ cup}} \times \frac{0.5\text{ cup}}{1} = 120\text{ mL}$

4 oz ice cream: $x\text{ mL} = \frac{30\text{ mL}}{1\text{ oz}} \times \frac{4\text{ oz}}{1} = 120\text{ mL}$

Solution using proportion method:

1 cup coffee	1 cup = 240 mL (no conversion needed)
6 oz milk	1 oz : 30 mL :: 6 oz : x mL x = 180 mL
2 cups coffee	1 cup : 240 mL :: 2 cups : x mL x = 480 mL
2 oz gelatin	1 oz : 30 mL :: 2 oz : x mL x = 60 mL
½ cup water	1 cup : 240 mL :: ½ cup : x mL x = 120 mL
4 oz ice cream	1 oz : 30 mL :: 4 oz : x mL x = 120 mL

Intake			**Output**
1 cup coffee	=	240 mL	240 mL
6 oz milk	=	180 mL	280 mL
2 cups coffee	=	480 mL	480 mL
2 oz gelatin	=	60 mL	360 mL
½ cup water	=	120 mL	1360 mL
4 oz ice cream	=	120 mL	
		1200 mL	

Therefore 1200 mL would be recorded for the intake and 1360 mL would be recorded for the output during the 6 AM to 6 PM shift.

EXAMPLE 3: (complex I&O): During the 6 AM to 6 PM shift, a patient has intravenous (IV) fluids of 0.9% normal saline infusing at 100 mL/h at 6 AM. After morning labs are reviewed, the IV fluids are decreased to 50 mL/h at 10 AM. The IV fluids are held for 2 hours while 1 unit of packed red blood cells (300 mL) is infused from 1 PM to 3 PM. The patient consumes 4 oz of orange juice for breakfast, 240 mL of milk for lunch, and 120 mL of coffee with dinner. At 1 PM, the patient has 200 mL of emesis. At 6 PM, the patient's Foley catheter is emptied of 1200 mL and a surgical drain is emptied of 50 mL. Calculate the I&O for this shift.

Solution using an I&O sheet:

	6-7	7-8	8-9	9-10	10-11	11-12	12-1	1-2	2-3	3-4	4-5	5-6	**Total**
Intake:													
Oral			120				240					120	480
IV	100	100	100	100	50	50	50	off	off	50	50	50	700
Blood								150	150				300
Shift Total:													**1480**
Output:													
Urine												1200	1200
Drains												50	50
Emesis								200					200
Shift Total:													**1450**

Therefore 1480 mL would be recorded for the intake and 1450 mL would be recorded for the output during the 6 AM to 6 PM shift. Note that all values entered into the I&O sheet are in milliliters.

CALCULATING PATIENT WEIGHT (FIG. 7-1)

EXAMPLE 1: 5.5 lb equals how many kilograms?

Dimensional Analysis Method

$$x \text{ kg} = \frac{1 \text{ kg}}{2.2 \text{ lb}}$$

$$x \text{ kg} = \frac{1 \text{ kg}}{2.2 \text{ lb}} \times \frac{5.5 \text{ lb}}{1}$$

$$x \text{ kg} = \frac{1 \text{ kg}}{2.2 \cancel{\text{lb}}} \times \frac{5.5 \cancel{\text{lb}}}{1} = 2.5 \text{ kg}$$

Proportion Method

1 kg : 2.2 lb : x kg : 5.5 lb

$2.2x = 5.5$

$$x = \frac{5.5}{2.2} = 2.5 \text{ kg}$$

EXAMPLE 2: 28 kg equals how many pounds?

Dimensional Analysis Method

$$x \text{ lb} = \frac{2.2 \text{ lb}}{1 \text{ kg}}$$

$$x \text{ lb} = \frac{2.2 \text{ lb}}{1 \text{ kg}} \times \frac{28 \text{ kg}}{1}$$

$$x \text{ lb} = \frac{2.2 \text{ lb}}{1 \cancel{\text{kg}}} \times \frac{28 \cancel{\text{kg}}}{1} = 61.6 \text{ lb}$$

Proportion Method

1 kg : 2.2 lb :: 28 kg : x lb

$x = 2.2 \times 28$

$x = 61.6$ lb

CALCULATING PATIENT LENGTHS (FIG. 7-2)

EXAMPLE 1: 62 inches equals how many centimeters?

Dimensional Analysis Method

$$x \text{ cm} = \frac{2.5 \text{ cm}}{1 \text{ inch}}$$

$$x \text{ cm} = \frac{2.5 \text{ cm}}{1 \text{ inch}} \times \frac{62 \text{ inches}}{1}$$

$$x \text{ cm} = \frac{2.5 \text{ cm}}{1 \cancel{\text{inch}}} \times \frac{62 \cancel{\text{inches}}}{1} = 155 \text{ cm}$$

Proportion Method

1 inch : 2.5 cm :: 62 inches : x cm

$x = 2.5 \times 62$

$x = 155$ cm

EXAMPLE 2: 10 cm equals how many inches?

Dimensional Analysis Method

$$x \text{ in} = \frac{1 \text{ inch}}{2.5 \text{ cm}}$$

$$x \text{ in} = \frac{1 \text{ inch}}{2.5 \text{ cm}} \times \frac{10 \text{ cm}}{1}$$

$$x \text{ in} = \frac{1 \text{ inch}}{2.5 \cancel{\text{cm}}} \times \frac{10 \cancel{\text{cm}}}{1} = 4 \text{ inches}$$

Proportion Method

2.5 cm : 1 inch :: 10 cm : x inches

$2.5x = 10$

$$x = \frac{10}{2.5} = 4 \text{ inches}$$

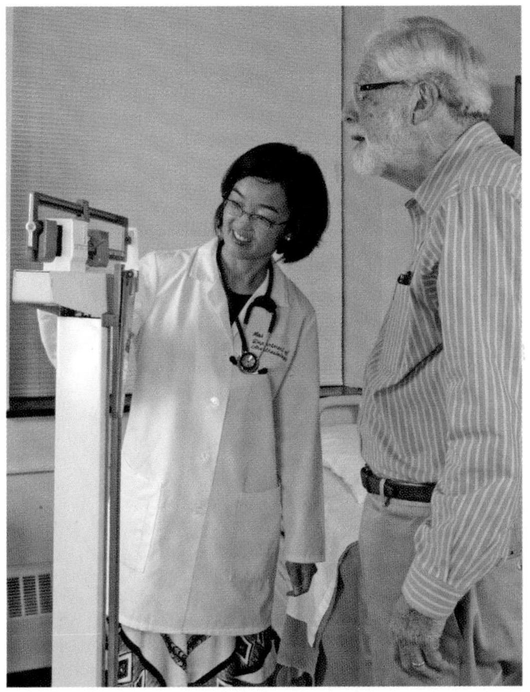

FIGURE 7-1 Weighing a patient. (From Jarvis C: *Physical examination & health assessment,* ed 7, St. Louis, 2015, Elsevier.)

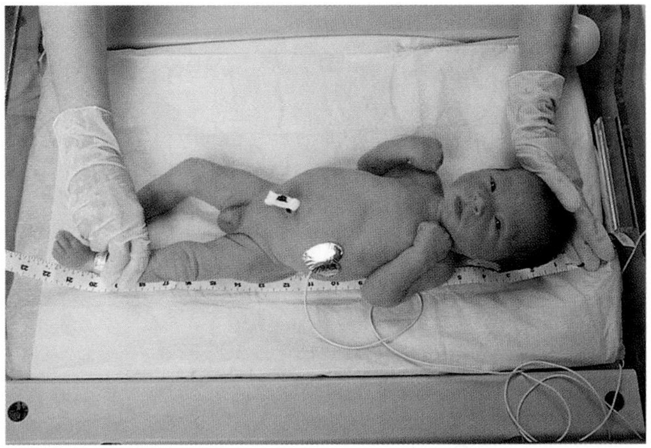

FIGURE 7-2 Measuring an infant's length. (From Potter P, Perry A, Stockert P, Hall A: *Fundamentals of nursing,* ed 9, St. Louis, 2016, Elsevier.)

APPROXIMATE EQUIVALENTS BETWEEN CELSIUS AND FAHRENHEIT MEASUREMENTS

Hospitals and health care centers use the metric system of measurement, including thermometers calibrated in the Celsius scale. It may be necessary for the nurse to convert the Celsius, or centigrade, scale to the Fahrenheit scale for patient or family information. Because not everyone concerned with patient care uses the same scale, it is also important for the nurse to be able to convert the Fahrenheit scale to the Celsius scale.

Most health care facilities now use digital thermometers rather than mercury thermometers. The following thermometers are included for illustration purposes only. Digital thermometers are available in the Fahrenheit or Celsius scale. Patients frequently ask for conversion charts at the time of discharge so that they can understand the readings if they are allowed to take their hospital thermometers home. The conversion charts are helpful for the nurse as well. However, the nurse should be able to convert from one scale to the other if necessary.

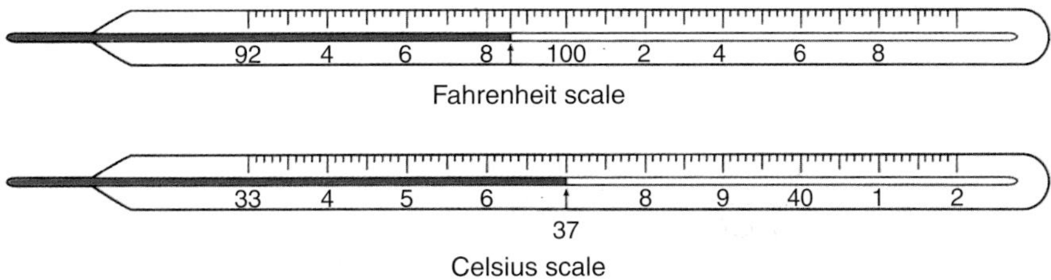

For conversion from one scale to another, the following proportion may be used:

Celsius : Fahrenheit − 32 :: 5 : 9
C : F − 32 :: 5 : 9

C or F will be the unknown.
Extend the decimal to hundredths; round to tenths.
Another means of converting Celsius and Fahrenheit temperatures to equivalents is given in Box 7-2.

BOX 7-2 CONVERTING CELSIUS AND FAHRENHEIT TEMPERATURES

Fahrenheit to Celsius	Celsius to Fahrenheit
Subtract 32	Multiply by 1.8
Divide by 1.8	Add 32

The following examples illustrate each method. (Round temperatures to nearest tenth.)

EXAMPLE 1: 100.6° F equals ______ ° C.

a. C : F − 32 :: 5 : 9
b. C : 100.6 − 32 :: 5 : 9
c. 9C = (100.6 − 32) × 5
d. 9C = 68.6 × 5
e. 9C = 343
f. $C = \frac{343}{9}$
g. C = 38.11
h. 100.6° F = 38.1° C.

a. 100.6 − 32 = 68.6
b. 68.6 ÷ 1.8 = 38.111, or 38.1° C

EXAMPLE 2: 37.6° C equals ______ ° F.

a. C : F − 32 :: 5 : 9
b. 37.6 : F − 32 :: 5 : 9
c. 5(F − 32) = 9 × 37.6
d. 5F − 160 = 338.4
e. 5F − 160 + 160 = 338.4 + 160
f. 5F = 498.4
g. $F = \frac{498.4}{5}$
h. F = 99.68
i. 37.6° C = 99.7° F.

a. 37.6 × 1.8 = 67.68
b. 67.68 + 32 = 99.68, or 99.7° F

Memorize the table of approximate equivalents (p. 135) for the household, apothecary, and metric systems of measure. Study the material on the calculations of I&O, lengths, weight, and temperature conversions. Complete the following work sheet, which provides for extensive practice. Check your answers. If you have difficulties, go back and review the necessary material. When you feel ready to evaluate your learning, take the first posttest. Check your answers. An acceptable score as indicated on the posttest signifies that you are ready for the next chapter. An unacceptable score signifies a need for further study before you take the second posttest.

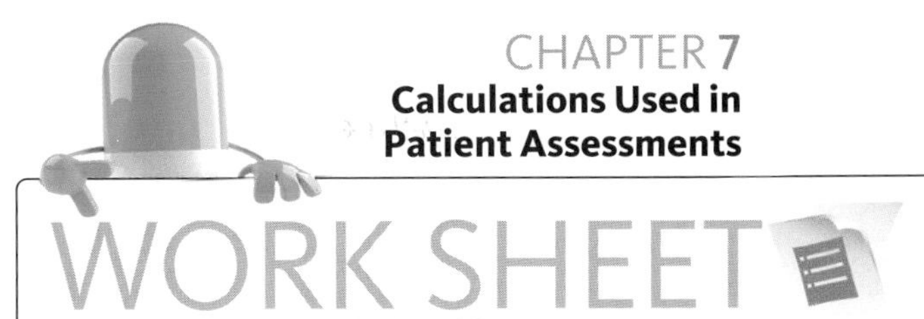

CHAPTER 7
Calculations Used in Patient Assessments

WORK SHEET

DIRECTIONS: Change to approximate equivalents as indicated. Solve the problems and show your work. Convert fractions to decimals before solving the problem.

1. 22 lb = ________ kg **2.** 3 cups = ________ mL **3.** 210 mL = ________ fl oz

4. 10 kg = ________ lb **5.** 1740 mL = ________ fl oz **6.** ½ fl oz = ________ mL

7. 4.2 inches = ________ cm **8.** 6 fl oz = ________ mL **9.** 3600 mL = ________ fl oz

10. 360 mL = ________ cups **11.** 3.3 kg = ________ lb **12.** 6 lb = ________ kg

13. 30 cm = ________ inches **14.** 5 lb = ________ kg **15.** 2400 mL = ________ cups

16. 2 cups = ________ mL **17.** 365 kg = ________ lb **18.** 4 fl oz = ________ mL

19. 12 lb = ________ g **20.** 75 lb = ________ kg **21.** 6 cups = ________ mL

22. 4500 g = ________ kg **23.** 25 kg = ________ lb **24.** 99.6° F = 37.6 ° C

25. 101.8° F = 38.8 ° C **26.** 40.4° C = 104.7 ° F **27.** 36.8° C = 98.2 ° F

28. 39.2° C = 102.6 ° F **29.** 98.4° F = 36.9 ° C **30.** 41.2° C = 106.2 ° F

31. 103.6° F = 39.8 ° C **32.** 102.2° F = 39 ° C **33.** 100.4° F = 38 ° C

34. During the 6 AM to 6 PM shift, a patient consumes 180 mL of apple juice and 120 mL of milk for breakfast, 240 mL of coffee and 120 mL of gelatin for lunch, and 120 mL of ice cream and 240 mL of tea for dinner. The patient voided four times during the shift for 340 mL, 220 mL, 440 mL, and 300 mL of urine. Calculate the I&O for this shift.

I ~ 1020
O ~ 1300

35. During the 7 AM to 7 PM shift, a patient has lactated Ringer's infusing at 125 mL/h. The patient consumed 180 mL of juice with breakfast, 120 mL of coffee and 80 mL of ice cream with lunch, and 360 mL of a soft drink with dinner. The patient also drank 8 oz of water. The patient voided 4 times during the shift for 440 mL, 280 mL, 200 mL, and 450 mL of urine. Calculate the I&O for this shift.

I ~ 2480
O ~ 1370

36. During the 6 AM to 6 PM shift, a patient consumes 2 cups of tea and 8 oz of milk for breakfast, 1 cup of coffee and 6 oz of gelatin for lunch, and ½ cup of broth and 4 oz of ice cream for dinner. The patient voided five times during the shift for 120 mL, 200 mL, 240 mL, 400 mL, and 320 mL of urine. Calculate the I&O for this shift.

I ~ 1380
O ~ 1280

37. During the 7 AM to 7 PM shift, a patient receives 4 oz of Glucerna every 3 hours followed by 2 oz of water per gastrostomy tube on an 8-11-2-5 schedule. The patient consumes 3 oz of ice pop over the shift. The chest tube drained 120 mL and the patient's indwelling urinary catheter is emptied of 1.5 L of urine at 7 PM. Calculate the I&O for this shift.

I ~ 810
O ~ 1620

38. During the 7 AM to 7 PM shift, a patient has total parenteral nutrition (TPN) infusing at 125 mL/h and IV fluids of NS infusing at 50 mL/h at 7 AM. An order is received to increase the IV fluids to 100 mL/h at 11 AM. The IV fluids are held for 2 hours while 40 mEq of potassium chloride in 150 mL of D_5W is infused from 9 AM to 11 AM. The patient consumes 4 oz of broth at 1 PM. At 7 PM, the patient's indwelling urinary catheter is emptied of 750 mL, the chest tube (CT) has drained 80 mL, and the nasogastric (NG) tube is emptied of 360 mL of gastric drainage. Calculate the I&O during this shift using the following I&O sheet.

	7-8	8-9	9-10	10-11	11-12	12-1	1-2	2-3	3-4	4-5	5-6	6-7	**Total**
Intake:													
Oral													
IV													
IV Meds													
TPN													
Shift Total:													
Output:													
Urine													
NG Tube													
CT													
Shift Total:													

39. During the 6 AM to 6 PM shift, a patient has intravenous (IV) fluids of D5 ½ NS with 20 mEq KCl infusing at 100 mL/h at 6 AM. An order is received to increase the IV fluids to 125 mL/h at 11 AM. The IV fluids are held for 2 hours while vancomycin 1 g in 250 mL of 0.9% NS is infused from 3 PM to 5 PM. The patient consumes 6 oz of broth and 3 oz of gelatin for breakfast, 240 mL of milk for lunch, and 120 mL of coffee with dinner. At 2 PM, the patient has 200 mL removed during a thoracentesis. At 6 PM, the patient's Foley catheter is emptied of 1100 mL and 150 mL is emptied from a surgical drain. Calculate the I&O for this shift using the following I&O sheet.

	6-7	7-8	8-9	9-10	10-11	11-12	12-1	1-2	2-3	3-4	4-5	5-6	**Total**
Intake:													
Oral													
IV													
IV Meds													
Shift Total:													
Output:													
Urine													
Drains													
Thora.													
Shift Total:													

ANSWERS ON PP. 156–157.

NAME ____________________

DATE ____________________

ACCEPTABLE SCORE **16**

YOUR SCORE ______

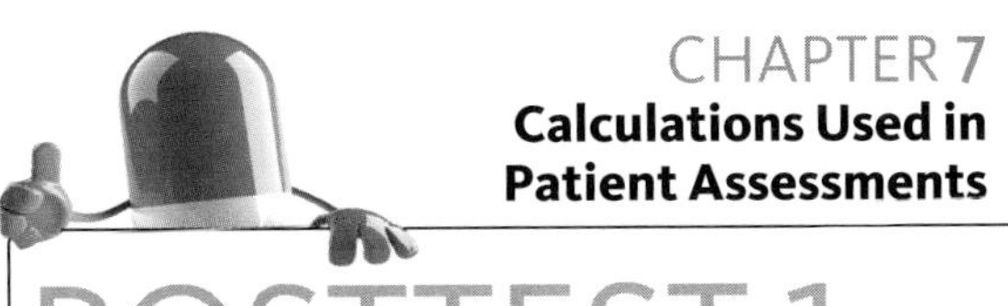

CHAPTER 7
Calculations Used in Patient Assessments

POSTTEST 1

DIRECTIONS: Change to approximate equivalents as indicated. Solve the problems and show your work. Convert fractions to decimals before solving the problem.

1. 3 fl oz = ________ mL

2. 1½ cups = ________ mL

3. 7½ lb = ________ g

4. 17 fl oz = ________ mL

5. 200 lb = ________ kg

6. 900 mL = ________ fl oz

7. 60 mL = ________ fl oz

8. 5 fl oz = ________ mL

9. 32 kg = ________ lb

10. 50 inches = ________ cm

11. 60 cm = ________ inches

12. 40.8° C = ________ ° F

13. 104.2° F = ________ ° C

14. 37.2° C = ________ ° F

15. 99.4° F = ________ ° C

16. During the 6 AM to 6 PM shift, a patient is nothing by mouth (NPO) and is receiving D5 ½ NS with 20 mEq KCl at 125 mL/h. The patient voided three times during the shift for 320 mL, 480 mL, and 320 mL of urine. Calculate the I&O for this shift.

17. During the 7 AM to 7 PM shift, a patient drinks 180 mL of cranberry juice and 240 mL of milk for breakfast, 240 mL of tea and 90 mL of gelatin for lunch, and 120 mL of ice cream and 240 mL of coffee for dinner. The patient voided 5 times during the shift for 120 mL, 240 mL, 260 mL, 340 mL, and 200 mL of urine. Calculate the I&O for this shift.

18. During the 6 AM to 6 PM shift, a patient receives 8 oz of Pulmocare every 6 hours followed by 4 oz of water per gastrostomy tube on an 8-2-8-2 schedule. The patient consumes 2 oz of ice pop one time. The patient's Foley catheter is emptied of 800 mL of urine at 6 PM. Calculate the I&O for this shift.

19. During the 7 AM to 7 PM shift, a patient drinks 4 oz of milk and 1 cup of coffee for breakfast, 1 cup of tea and 3 oz of pudding for lunch, and ¾ cup of broth and 6 oz of ice cream for dinner and 480 mL of water with medications. The patient voided 3 times during the shift for 240 mL, 400 mL, and 540 mL of urine. Calculate the I&O for this shift.

20. During the 7 AM to 7 PM shift, a patient has lactated Ringer's infusing at 75 mL/h beginning at 7 AM. At 10 AM, an order is received to increase the IV fluids to 125 mL/h. The IV fluids are held for 2 hours while potassium 20 mEq 100 mL NaCl is infused from 1 PM to 3 PM. The patient drinks 4 oz of broth and 6 oz of gelatin for breakfast, 120 mL of milk for lunch, and 240 mL of coffee with dinner. At 5 PM, the patient has 200 mL removed during a paracentesis. At 7 PM, the patient's indwelling urinary catheter is emptied of 1250 mL, and 200 mL is emptied from a surgical drain. Calculate the I&O for this shift using the following I&O sheet.

	7-8	8-9	9-10	10-11	11-12	12-1	1-2	2-3	3-4	4-5	5-6	6-7	**Total**
Intake:													
Oral													
IV													
IV Meds													
Shift Total:													
Output:													
Urine													
Drains													
Parac.													
Shift Total:													

21. During the 6 AM to 6 PM shift, a patient has total parenteral nutrition (TPN) infusing at 80 mL/h and IV fluids of normal saline (NS) infusing at 50 mL/h at 6 AM. An order is received to increase the IV fluids to 75 mL/h at 2 PM. The IV fluids are held for 2 hours while 20 mEq KCl in 50 mL of D5W is infused from 9 AM to 11 AM. The patient consumes 6 oz of ice pop at 10:30 AM. The patient has 200 mL of emesis at 2 PM. At 6 PM, the patient's Foley catheter is emptied of 900 mL, and 60 mL is emptied from a surgical drain. Calculate the I&O for this shift using the following I&O sheet.

	6-7	7-8	8-9	9-10	10-11	11-12	12-1	1-2	2-3	3-4	4-5	5-6	**Total**
Intake:													
Oral													
IV													
IV Med													
TPN													
Shift Total:													
Output:													
Urine													
Drains													
Emesis													
Shift Total:													

ANSWERS ON PP. 157–158.

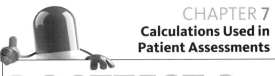

CHAPTER 7
Calculations Used in Patient Assessments

NAME ______________________

DATE ______________________

ACCEPTABLE SCORE **16**

YOUR SCORE ______

POSTTEST 2

DIRECTIONS: Change to approximate equivalents as indicated. Solve the problems and show your work. Convert fractions to decimals before solving the problem.

1. 60 lb = ________ kg

2. 2100 mL = ________ fl oz

3. 20 lb = ________ kg

4. 3.5 cups = ________ mL

5. 15 fl oz = ________ mL

6. 1200 g = ________ lb

7. 42 kg = ________ lb

8. 7 kg = ________ lb

9. 3½ lb = ________ g

10. 100 cm = ________ inches

11. 12 inches = ________ cm

12. 97.8° F = ________ ° C

13. 40.4° C = ________ ° F

14. 100.8° F = ________ ° C

15. 103.2° F = ________ ° C

16. During the 6 AM to 6 PM shift, a patient has lactated Ringer's solution (LR) infusing at 100 mL/h. The patient consumes 120 mL of juice with breakfast, 240 mL of coffee and 120 mL of ice cream with lunch, and 240 mL of milk with dinner. The patient also drank half of the water in the 900-mL water pitcher. The patient voided three times during the shift for 340 mL, 480 mL, and 540 mL of urine. Calculate the I&O for this shift

17. During the 7 AM to 7 PM shift a patient is nothing by mouth (NPO) and is receiving D5NS with 20 mEq KCl at 150 mL/h. The patient voided 4 times during the shift for 260 mL, 380 mL, 160 mL, and 320 mL of urine. Calculate the I&O for this shift.

18. During the 6 AM to 6 PM shift, a patient receives 6 oz of Glucerna every 4 hours followed by 3 oz of water per gastrostomy tube on an 8-12-4-8-12-4 schedule. The patient consumes 4 oz of ice pop over the shift. The patient's Foley catheter is emptied of 1 L of urine at 6 PM. Calculate the I&O for this shift.

19. During the 7 AM to 7 PM shift a patient receives 6 oz of Pulmocare every 6 hours followed by 3 oz of water per G-Tube on an 8-2-8-2 schedule. The patient consumes 4 oz of ice pop one time. The patient's indwelling urinary catheter is emptied of 600 mL of urine at 6 PM. Calculate the I&O for this shift.

20. During the 7 AM to 7 PM shift, a patient has intralipids 10%, 250 mL infusing over 5 hours, and continuous IV fluids of normal saline infusing at 50 mL/h. At 10 AM, an order is received to increase the IV fluids to 75 mL/h. The IV fluids are held for 1 hour while 1 g magnesium in 50 mL of D_5W is infused from 8 AM to 9 AM. The patient consumes 2 oz of ice pop at 10:30 AM. The patient has 350 mL of emesis at 1 PM. At 7 PM, the patient's indwelling urinary catheter is emptied of 820 mL, and 80 mL is emptied from a surgical drain. Calculate the I&O for this shift using the following I&O sheet.

	7-8	8-9	9-10	10-11	11-12	12-1	1-2	2-3	3-4	4-5	5-6	6-7	**Total**
Intake:													
Oral													
IV													
IV Meds													
Liquids													
Shift Total:													
Output:													
Urine													
Drains													
Emesis													
Shift Total:													

21. During the 6 AM to 6 PM shift, a patient has total parenteral nutrition (TPN) infusing at 75 mL/h and IV fluids of normal saline (NS) infusing at 100 mL/h at 6 AM. An order is received to decrease the IV fluids to 50 mL/h at 1 PM. The IV fluids are held for 1 hour while 1 g of magnesium in 50 mL of D5Q is infused from 9 AM to 10 AM. The patient consumes 8 oz of broth at 2 PM. At 6 PM, the patient's Foley catheter is emptied of 750 mL, the chest tube (CT) has drained 120 mL, and the nasogastric (NG) tube is emptied of 240 mL of gastric drainage. Calculate the I&O for this shift using the following I&O sheet.

	6-7	7-8	8-9	9-10	10-11	11-12	12-1	1-2	2-3	3-4	4-5	5-6	**Total**
Intake:													
Oral													
IV													
IV Med													
TPN													
Shift Total:													
Output:													
Urine													
NG Tube													
CT													
Shift Total:													

ANSWERS ON PP. 158–159.

evolve For additional practice problems, refer to the Conversions and Equivalents section of *Elsevier's Interactive Drug Calculation Application*, version 1.

ANSWERS

CHAPTER 7 Calculations Used in Patient Assessments—Pretest, p. 137

1. 50 kg
2. 2 cups
3. 79⅕ lb or 79.2 lb
4. 3 fl oz
5. 720 mL
6. 18 lb
7. 2.5 cups
8. 480 mL
9. 210 mL
10. 12 fl oz
11. 38.6363 or 38.6 kg
12. 45 mL
13. 37.1° C
14. 105.8° F
15. 36.4° C
16. 101.3° F
17. 8 inches
18. 125 cm

CHAPTER 7 Calculations Used in Patient Assessments—Work Sheet, pp. 145–147

1. 10 kg
2. 720 mL
3. 7 fl oz
4. 22 lb
5. 58 fl oz
6. 15 mL
7. 10.5 cm
8. 180 mL
9. 120 fl oz
10. 1.5 cups
11. 7.26, 7.3 lb
12. 2.7272 or 2.7 kg
13. 12 inches
14. 2.2727 or 2.3 kg
15. 10 cups
16. 480 mL
17. 803 lb
18. 120 mL
19. 5454.5454 or 5454.5 kg
20. 34.0909 or 34.1 kg
21. 1440 mL
22. 4.5 kg
23. 55 lb
24. 37.6° C
25. 38.8° C
26. 104.7° F
27. 98.2° F
28. 102.6° F
29. 36.9° C
30. 106.2° F
31. 39.8° C
32. 39° C
33. 38° C

34.

Intake	Output
180 mL	340 mL
120 mL	220 mL
240 mL	440 mL
120 mL	300 mL
120 mL	1300 mL
240 mL	
1020 mL	

35.

		Intake	Output
125 mL × 12 h	=	1500 mL	440 mL
	=	180 mL	280 mL
	=	120 mL	200 mL
	=	80 mL	450 mL
	=	360 mL	1370 mL
	=	240 mL	
		2480 mL	

36.

		Intake	Output
2 cups tea	=	480 mL	120 mL
8 oz milk	=	240 mL	200 mL
1 cup coffee	=	240 mL	240 mL
6 oz gelatin	=	180 mL	400 mL
½ cup broth	=	120 mL	320 mL
4 oz ice cream	=	120 mL	1280 mL
		1380 mL	

37.

		Intake	Output
4 oz Glucerna	=	120 mL	1500 mL
2 oz water	=	60 mL	120 mL
4 oz Glucerna	=	120 mL	1620 mL
2 oz water	=	60 mL	
4 oz Glucerna	=	120 mL	
2 oz water	=	60 mL	
4 oz Glucerna	=	120 mL	
2 oz water	=	60 mL	
3 oz ice pop	=	90 mL	
		810 mL	

38.

	7-8	8-9	9-10	10-11	11-12	12-1	1-2	2-3	3-4	4-5	5-6	6-7	Total
Intake:													
Oral							120						120
IV	50	50	off	off	100	100	100	100	100	100	100	100	900
IV Meds			75	75									150
TPN	125	125	125	125	125	125	125	125	125	125	125	125	1500
Shift Total:													**2670**
Output:													
Urine												750	750
NG Tube												360	360
CT												80	80
Shift Total:													**1190**

39.

	6-7	7-8	8-9	9-10	10-11	11-12	12-1	1-2	2-3	3-4	4-5	5-6	Total
Intake:													
Oral			270				240					120	630
IV	100	100	100	100	100	125	125	125	125	off	off	125	1125
IV Meds										125	125		250
Shift Total:													**2005**
Output:													
Urine												1100	1100
Drains												150	150
Thora.									200				200
Shift Total:													**1450**

CHAPTER 7 Calculations Used in Patient Assessments—Posttest 1, pp. 149–151

1. 90 mL
2. 360 mL
3. 3409.0909, 3409.1 g
4. 510 mL
5. 90.9090, 90.9 kg
6. 30 fl oz
7. 2 fl oz
8. 150 mL
9. $70\frac{2}{5}$, 70.4 lb
10. 125 cm
11. 24 inches
12. 105.4° F
13. 40.1° C
14. 99° F
15. 37.4° C

16.

Intake	Output
125 mL	320 mL
× 12 h	480 mL
1500 mL	320 mL
	1120 mL

17.

Intake	Output
180 mL	120 mL
240 mL	240 mL
240 mL	260 mL
90 mL	340 mL
120 mL	200 mL
240 mL	1160 mL
1110 mL	

ANSWERS

18.

		Intake	Output
8 oz Pulmocare	=	240 mL	800 mL
4 oz water	=	120 mL	
8 oz Pulmocare	=	240 mL	
4 oz water	=	120 mL	
2 oz ice pop	=	60 mL	
		780 mL	

19.

		Intake	Output
4 oz milk	=	120 mL	240 mL
1 cup coffee	=	240 mL	400 mL
1 cup tea	=	240 mL	540 mL
3 oz gelatin	=	90 mL	1180 mL
¾ cup broth	=	180 mL	
6 oz ice cream	=	180 mL	
Water	=	480 mL	
		1530 mL	

20.

	7-8	8-9	9-10	10-11	11-12	12-1	1-2	2-3	3-4	4-5	5-6	6-7	Total
Intake:													
Oral			300				120					240	660
IV	75	75	75	125	125	125	off	off	125	125	125	125	1100
IV Meds							50	50					100
Shift Total:													**1860**
Output:													
Urine												1250	1250
Drains												200	200
Parac.											200		200
Shift Total:													**1650**

21.

	6-7	7-8	8-9	9-10	10-11	11-12	12-1	1-2	2-3	3-4	4-5	5-6	Total
Intake:													
Oral					180								180
IV	50	50	50	off	off	50	50	50	75	75	75	75	600
IV Med				25	25								50
TPN	80	80	80	80	80	80	80	80	80	80	80	80	960
Shift Total:													**1790**
Output:													
Urine												900	900
Drains												60	60
Emesis									200				200
Shift Total:													**1160**

CHAPTER 7 Calculations Used in Patient Assessments—Posttest 2, pp. 153–155

1. 27.2727, 27.3 kg
2. 70 fl oz
3. 9.09, 9.1 kg
4. 840 mL
5. 450 mL
6. 2.64, 2.6 lb
7. 92⅖, 92.4 lb
8. 15⅖, 15.4 lb
9. 1590.909, 1590.9 g
10. 40 inches
11. 30 cm
12. 36.6° C
13. 104.7° F
14. 38.2° C
15. 39.6° C

16.

	Intake	Output
100 mL × 12 h =	1200 mL	340 mL
	120 mL	480 mL
	240 mL	540 mL
	120 mL	1360 mL
	240 mL	
	450 mL	
	2370 mL	

17.

Intake	Output
150 mL	260 mL
× 12 h	380 mL
1800 mL	160 mL
	320 mL
	1120 mL

18.

		Intake	Output
6 oz Glucerna	=	180 mL	1000 mL
3 oz water	=	90 mL	
6 oz Glucerna	=	180 mL	
3 oz water	=	90 mL	
6 oz Glucerna	=	180 mL	
3 oz water	=	90 mL	
4 oz ice pop	=	120 mL	
		930 mL	

19.

		Intake	Output
6 oz Pulmocare	=	180 mL	600 mL
3 oz water	=	90 mL	
6 oz Pulmocare	=	180 mL	
3 oz water	=	90 mL	
4 oz ice pop	=	120 mL	
		660 mL	

20.

	7-8	8-9	9-10	10-11	11-12	12-1	1-2	2-3	3-4	4-5	5-6	6-7	**Total**
Intake:													
Oral				60									60
IV	50	off	50	75	75	75	75	75	75	75	75	75	775
IV Meds		50											50
Lipids	50	50	50	50	50	off							250
Shift Total:													1135
Output:													
Urine												820	820
Drains												80	80
Emesis							350						350
Shift Total:													1250

21.

	6-7	7-8	8-9	9-10	10-11	11-12	12-1	1-2	2-3	3-4	4-5	5-6	**Total**
Intake:													
Oral									240				240
IV	100	100	100	off	100	100	100	50	50	50	50	50	850
IV Med				50									50
TPN	75	75	75	75	75	75	75	75	75	75	75	75	900
Shift Total:													2040
Output:													
Urine												750	750
NG Tube												240	240
CT												120	120
Shift Total:													1110

PART THREE

PREPARATION for CALCULATION of DRUG DOSAGES

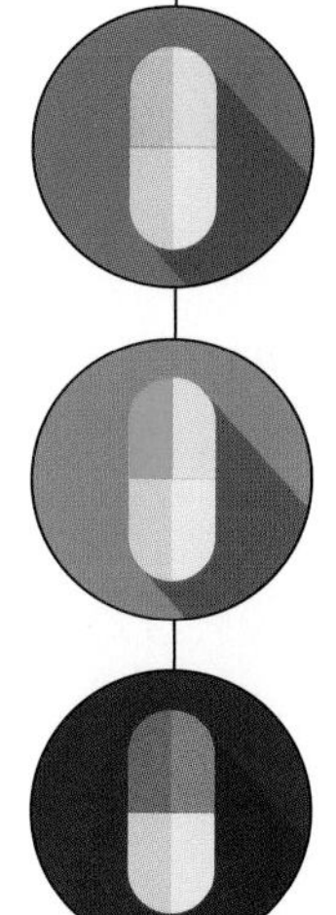

CHAPTERS

CHAPTER **8**

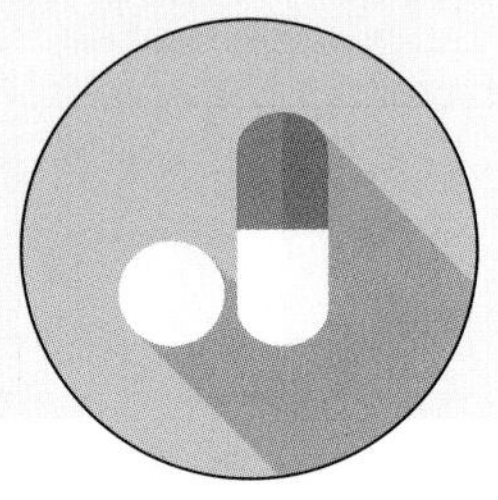

Safety in Medication Administration

LEARNING OBJECTIVES

Upon completion of the materials provided in this chapter, you will be able to:

1. Explain the fundamental need for patient safety programs
2. Describe the impact of medical errors on patient outcomes
3. Describe strategies to maintain patient and staff safety during medication administration
4. Identify the special problems and issues of the elderly population related to medication administration

The concept of safety in health care is applicable to both patient populations and health care workers. Both groups are susceptible to injury unless measures are taken that maximize prevention while minimizing the likelihood that a medical error or injury will occur. The following sections relate to both patient and personal safety.

PATIENT SAFETY

Patient safety has never been more important. It is linked directly to a health care organization's ability to attract patients, to fund services that are market competitive, and to meet the requirements for accreditation by regulatory agencies. Additionally, it is important in the delivery of high-quality patient care outcomes, which are of interest to third-party payers for reimbursement and to external agencies monitoring quality. These parties include the federal government through the Centers for Medicare & Medicaid Services (CMS), the Joint Commission, the Leapfrog Group, and some state governments. All these agencies require reporting of significant or sentinel events that result in patient harm.

The risk associated with delivery of health services to patients creates a sense of urgency in the monitoring of safety. Health care as an industry is considered at high risk in regard to its ability to deliver safe patient care. In this people-to-people business, the likelihood of errors related to medications and procedures is greater than the likelihood of a product error in the manufacturing industry. This is believed to be due to many factors that are present in the health care culture today, such as

- The fast-paced environment in which patient care activities occur
- Advanced technologies that require more attention and skills
- Possible decreases in staffing in critical positions, such as nursing and pharmacy
- A sicker and older patient population
- Declining financial resources

■ Content in this chapter was written by Ruth Anne Burris, MBA, RN, for previous editions of this text.

These factors create a more complex environment for both patients and health care workers. The potential for negative patient outcomes increases as workers become more stressed in terms of management of time, patient needs for medication and treatments, and equipment. Negative outcomes can result in

- Increases in the costs of care
- Complications that affect patients' ability to get well and go home
- Serious physical or psychological harm
- Death

How does this information relate to medication calculations and delivery? Let's examine the outcomes to two different scenarios in which a medication error has occurred. Both scenarios describe the care that was ordered by a licensed prescriber, the events that occurred, and the outcome for the patient in terms of recovery, cost, and long-term needs.

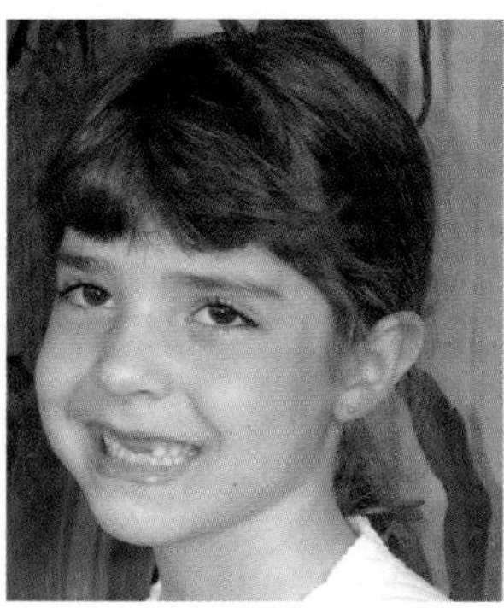

Scenario A: A 6-year-old girl has come into the hospital for suspected pyelonephritis and dehydration due to nausea and vomiting (N&V). She complains of pain in her back and side and is unable to sit or lie down comfortably. The licensed prescriber suspects a kidney stone may be present and wishes to run diagnostic tests to evaluate kidney function and to determine if there is blockage of the ureters. Tests are ordered that require a specific medication to be given before testing. The nurse assigned to this child gives the medication within the prescribed time frame before the test. However, she does not read the name of the drug correctly on the medication label (it is similar to a cardiac medication) and does not calculate the right dosage based on the child's weight. The child suffers a cardiac arrest after administration of the wrong medication at the wrong dose. The child survives but experiences severe brain damage and is determined to be mentally and physically disabled for life.

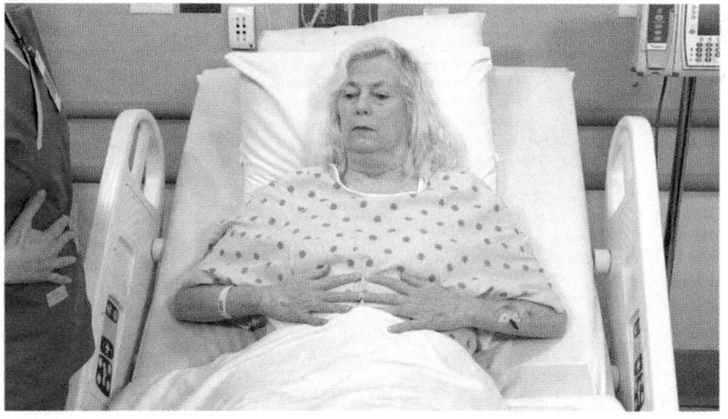

Scenario B: A 46-year-old woman is post-op following surgery. Her admission history includes a list of allergies to medications, including antibiotics. Orders are written, which include an antibiotic to reduce surgical site infection. The nurse caring for this patient receives the order but does not review the list of allergies before giving the medication. The patient has an allergic reaction that causes her to have a cardiac arrest and die.

Both of these scenarios are real-life events that have resulted in harm to a patient somewhere in the United States. There are no substitutes for attention to patient safety, because patients turn over their well-being to virtual strangers when they come into our institutions for care. With adverse drug events topping the list as the most frequently occurring type of medical error, the Joint Commission has taken a strong stance on establishing standards that address potential sources for error, especially abbreviations that are easily misread or confused in written form and drug names that sound and look alike.

Health care workers owe it to their patients to be vigilant, detail oriented, and mentally present when directing or delivering care. This is especially true when calculating or administering medications. Medications that are inaccurately dosed, inaccurately delivered, or omitted create outcomes that may cost patients the ultimate price—their lives. At the very least, these errors can affect the patient's ability to recover in a timely fashion and return to his or her life. Armed with this knowledge, each of us should begin and end our work shifts with one question in mind: Did I do all that I could from a safe practice perspective to protect my patients today?

QUALITY AND SAFETY EDUCATION FOR NURSES

The Quality and Safety Education for Nurses (QSEN) project has the goal of preparing student nurses with the knowledge, skills, and attitudes needed to improve the quality and safety of patient care. The QSEN project looks at six areas of patient care. Two of those areas are safety and informatics. *Safety* refers to reducing the risk of harm to patients and health care providers, and *informatics* refers to the technology used to mitigate errors.

METHODS TO PROMOTE SAFETY IN MEDICATION ADMINISTRATION

The reduction in medical errors is highly reliant on each individual health care provider's commitment to practicing within the scope of his or her position, observing correct safety practices, and adhering to established standards of care.

Six Rights of Medication Administration

BOX 8-1 SIX RIGHTS OF MEDICATION ADMINISTRATION

1. Drug
2. Dose
3. Patient
4. Route
5. Time
6. Documentation

Health care workers who are administering medications to patients have the legal responsibility to ensure that the right ***medication*** is delivered to the right ***patient*** in the right ***dose*** and right ***route*** at the right ***time***. Right ***documentation*** in the patient's medical record is the sixth right (Box 8-1). The health care provider performs "three checks" to ensure the first five rights are met by comparing the medication package to the medication administration record (MAR) three times (Figure 8-1). One way to ensure right documentation is an electronic MAR (eMAR), through which the medications appear on a computer screen. When the drug is scanned using the eMAR system, documentation of drug administration is complete (Figure 8-2).

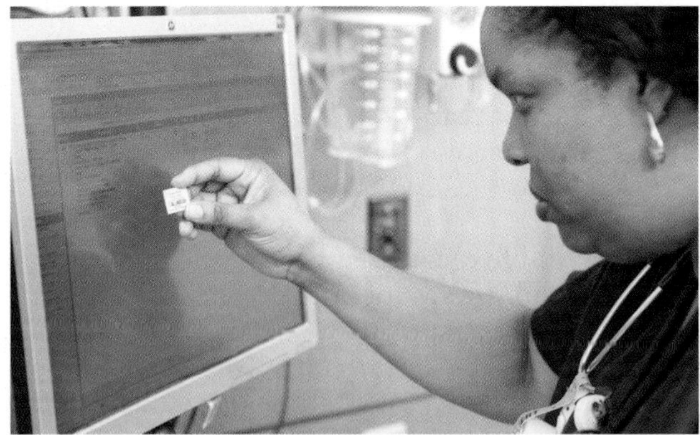

FIGURE 8-1 A nurse comparing the drug package information with the *e*MAR. (From Perry AG, Potter PA, Ostendorf WR: *Nursing interventions & clinical skills,* ed. 6, St. Louis, 2016, Elsevier.)

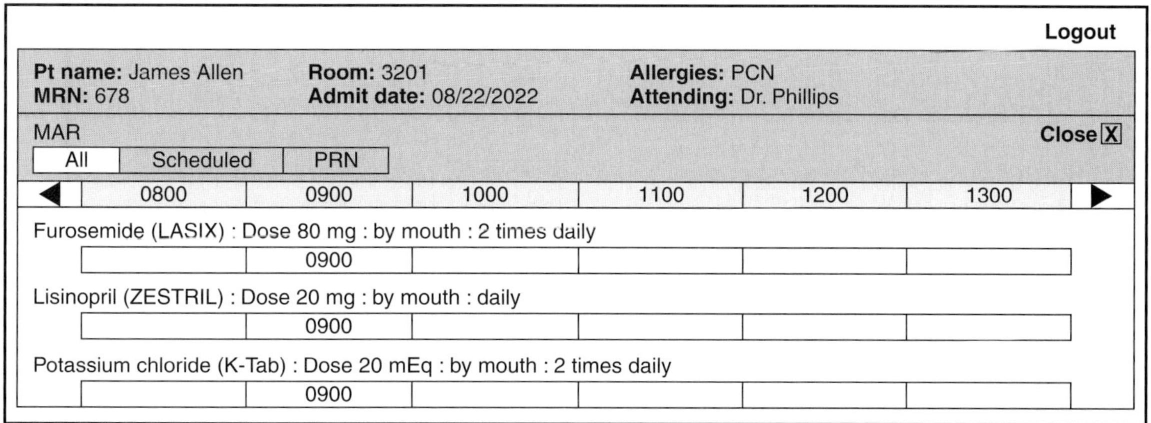

FIGURE 8-2 An example of an electronic medication administration record (eMar) that would appear on the computer screen.

Knowledge

A thorough knowledge of the patient's medical history, including drug allergies and medications the patient has previously taken, is necessary to safeguard against medication interactions and anaphylactic reactions. It is also important for the health care provider to have knowledge of every medication's intended action, how it is to be safely delivered, and the potential effects (both therapeutic and side effects) it can have on the patient.

"Do Not Use" Abbreviations

Health care providers involved in medication administration need to be aware of "do not use" abbreviations that can increase the potential for medication errors. The Joint Commission's "Do Not Use" list is shown in Table 8-1. Another resource, the Institute for Safe Medication Practices (ISMP), has a website (www.ismp.org) dedicated to education, awareness, and tools for prevention of medication errors (Figure 8-3).

TABLE 8-1 THE JOINT COMMISSION'S OFFICIAL "DO NOT USE" ABBREVIATIONS LIST[1]

Do Not Use	*Potential Problem*	Use Instead
U, u (unit)	Mistaken for "0" (zero), the number "4" (four) or "cc"	Write "unit"
IU (International Unit)	Mistaken for IV (intravenous) or the number 10 (ten)	Write "International Unit"
Q.D., QD, q.d., qd (daily)	Mistaken for each other	Write "daily"
Q.O.D., QOD, q.o.d, qod (every other day)	Period after the Q mistaken for "I" and the "O" mistaken for "I"	Write "every other day"
Trailing zero (X.0 mg)*	Decimal point is missed	Write X mg
Lack of leading zero (.X mg)		Write 0.X mg
MS	Can mean morphine sulfate or magnesium sulfate	Write "morphine sulfate" Write "magnesium sulfate"
MSO_4 and $MgSO_4$	Confused for one another	

[1] Applies to all orders and all medication-related documentation that is handwritten (including free-text computer entry) or on pre-printed forms.

***Exception:** A "trailing zero" may be used only where required to demonstrate the level of precision of the value being reported, such as for laboratory results, imaging studies that report size of lesions, or catheter/tube sizes. It may not be used in medication orders or other medication-related documentation.

Institute for Safe Medication Practices

ISMP's List of *Error-Prone Abbreviations, Symbols,* and *Dose Designations*

The abbreviations, symbols, and dose designations found in this table have been reported to ISMP through the ISMP National Medication Errors Reporting Program (ISMP MERP) as being frequently misinterpreted and involved in harmful medication errors. They should **NEVER** be used when communicating medical information. This includes internal communications, telephone/verbal prescriptions, computer-generated labels, labels for drug storage bins, medication administration records, as well as pharmacy and prescriber computer order entry screens.

Abbreviations	Intended Meaning	Misinterpretation	Correction
µg	Microgram	Mistaken as "mg"	Use "mcg"
AD, AS, AU	Right ear, left ear, each ear	Mistaken as OD, OS, OU (right eye, left eye, each eye)	Use "right ear," "left ear," or "each ear"
OD, OS, OU	Right eye, left eye, each eye	Mistaken as AD, AS, AU (right ear, left ear, each ear)	Use "right eye," "left eye," or "each eye"
BT	Bedtime	Mistaken as "BID" (twice daily)	Use "bedtime"
cc	Cubic centimeters	Mistaken as "u" (units)	Use "mL"
D/C	Discharge or discontinue	Premature discontinuation of medications if D/C (intended to mean "discharge") has been misinterpreted as "discontinued" when followed by a list of discharge medications	Use "discharge" and "discontinue"
IJ	Injection	Mistaken as "IV" or "intrajugular"	Use "injection"
IN	Intranasal	Mistaken as "IM" or "IV"	Use "intranasal" or "NAS"
HS **hs**	Half-strength At bedtime, hours of sleep	Mistaken as bedtime Mistaken as half-strength	Use "half-strength" or "bedtime"
IU**	International unit	Mistaken as IV (intravenous) or 10 (ten)	Use "units"
o.d. or OD	Once daily	Mistaken as "right eye" (OD-oculus dexter), leading to oral liquid medications administered in the eye	Use "daily"
OJ	Orange juice	Mistaken as OD or OS (right or left eye); drugs meant to be diluted in orange juice may be given in the eye	Use "orange juice"
Per os	By mouth, orally	The "os" can be mistaken as "left eye" (OS-oculus sinister)	Use "PO," "by mouth," or "orally"
q.d. or QD**	Every day	Mistaken as q.i.d., especially if the period after the "q" or the tail of the "q" is misunderstood as an "i"	Use "daily"
qhs	Nightly at bedtime	Mistaken as "qhr" or every hour	Use "nightly"
qn	Nightly or at bedtime	Mistaken as "qh" (every hour)	Use "nightly" or "at bedtime"
q.o.d. or QOD**	Every other day	Mistaken as "q.d." (daily) or "q.i.d. (four times daily) if the "o" is poorly written	Use "every other day"
q1d	Daily	Mistaken as q.i.d. (four times daily)	Use "daily"
q6PM, etc.	Every evening at 6 PM	Mistaken as every 6 hours	Use "daily at 6 PM" or "6 PM daily"
SC, SQ, sub q	Subcutaneous	SC mistaken as SL (sublingual); SQ mistaken as "5 every;" the "q" in "sub q" has been mistaken as "every" (e.g., a heparin dose ordered "sub q 2 hours before surgery" misunderstood as every 2 hours before surgery)	Use "subcut" or "subcutaneously"
ss	Sliding scale (insulin) or ½ (apothecary)	Mistaken as "55"	Spell out "sliding scale;" use "one-half" or "½"
SSRI **SSI**	Sliding scale regular insulin Sliding scale insulin	Mistaken as selective-serotonin reuptake inhibitor Mistaken as Strong Solution of Iodine (Lugol's)	Spell out "sliding scale (insulin)"
i/d	One daily	Mistaken as "tid"	Use "1 daily"
TIW or tiw	3 times a week	Mistaken as "3 times a day" or "twice in a week"	Use "3 times weekly"
U or u**	Unit	Mistaken as the number 0 or 4, causing a 10-fold overdose or greater (e.g., 4U seen as "40" or 4u seen as "44"); mistaken as "cc" so dose given in volume instead of units (e.g., 4u seen as 4cc)	Use "unit"
UD	As directed ("ut dictum")	Mistaken as unit dose (e.g., diltiazem 125 mg IV infusion "UD" misinterpreted as meaning to give the entire infusion as a unit [bolus] dose)	Use "as directed"
Dose Designations and Other Information	**Intended Meaning**	**Misinterpretation**	**Correction**
Trailing zero after decimal point (e.g., 1.0 mg)**	1 mg	Mistaken as 10 mg if the decimal point is not seen	Do not use trailing zeros for doses expressed in whole numbers
"Naked" decimal point (e.g., .5 mg)**	0.5 mg	Mistaken as 5 mg if the decimal point is not seen	Use zero before a decimal point when the dose is less than a whole unit
Abbreviations such as mg. or mL. with a period following the abbreviation	mg mL	The period is unnecessary and could be mistaken as the number 1 if written poorly	Use mg, mL, etc. without a terminal period

FIGURE 8-3 ISMP's list of error-prone abbreviations, symbols, and dose designations. (© ISMP 2013. Reprinted with permission.)

ISMP's List of *Error-Prone Abbreviations, Symbols,* and *Dose Designations* (continued)

Dose Designations and Other Information	Intended Meaning	Misinterpretation	Correction
Drug name and dose run together (especially problematic for drug names that end in "l" such as Inderal40 mg; Tegretol300 mg)	Inderal 40 mg Tegretol 300 mg	Mistaken as Inderal 140 mg Mistaken as Tegretol 1300 mg	Place adequate space between the drug name, dose, and unit of measure
Numerical dose and unit of measure run together (e.g., 10mg, 100mL)	10 mg 100 mL	The "m" is sometimes mistaken as a zero or two zeros, risking a 10- to 100-fold overdose	Place adequate space between the dose and unit of measure
Large doses without properly placed commas (e.g., 100000 units; 1000000 units)	100,000 units 1,000,000 units	100000 has been mistaken as 10,000 or 1,000,000; 1000000 has been mistaken as 100,000	Use commas for dosing units at or above 1,000, or use words such as 100 "thousand" or 1 "million" to improve readability
Drug Name Abbreviations	**Intended Meaning**	**Misinterpretation**	**Correction**
To avoid confusion, do not abbreviate drug names when communicating medical information. Examples of drug name abbreviations involved in medication errors include:			
APAP	acetaminophen	Not recognized as acetaminophen	Use complete drug name
ARA A	vidarabine	Mistaken as cytarabine (ARA C)	Use complete drug name
AZT	zidovudine (Retrovir)	Mistaken as azathioprine or aztreonam	Use complete drug name
CPZ	Compazine (prochlorperazine)	Mistaken as chlorpromazine	Use complete drug name
DPT	Demerol-Phenergan-Thorazine	Mistaken as diphtheria-pertussis-tetanus (vaccine)	Use complete drug name
DTO	Diluted tincture of opium, or deodorized tincture of opium (Paregoric)	Mistaken as tincture of opium	Use complete drug name
HCl	hydrochloric acid or hydrochloride	Mistaken as potassium chloride (The "H" is misinterpreted as "K")	Use complete drug name unless expressed as a salt of a drug
HCT	hydrocortisone	Mistaken as hydrochlorothiazide	Use complete drug name
HCTZ	hydrochlorothiazide	Mistaken as hydrocortisone (seen as HCT250 mg)	Use complete drug name
MgSO4**	magnesium sulfate	Mistaken as morphine sulfate	Use complete drug name
MS, MSO4**	morphine sulfate	Mistaken as magnesium sulfate	Use complete drug name
MTX	methotrexate	Mistaken as mitoxantrone	Use complete drug name
PCA	procainamide	Mistaken as patient controlled analgesia	Use complete drug name
PTU	propylthiouracil	Mistaken as mercaptopurine	Use complete drug name
T3	Tylenol with codeine No. 3	Mistaken as liothyronine	Use complete drug name
TAC	triamcinolone	Mistaken as tetracaine, Adrenalin, cocaine	Use complete drug name
TNK	TNKase	Mistaken as "TPA"	Use complete drug name
ZnSO4	zinc sulfate	Mistaken as morphine sulfate	Use complete drug name
Stemmed Drug Names	**Intended Meaning**	**Misinterpretation**	**Correction**
"Nitro" drip	nitroglycerin infusion	Mistaken as sodium nitroprusside infusion	Use complete drug name
"Norflox"	norfloxacin	Mistaken as Norflex	Use complete drug name
"IV Vanc"	intravenous vancomycin	Mistaken as Invanz	Use complete drug name
Symbols	**Intended Meaning**	**Misinterpretation**	**Correction**
ʒ ♏	Dram Minim	Symbol for dram mistaken as "3" Symbol for minim mistaken as "mL"	Use the metric system
x3d	For three days	Mistaken as "3 doses"	Use "for three days"
> and <	Greater than and less than	Mistaken as opposite of intended; mistakenly use incorrect symbol; "< 10" mistaken as "40"	Use "greater than" or "less than"
/ (slash mark)	Separates two doses or indicates "per"	Mistaken as the number 1 (e.g., "25 units/10 units" misread as "25 units and 110" units)	Use "per" rather than a slash mark to separate doses
@	At	Mistaken as "2"	Use "at"
&	And	Mistaken as "2"	Use "and"
+	Plus or and	Mistaken as "4"	Use "and"
°	Hour	Mistaken as a zero (e.g., q2° seen as q 20)	Use "hr," "h," or "hour"
Φ or ø	zero, null sign	Mistaken as numerals 4, 6, 8, and 9	Use 0 or zero, or describe intent using whole words

**These abbreviations are included on The Joint Commission's "minimum list" of dangerous abbreviations, acronyms, and symbols that must be included on an organization's "Do Not Use" list, effective January 1, 2004. Visit www.jointcommission.org for more information about this Joint Commission requirement.

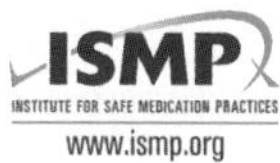

FIGURE 8-3—CONT'D ISMP's list of error-prone abbreviations, symbols, and dose designations. (© ISMP 2013. Reprinted with permission.)

Look-alike/Sound-alike Medications

Health care providers involved in medication administration also need to be aware of look-alike/sound-alike medication names that can increase the potential for medication errors. An example is dopamine and dobutamine. Both medications look alike and sound alike but have very different actions. Using the *Tall Man Letters* can reduce errors for look-alike and sound-alike medications. The Tall Man Lettering system differentiates the drugs by capitalizing the letters that are different. For example: DOPamine and DOBUTamine. See the ISMP website, www.ismp.org/tools/tallmanletters.pdf, for more examples of *Tall Man Letters*.

Electronic IV Pumps

The use of electronic intravenous (IV) pumps assists with the safe administration of IV fluids and medications. Many devices come with the capability of drug calculation and safeguard parameters (Figure 8-4).

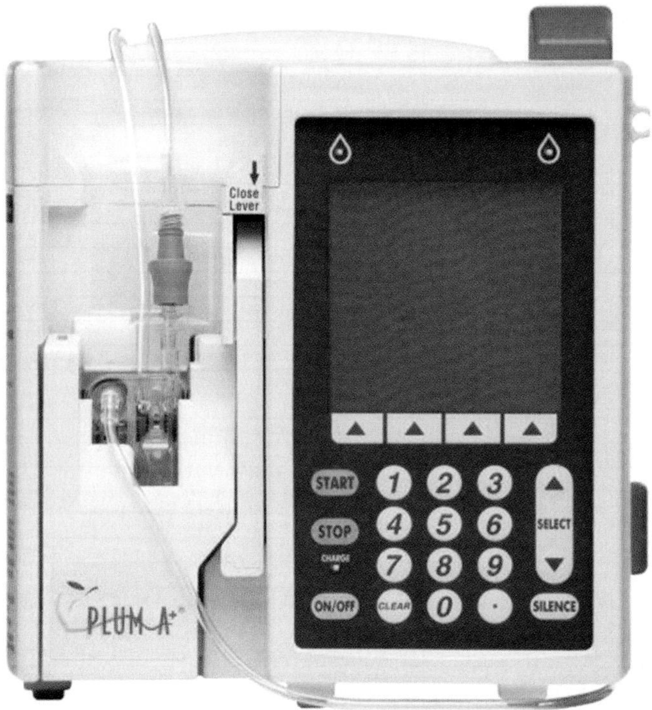

FIGURE 8-4 Plum A+ ® Drug infusion pump and confirmation screen. (From Hospira, Inc., Lake Forest, IL.)

Personal Safety

The use of personal protective equipment (PPE) such as gloves, goggles, and gowns can protect a health care provider from a hazardous substance, such as a medication that may be toxic or damaging to the eyes, mucous membranes, or skin (Figure 8-5). The use of safety devices during the administration of injectable medications or when starting IV lines minimizes the likelihood of an injury from a contaminated needle (Figure 8-6). Practice standards—including the proper use and disposal of medications, their containers (especially glass), and delivery devices into specified containers such as needle boxes—provide a level of safety if stringent adherence is the normal pattern of practice (Figure 8-7).

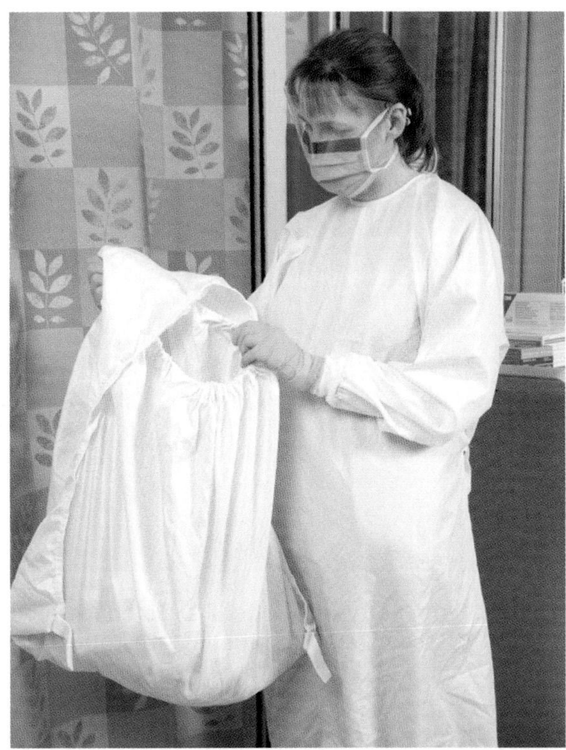

FIGURE 8-5 Health care provider wearing gown, gloves, mask and goggles for personal safety. (From Perry AG, Potter PA, Ostendorf WR: *Nursing interventions and clinical skills*, ed 6, St Louis, 2016, Elsevier.)

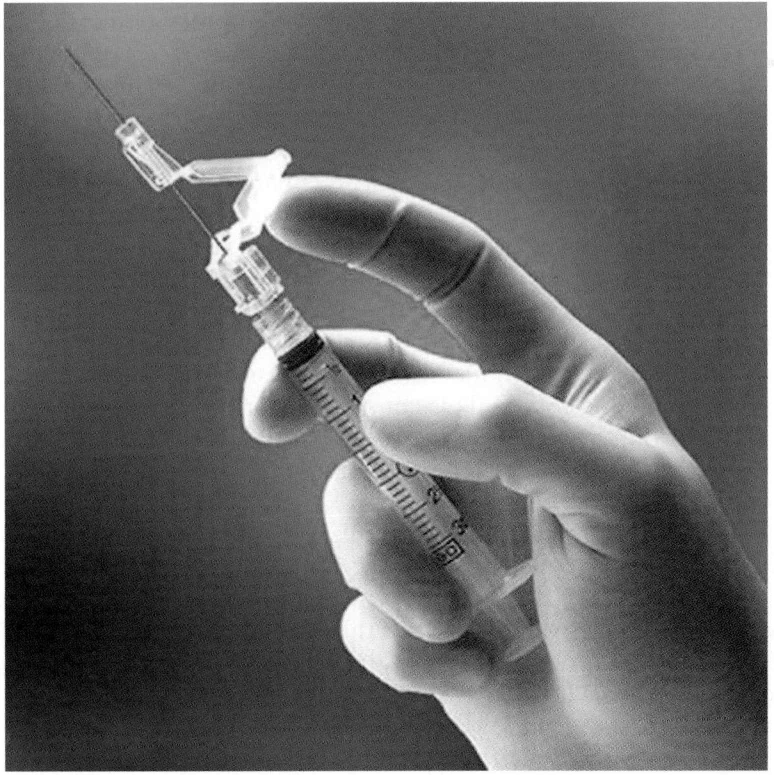

FIGURE 8-6 Safety syringe with needle guard. (From Becton, Dickinson, and Company, Franklin Lakes, NJ.)

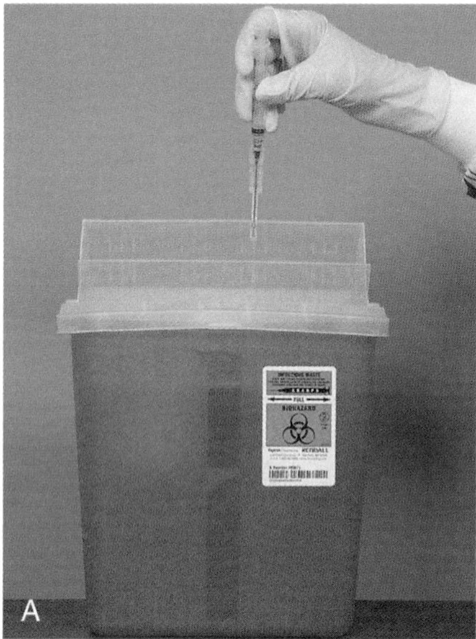
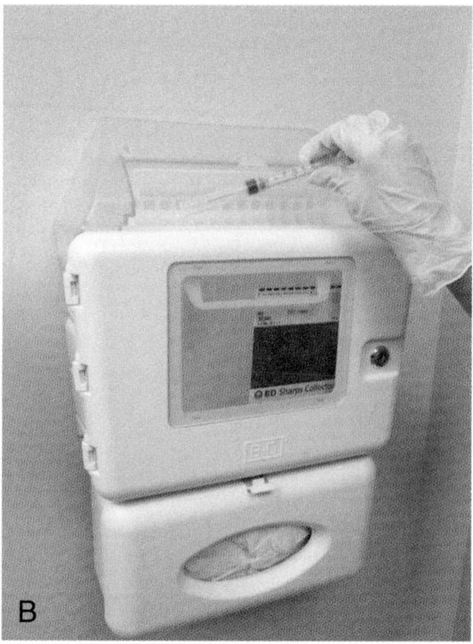

FIGURE 8-7 Safety containers. (**A,** From Perry AG, Potter PA, Ostendorf WR: *Nursing interventions and clinical skills,* ed 6, St Louis, 2016, Elsevier. **B,** From Potter AG, Potter PA, Stockert PA, Hall AM: *Fundamentals in nursing,* ed 9, St. Louis, 2017; Elsevier.)

AUTOMATED MEDICATION DISPENSING SYSTEMS

Health care delivery systems continue to strive to improve the accuracy and efficiency of the delivery of medications to patients. Each patient care unit is provided with a special cabinet that houses the medications that will be dispensed from that unit. The medications in the machine are usually listed by both their trade and generic names. This feature helps expedite location of the medications by the nurse. These cabinets are connected to the central pharmacy for order verifications and accuracy, as well as for automation of usage reports that are provided for many facets of the medication process.

An automated medication dispensing system leads to a reduction in medication errors. This is especially true as vendors market new options that allow only the designated drawer housing the medication that is being given at that time to open.

The automated medication dispensing system also enhances patient satisfaction. With an automated system, the nurse is able to access the medication from the cabinet and confirm the accuracy of the controlled substance count immediately. The medication may then be given to the patient in a timely manner. All these systems are password secured. Each nurse has a password or ID number. Some systems also use biometric fingerprint scanning. Continuous documentation occurs while the cabinet is in use.

Another advantage of an automated medication dispensing system is reduction in the time required for end-of-shift narcotic counts. This count is performed by two nurses, usually one from the ending shift and one from the starting shift. It is also standard practice that until the narcotic count is completed and correct, all staff who are ending their shift may not leave. This results in staff dissatisfaction and unnecessary overtime costs that can be better spent on actual patient care. This scenario is prevented because automated systems require the confirmation of the count of controlled substance medications after each withdrawal.

To aid in the six rights of medication administration, many facilities are transitioning to a system that allows the licensed prescriber to enter the orders for the patient. Also, medication storage/delivery systems allow bar code scanning, in which the nurse scans a bar code on the patient's armband and on the medication package (Figure 8-8).

Some systems currently on the market interface with the health care system's program for charting medications. With some dispensing systems, charting is done at the cabinet in the unit, whereas other manufacturers are designing programs to document the administration of medication at the bedside. With the automated documentation of the administration of the patient's medications, the nurse is not required to return to the paper medication administration record and manually chart that the medicine has been given.

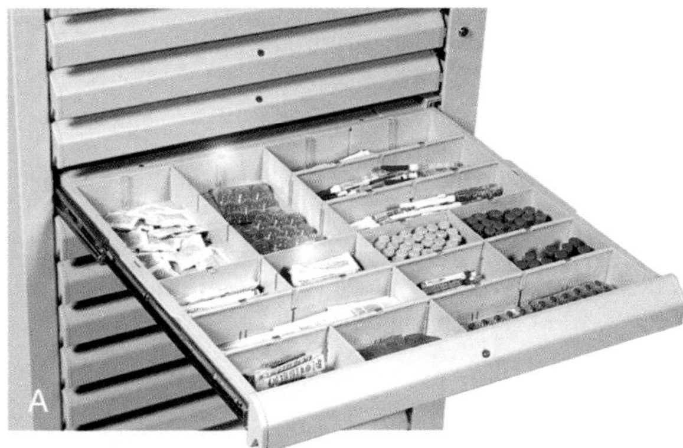

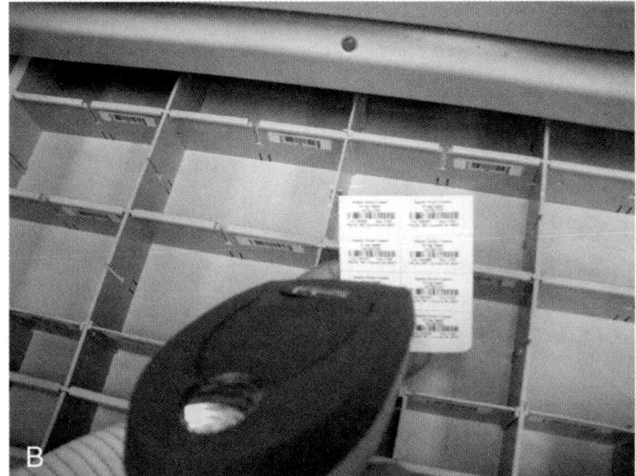

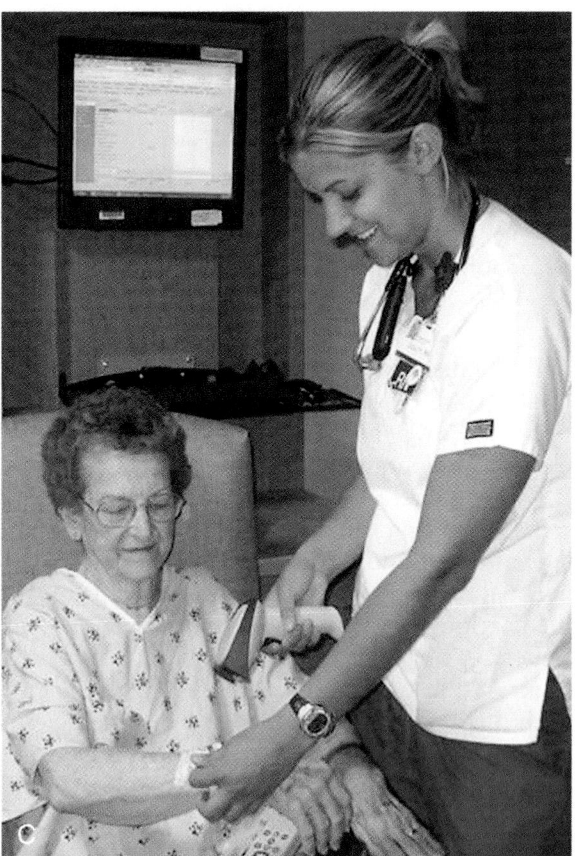

FIGURE 8-8 **A,** Example of a medication drawer from the Omnicell medication storage/delivery system. **B,** Bar code scanning of the medication package. **C,** Bar code scanning of the patient's armband. (**A** and **B** Images courtesy of Omnicell, Inc., Mountain View, CA. **C** from Potter PA, Perry AG, Stockert P, Hall A: *Fundamentals of nursing*, ed 9, St Louis, 2017, Elsevier.)

There are some disadvantages to the automated dispensing systems. Because some of the drawers have open compartments, it is possible for the wrong medication to be placed in the drawer. This makes the three medicine checks the nurse performs when he or she prepares a patient's medicines absolutely paramount. Technology is *not* perfect, and mistakes can and do occur in the delivery of medication. The pharmacy, as the cabinet is being restocked, or another nurse may have mishandled the medications while searching the drawers. If the machine houses all the patient medications, lines may form when several nurses need to obtain patient medications at the same time. The nurse needs to be well organized and plan ahead for access to the cabinet.

As health care facilities continue to monitor costs and at the same time strive to improve patient and staff satisfaction, the use of automated medication dispensing systems will become more widespread. This is an area in which nursing students will need to become knowledgeable and competent because the accurate and efficient delivery of medications is one of the most important tasks of patient care that the nurse is required to perform.

MINIMIZING MEDICATION ERRORS FOR OLDER ADULTS

Older adults at home are more prone to medication errors than those in health care facilities. The most common error is omission, often relating to the cost of the medication or the person's forgetfulness. Other medication errors involve the incorrect dosage, wrong administration time, or a misunderstanding of directions.

A decrease in gross and fine motor skills may affect how well a patient can handle the packaging of medications. For example, arthritis may make it difficult for a patient with Type 1

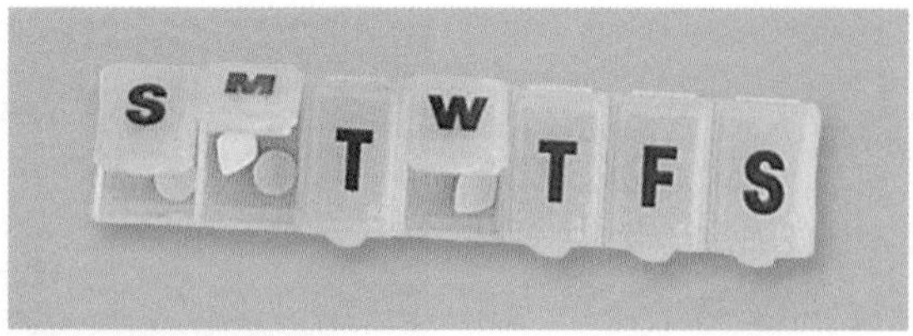

FIGURE 8-9 Example of a container that holds medications for a week. (From Perry AG, Potter PA, Ostendorf WR: *Nursing interventions and clinical skills,* ed 6, St Louis, 2016, Elsevier.)

diabetes mellitus to draw up and self-administer the correct dose of insulin. If the patient is unable to self-administer, then a family member, friend, or caretaker will need to be taught the procedure. When purchasing medications from a pharmacy, older adults should request that childproof containers *not* be used.

It is important for the nurse to make certain that older adult patients understand the directions for taking their medications safely. Many older adults are hearing impaired to some degree. The nurse should ask the patient to verbally repeat the instructions. Older adults may also have a visual impairment. It is necessary to make sure that older patients can read the labels of their medications and that any written directions are printed in a large, easy-to-read format. Containers or pill organizers are available to prepare medications for a day or a week at a time (see Figure 8-9). An appointment book with the day and date, a spiral notebook, or a writing tablet with the day and date added can be an efficient and safe way to plan medications taken in the home. The medications and the times they are to be taken each day are listed. The entry is crossed off after the medication has been taken (Box 8-2).

BOX 8-2 MEDICATION SHEET EXAMPLE

Thursday, March 25
Motrin 300 mg after each meal
~~8:00~~ AM 1:00 PM 6:00 PM
Naprosyn 250 mg two times a day
~~8:00~~ AM 4:00 PM
Persantin 25 mg two times a day
10:00 AM 6:00 PM
Lasix 40 mg daily
10:00 AM
Mylanta 2 tablespoons after meals

Medication errors among older adults can be reduced if time is taken to explain the reason for the medication, its importance, and how it works. This is especially important if timing is crucial in maintaining a therapeutic blood level of the medication.

The health care worker should also assess the person's alcohol use because alcohol is one of the most abused drugs in the older adult population. The combination of alcohol and certain medications may be a problem with the occasional or chronic drinker.

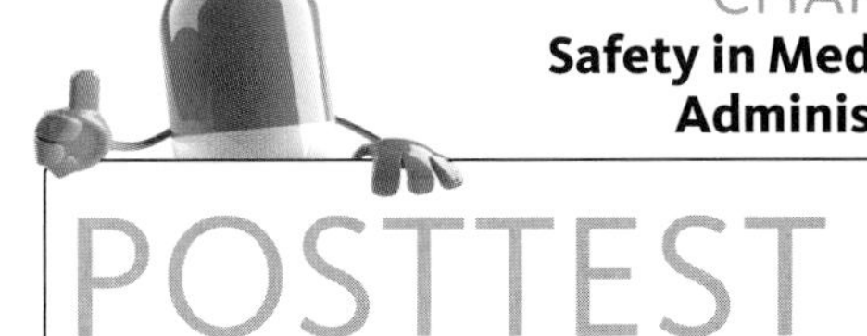

NAME ______________________

DATE ______________________

ACCEPTABLE SCORE **8**

YOUR SCORE ______

POSTTEST

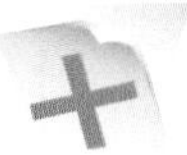

DIRECTIONS: Answer the following questions.

1. A nurse checking a patient's medication record notices a change in the dose and route for a medication given earlier in the day. What would be the appropriate action by the nurse?
   a. Administer the medication as it appears on the medication record.
   b. Check for new orders by the licensed prescriber.
   c. Change the medication record back to the dose and route that was administered with the morning dose.
   d. Ask the patient to verify the change in the order.
2. While the nurse is administering morning medications, the patient asks, "What is the pill for?" When the nurse explains the pill is for high cholesterol, the patient responds, "I have never had a problem with high cholesterol." What is the appropriate action by the nurse?
   a. Encourage the patient to take the medication.
   b. Leave a note in the patient's chart for the licensed prescriber.
   c. Repeat the three checks for the medication.
   d. Review the original order for the medication.
3. Which of the following are examples of using technology for safe medication administration? (Select all that apply.)
   a. Electronic medication administration record (eMAR).
   b. Scanning procedures of the medication package and patient armband.
   c. Safeguard parameters on the IV pump.
   d. Automated medication dispensing machines.
4. Which of the following is an example of an appropriate order?
   a. Furosemide 40 mg by mouth qd
   b. Furosemide 40 mg by mouth Q.D.
   c. Furosemide 40 mg by mouth daily
   d. Furosemide 40 mg by mouth QD
5. The nurse needs to administer a medication that can be toxic to the skin and mucous membranes. Which of the following PPE would be appropriate for the nurse to don? (Select all that apply.)
   a. Gown
   b. Gloves
   c. Mask
   d. Goggles
   e. Shoe protectors
6. Which of the following are actions in verifying the "right patient" before medication administration? (Select all that apply.)
   a. Ask the patient to state his or her name and date of birth.
   b. Scan the bar code on the patient's armband.
   c. Compare the patient's name with the eMAR.
   d. Skip this step if the patient is asleep.
7. The nurse is preparing DULoxetine. How do the capital letters "DUL" assist the nurse in safe medication administration?
   a. They help in alphabetizing the medications in the automated medication dispensing machine.
   b. They alert the nurse of a sound-alike/look-alike medication.
   c. They are the initials for the medication classification.
   d. They are the letters that start both the generic and trade name for the medication.
8. A dosage calculation answer is 5.02 mcg with directions to round to the nearest tenth place. How would the final answer be documented? ____________ mcg

ANSWERS ON P. 174.

ANSWERS

CHAPTER 8 Safety in Medication Administration—Posttest, p. 173

1. b
2. d
3. a, b, c, d
4. c
5. a, b, c, d
6. a, b, c
7. b
8. 5

CHAPTER 9

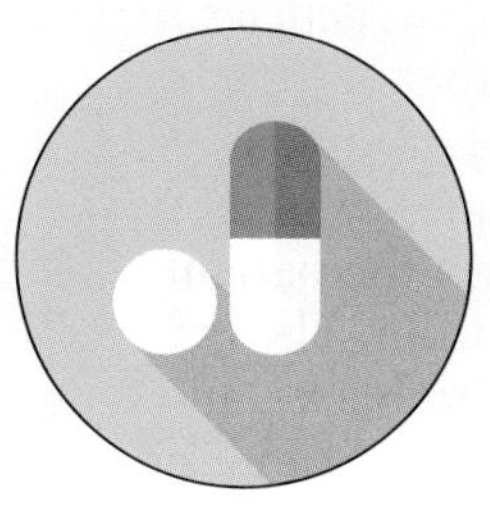

Interpretation of the Licensed Prescriber's Orders

LEARNING OBJECTIVES

Upon completion of the materials provided in this chapter, you will be able to:

1. Discuss electronic health records
2. Successfully complete a patient's medication administration record (MAR) based on a licensed prescriber's order
3. Convert from 24-hour clock time to AM-PM time
4. Identify the five components of an MAR
5. Demonstrate proper documentation on the MAR

Administration of medications is one of the nurse's most important responsibilities. For medications to be administered safely and effectively, the nurse must know how to interpret the licensed prescriber's medication orders.

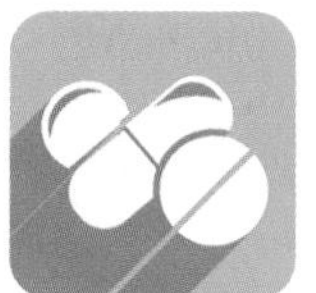

ORDERS

In hospitals and other health care centers, a licensed prescriber orders medications and makes other orders for a patient using either an electronic health care record (EHR) or a handwritten form. Advantages to the EHR is that the computer automatically records some of the needed information (the date of the original order and the prescriber's name) and uses terminology that meets safety guidelines for medication administration. Both the EHR and handwritten methods are shown in this chapter. Regardless of the system, the basic rules for orders apply to both EHRs and handwritten orders. When a medication is prescribed for a patient, the order must contain the following information to be considered complete:

- The date the medication was prescribed
- Name of the medication
- Dose of the medication
- Route of administration
- Frequency of administration
- Special instructions
- Purpose for administration when the medication is ordered as needed (prn)
- Length of time the patient is to receive the medication

To interpret electronic orders (Figure 9-1, *A*) and handwritten orders (Figure 9-2, *A*), the nurse must know the terminology, abbreviations, and symbols used in writing orders for medications. A list of the most frequently used abbreviations relating to medications can be found in Table 9-2. Memorize this list; also refer to the Glossary for help with unfamiliar terms.

The nurse should always be knowledgeable about the laws governing practice in his or her state and facility. In all institutions, nurses should have access to the most current listing of individuals credentialed for prescriptive authority.

VERBAL ORDERS

Although verbal orders are discouraged as routine policy, certain situations or emergencies may require telephone orders. Such orders are generally initiated by the nurse. Whether electronic or handwritten, the order must include the same information as the written order: the date and time the order is recorded, the name and dosage of the drug, the route and frequency of administration, and any special instructions. After the nurse has recorded the orders on the patient's health record, the orders must be repeated to the licensed prescriber for verification. The licensed prescriber's name, a notation that this is a verbal order (VORB, verbal order read back), and the nurse's signature are required. The licensed prescriber should sign handwritten notes or electronically verify the verbal orders as soon as possible. The nurse should follow his or her institution's policy.

HANDWRITTEN EXAMPLE:	1/18/22 1400	Morphine sulfate 8 mg IM q4 h prn for pain VORB Dr. James T. Smith/Helen Alexander, RN

ELECTRONIC EXAMPLE:

			Logout
Pt name: James Allen **MRN:** 678	**Room:** 3201 **Admit date:** 08/22/2022	**Allergies:** NKDA **Attending:** Dr. Phillips	
Orders Active Orders Pain medication			**Close** X
Morphine sulfate	8 mg IM q4h prn for pain	Modify	Discontinue

SCHEDULING THE ADMINISTRATION OF MEDICATIONS

The licensed prescriber's orders provide guidelines for the nurse in planning when each medication will be given to the patient. The purpose for prescribing the medication, drug interactions, absorption of the drug, or side effects caused by the drug may determine when the drug is given. The prescribed order may be very specific or may give the nurse latitude in scheduling.

The majority of hospitals use 24-hour clock time rather than ante meridiem (AM) and post meridiem (PM) time. Table 9-1 will assist in conversion to 24-hour clock time. Twenty-four–hour clock time can be computed quickly by adding 12 to PM time—for example, 12 + 3 = 1500 hours.

Most hospitals and health care centers have routine times for administering medications. These times may differ from one hospital to another. The nurse should review the policy and procedure for medication administration at each facility where he or she is employed to determine the appropriate schedule. The guidelines assist the nurse in planning a medication routine that is safe for the patient. Table 9-2 provides examples of planning times for administering each medication at one institution.

TABLE 9-1 CONVERSION FROM 24-HOUR CLOCK TIME TO AM–PM TIME

0100—1:00 AM	0900—9:00 AM	1700—5:00 PM
0200—2:00 AM	1000—10:00 AM	1800—6:00 PM
0300—3:00 AM	1100—11:00 AM	1900—7:00 PM
0400—4:00 AM	1200—12:00 noon	2000—8:00 PM
0500—5:00 AM	1300—1:00 PM	2100—9:00 PM
0600—6:00 AM	1400—2:00 PM	2200—10:00 PM
0700—7:00 AM	1500—3:00 PM	2300—11:00 PM
0800—8:00 AM	1600—4:00 PM	2400/0000—12:00 midnight*

*Hospitals and 24-hour clock time use 2400 for midnight. Digital clocks use 0000.

TABLE 9-2 ABBREVIATIONS AND EXAMPLES OF TIMES FOR ADMINISTERING MEDICATIONS

Abbreviations	Definition	Example Times of Administration	# Doses/ 24 Hours
ac*	Before meals	0730-1130-1730	3
AM	Morning, before noon	0900	1
pc*	After meals	0830-1230-1830	3
PM	Evening, before midnight	2100	1
prn	As needed		
qh	Every hour	0800-0900-1000-etc.	24
q2 h	Every 2 hours	0800-1000-1200-etc.	12
q3 h	Every 3 hours	0900-1200-1500-etc.	8
q4 h	Every 4 hours	0800-1200-1600-etc.	6
q6 h	Every 6 hours	0600-1200-1800-2400	4
q8 h	Every 8 hours	0800-1600-2400	3
q12 h	Every 12 hours	0800-2000	2
stat	Immediately		1

*Providing that meals are served at 0800, 1200, and 1800.

It is the nurse's responsibility to administer medications at the times that will provide the optimal therapeutic effect. For some drugs, following the facility's routine administration schedule would not provide the optimal benefit to the patient.

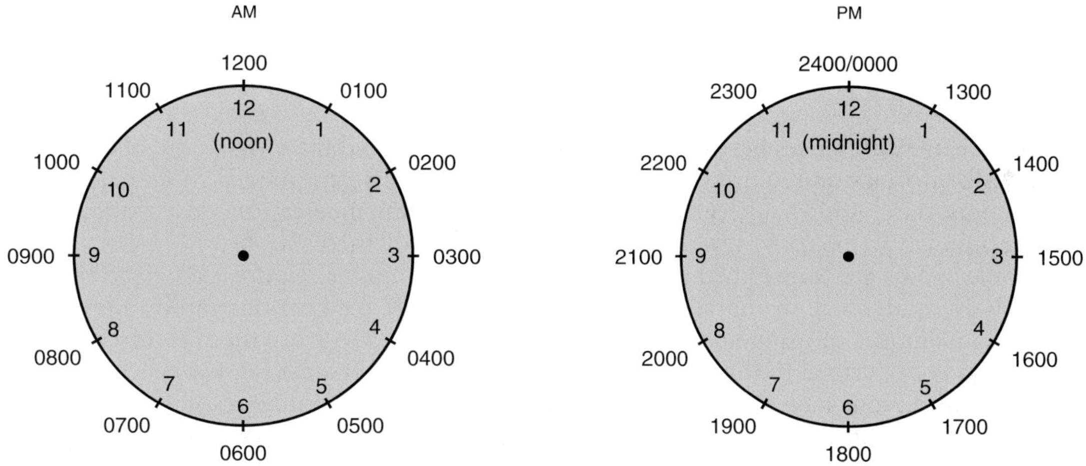

For example, if sucralfate is ordered q 4 h and plugged into a schedule of 0900-1300-1700-2100, the patient would receive the medication *after* breakfast and *after* lunch. This is a medication that needs to be given *before* a meal or other medicines. The nurse must be the advocate for patients to receive their medications at the optimal time of day.

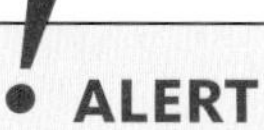

ALERT

The nurse has the responsibility to *always* schedule all medications at times that will provide the optimal effect for patient outcomes.

INTRODUCTION TO DRUG DOSAGES

The nurse obtains the medication from the pharmacy or from an available supply in the clinical unit, prepares the dose, and administers the medication. Unit dosages are prepared in individual doses by the manufacturer or hospital pharmacy and are ready for the nurse to administer.

Most medications are secured in the required dosage. However, problems of drug calculation arise when a drug is not manufactured in the strength required by the patient, the drug is not available in the strength ordered, or the drug is ordered in one system of measurement but is available only in another system of measurement.

When you change from one system of measurement to another, you have an equivalent measure that may or may not be exact. Therefore the answer to your problem may vary according to the system of measurement used. For example, if you change the required dosage to the available dosage, the equivalent dosage may be different than if you changed the available dosage to the required dosage. All problems in this book are calculated by changing the required dosage to the available dosage. The answers reflect this method of calculation. This is good practice because you have the medication on hand in the dosage provided.

The nurse is ethically and legally responsible for the medications administered to the patient. Even though the licensed prescriber writes the order for the medication to be given to the patient and even though the pharmacy may prepare the wrong medication, the nurse who administers the medication is ultimately responsible for the error. Before preparing the drug, the nurse *must know* the maximum and minimum dosages and the actions of and contraindications for each administered drug. In addition, the nurse should consult the patient and the patient's medical record for any known allergies.

HANDWRITTEN MEDICATION ADMINISTRATION RECORD (MAR) AND ELECTRONIC MEDICATION ADMINISTRATION RECORD (eMAR)

Although there are differences between the handwritten MAR and the eMAR, they both contain the same basic information required for safe medication administration: patient name, medical record numbers, date of birth, allergies, admit date, name of the medication, dose, route, frequency, special instructions, and the reason for the "as needed" medications.

Electronic orders are transcribed to the eMAR by the computer (Figure 9-1). Even though the system is computerized, the nurse still verifies orders before medications can be administered. Some of the advantages of using an eMAR over a handwritten MAR are the speed from the time the medication is prescribed to the time the patient receives the medication; the space for added medication information, such as common adverse effects; access to online resources, such as a link to a medication formulary; and instant documentation when the eMAR screen information is accepted.

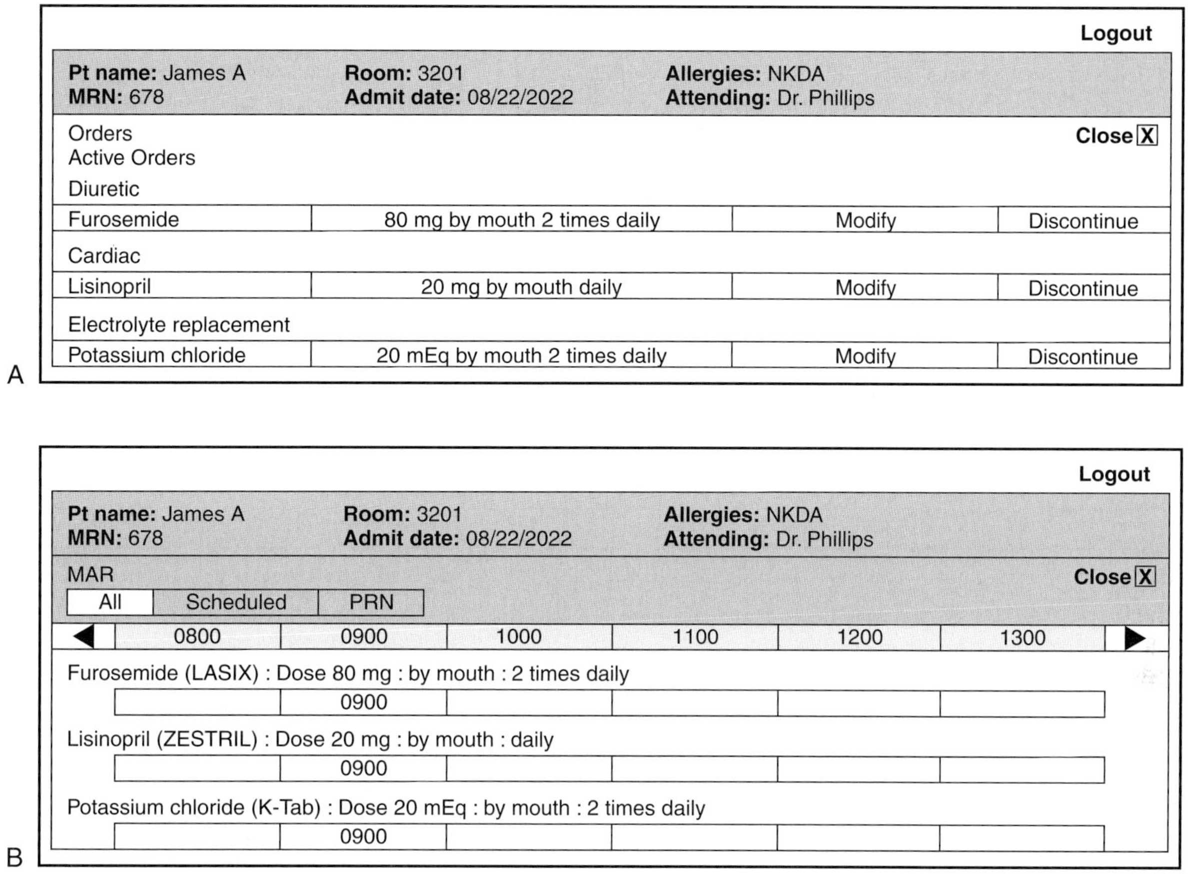

Logout

Pt name: James A **MRN:** 678 | **Room:** 3201 **Admit date:** 08/22/2022 | **Allergies:** NKDA **Attending:** Dr. Phillips

Orders
Active Orders

Close [X]

Diuretic			
Furosemide	80 mg by mouth 2 times daily	Modify	Discontinue
Cardiac			
Lisinopril	20 mg by mouth daily	Modify	Discontinue
Electrolyte replacement			
Potassium chloride	20 mEq by mouth 2 times daily	Modify	Discontinue

A

Logout

Pt name: James A **MRN:** 678 | **Room:** 3201 **Admit date:** 08/22/2022 | **Allergies:** NKDA **Attending:** Dr. Phillips

MAR

Close [X]

All | Scheduled | PRN

◀ 0800	0900	1000	1100	1200	1300 ▶
Furosemide (LASIX) : Dose 80 mg : by mouth : 2 times daily					
	0900				
Lisinopril (ZESTRIL) : Dose 20 mg : by mouth : daily					
	0900				
Potassium chloride (K-Tab) : Dose 20 mEq : by mouth : 2 times daily					
	0900				

B

FIGURE 9-1 Example of electronic licensed prescriber orders **(A)** and a patient's electronic medication administration record **(B)**.

Handwritten orders are transcribed onto the patient's MAR by nonnursing personnel. Nurses are required to verify the transcription was correctly completed before a medication can be administered. Although there are many different types of handwritten MARs, they contain the same information. The MAR in Figure 9-2, *B*, is only one example. The advantages to using a handwritten MAR are the economical cost, the ability to view multiple days (3 to 30) of medication administration at a glance, and the minimal amount of training required to use the MAR.

As you review the eMAR and handwritten MAR examples, notice the appropriate drug information, including the patient's name, name of the medication, dose, route, and frequency.

PHYSICIAN'S ORDERS

1. LABEL BEFORE PLACING IN PATIENT'S CHART ▶
2. INITIAL AND DETACH COPY EACH TIME PHYSICIAN WRITES ORDERS
3. TRANSMIT COPY TO PHARMACY
4. ORDERS MUST BE DATED AND TIMED

Patient, James A.

DATE	ORDERS	TRANS BY
	Diagnosis: Weight: Height:	
	Sensitivities/Drug Allergies:	
1/12/22	0900 Furosemide 80 mg. p.o. twice a day	
	Lisinopril 20 mg by mouth daily	
	Potassium chloride 20 mEq by mouth 2 times daily	
	A. Physician, M.D.	

MEDICAL RECORDS COPY **PHYSICIAN'S ORDERS** T-5

B-CLIN. NOTES	E-LAB	G-X-RAY	K-DIAGNOSTIC	M-SURGERY	Q-THERAPY	T-ORDERS	W-NURSING	Y-MISC.

A

Transcription of Med Sheet by: ______

Reviewed by: ______ Page ___ of ___

Initials	Signature
NJ	N. Jones R.N.
AN	A. Nurse R.N.

Allergies: ☑ NKDA

Injection Sites: A = RUE, B = LUE, C = RLE, D = LLE, E = Abdomen, F = R Glut, G = L Glut

Special Notes:

Patient, James A.

☐ Inpatient ☐ Outpatient

See Legend on Back

DATE	DRUG	08 09 10 11	12 13 14 15	16 17 18 19	20 21 22 23	24 01 02 03	04 05 06 07	1/12/19	1/13/19	1/14/19	1/15/19	1/16/19
1 1/12/22	Furosemide							09 AN; 21 NJ	09 AN; 21 NJ			
	80 mg dose, p.o. route, twice a day interval	09		17								
2 1/12/22	Lisinopril							09 AN	09 AN			
	20 mg dose, p.o. route, once a day interval	09										
3 1/12/22	Potassium chloride							08 AN; 12 NJ	08 AN; 12 NJ			
	20 mEq dose, p.o. route, breakfast & lunch interval	08	17									
4												
	dose, route, interval											
5												
	dose, route, interval											

MEDICATION PROFILE

B-CLIN. NOTES	E-LAB	G-X-RAY	K-DIAGNOSTIC	M-SURGERY	Q-THERAPY	T-ORDERS	W-NURSING	Y-MISC.

B

FIGURE 9-2 Example of handwritten licensed prescriber's orders **(A)** and a handwritten patient medication administration record **(B)** with appropriate drug interpretations.

NAME ______________________

DATE ______________________

ACCEPTABLE SCORE 19

YOUR SCORE ______

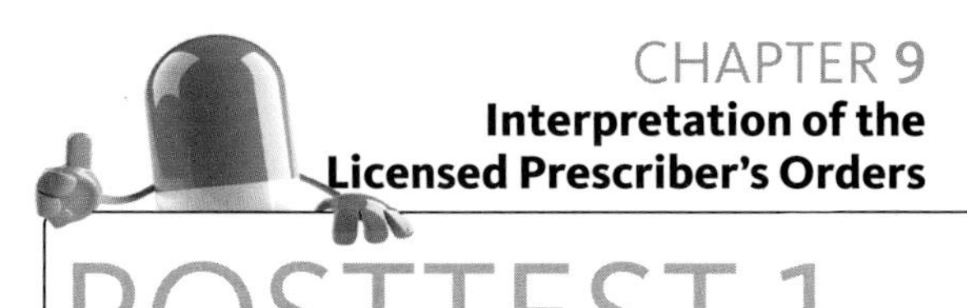

CHAPTER 9
Interpretation of the Licensed Prescriber's Orders

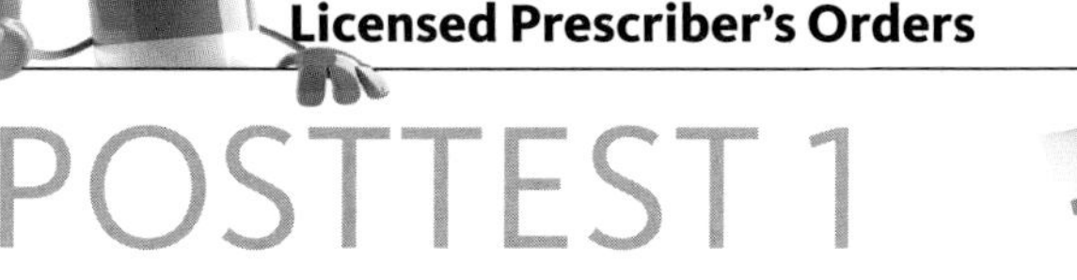

POSTTEST 1

DIRECTIONS: Change to equivalents between 24-hour clock time and AM/PM times.

1. 2:30 PM ______________________
2. 10:30 AM ______________________
3. 5:00 PM ______________________
4. Midnight ______________________
5. 8:00 AM ______________________
6. 3:45 AM ______________________
7. 9:30 PM ______________________
8. 4:00 AM ______________________
9. 6:30 PM ______________________
10. 10:15 PM ______________________
11. 2315 ______________________
12. 0440 ______________________
13. 1745 ______________________
14. 0920 ______________________
15. 1845 ______________________
16. 1630 ______________________
17. 1900 ______________________
18. 2230 ______________________
19. 0750 ______________________
20. 0115 ______________________

ANSWERS ON P. 185.

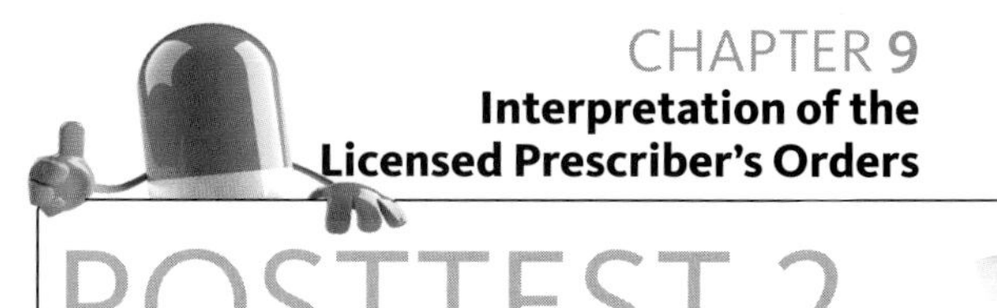

POSTTEST 2

NAME ______________________

DATE ______________________

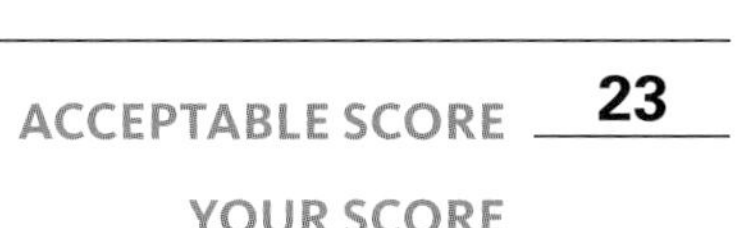

ACCEPTABLE SCORE **23**

YOUR SCORE ______

DIRECTIONS: Answer the following questions using the eMAR below.

Logout

Pt name: James A
MRN: 678
DOB: 05/09/1958

Room: 3201
Admit date: 08/22/2022

Allergies: Vancomycin
Attending: Dr. Phillips

MAR — Close X

All | Scheduled | PRN

◀	0600	0700	0800	0900	1000	1100	▶
Clopidogrel (PLAVIX) : Dose 75 mg : by mouth : daily							
				0900			
Carvedilol (Coreg) : Dose 12.5 mg : by mouth : twice daily							
			0800				
Levothyroxine (SYNTHROID) : Dose 250 mcg : by mouth : before breakfast							
	0600						

1. When asking the patient's date of birth (DOB), what answer is the nurse expecting to hear? ______________________
2. What allergies are listed on the eMAR? ______________________
3. What is the dose of clopidogrel? ______________________
4. What route would the nurse use to administer the carvedilol? __________
5. What time would the nurse administer the levothyroxine? __________

ANSWERS ON P. 185.

DIRECTIONS: Copy the following licensed prescriber's orders onto the medication administration record sheet below. Be sure to schedule the times for each drug administration.

PHYSICIAN'S ORDERS

1. LABEL BEFORE PLACING IN PATIENT'S CHART ▶
2. INITIAL AND DETACH COPY EACH TIME PHYSICIAN WRITES ORDERS
3. TRANSMIT COPY TO PHARMACY
4. ORDERS MUST BE DATED AND TIMED

Patient, James A.

DATE	ORDERS	TRANS BY
	Diagnosis: Weight: Height:	
	Sensitivities/Drug Allergies:	
1/12/22	0800 Cefuroxime 1 g IV q8 h	
	Furosemide 40 mg po twice a day	
	Potassium chloride 10 mEq po twice a day	
	A. Physician, M.D.	

Transcription of Med Sheet by: ______

Reviewed by: ______ Page ___ of ___

Initials ___ Signature ___

Allergies: ☐ NKDA

Injection Sites: A = RUE, B = LUE, C = RLE, D = LLE, E = Abdomen, F = R Glut, G = L Glut

Special Notes:

See Legend on Back

Patient, James A.

☐ Inpatient ☐ Outpatient

DATE	DRUG			08 09 10 11	12 13 14 15	16 17 18 19	20 21 22 23	24 01 02 03	04 05 06 07	DATES														
1																								
	dose	route	interval																					
2																								
	dose	route	interval																					
3																								
	dose	route	interval																					
4																								
	dose	route	interval																					
5																								
	dose	route	interval																					

ANSWERS ON P. 185.

ANSWERS

CHAPTER 9 Interpretation of the Licensed Prescriber's Orders—Posttest 1, p. 181

1. 1430
2. 1030
3. 1700
4. 2400, or 0000
5. 0800
6. 0345
7. 2130
8. 0400
9. 1830
10. 2215
11. 11:15 PM
12. 4:40 AM
13. 5:45 PM
14. 9:20 AM
15. 6:45 PM
16. 4:30 PM
17. 7:00 PM
18. 10:30 PM
19. 7:50 AM
20. 1:15 AM

CHAPTER 9 Interpretation of the Licensed Prescriber's Orders—Posttest 2, p. 183

1. May 9, 1958
2. Vancomycin
3. 75 mg
4. Oral/by mouth
5. 0600

1 1/12/22	Cefuroxime																							
	1 g dose	IV route	q8 h interval	08		16		24																
2 1/12/22	Furosemide																							
	40 mg dose	po route	twice daily interval		09		21																	
3 1/12/22	Potassium chloride																							
	10 mEq dose	po route	twice daily interval		09		21																	

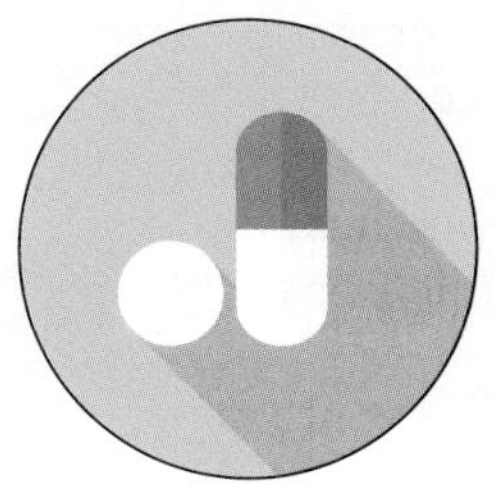

Reading Medication Labels

LEARNING OBJECTIVES

Upon completion of the materials provided in this chapter, you will be able to identify the following parts of each drug label:

1. Trade name of the medication
2. Generic name of the medication
3. Strength of the medication dosage
4. Form in which the medication is provided
5. Route of administration
6. Total amount or volume of the medication provided in the container
7. Directions for mixing or preparation of the medication if required

The safe administration of medications to patients begins with the nurse accurately reading and interpreting the drug label. Thus it is important for the nurse to be familiar and comfortable with the information that is found on the drug label.

PARTS OF A DRUG LABEL

1. TRADE NAME. The trade name (also known as the brand or proprietary name) is usually capitalized and written in bold print. It is the first name written on the label. The trade name is always followed by the ® registration symbol. Different manufacturers market the same medication under different trade names.

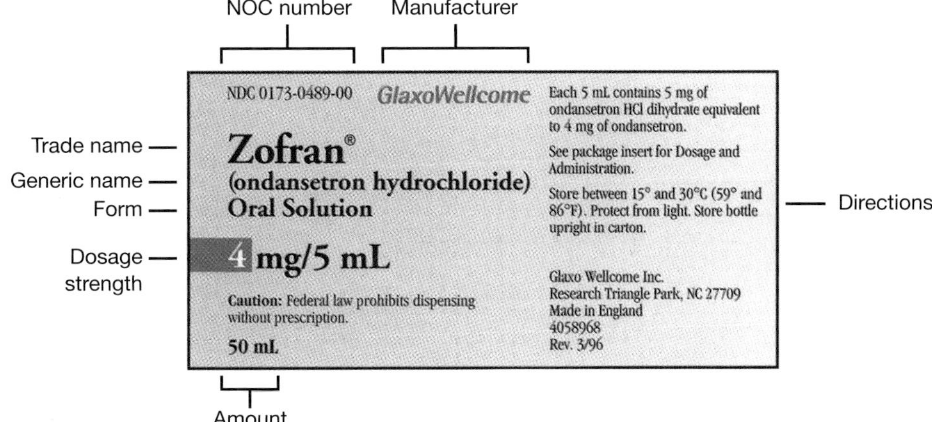

NOC number
Manufacturer
Trade name
Generic name
Form
Dosage strength
Directions
Amount
NDC 0173-0489-00
GlaxoWellcome
Zofran®
(ondansetron hydrochloride)
Oral Solution
4 mg/5 mL
Caution: Federal law prohibits dispensing without prescription.
50 mL
Each 5 mL contains 5 mg of ondansetron HCl dihydrate equivalent to 4 mg of ondansetron.
See package insert for Dosage and Administration.
Store between 15° and 30°C (59° and 86°F). Protect from light. Store bottle upright in carton.
Glaxo Wellcome Inc.
Research Triangle Park, NC 27709
Made in England
4058968
Rev. 3/96

2. GENERIC NAME. The generic name is the official name of the drug. Each drug has only *one* generic name. This name appears directly under the trade name, usually in smaller or different type letters. Licensed prescribers may order a patient's medication by generic or trade name. Nurses need to be familiar with both names and cross-check references as needed. Occasionally, only the generic name will appear on the label.
3. DOSAGE STRENGTH. The strength indicates the amount or weight of the medication that is supplied in the specific unit of measure. This amount may be per capsule, tablet, or milliliter, for example.
4. FORM. The form indicates how the drug is supplied. Examples of various forms are tablets, capsules, liquids, suppositories, and ointments.
5. ROUTE. The label will indicate how the drug is to be administered. The route can be oral, topical, injection (subcutaneous, intradermal, intramuscular), or intravenous.
6. AMOUNT. The total amount or volume of the medication may be indicated. Some examples are 250 mL of oral suspension and a bottle that contains 50 capsules.
7. DIRECTIONS. Some medications must be mixed before use. The amounts and types of diluent required will be listed along with the resulting strengths of the medication. This information may also be found on package inserts.

Other information may be found on drug labels: the name of the manufacturer, expiration date, special instructions for storage, a National Drug Code (NDC) number, and contraindications.

EXAMPLES FOR PRACTICE IN READING DRUG LABELS

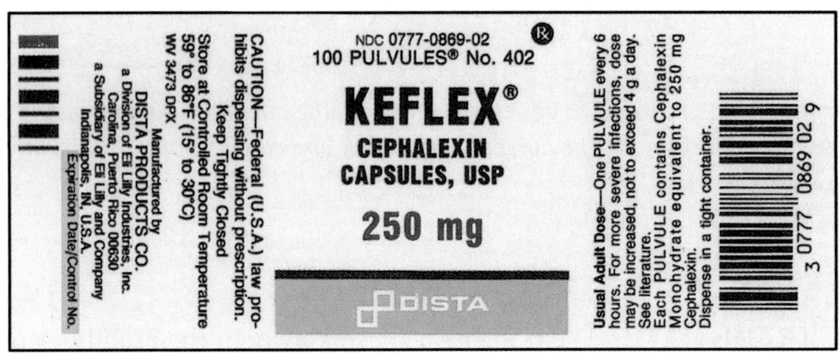

1. Trade name .... Keflex
2. Generic name .... cephalexin
3. Dosage strength .... 250 mg
4. Form .... Capsules
5. Amount.................................... 100
6. Directions .... Keep tightly closed. Store at controlled room temperature 59° to 86° F (15° to 30° C).
7. NDC number 0777-0869-02
8. Manufacturer........................... DISTA
9. Expiration date .... (Yellow highlight)

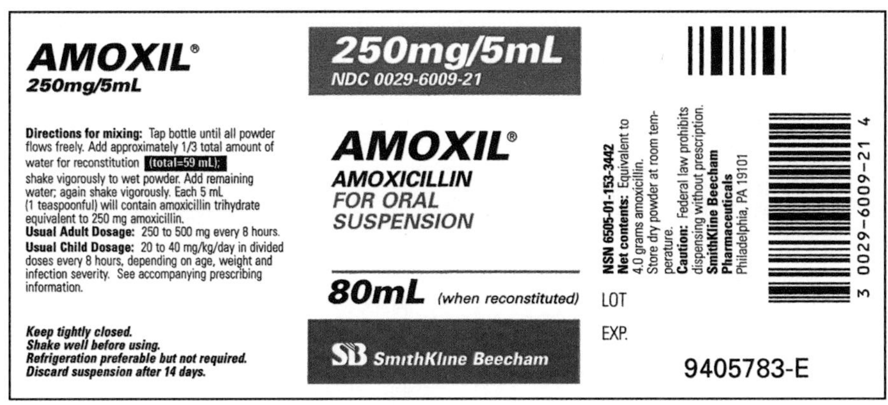

1. Trade name .... AMOXIL
2. Generic name .... amoxicillin
3. Dosage strength...................... 250 mg/5 mL
4. Form .... Suspension
5. Route .... Oral
6. Amount................................... 80 mL
7. Directions............................... Keep tightly closed. Shake well before using. Refrigeration preferable but not required. Discard suspension after 14 days.
8. Direction for mixing............... Tap bottle until all powder flows freely. Add approximately 1/3 total amount of water for reconstitution (TOTAL = 59 mL). Shake vigorously.
9. NDC number 0029-6009-21
10. Manufacturer......................... SmithKline Beecham
11. Expiration date .... Found after EXP
12. Usual adult dosage .... 250-500 mg every 8 hours

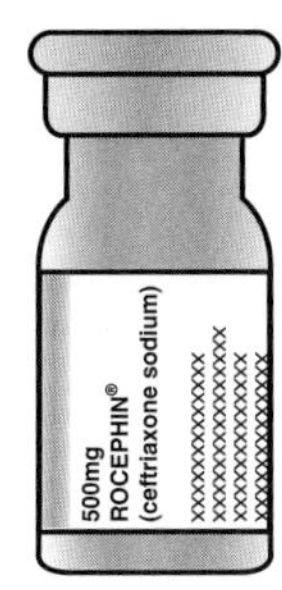

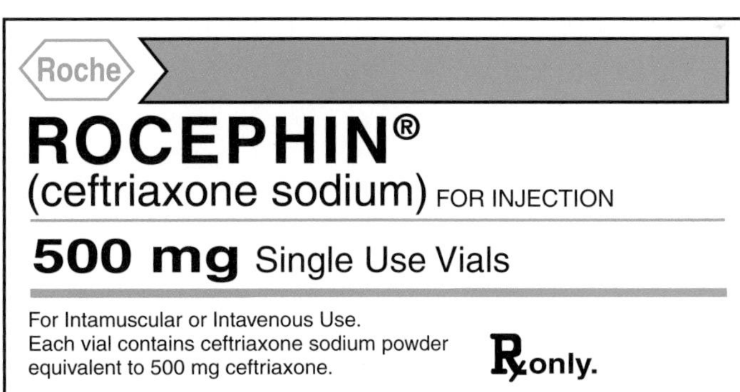

1. Trade name .... Rocephin
2. Generic name .... Ceftriaxone
3. Dosage strength .... 500 mg
4. Route .... Intramuscular or intravenous
5. Directions .... Single-use vial
6. Manufacturer........................... Roche

Occasionally, a drug label will have only one name listed. The one name is the generic name. These are drugs that have been in use for many years and are very well known. The drug companies do not market them under different trade names. They all simply use the generic name.

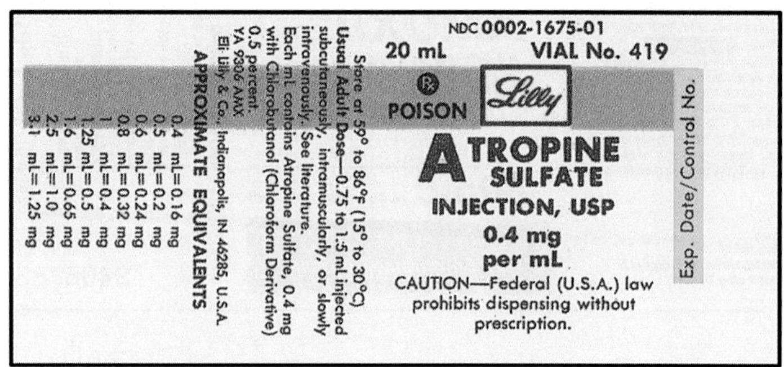

1. Trade name .... None
2. Generic name .... atropine sulfate
3. Dosage strength....................... 0.4 mg per mL
4. Form .... Liquid
5. Route .... Injection
6. Amount................................... 20 mL
7. NDC number 0002-1675-01
8. Expiration date .... (Yellow highlight)
9. Manufacturer .... Lilly
10. Caution .... Federal (U.S.) law prohibits dispensing without prescription.

Study the material and examples for practice in reading drug labels. When you feel ready to evaluate your learning, take the first posttest. Check your answers. An acceptable score as indicated on the posttest signifies that you are ready for the next chapter. An unacceptable score signifies a need for further study before you take the second posttest.

NAME ______________________

DATE ______________________

ACCEPTABLE SCORE 19

YOUR SCORE ______

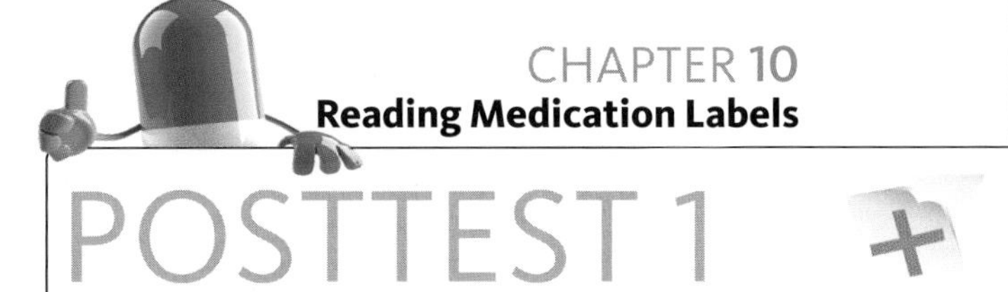

CHAPTER 10
Reading Medication Labels

POSTTEST 1

DIRECTIONS: Identify the requested parts of each of the following medication labels.

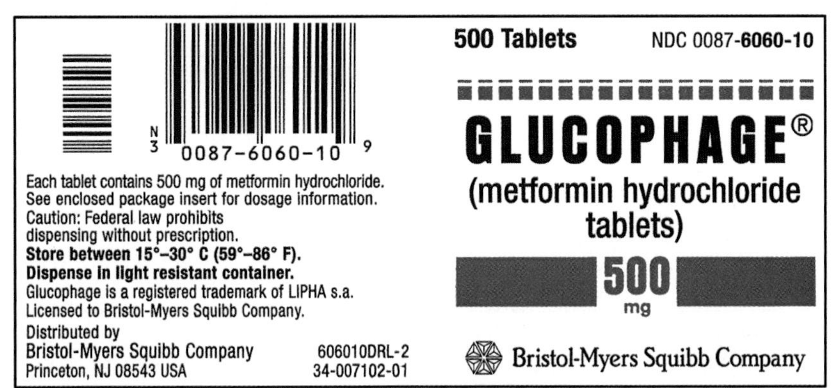

500 Tablets
NDC 0087-6060-10
GLUCOPHAGE®
(metformin hydrochloride tablets)
500 mg
Bristol-Myers Squibb Company
N 3 0087-6060-10 9
Each tablet contains 500 mg of metformin hydrochloride.
See enclosed package insert for dosage information.
Caution: Federal law prohibits dispensing without prescription.
Store between 15°–30° C (59°–86° F).
Dispense in light resistant container.
Glucophage is a registered trademark of LIPHA s.a.
Licensed to Bristol-Myers Squibb Company.
Distributed by
Bristol-Myers Squibb Company
Princeton, NJ 08543 USA
606010DRL-2
34-007102-01

1. a. Trade name ______________________
   b. Generic name ______________________
   c. Dosage strength ______________________
   d. Form ______________________
   e. Amount ______________________

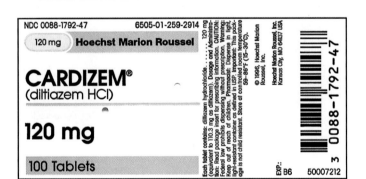

2. a. Trade name ______________________
   b. Generic name ______________________
   c. Dosage strength ______________________
   d. Form ______________________
   e. Amount ______________________

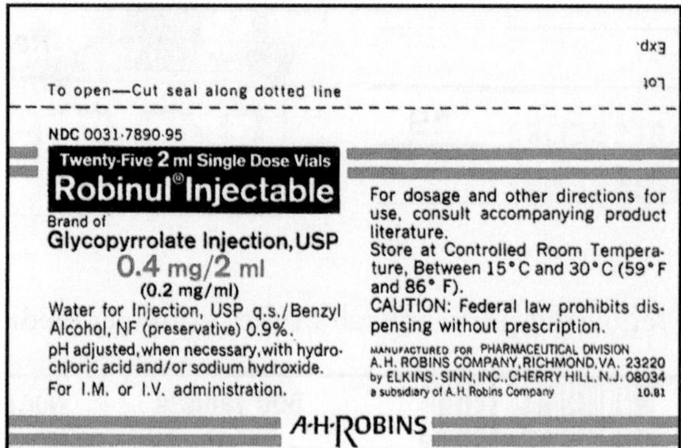

3. a. Trade name __________
   b. Generic name __________
   c. Dosage strength __________
   d. Form __________
   e. Route __________

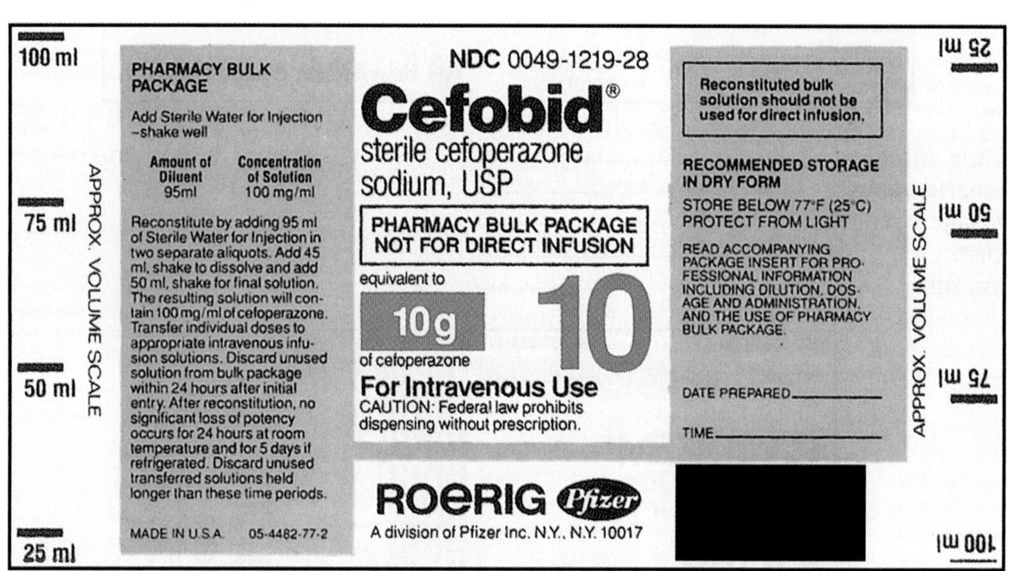

4. a. Trade name __________
   b. Generic name __________
   c. Dosage strength __________
   d. Form __________
   e. Route __________

ANSWERS ON P. 195.

NAME ______________________

DATE ______________________

ACCEPTABLE SCORE 19

YOUR SCORE ______

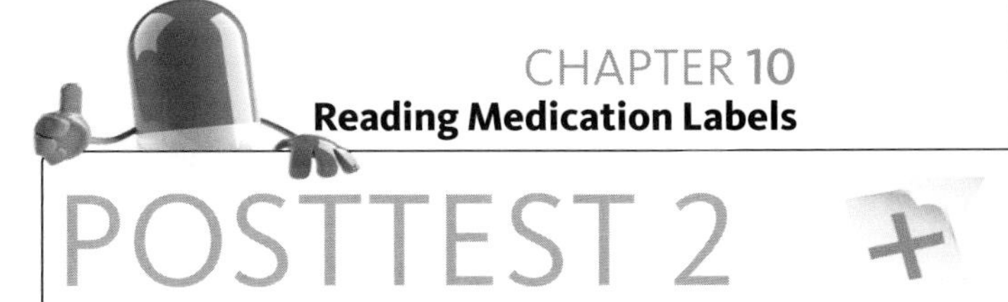

POSTTEST 2

DIRECTIONS: Identify the requested parts of each of the following medication labels.

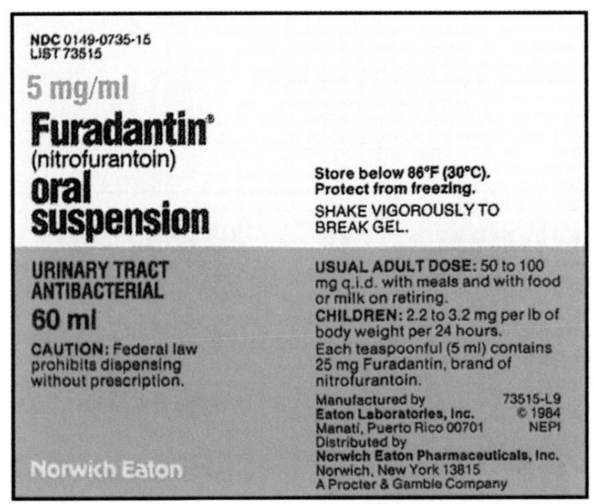

NDC 0149-0735-15
LIST 73515
5 mg/ml
Furadantin®
(nitrofurantoin)
oral suspension
Store below 86°F (30°C).
Protect from freezing.
SHAKE VIGOROUSLY TO BREAK GEL.
URINARY TRACT ANTIBACTERIAL
60 ml
CAUTION: Federal law prohibits dispensing without prescription.
USUAL ADULT DOSE: 50 to 100 mg q.i.d. with meals and with food or milk on retiring.
CHILDREN: 2.2 to 3.2 mg per lb of body weight per 24 hours.
Each teaspoonful (5 ml) contains 25 mg Furadantin, brand of nitrofurantoin.
Manufactured by Eaton Laboratories, Inc. Manati, Puerto Rico 00701
73515-L9 © 1984 NEPI
Distributed by Norwich Eaton Pharmaceuticals, Inc. Norwich, New York 13815
A Procter & Gamble Company
Norwich Eaton

1. a. Trade name ______________
   b. Generic name ______________
   c. Dosage strength ______________
   d. Form ______________
   e. Route ______________
   f. Amount ______________

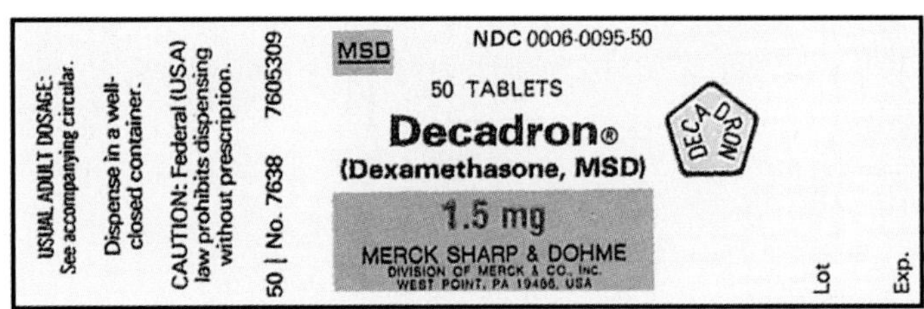

USUAL ADULT DOSAGE: See accompanying circular.
Dispense in a well-closed container.
CAUTION: Federal (USA) law prohibits dispensing without prescription.
50 | No. 7638 7605309
MSD
NDC 0006-0095-50
50 TABLETS
Decadron®
(Dexamethasone, MSD)
DECADRON
1.5 mg
MERCK SHARP & DOHME
DIVISION OF MERCK & CO., INC.
WEST POINT, PA 19486, USA
Lot
Exp.

2. a. Trade name ______________
   b. Generic name ______________
   c. Dosage strength ______________
   d. Form ______________

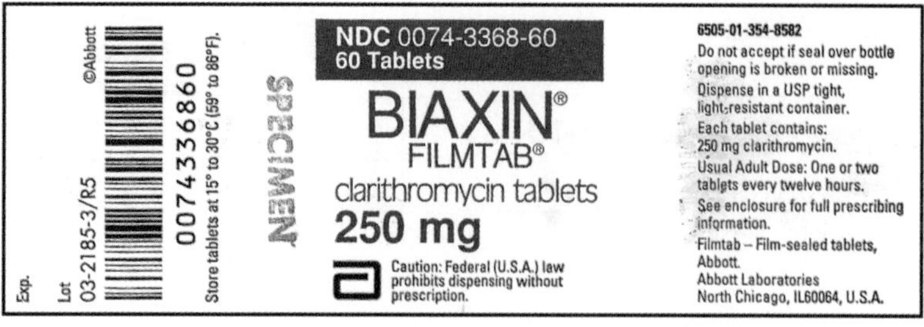

3. a. Trade name ____________
   b. Generic name ____________
   c. Dosage strength ____________
   d. Form ____________
   e. Amount ____________

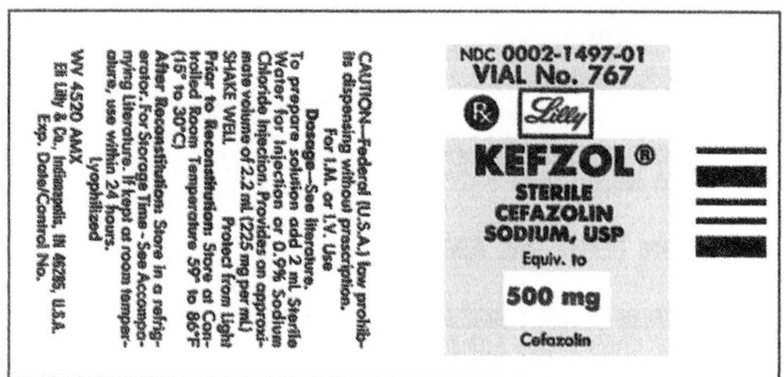

4. a. Trade name ____________
   b. Generic name ____________
   c. Dosage strength ____________
   d. Form ____________
   e. Route ____________

ANSWERS ON P. 195.

ANSWERS

CHAPTER 10 Reading Medication Labels—Posttest 1, pp. 191–192

1. a. Glucophage
   b. metformin hydrochloride
   c. 500 mg
   d. tablets
   e. 500 tablets
2. a. Cardizem
   b. diltiazem
   c. 120 mg
   d. tablets
   e. 100 tablets
3. a. Robinul
   b. glycopyrrolate
   c. 0.4 mg/2 mL or 0.2 mg/mL
   d. milliliters, liquid
   e. IM or IV
4. a. Cefobid
   b. cefoperazone sodium
   c. 10 g or 100 mg/mL
   d. milliliters, powder reconstituted into liquid
   e. IV

CHAPTER 10 Reading Medication Labels—Posttest 2, pp. 193–194

1. a. Furadantin
   b. nitrofurantoin
   c. 5 mg/mL
   d. suspension
   e. oral
   f. 60 mL
2. a. Decadron
   b. dexamethasone
   c. 1.5 mg
   d. tablets
3. a. Biaxin
   b. clarithromycin
   c. 250 mg
   d. tablet
   e. 60 tablets
4. a. Kefzol
   b. cefazolin sodium
   c. 225 mg/mL
   d. milliliters, powder reconstituted into liquid
   e. IM or IV

PART **FOUR**

CALCULATION of **DRUG DOSAGES**

CHAPTERS

CHAPTER 11

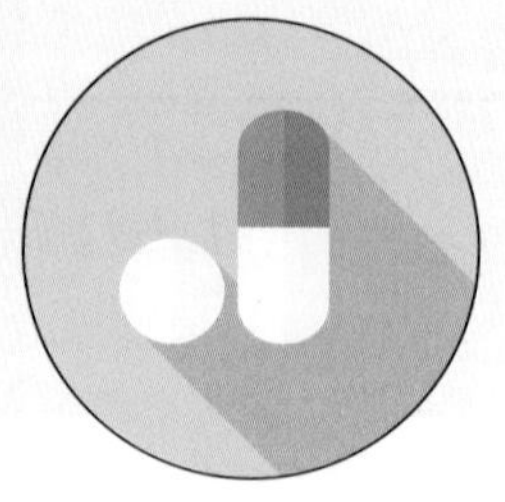

Oral Dosages

LEARNING OBJECTIVES

Upon completion of the materials provided in this chapter, you will be able to perform computations accurately by mastering the following mathematical concepts:

1. Using the dimensional analysis method to solve problems of oral dosages involving tablets, capsules, liquid medications, and those measured in milliequivalents
2. Converting all measures within the problem to equivalent measures in one system of measurement if required
3. Using a proportion to solve problems of oral dosages involving tablets, capsules, liquid medications, and those measured in milliequivalents
4. Using the stated formula as an alternative method of solving problems of oral dosages involving tablets, capsules, liquid medications, and those measured in milliequivalents

Oral drugs are preferred for administration of medications because they are easy to take and convenient for the patient. Oral medications are absorbed through the gastrointestinal tract; therefore the skin is not interrupted. Oral medications may be more economical because the production cost is usually lower than for other forms of medication.

Oral medications are absorbed primarily in the small intestine. Because of the differences in absorption factors, they might not be as effective as other forms of medication. Some oral medications are irritating to the alimentary canal and must be given with meals or a snack. Others may be harmful to the teeth and should be taken through a straw or feeding tube.

Oral medications are supplied in a variety of forms (Figure 11-1). The most common form is a tablet. Tablets come in many colors, sizes, and shapes. A tablet is produced from a drug powder. The tablet may be grooved for ease in administering only a fraction of the whole tablet. Some tablets are scored into halves, and others are divided into fourths (Figure 11-2).

Many licensed prescribers order medications that allow their patients to cut the tablets in half at home. With the rising cost of medications, this strategy helps to decrease the cost for the patient and encourages compliance in taking the medication.

If a patient has difficulty swallowing pills, some pills may be crushed using a mortar and pestle (Figure 11-3). Before crushing any medication in pill form, verify that the medication can be crushed. Some medications, such as those that are enteric coated or sustained or extended release, should not be crushed.

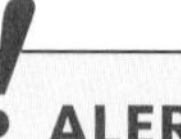

ALERT

Before crushing, verify from the pharmacist that the medication may be crushed and the instructions for crushing.

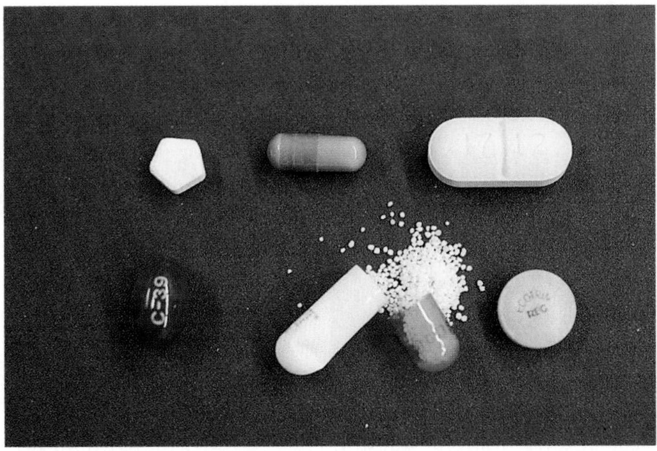

FIGURE 11-1 Forms of solid oral medication. *Top row:* Uniquely shaped tablet, capsule, scored tablet. *Bottom row:* Gelatin-coated liquid, extended-release capsule, and enteric-coated tablet. (From Potter PA, Perry AG, Stockert PA, Hall AM: *Fundamentals of nursing,* ed 8, St Louis, 2013, Mosby.)

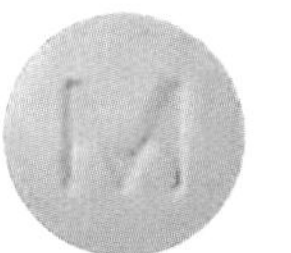

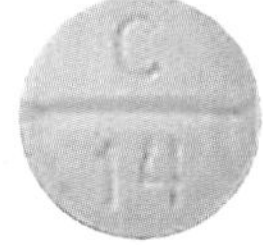

FIGURE 11-2 Scored medication tablet. (From *Mosby's drug consult 2007,* St Louis, 2007, Mosby.)

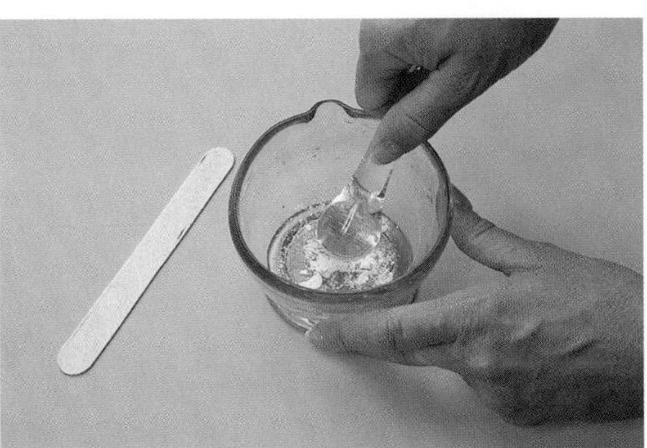

FIGURE 11-3 Mortar and pestle. (From Perry AG, Potter PA, Elkin MK: *Nursing interventions and clinical skills,* ed 5, St Louis, 2012, Mosby.)

Oral medications may also be supplied in capsule form. A capsule is a hard or soft gelatin that houses a powder, liquid, or granular form of a specific medicine(s). Capsules are produced in a variety of sizes and colors (Figure 11-4). Capsules cannot be divided or crushed.

Oral medications may also be administered in liquid form such as an elixir or an oral suspension. Oral liquid medications can be measured with a medication cup, oral syringe (syringe without the needle attached), or dropper (Figures 11-5 to 11-7).

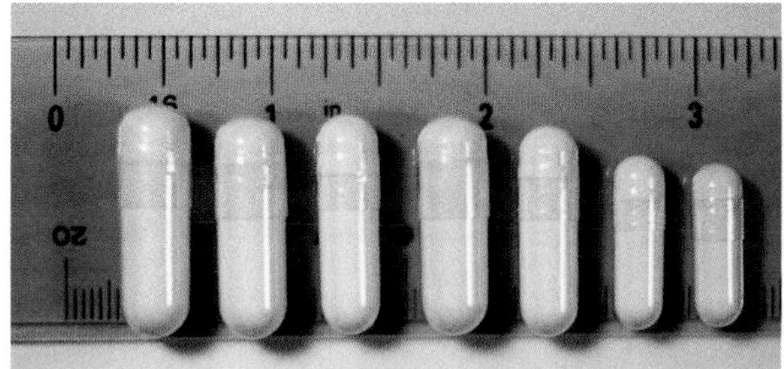

FIGURE 11-4 Various sizes and numbers of gelatin capsules (actual size). (From Clayton BD, Willihnganz M: *Basic pharmacology for nurses,* ed 17, St Louis, 2017, Elsevier.)

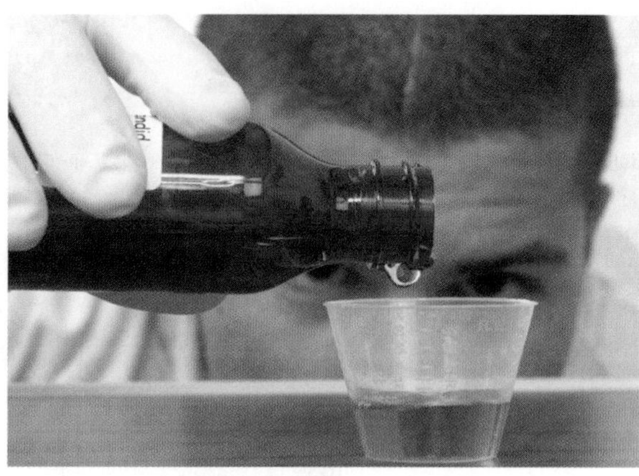

FIGURE 11-5 Oral liquid medication measured with a medication cup. (From Potter PA, Perry AG, Stokert PA, Hall AM: *Fundamentals of Nursing,* ed 9, St Louis, 2017, Elsevier.)

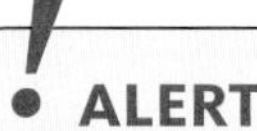

ALERT

Check accuracy of liquid measurement with the cup at eye level, on a hard surface.

An oral syringe or a calibrated dropper may be provided for oral medications to ensure accurate measurement of the medication for administration.

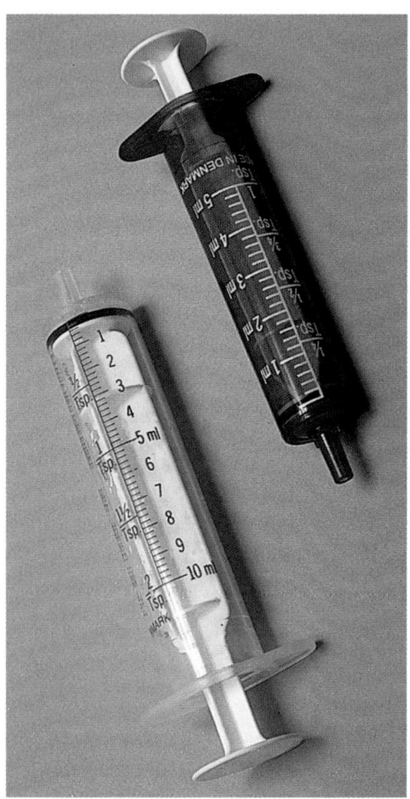

FIGURE 11-6 Plastic oral syringe. (From Clayton BD, Willihnganz M: *Basic pharmacology for nurses,* ed 17, St Louis, 2017, Elsevier.)

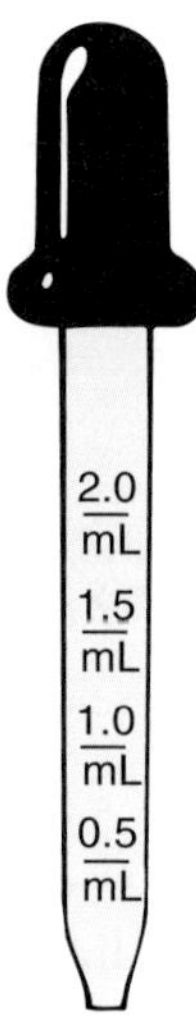

FIGURE 11-7 Medicine dropper. (From Clayton BD, Willihnganz M: *Basic pharmacology for nurses,* ed 17, St Louis, 2017, Elsevier.)

ORAL MEDICATIONS AND ROUNDING

Liquids

Liquid medications supplied in millimeters may need to be rounded based upon the order and the device used for measuring. Oral liquid medications greater than 1 mL may be rounded to the nearest tenth of a milliliter.

Practice Problems. Round the following amounts to the nearest tenth of a milliliter.

1. 1.34 mL = _____ mL
2. 1.75 mL = _____ mL
3. 2.93 mL = _____ mL
4. 1.16 mL = _____ mL
5. 4.17 mL = _____ mL
6. 3.87 mL = _____ mL
7. 2.27 mL = _____ mL
8. 3.54 mL = _____ mL
9. 1.05 mL = _____ mL
10. 1.45 mL = _____ mL

Answers

1. 1.3 mL
2. 1.8 mL
3. 2.9 mL
4. 1.2 mL
5. 4.2 mL
6. 3.9 mL
7. 2.3 mL
8. 3.5 mL
9. 1.1 mL
10. 1.5 mL

Tables and Capsules

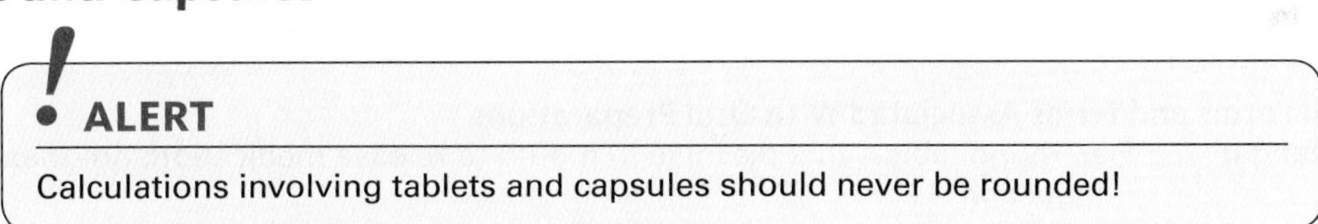
ALERT

Calculations involving tablets and capsules should never be rounded!

Tablets may be split in half to provide the correct dosage of a drug to be administered. An example would be a patient who has 25 mg of a drug ordered. You have 50 mg scored tablets available. The tablet can be split in half with a pill cutter (Figure 11-8). Then ½ of the tablet would be given to the patient.

Table 11-1 describes the forms of a variety of medications.

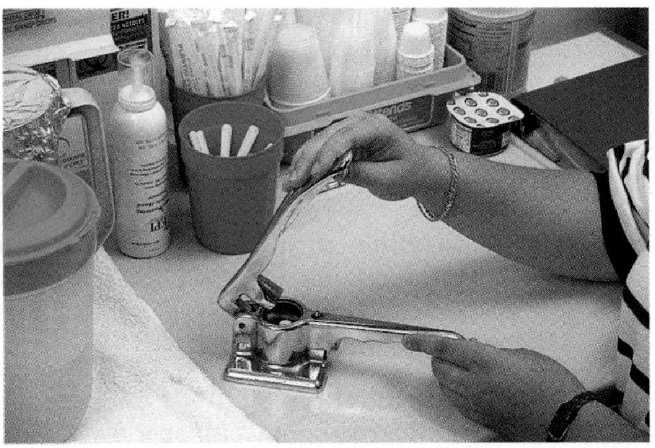

FIGURE 11-8 Pill crusher. (From Perry AG, Potter PA, Elkin MK: *Nursing interventions and clinical skills,* ed 5, St Louis, 2012, Elsevier.)

TABLE 11-1 FORMS OF MEDICATION

Form	Description
Medication Forms Commonly Prepared for Administration by Oral Route	
Solid Forms	
Caplet	Solid dosage form for oral use; shaped like capsule and coated for ease of swallowing
Capsule	Medication encased in gelatin shell
Tablet	Powdered medication compressed into hard disk or cylinder; in addition to primary medication, contains binders (adhesive to allow powder to stick together), disintegrators (to promote tablet dissolution), lubricants (for ease of manufacturing), and fillers (for convenient tablet size)
Enteric-coated tablet	Coated tablet that does not dissolve in stomach; coating dissolves in intestine, where medication is absorbed
Liquid Forms	
Elixir	Clear fluid containing water and/or alcohol; often sweetened
Extract	Concentrated medication form made by removing the active part of medication from its other components
Aqueous solution	Substance dissolved in water and syrups
Aqueous suspension	Finely dissolved drug particles dispersed in liquid medium; when suspension is left standing, particles settle to bottom of container
Syrup	Medication dissolved in a concentrated sugar solution
Other Oral Forms and Terms Associated With Oral Preparations	
Troche (lozenge)	Flat, round tablets that dissolve in mouth to release medication; not meant for ingestion
Aerosol	Aqueous medication sprayed and absorbed in mouth and upper airway; not meant for ingestion
Sustained release	Tablet or capsule that contains small particles of a medication coated with material that requires a varying amount of time to dissolve
Medication Forms Commonly Prepared for Administration by Topical Route	
Ointment (salve or cream)	Semisolid, externally applied preparation, usually containing one or more medications
Liniment	Usually contains alcohol, oil, or soapy emollient applied to skin
Lotion	Semiliquid suspension that usually protects, cools, or cleanses skin
Paste	Thick ointment; absorbed through skin more slowly than ointment; often used for skin protection
Transdermal disk or patch	Medicated disk or patch absorbed through skin slowly over long period of time (e.g., 24 hours)
Medication Forms Commonly Prepared for Administration by Parenteral Route	
Solution	Sterile preparation that contains water with one or more dissolved compounds
Powder	Sterile patches of medication that are dissolved in a sterile liquid (e.g., water, normal saline) before administration
Medication Forms Commonly Prepared for Instillation Into Body Cavities	
Intraocular disk	Small, flexible oval (similar to contact lens) consisting of two soft outer layers and a middle layer containing medication; slowly releases medication when moistened by ocular fluid
Suppository	Solid dosage form mixed with gelatin and shaped in form of pellet for insertion into body cavity (rectum or vagina); melts when it reaches body temperature, releasing medication for absorption

From Potter PA, Perry AG, Stockert PA, Hall AM: *Fundamentals of nursing,* ed 9, St Louis, 2017, Elsevier.

Oral Dosages Involving Capsules and Tablets: Dimensional Analysis Method

Dimensional analysis is another method for setting up problems to calculate drug dosages. The advantage of dimensional analysis is that only one equation is needed. This is true even if the information supplied indicates a need to convert to like units before setting up the proportion to perform the actual calculation of the amount of medication to be given to the patient.

EXAMPLE 1: The order states Augmentin 500 mg po daily. The drug is supplied in 250-mg tablets. How many tablets will the nurse administer?

Step 1. On the left side of the equation, place the name or abbreviation of the drug form of x, or what you are solving for.

$$x \text{ tablet} =$$

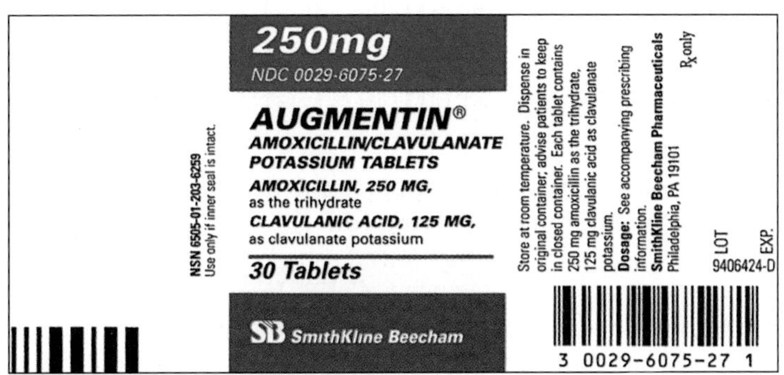

Step 2. On the right side of the equation, place the available information related to the measurement or abbreviation that was placed on the left side. In this example that is *tablet*. This information is placed in the equation as a common fraction; match the appropriate abbreviation or measurement. Thus the abbreviation that matches the x quantity must be placed in the numerator. We also know from the problem that each tablet contains 250 mg of Augmentin. This information is the denominator of our fraction.

$$x \textbf{ tablet} = \frac{\textbf{1 tablet}}{250 \text{ mg}}$$

Step 3. Next, find the information that matches the measurement or abbreviation used in the denominator of the fraction you created. In this example *mg* is in the denominator and our order is for 500 mg. Therefore the full equation is

$$x \text{ tablet} = \frac{1 \text{ tablet}}{250 \textbf{ mg}} \times \frac{500 \textbf{ mg}}{1}$$

Step 4. Now cancel out the like abbreviations on the right side of the equation. If you have set up the problem correctly, the remaining measurement or abbreviation should match that used on the left side of the equation. You are now ready to solve for x.

$$x \text{ tablet} = \frac{1 \text{ tablet}}{250 \cancel{\text{mg}}} \times \frac{500 \cancel{\text{mg}}}{1}$$

$$x = \frac{500}{250}$$

$$x = 2 \text{ tablets}$$

The answer to the problem is 2 tablets.

EXAMPLE 2: The licensed prescriber orders aspirin 975 mg po four times a day. Aspirin 325-mg tablets are available. How many tablets will the nurse administer? _______

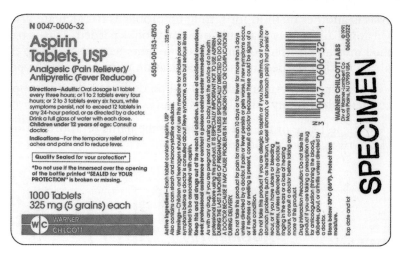

Step 1. On the left side of the equation, place the name or abbreviation of the drug form of x, or what you are solving for.

$$x \text{ tablet} =$$

Step 2. On the right side of the equation, place the available information related to the measurement or abbreviation that was placed on the left side. In this example that is *tablet*. This information is placed in the equation as a common fraction; match the appropriate abbreviation or measurement. Thus the abbreviation that matches the x quantity must be placed in the numerator. We also know from the problem that each tablet contains 325 mg of aspirin. This information is the denominator of our fraction.

$$x \text{ tablet} = \frac{1 \text{ tablet}}{325 \text{ mg}}$$

Step 3. Next, find the information that matches the measurement or abbreviation used in the denominator of the fraction you created. In this example *mg* is in the denominator and our order is for 975 mg. Therefore the full equation is

$$x \text{ tablet} = \frac{1 \text{ tablet}}{325 \text{ mg}} \times \frac{975 \text{ mg}}{1}$$

Step 4. Now cancel out the like abbreviations on the right side of the equation. If you have set up the problem correctly, the remaining measurement or abbreviation should match that used on the left side of the equation. You are now ready to solve for x.

$$x \text{ tablet} = \frac{1 \text{ tablet}}{\underset{1}{\cancel{325}}\ \cancel{\text{mg}}} \times \frac{\overset{3}{\cancel{975}}\ \cancel{\text{mg}}}{1}$$

$$x = \frac{975}{325} = \frac{3}{1}$$

$$x = 3 \text{ tablets}$$

The answer to the problem is 3 tablets.

Oral Dosages Involving Liquids: Dimensional Analysis Method

EXAMPLE 1: The licensed prescriber orders phenobarbital 45 mg po two times a day. Phenobarbital elixir, 20 mg/5 mL, is available. How many milliliters will the nurse administer? _______

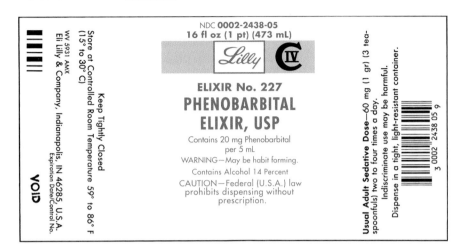

Step 1. On the left side of the equation, place the name or abbreviation of the drug form of x, or what you are solving for. (NOTE: We are now calculating the volume to be administered.)

$$x \text{ mL} =$$

Step 2. On the right side of the equation, place the available information related to the measurement or abbreviation that was placed on the left side. In this example, that is *mL*. This information is placed in the equation as a common fraction; match the appropriate abbreviation or measurement. Thus the abbreviation that matches the x quantity must be placed in the numerator. We also know from the problem that each 5 *mL* contains 20 mg of phenobarbital elixir. This information is the denominator of our fraction.

$$x \text{ mL} = \frac{5 \text{ mL}}{20 \text{ mg}}$$

Step 3. Next, find the information that matches the measurement or abbreviation used in the denominator of the fraction you created. In this example *mg* is in the denominator and our order is for 45 mg. Therefore the full equation is

$$x \text{ mL} = \frac{5 \text{ mL}}{20 \text{ mg}} \times \frac{45 \text{ mg}}{1}$$

Step 4. Now cancel out the like abbreviations on the right side of the equation. If you have set up the problem correctly, the remaining measurement or abbreviation should match that used on the left side of the equation. You are now ready to solve for x.

$$x \text{ mL} = \frac{5 \text{ mL}}{\underset{4}{\cancel{20}} \ \cancel{\text{mg}}} \times \frac{\overset{9}{\cancel{45}} \ \cancel{\text{mg}}}{1}$$

$$x = \frac{5 \times 9}{4 \times 1} = \frac{45}{4}$$

$$x = 11.25 \text{ mL}$$

The answer to the problem is 11.25 mL.

EXAMPLE 2: The licensed prescriber orders Thorazine 20 mg po q 4 h. The drug is available in 120-mL bottles of Thorazine syrup containing 10 mg/5 mL. How many milliliters will the nurse administer? _______

Step 1. On the left side of the equation, place the name or abbreviation of the drug form of x, or what you are solving for.

$$x \text{ mL} =$$

Step 2. On the right side of the equation, place the available information related to the measurement or abbreviation that was placed on the left side. In this example that is *mL*. This information is placed in the equation as a common fraction; match the appropriate abbreviation or measurement. Thus the abbreviation that matches the x quantity must be placed in the numerator. We also know from the problem that each 5 mL contains 10 mg of Thorazine. This information is the denominator of our fraction.

$$x \text{ mL} = \frac{5 \text{ mL}}{10 \text{ mg}}$$

Step 3. Next, find the information that matches the measurement or abbreviation used in the denominator of the fraction you created. In this example *mg* is in the denominator and our order is for 20 mg. Therefore the full equation is

$$x \text{ mL} = \frac{5 \text{ mL}}{10 \text{ mg}} \times \frac{20 \text{ mg}}{1}$$

Step 4. Now cancel out the like abbreviation on the right side of the equation. If you have set up the problem correctly, the remaining measurement or abbreviation should match that used on the left side of the equation. You are now ready to solve for x.

$$x \text{ mL} = \frac{5 \text{ mL}}{\underset{1}{\cancel{10}} \cancel{\text{mg}}} \times \frac{\overset{2}{\cancel{20}} \cancel{\text{mg}}}{1}$$

$$x = \frac{5 \times 2}{1} = \frac{10}{1}$$

$$x = 10 \text{ mL}$$

The answer to the problem is 10 mL.

Oral Dosages Involving Milliequivalents: Dimensional Analysis Method

EXAMPLE: The licensed prescriber orders potassium chloride (KCl) 60 mEq three times a day with meals. KCl 40 mEq/30 mL is available. How many milliliters will the nurse administer? _______

A **milliequivalent** is the number of grams of a solute contained in 1 mL of a normal solution. The milliequivalent is used in a drug dosage proportion, the same as a form of measurement in the metric system.

Step 1. On the left side of the equation, place the name or abbreviation of the drug form of x, or what you are solving for. (NOTE: We are now calculating the volume to be administered.)

$$x \text{ mL} =$$

Step 2. On the right side of the equation, place the available information related to the measurement or abbreviation that was placed on the left side. In this example that is *mL*. This information is placed in the equation as a common fraction; match the appropriate abbreviation or measurement. Thus the abbreviation that matches the x quantity must be placed in the numerator. We also know from the problem that each 30 mL contains 40 mEq of potassium chloride (KCl). This information is the denominator of our fraction.

$$x \text{ mL} = \frac{30 \text{ mL}}{40 \text{ mEq}}$$

Step 3. Next, find the information that matches the measurement or abbreviation used in the denominator of the fraction you created. In this example *mEq* is in the denominator and our order is for 60 mEq. Therefore the full equation is

$$x \text{ mL} = \frac{30 \text{ mL}}{40 \text{ mEq}} \times \frac{60 \text{ mEq}}{1}$$

Step 4. Now cancel out the like abbreviations on the right side of the equation. If you have set up the problem correctly, the remaining measurement or abbreviation should match that used on the left side of the equation. You are now ready to solve for x.

$$x \text{ mL} = \frac{30 \text{ mL}}{\underset{2}{\cancel{40}} \ \cancel{\text{mEq}}} \times \frac{\overset{3}{\cancel{60}} \ \cancel{\text{mEq}}}{1}$$

$$x = \frac{30 \times 3}{2 \times 1} = \frac{90}{2}$$

$$x = 45 \text{ mL}$$

The answer to the problem is 45 mL.

Oral Dosages Involving Capsules and Tablets: Proportion Method

Sometimes the licensed prescriber's order is in one strength of measurement, and the drug is supplied in another strength of measurement. It is therefore necessary to convert one of the measurements so that they are both in the same strength of measurement. After this is done, another proportion will be written to calculate the actual drug dosage.

EXAMPLE 1: The licensed prescriber orders ampicillin 0.5 g po four times a day. The drug is supplied in 250-mg capsules. How many capsules will the nurse administer? _______

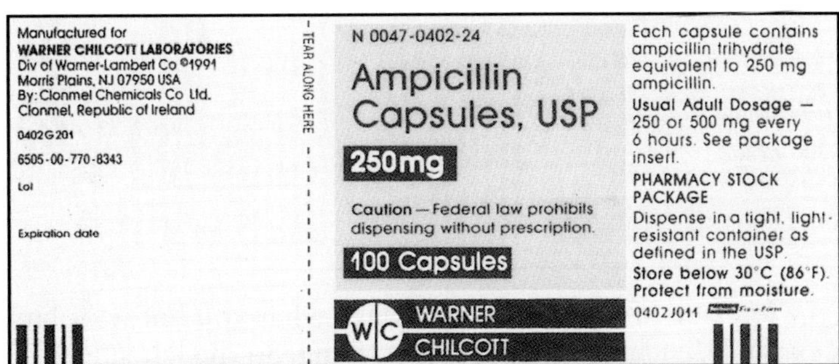

The licensed prescriber's order is in grams and the drug is supplied in milligrams. The order and the supplied drug must be in the same strength of measurement because only two different abbreviations can be used in each proportion. Therefore first convert 0.5 g to milligrams.

$$1000 \text{ mg} : 1 \text{ g} :: x \text{ mg} : 0.5 \text{ g}$$

$$1000 : 1 :: x : 0.5$$

$$1x = 1000 \times 0.5$$

$$x = 500 \text{ mg}$$

$$0.5 \text{ g} = 500 \text{ mg}$$

Now that the order and the supplied drug are in the same strength of measurement, a proportion may be written to calculate the amount of the drug to be given.

Step 1. 250 mg : 1 capsule ::

Step 2. 250 mg : 1 capsule :: _______ mg : _______ capsule

250 mg : 1 capsule :: 500 mg : x capsule

Step 3. 250 : 1 :: 500 : x

Step 4. $250x = 1 \times 500$

$$250x = 500$$

$$x = \frac{500}{250}$$

$$x = 2$$

Step 5. $x = 2$ capsules. Therefore to give 0.5 g of the medication, the nurse will administer 2 capsules.

How many capsules will be given in 1 day? _______

The drug is to be given four times a day.

Step 1. 2 capsules : 1 dose ::

Step 2. 2 capsules : 1 dose :: _______ capsules : _______ dose

2 capsules : 1 dose :: x capsules : 4 doses

Step 3. 2 : 1 :: x : 4

Step 4. $1x = 2 \times 4$

$x = 8$

Step 5. 8 capsules will be given each day.

EXAMPLE 2: The licensed prescriber orders aspirin 975 mg po four times a day. Aspirin 325-mg tablets are available. How many tablets will the nurse administer? _______

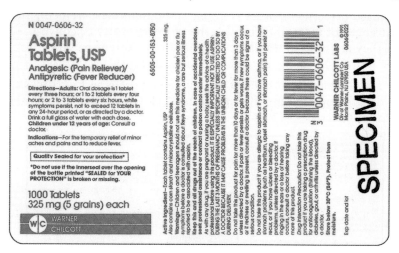

Step 1. On the left side of the proportion place what you know or have available. In this example, each tablet contains 325 mg. So the left side of the proportion is

1 tablet : 325 mg ::

Step 2. The right side of the proportion is determined by the licensed prescriber's order and the abbreviations used on the left side of the proportion. Only *two* different abbreviations may be used in a single proportion. The abbreviations must be in the same position on the right as they are on the left.

1 tablet : 325 mg :: _______ tablet : _______ mg

In the example, the licensed prescriber has ordered 975 mg.

1 tablet : 325 mg :: _______ tablet : 975 mg

We need to find the number of tablets to be given, so we use the symbol x to represent the unknown. Therefore the full proportion is

$$1 \text{ tablet} : 325 \text{ mg} :: x \text{ tablet} : 975 \text{ mg}$$

Step 3. Rewrite the proportion without using the abbreviations.

$$1 : 325 :: x : 975$$

Step 4. Solve for x.

$$325x = 1 \times 975$$

$$325x = 975$$

$$x = \frac{975}{325}$$

$$x = 3$$

Step 5. Label your answer as determined by the abbreviation placed next to x in the original proportion.

$$975 \text{ mg} = 3 \text{ tablets}$$

Oral Dosages Involving Liquids: Proportion Method

EXAMPLE 1: The licensed prescriber orders phenobarbital 45 mg po two times a day. Phenobarbital elixir, 20 mg/5 mL, is available. How many milliliters will the nurse administer? _______

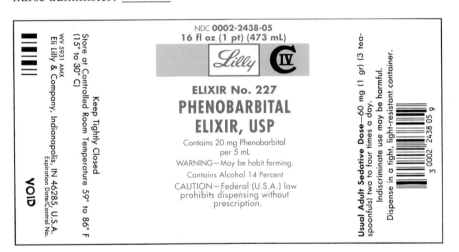

A proportion can be written to calculate the actual volume amount of the drug to be administered.

Step 1. 20 mg : 5 mL ::

Step 2. 20 mg : 5 mL :: _______ mg : _______ mL

20 mg : 5 mL :: 45 mg : x mL

Step 3. $20 : 5 :: 45 : x$

Step 4. $20x = 5 \times 45$

$$20x = 225$$

$$x = \frac{225}{20}$$

$$x = 11.25$$

Step 5. $x = 11.25$ mL. Therefore 11.25 mL is the amount of each individual dose twice a day.

EXAMPLE 2: The licensed prescriber orders Thorazine 20 mg po q 4 h. The drug is available in 120-mL bottles of Thorazine syrup containing 10 mg/5 mL. How many milliliters will the nurse administer? _______ How many doses are available in 120 mL? _______

Step 1. 10 mg : 5 mL ::
Step 2. 10 mg : 5 mL :: _______ mg : _______ mL
10 mg : 5 mL :: 20 mg : x mL
Step 3. $10 : 5 :: 20 : x$
Step 4. $10x = 5 \times 20$

$$10x = 100$$

$$x = \frac{100}{10}$$

$$x = 10$$

Step 5. $x = 10$ mL. Therefore 10 mL is the amount of each individual dose q 4 h.

A proportion can be written to calculate the number of doses in a 120-mL bottle.

Step 1. 10 mL : 1 dose ::
Step 2. 10 mL : 1 dose :: _______ mL : _______ dose
10 mL : 1 dose :: 120 mL : x dose
Step 3. $10 : 1 :: 120 : x$
Step 4. $10x = 120$

$$x = \frac{120}{10}$$

$$x = 12$$

Step 5. $x = 12$ doses. Therefore each 120-mL bottle contains 12 doses.

Oral Dosages Involving Milliequivalents: Proportion Method

EXAMPLE: The licensed prescriber orders potassium chloride (KCl) 60 mEq three times a day with meals. KCl 40 mEq/30 mL is available. How many milliliters will the nurse administer? _______

A **milliequivalent** is the number of grams of a solute contained in 1 mL of a normal solution. The milliequivalent is used in a drug dosage proportion, the same as a form of measurement in the apothecary or metric system. (NOTE: We are now calculating the volume to be administered.)

Step 1. 40 mEq : 30 mL ::
Step 2. 40 mEq : 30 mL :: _______ mEq : _______ mL
40 mEq : 30 mL :: 60 mEq : x mL
Step 3. $40 : 30 :: 60 : x$
Step 4. $40x = 30 \times 60$

$$40x = 1800$$

$$x = \frac{1800}{40}$$

$$x = 45$$

Step 5. $x = 45$ mL. Therefore to give 60 mEq of the medication, the nurse will administer 45 mL.

Alternative Formula Method of Oral Drug Dosage Calculation

A formula has been used for many years in the calculation of drug dosages by nurses. The formula method may be the method that some students learned first in an earlier nursing role (e.g., for a nurse who was a licensed practical nurse or who is returning to work in the area of direct patient care). If this is the case and the student accurately uses the formula method, we do not recommend changing to dimensional analysis or the proportion method. Remember, choose the method that you feel is best for you and consistently use the chosen method. We do not recommend switching back and forth between the formula method and the proportion method. When you use the formula method, the *desired and available amounts must be in the same units of measurement.*

$$\text{Formula: } \frac{D}{A} \times Q = x$$

D represents the **desired** amount of the medication that has been ordered by the licensed prescriber.

A represents the strength of the medication that is **available.**

Q represents the **quantity** or amount of the medication that contains the available strength.

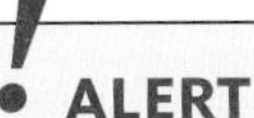

ALERT

When the medication is a solid such as a tablet, capsule, or caplet, the quantity will always be 1. If the medication is in liquid form, the number will vary. Remember from the math review, the denominator of a whole number is always one: $\frac{1}{1}, \frac{2}{1}, \frac{3}{1}$, etc.

x represents the dose that is unknown.

This formula can be read as:

Desired over (or divided by) available multiplied by the quantity available equals *x*, or the amount to be given to the patient.

Oral Dosages Involving Capsules and Tablets: Alternative Formula

If the licensed prescriber's order is in one strength of measurement and the drug is supplied in another strength of measurement, it will still be necessary to convert one of the measurements so that both are expressed in the same system. After this is done, the formula may be used to calculate the drug dose to be administered.

EXAMPLE 1: The licensed prescriber orders ampicillin 0.5 g po four times a day. The drug is supplied in 250-mg capsules. How many capsules will the nurse administer? _______

The licensed prescriber's order is expressed in grams and the drug is supplied in milligrams. Therefore convert the order to milligrams as outlined in Chapter 6.

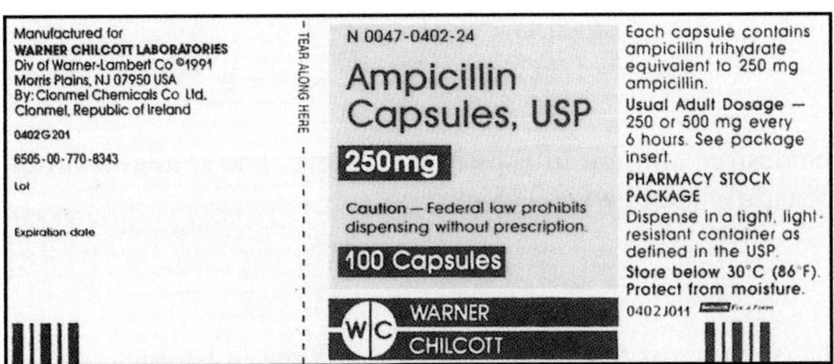

$$1000\text{ mg} : 1\text{ g} :: x\text{ mg} : 0.5\text{ g}$$

$$1000 : 1 :: x : 0.5$$

$$x = 1000 \times 0.5$$

$$x = 500\text{ mg}$$

Now the numbers may be filled into the formula $\frac{D}{A} \times Q = x$

Step 1. The desired amount of ampicillin is 500 mg. The available amount or strength of ampicillin supplied is 250 mg.

$$\frac{500\text{ mg}}{250\text{ mg}}$$

Step 2. The quantity available is in capsule form, or 1.

$$\frac{500\text{ mg}}{250\text{ mg}} \times \frac{1}{1}$$

Step 3. Rewrite the problem with the abbreviations canceled.

$$\frac{500\ \cancel{\text{mg}}}{250\ \cancel{\text{mg}}} \times \frac{1}{1}$$

Step 4. Solve for x.

$$x = \frac{500 \times 1}{250 \times 1}$$

$$x = \frac{500}{250}$$

$$x = 2$$

Step 5. Label your answer as determined by the quantity.

500 mg = 2 capsules

EXAMPLE 2: The licensed prescriber orders aspirin 975 mg po four times a day. Aspirin is available in 325-mg tablets. How many tablets will the nurse administer? _______

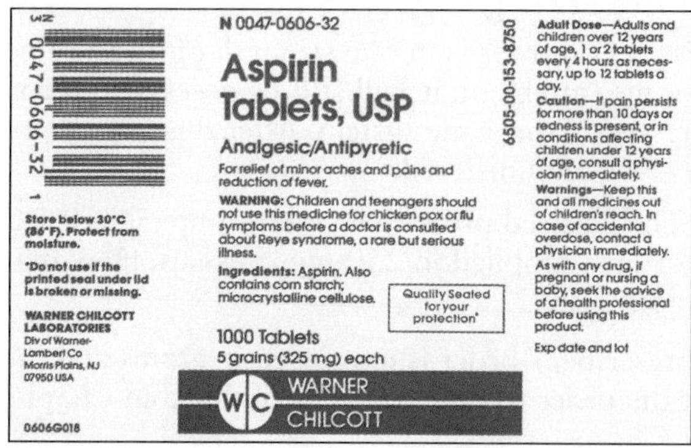

$$\frac{D}{A} \times Q = x$$

Step 1. The desired amount of aspirin is 975 mg. The available amount or strength of the aspirin supplied is 325 mg.

$$\frac{975\text{ mg}}{325\text{ mg}}$$

Step 2. The quantity of the medication for 325 mg is 1 tablet.

$$\frac{975\text{ mg}}{325\text{ mg}} \times \frac{1}{1}$$

Step 3. Rewrite the problem with the abbreviations canceled.

$$\frac{975 \cancel{mg}}{325 \cancel{mg}} \times \frac{1}{1}$$

Step 4. Solve for x.

$$x = \frac{975}{325} \times \frac{1}{1}$$

$$x = \frac{975 \times 1}{325 \times 1}$$

$$x = \frac{975}{325}$$

$$x = 3$$

Step 5. Label your answer as determined by the quantity.

975 mg = 3 tablets

Oral Dosages Involving Liquids: Alternative Formula

EXAMPLE: The licensed prescriber orders phenobarbital 45 mg po two times a day. Phenobarbital elixir, 20 mg/5 mL, is available. How many milliliters will the nurse administer? _______

The numbers may be filled into the formula $\frac{D}{A} \times Q = x$.

Step 1. The desired amount is 45 mg. The available amount or strength of phenobarbital is 20 mg.

$$\frac{45 \text{ mg}}{20 \text{ mg}}$$

Step 2. The quantity available is 5 mL.

$$\frac{45 \text{ mg}}{20 \text{ mg}} \times \frac{5 \text{ mL}}{1 \text{ mL}}$$

Step 3. Rewrite the problem with the abbreviations canceled.

$$\frac{45 \cancel{mg}}{20 \cancel{mg}} \times \frac{5 \cancel{mL}}{1 \cancel{mL}}$$

Step 4. Solve for x.

$$x = \frac{45}{20} \times \frac{5}{1}$$

$$x = \frac{45}{\underset{4}{\cancel{20}}} \times \frac{\overset{1}{\cancel{5}}}{1}$$

$$x = \frac{45 \times 1}{4 \times 1}$$

$$x = \frac{45}{4}$$

$$x = 11.25$$

Step 5. Label your answer as determined by the quantity.

45 mg = 11.25 mL

Complete the following work sheet, which provides for extensive practice in the calculation of oral dosage problems. Check your answers. It is sometimes impossible to administer the exact amount ordered. All capsules and tablets that are not scored are impossible to divide accurately. If you have difficulties, go back and review the necessary material. When you feel ready to evaluate your learning, take the first posttest. Check your answers. An acceptable score as indicated on the posttest signifies that you are ready for the next chapter. An unacceptable score signifies a need for further study before taking the second posttest.

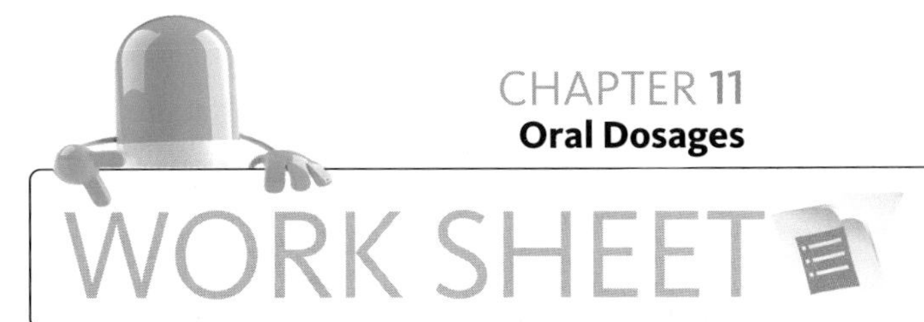

CHAPTER 11
Oral Dosages

WORK SHEET

DIRECTIONS: The medication order is listed at the beginning of each problem. Calculate the oral doses. Show your work. Shade each medicine cup or oral syringe when provided to indicate the correct dose.

1. The licensed prescriber orders Minipress 2 mg po two times a day for Mr. Shaw's high blood pressure. How many capsules will the nurse administer per dose? _______

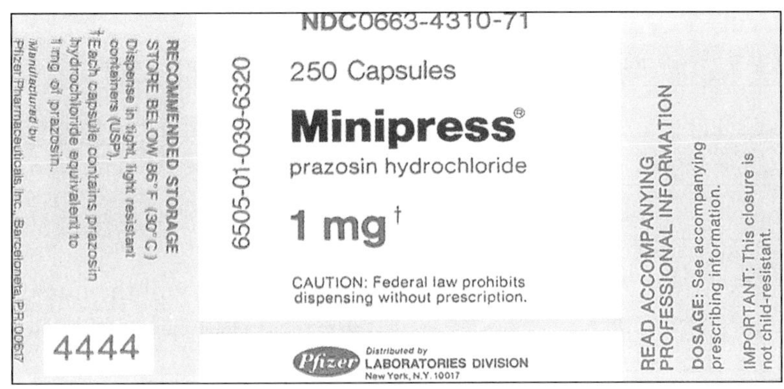

NDC0663-4310-71
250 Capsules

prazosin hydrochloride
1 mg†
CAUTION: Federal law prohibits dispensing without prescription.
Distributed by Pfizer LABORATORIES DIVISION New York, N.Y. 10017
6505-01-039-6320
RECOMMENDED STORAGE
STORE BELOW 86° F (30° C)
Dispense in tight, light resistant containers (USP).
†Each capsule contains prazosin hydrochloride equivalent to 1 mg of prazosin.
Manufactured by Pfizer Pharmaceuticals Inc. Barceloneta, P.R. 00617
4444
READ ACCOMPANYING PROFESSIONAL INFORMATION
DOSAGE: See accompanying prescribing information.
IMPORTANT: This closure is not child-resistant.

2. Mrs. Taylor has a long history of seizures. Elixir of phenobarbital 30 mg po q 12 h is ordered. How many milliliters will the nurse administer per dose? _______

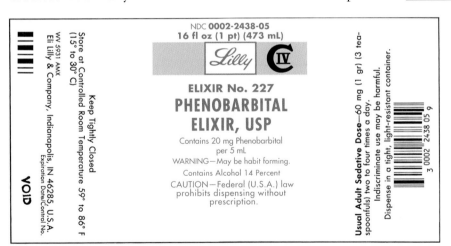

NDC 0002-2438-05
16 fl oz (1 pt) (473 mL)
Lilly
CIV
ELIXIR No. 227
PHENOBARBITAL ELIXIR, USP
Contains 20 mg Phenobarbital per 5 mL
WARNING—May be habit forming.
Contains Alcohol 14 Percent
CAUTION—Federal (U.S.A.) law prohibits dispensing without prescription.
Keep Tightly Closed
Store at Controlled Room Temperature 59° to 86° F (15° to 30° C)
WV 5931 AMX
Eli Lilly & Company, Indianapolis, IN 46285, U.S.A.
Expiration Date/Control No.
VOID
Usual Adult Sedative Dose—60 mg (1 gr) (3 teaspoonfuls) two to four times a day.
Indiscriminate use may be harmful.
Dispense in a tight, light-resistant container.
3 0002 2438 05 9

3. The licensed prescriber orders Crystodigin 0.2 mg po two times a day for 4 days, then 0.15 mg po two times a day. You have Crystodigin 0.05-mg tablets available. How many tablets will you give for each dose the first 4 days? _______ How many tablets will you give for each dose thereafter? _______

4. Mr. Davis has a diagnosis of acute maxillary sinusitis. His licensed prescriber orders Biaxin 500 mg q 12 h × 10 days. How many tablets will the nurse administer per dose? _______

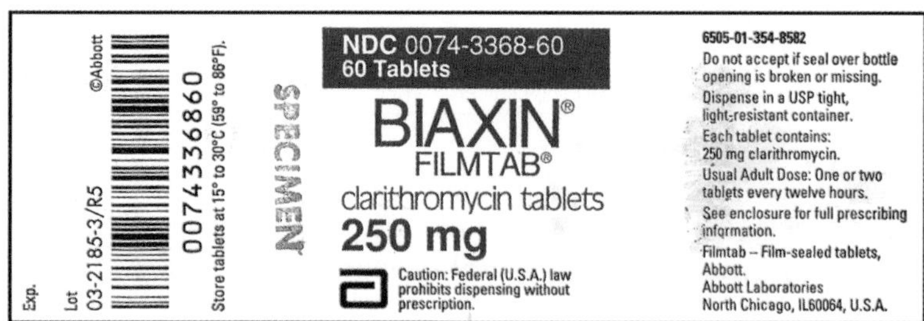

5. Mrs. Rios complains of nausea. Compazine 2.5 mg po three times a day is ordered. The stock supply is Compazine syrup 5 mg/5 mL. How many milliliters will the nurse administer per dose? _______

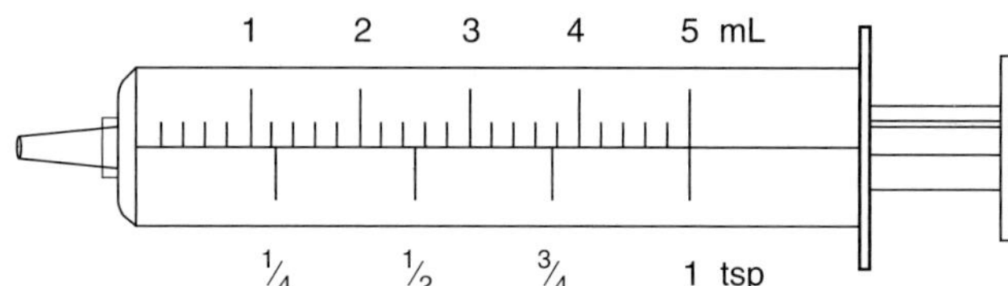

6. The licensed prescriber orders Ativan 2 mg at bedtime. How many tablets will the nurse administer per dose? _______

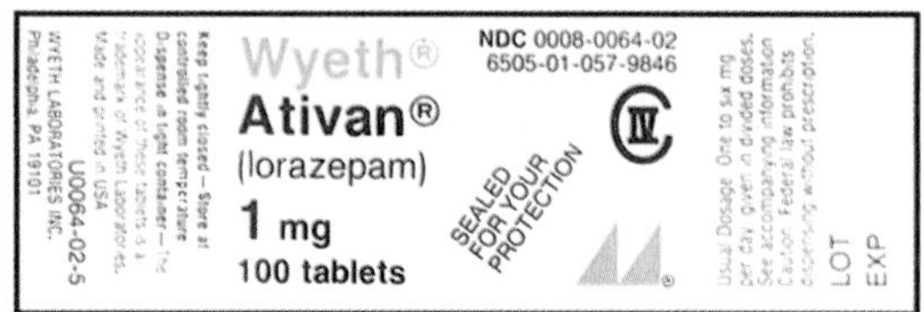

7. The licensed prescriber orders Pravachol 20 mg po at bedtime. How many tablets will the nurse administer per dose? _______

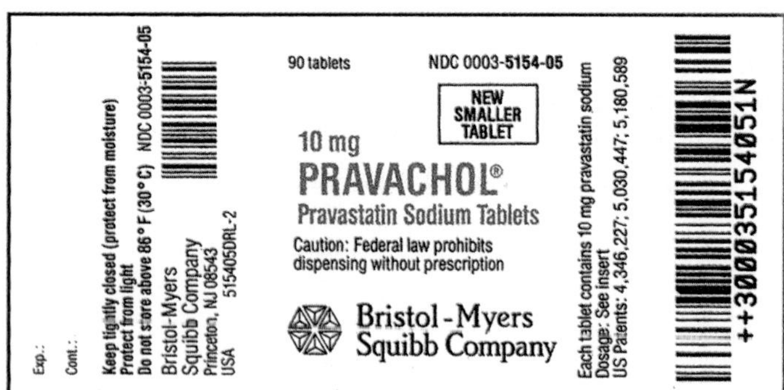

8. Mandelamine 1 g po four times a day is scheduled for Mr. Eaton to treat his urinary tract infection. You have 0.5-g tablets available. How many tablets will you administer per dose? _______

9. The licensed prescriber orders Prozac 40 mg po daily in AM. How many milliliters will the nurse administer per dose? _______

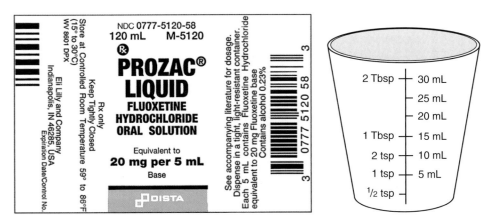

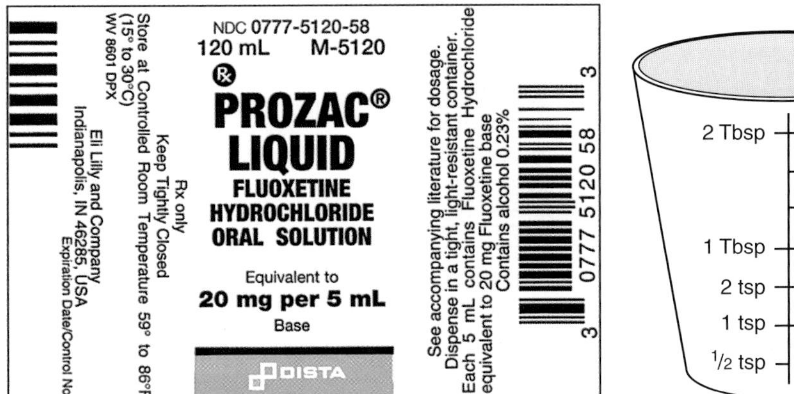

10. Mr. Chang has Parkinson's disease and is to receive Cogentin 1 mg po at 1900. How many tablets will the nurse administer per dose? _______

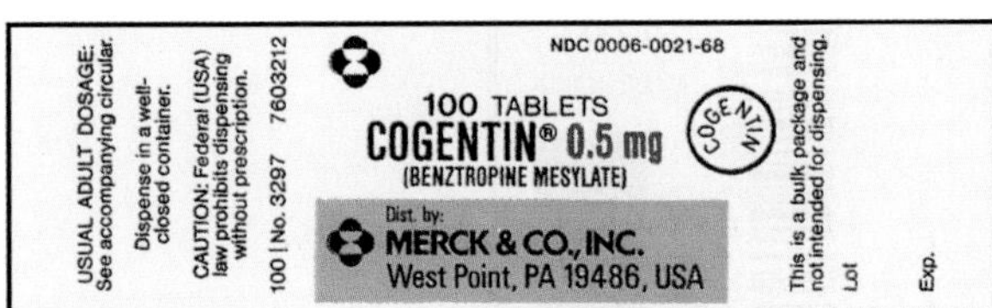

11. Mrs. Martin receives Motrin 800 mg po three times a day for arthritis pain. The drug is supplied in 400-mg tablets. How many tablets will the nurse administer per dose? _______

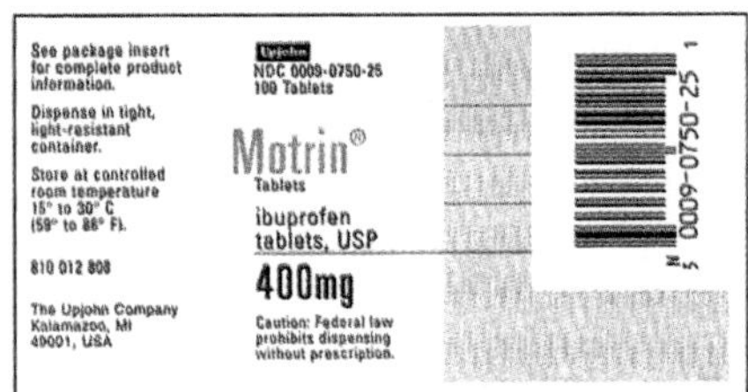

12. The licensed prescriber orders lithium carbonate 0.6 g po two times a day. The drug is supplied in 300-mg scored tablets. How many tablets will the nurse administer per dose? _______ How many milligrams will be given each day? _______

13. Your patient is taking minoxidil 30 mg daily for hypertension. How many tablets will you administer per dose? _______

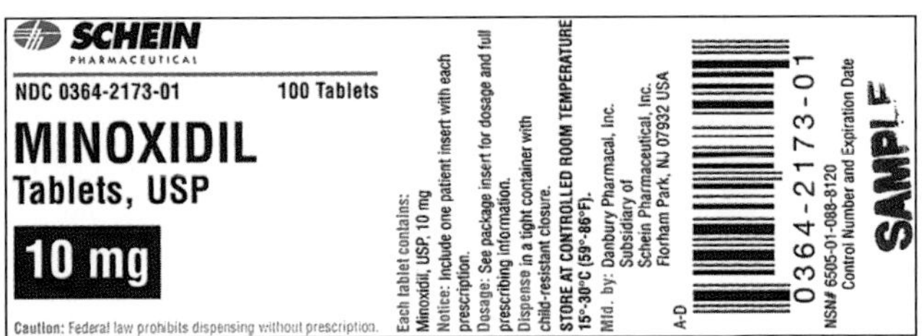

14. Mr. Hill is to receive Cipro 0.75 g q 12 h for a knee infection. How many tablets will the nurse administer per dose? _______

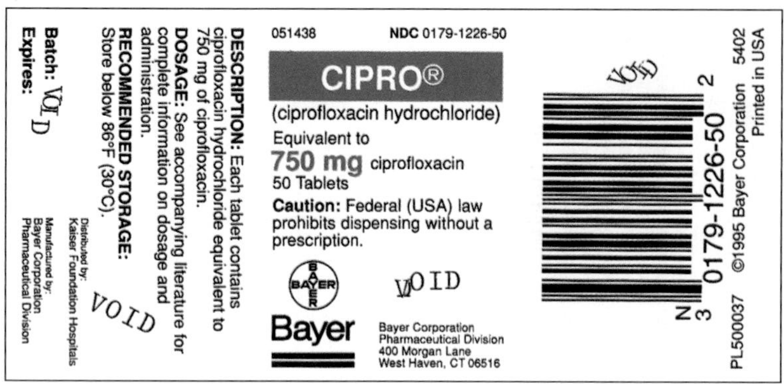

15. The licensed prescriber orders Geodon 80 mg bid to treat Mrs. Basey's acute agitation. You have 40-mg capsules available. How many capsules will you administer per dose? _______

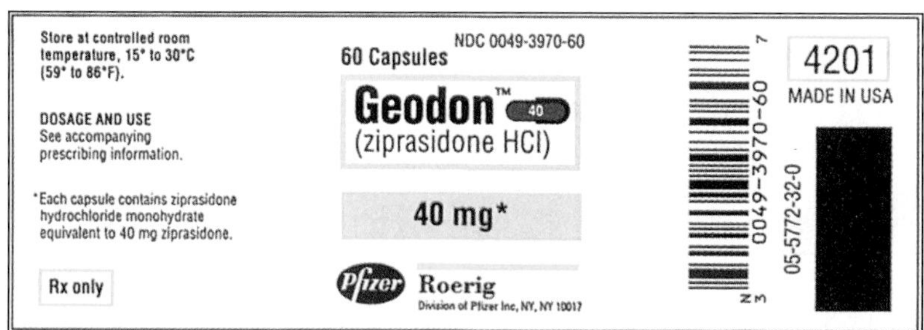

16. The licensed prescriber orders Gantrisin 4 g po STAT, then 2 g q 6 h. How many tablets will be given for the STAT dose? _______ How many tablets will be given for each of the 2-g doses? _______

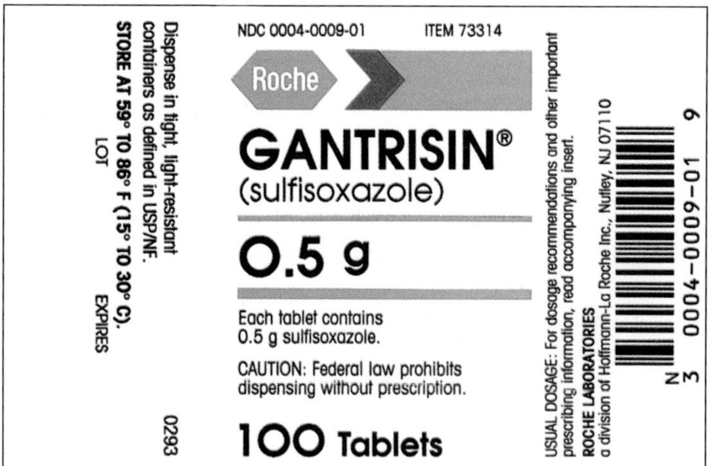

17. The licensed prescriber orders acyclovir 800 mg po q 4 h while the patient is awake. Acyclovir 400-mg tablets are available. How many tablets will the nurse administer per dose? _______

18. The licensed prescriber orders Gaviscon 30 mL po four times a day. Gaviscon is supplied in 360-mL bottles. How many mLs will be given in 1 day? _______

19. Ms. Vega complains of a rash on her abdomen, and the licensed prescriber orders Benadryl 30 mg po three times a day. How many milliliters will the nurse administer per dose? _______

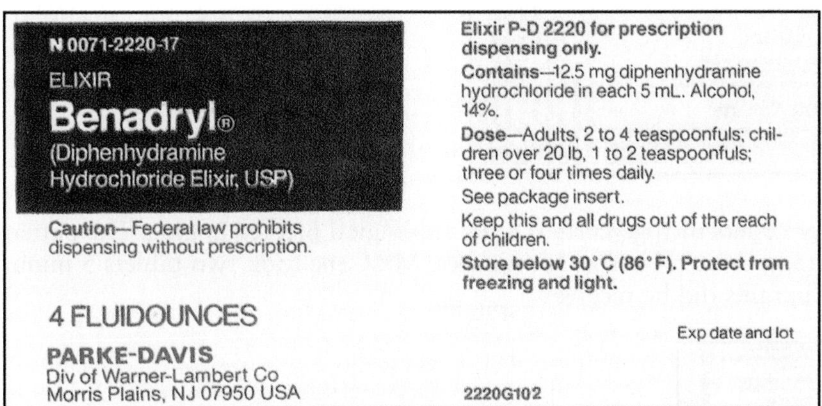

20. Mr. Gifford has had a lumbar laminectomy and requires pain medication. The patient has an order for codeine 60 mg po q 3 h prn. How many tablets will the nurse administer per dose? _______

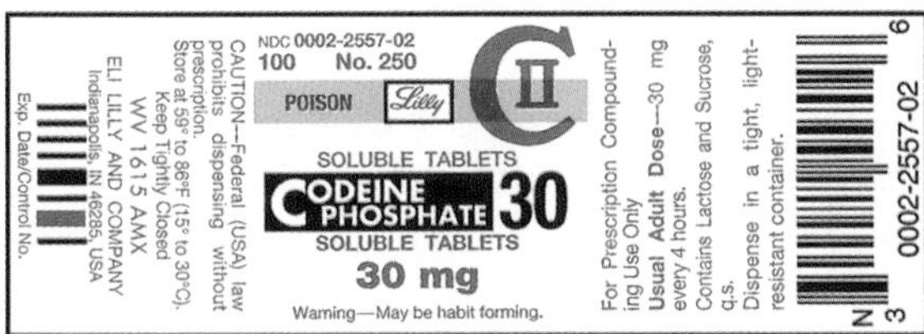

21. The licensed prescriber orders Amoxil suspension 5.5 mL (125 mg/5 mL strength) po q 6 h for your patient who had a tonsillectomy. How many milligrams will you administer every 6 hours? _______

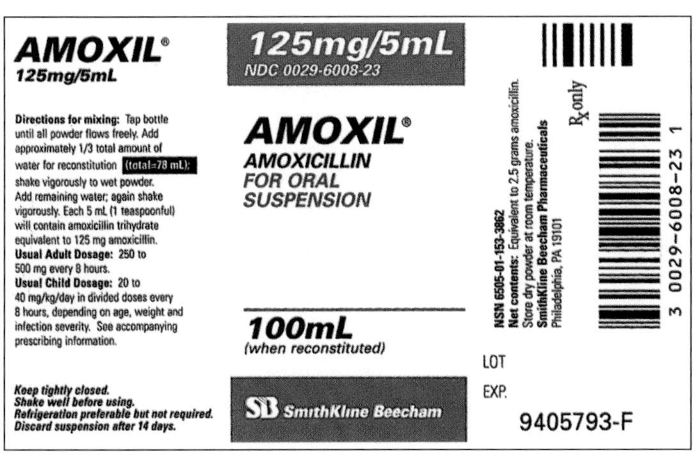

22. Mr. Sawyer is admitted with congestive heart failure. His orders require Lasix 80 mg po daily. How many tablets will the nurse administer per dose? _______

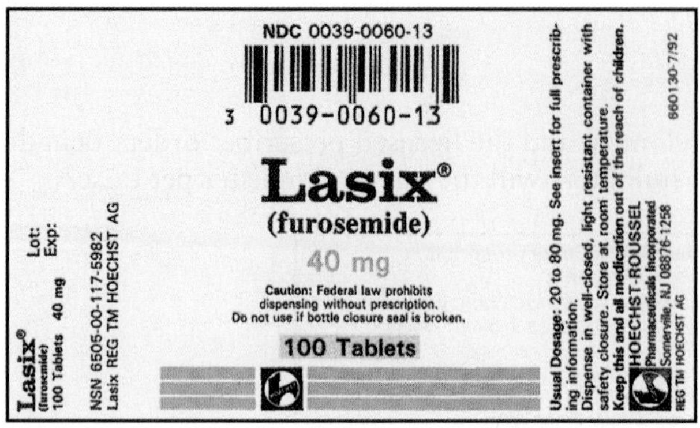

23. The licensed prescriber orders nitroglycerin 0.4 mg sublingual prn for angina. The patient should take no more than three tablets in 15 minutes. Mr. Cane took two tablets 5 minutes apart. How many milligrams did he receive? _______

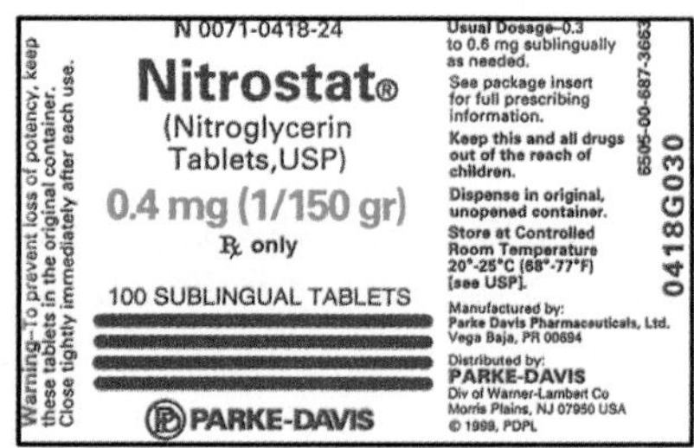

24. Mr. Koehler has rheumatoid arthritis and has Decadron 1.5 mg po q 12 h ordered. You have Decadron elixir 0.5 mg/5 mL. How many milliliters will you administer per dose? _______ How many ounces will you administer per dose? _______

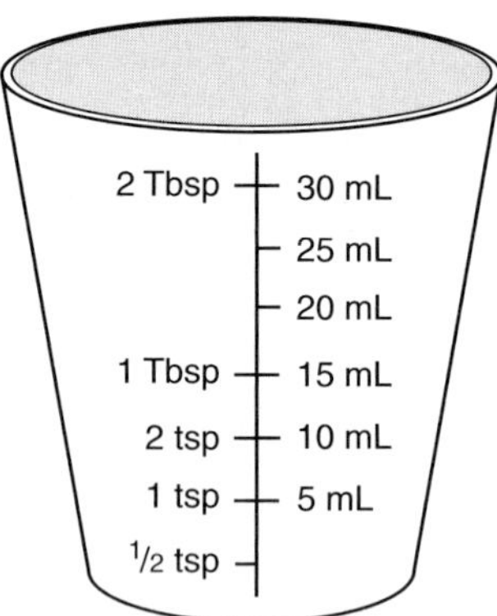

25. Your adult patient has acute bronchitis and has cefaclor 500 mg po q 12 h ordered. How many milliliters will you administer per dose? _______

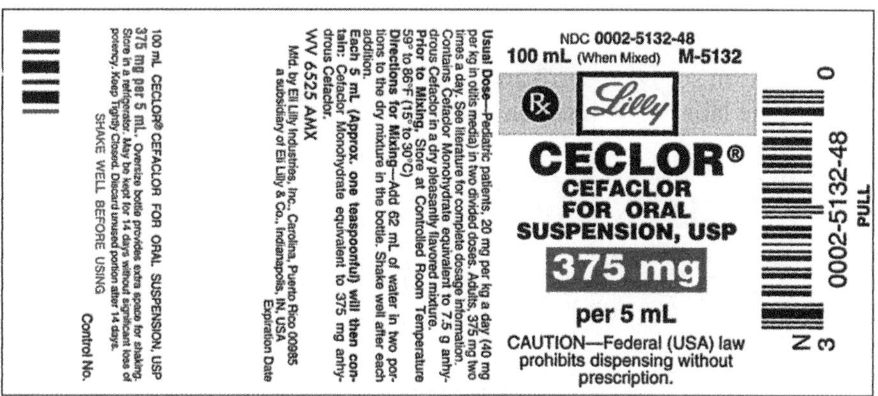

26. Mrs. Turner is admitted with hypertension. Apresoline 25 mg po four times a day is ordered. You have 50-mg scored tablets available. How many tablets will you administer per dose? _______

27. Your patient complains of indigestion during meals. Mylanta 30 mL po pc four times a day is ordered. Mylanta is supplied in a 360-mL bottle. There are _______ doses in one 360-mL bottle.

28. The licensed prescriber orders Halcion 0.25 mg po at bedtime. How many tablets will the nurse administer per dose? _______

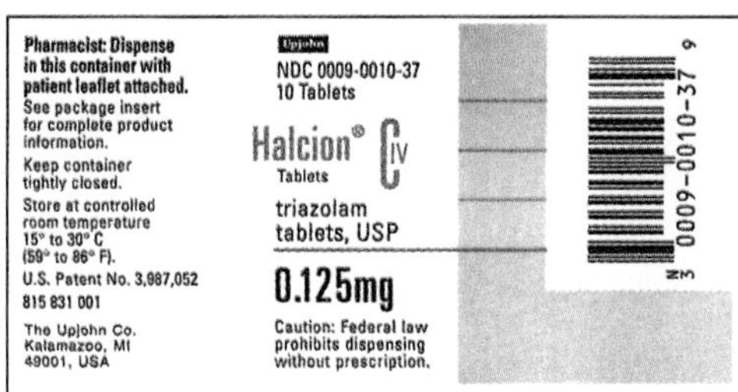

29. Mr. Bates has a history of seizure activity. Phenobarbital 15 mg po q 3 h is ordered. How many tablets will the nurse administer per dose? _______

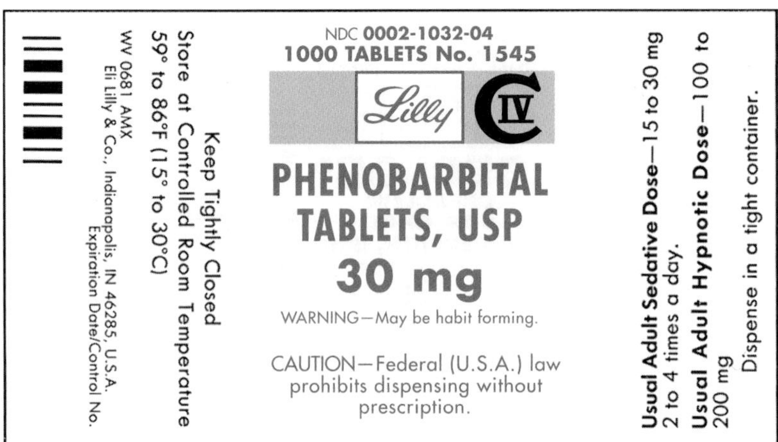

30. Mrs. Ortega has chronic sinusitis. Her licensed prescriber orders amoxicillin 125 mg po q 8 h. How many milliliters will the nurse administer per dose? _______

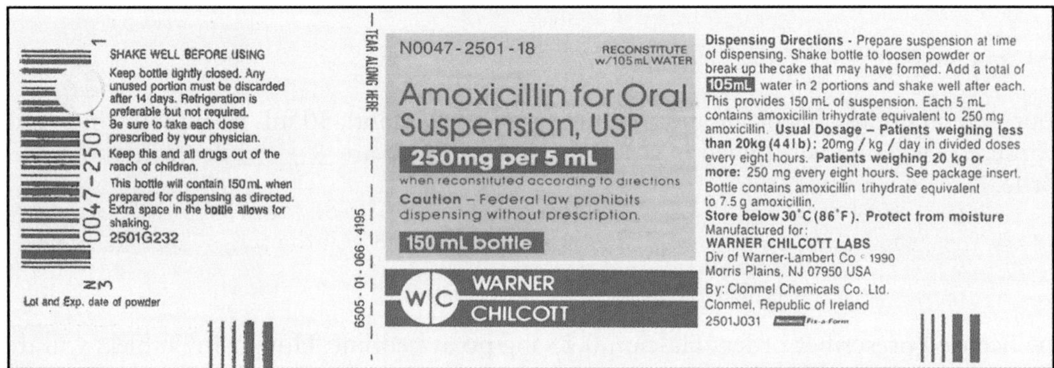

31. The licensed prescriber prescribes Tenormin 25 mg po q 4 h for Mr. Hutton's high blood pressure. How many tablets will you administer per dose? _______

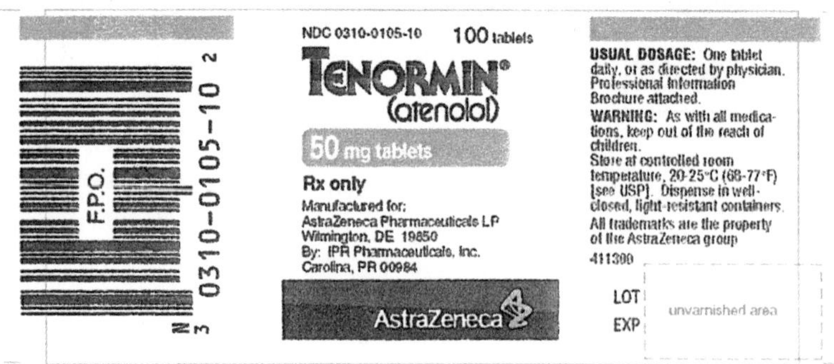

32. The licensed prescriber orders quinidine 0.6 g po q 4 h. Quinidine is supplied in 200-mg tablets. How many tablets will you give for one dose? _______ How many tablets will you give in 24 hours? _______

33. Mrs. Farmer has Zofran 8 mg po three times a day ordered for relief of nausea. How many milliliters will the nurse administer per dose? _______

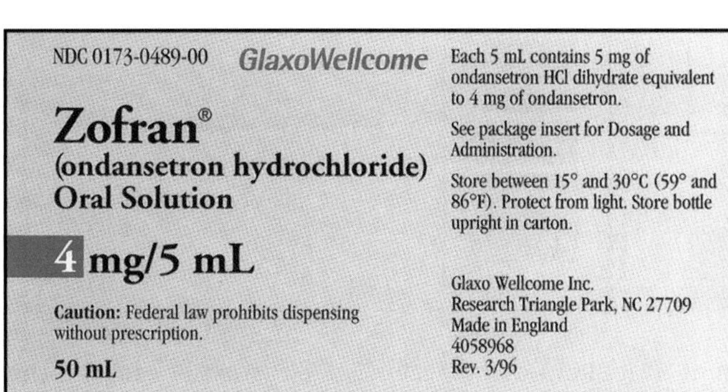

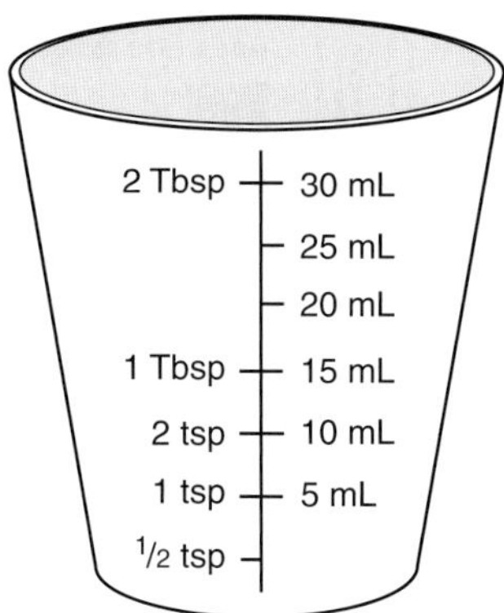

34. Your patient has Cipro 750 mg po q 12 h ordered for a severe respiratory tract infection. You have Cipro oral suspension 500 mg/5 mL available. How many milliliters will you administer per dose? _______

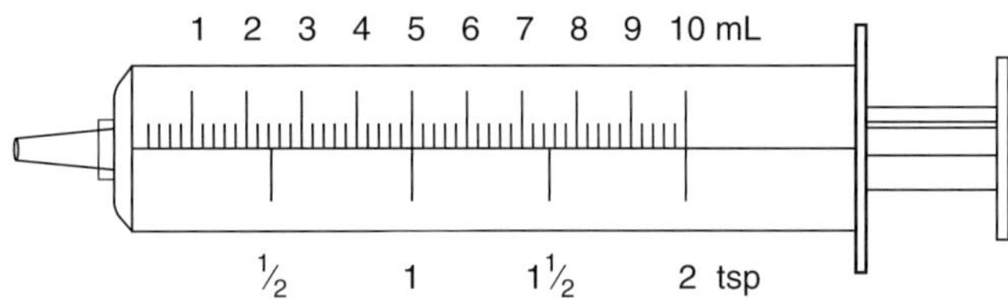

35. Mr. Golden, recovering from a left great toe amputation, has Colace elixir 100 mg po at bedtime ordered for constipation. How many milliliters will the nurse administer per dose? _______

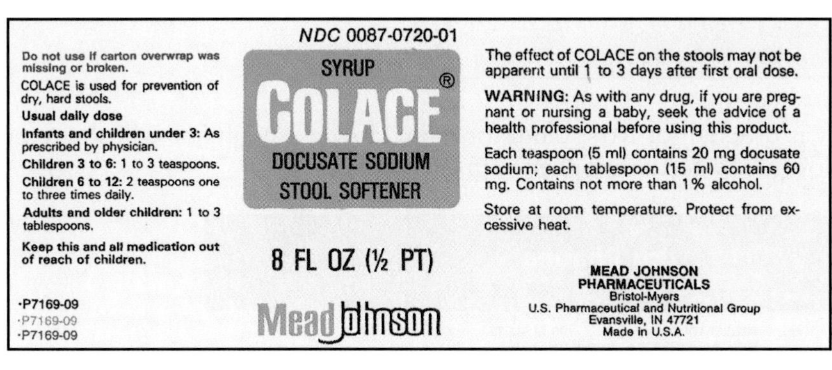

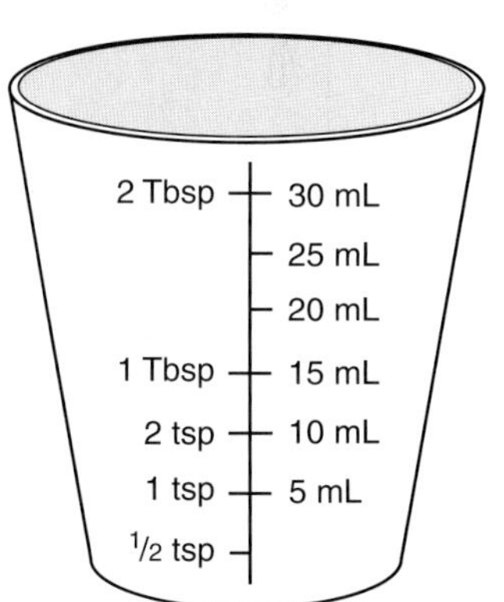

36. Mr. Malito is to receive Procanbid 1 g po now. How many tablets will you administer per dose? _______

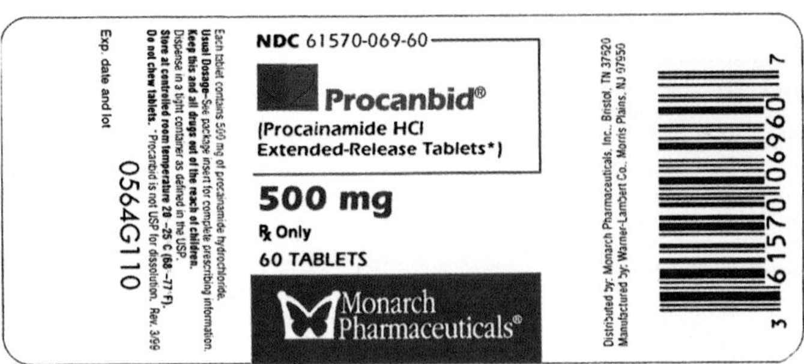

37. Mr. Mikal was admitted for treatment of leukemia and receives Deltasone 7.5 mg po three times a day as part of his chemotherapy. The drug is available in 2.5-mg tablets. How many tablets will the nurse administer per dose? _______

38. The licensed prescriber orders Tegretol 0.2 g po three times a day for Mr. Pine's epilepsy. How many tablets will the nurse administer per dose? _______

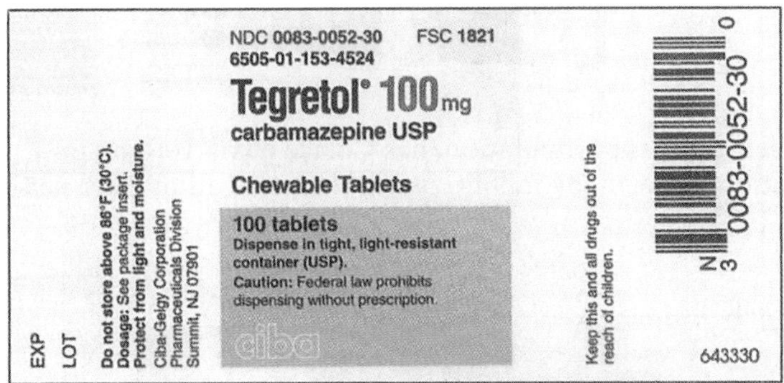

39. Lortab 5/500 po now is ordered for Mrs. Lindl for pain. How many tablets will she receive per dose? _______ How much acetaminophen is in each tablet? _______

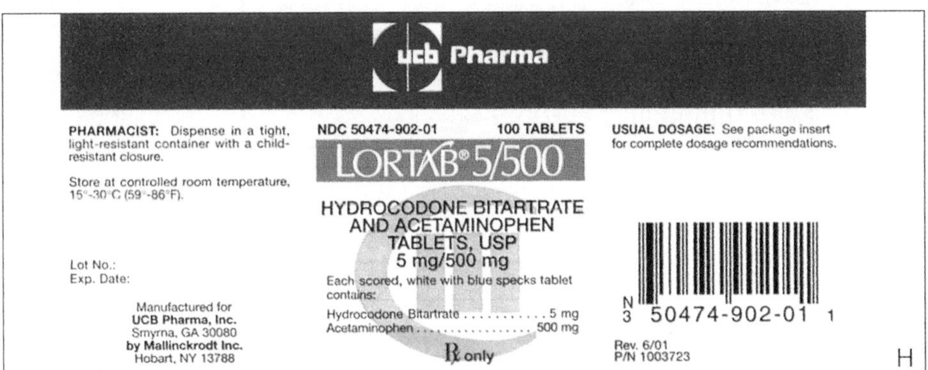

40. Mrs. Cross was admitted with a myasthenia crisis. Decadron 0.5 mg po q 12 h is ordered. How many tablets will the nurse administer per dose? _______

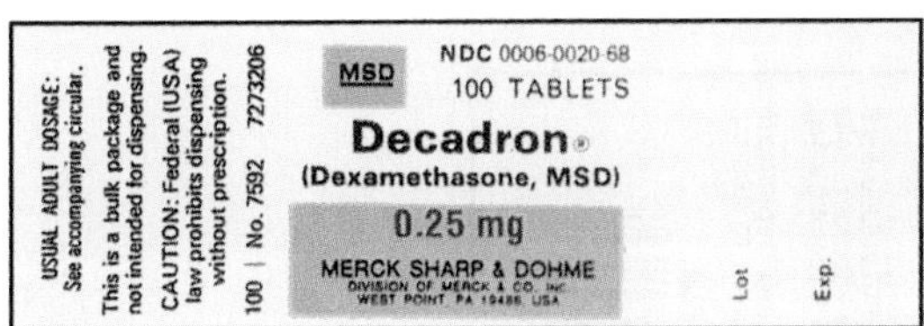

41. Mr. Cook requires medication for nausea. Compazine 10 mg po q 4 h prn is ordered. You have Compazine 5-mg tablets available. How many tablets will you administer per dose? _______

42. Mr. Pace receives Atarax 100 mg po at bedtime prn to relieve anxiety. You have 50-mg tablets available. How many tablets will you administer per dose? _______

43. The licensed prescriber orders Rifadin 600 mg po 1 hour before dinner daily. How many capsules will the nurse administer per dose? _______

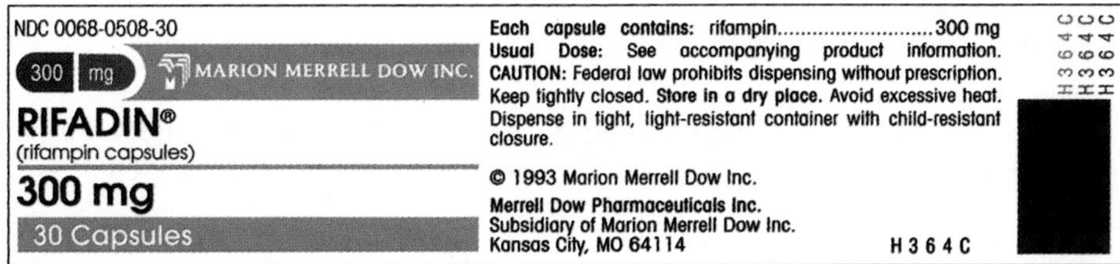

44. Mr. Day receives Lanoxin 0.25 mg po daily for atrial fibrillation. How many tablets will the nurse administer per dose? _______

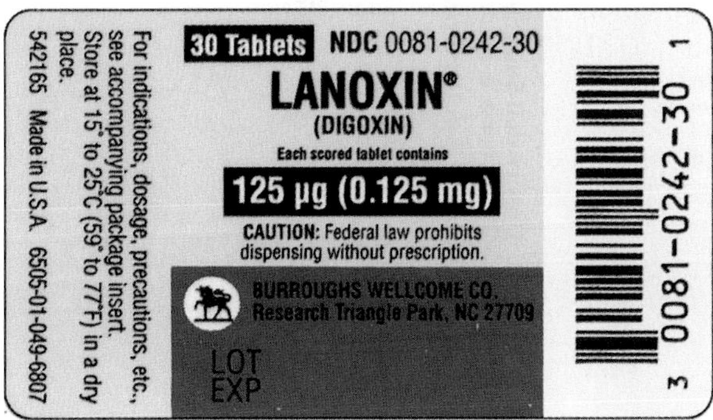

45. Mr. Payne receives Keflex 500 mg po four times a day before his dental extraction. How many capsules will the nurse administer in each dose? _______ How many capsules will the nurse administer for 1 day? _______

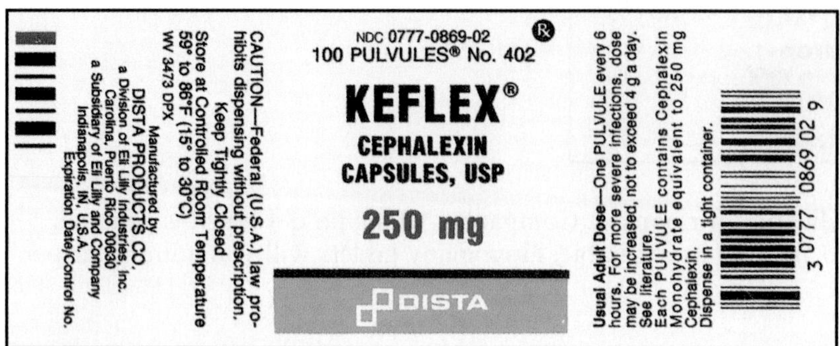

46. Mr. Tune is experiencing gastroesophageal reflux. The licensed prescriber orders Nexium 40 mg po daily for 3 days. How many capsules will the nurse administer per dose? _______

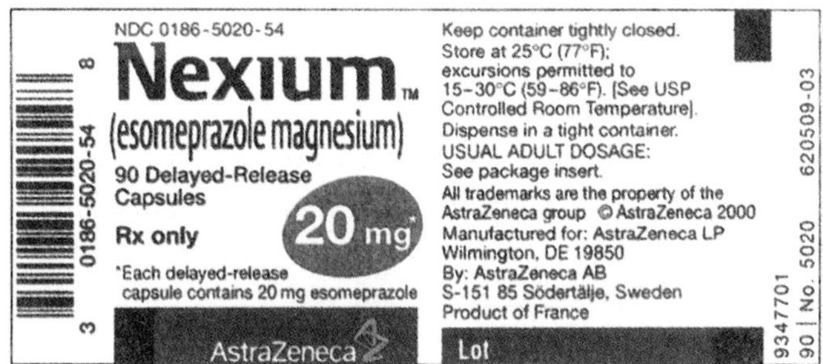

47. Mrs. Graves receives phenobarbital tablets 90 mg po q 3 h prn for seizure activity. How many tablets will the nurse administer per dose? _______

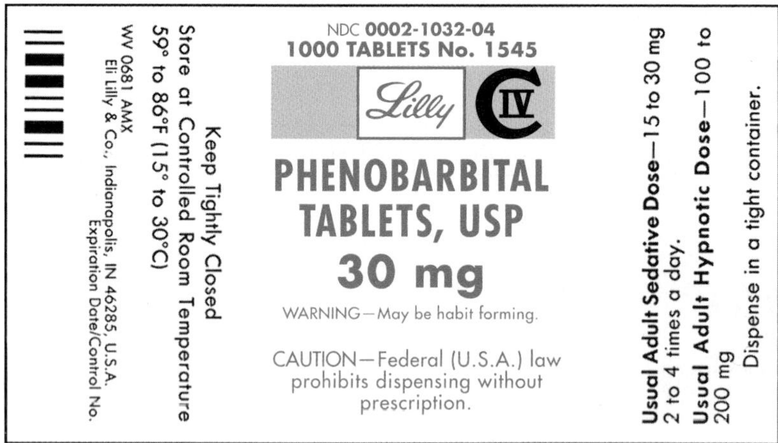

48. Mr. Vee is enrolled in a smoking-cessation program. He is to begin with Wellbutrin 150 mg po daily for 3 days. How many tablets will the nurse administer per dose? _______

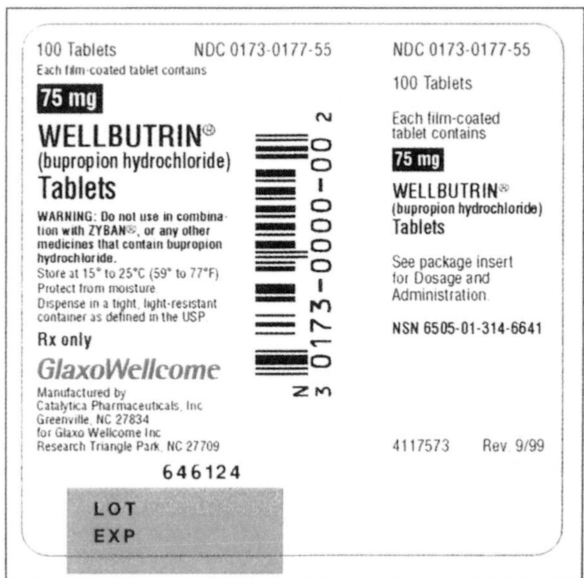

49. Mr. Sahl, recovering from a coronary artery bypass graft, receives Capoten 25 mg po twice a day. How many tablets will the nurse administer per dose? _______

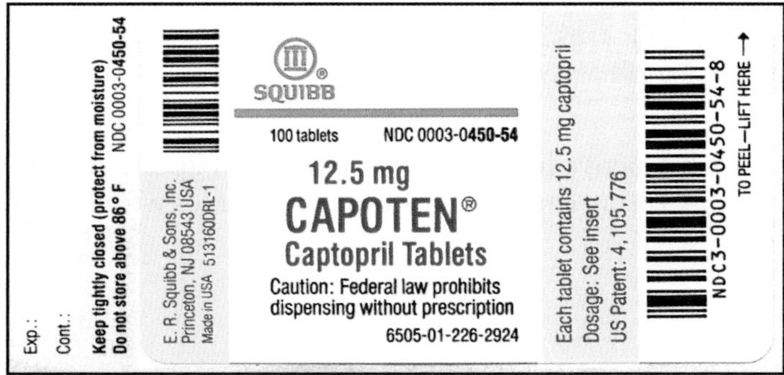

50. Mr. Dale receives Zantac 150 mg two times a day as part of his treatment for esophagitis. How many milliliters will the nurse administer per dose? _______

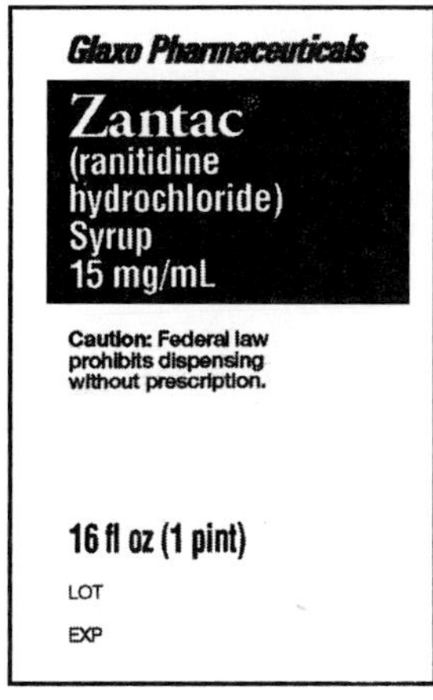

51. Mrs. Line has erythromycin 500 mg po q 6 h prescribed for treatment of her strep throat. How many tablets will you administer per dose? _______

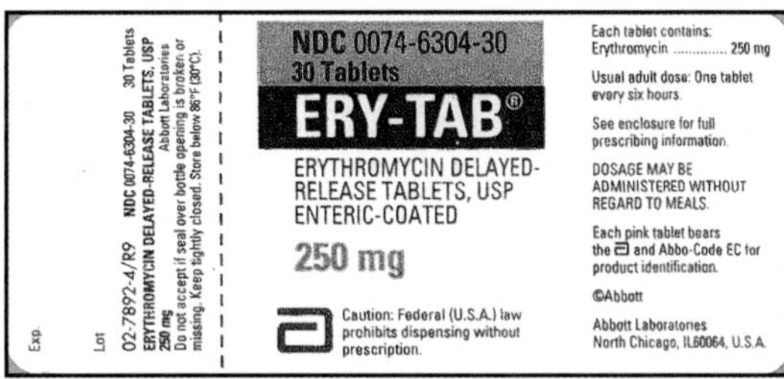

52. The licensed prescriber has prescribed Cytotec 0.2 mg po four times daily with meals and at bedtime for a patient with a history of gastric ulcers. How many tablets will the patient receive for each dose? _______

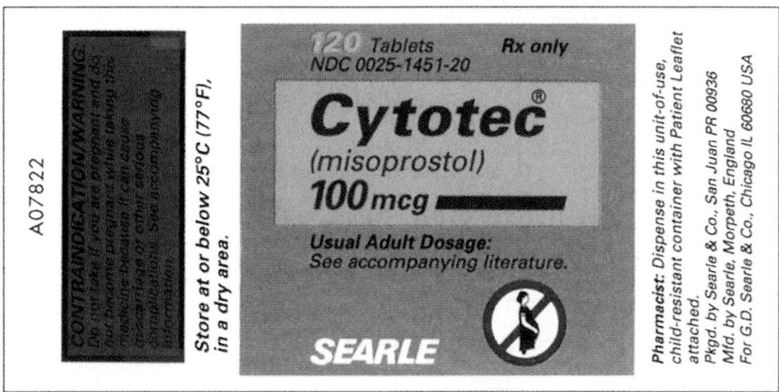

53. Mr. Romero, admitted with chronic obstructive lung disease, takes Bentyl 20 mg po three times a day ac. The drug is available in 10-mg capsules. How many capsules will the nurse administer per dose? _______

54. Mrs. Tyth has pruritic dermatosis. The licensed prescriber prescribes Atarax 30 mg po two times daily as part of her therapy. The drug is supplied in syrup containing 10 mg/5 mL. How many milliliters will the nurse administer per dose? _______

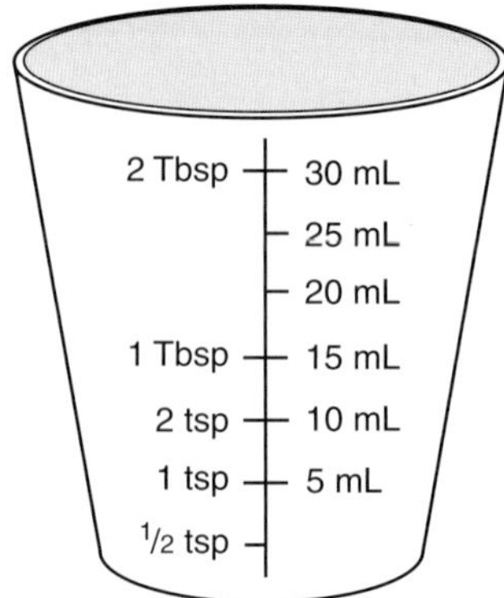

55. Mrs. Gale, admitted for alcohol abuse, has an order for ascorbic acid 0.75 g po daily while hospitalized. You have 250-mg tablets available. How many tablets will you administer per dose? _______

56. Your patient who is receiving chemotherapy has an order for Zofran 8 mg po ½ hour before chemotherapy for relief of nausea. How many milliliters will the nurse administer per dose? _______

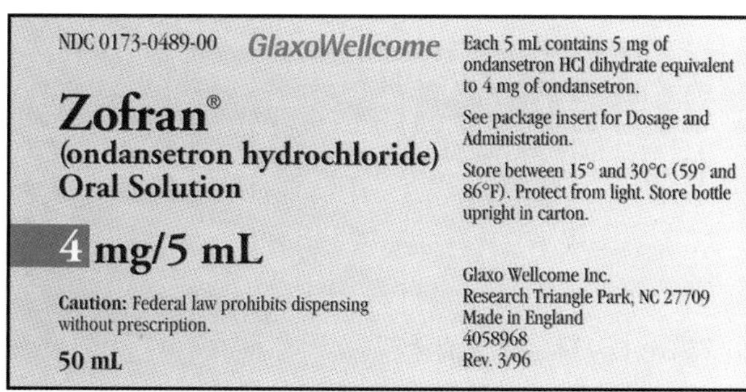
NDC 0173-0489-00
GlaxoWellcome
Zofran®
(ondansetron hydrochloride)
Oral Solution
4 mg/5 mL
Caution: Federal law prohibits dispensing without prescription.
50 mL
Each 5 mL contains 5 mg of ondansetron HCl dihydrate equivalent to 4 mg of ondansetron.
See package insert for Dosage and Administration.
Store between 15° and 30°C (59° and 86°F). Protect from light. Store bottle upright in carton.
Glaxo Wellcome Inc.
Research Triangle Park, NC 27709
Made in England
4058968
Rev. 3/96

57. Mr. Nade, hospitalized for a radical neck dissection, has Vistaril 15 mg po four times a day ordered to suppress nausea. You have Vistaril 25 mg/5 mL available. How many milliliters will you administer per dose? _______

58. Mrs. Snell requires Lopressor 100 mg po two times daily. How many tablets will the nurse administer per dose? _______

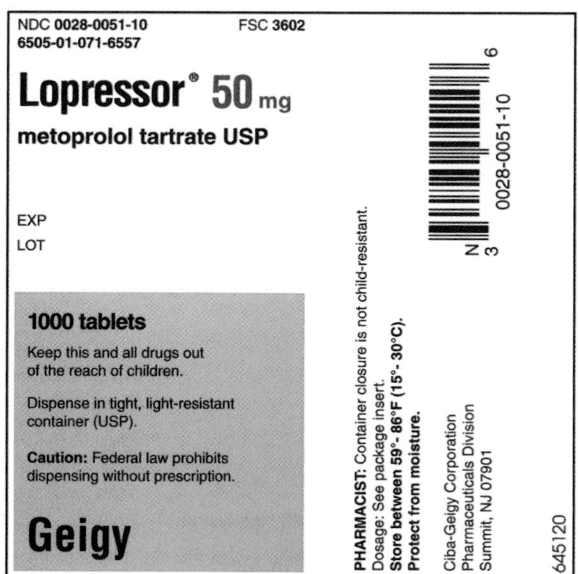
NDC 0028-0051-10
6505-01-071-6557
FSC 3602
Lopressor® 50 mg
metoprolol tartrate USP
EXP
LOT
1000 tablets
Keep this and all drugs out of the reach of children.
Dispense in tight, light-resistant container (USP).
Caution: Federal law prohibits dispensing without prescription.
Geigy
PHARMACIST: Container closure is not child-resistant.
Dosage: See package insert.
Store between 59°- 86°F (15°- 30°C).
Protect from moisture.
Ciba-Geigy Corporation
Pharmaceuticals Division
Summit, NJ 07901
N 3 0028-0051-10 6
645120

59. Your patient with type 2 adult-onset diabetes mellitus receives metformin hydrochloride 1 g po twice daily. How many tablets will the nurse administer per dose? _______

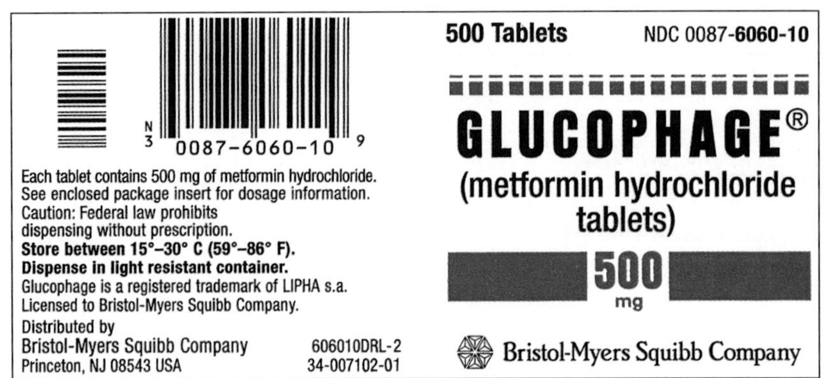

60. Mr. Aden requires Chloromycetin 250 mg po q 6 h for treatment of a *Salmonella* infection. You have Chloromycetin 150 mg/5 mL available. How many milliliters will you administer per dose? _______

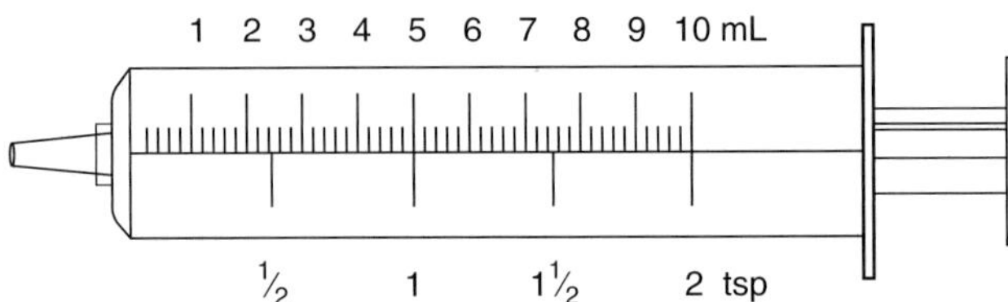

61. Mr. Scheottle receives Vibramycin 100 mg po q 12 h for treatment of inclusion conjunctivitis. How many milliliters will the nurse administer per dose? _______

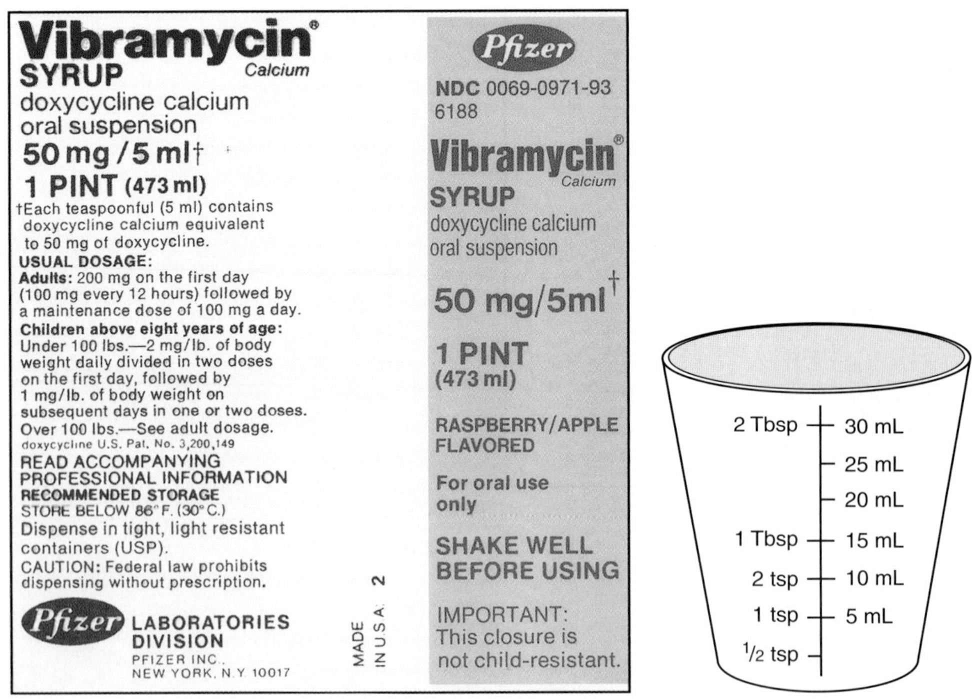

62. Your patient, admitted for cardiac catheterization, receives HydroDIURIL 25 mg po two times a day for hypertension. You have 50-mg scored tablets available. How many tablets will you administer per dose? _______

63. Tylenol 240 mg po q 4 h is ordered for a temperature of 38.9° C. You have Tylenol 80-mg chewable tablets available. How many tablets will be required for each dose? _______

64. The licensed prescriber prescribes Lanoxin elixir 90 mcg po two times a day for your patient with atrial fibrillation. How many milliliters will you administer per dose? _______

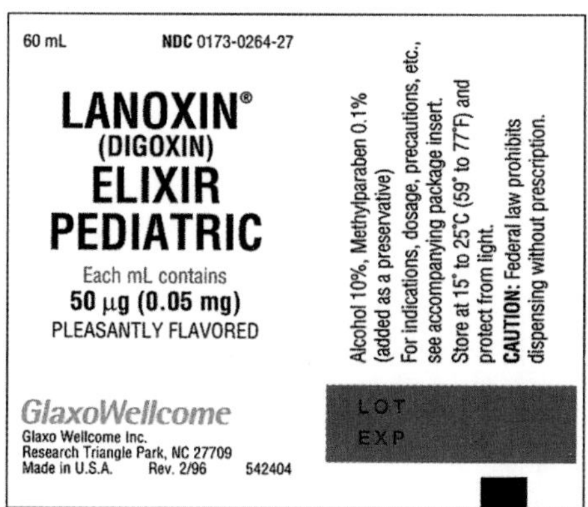
60 mL
NDC 0173-0264-27
LANOXIN®
(DIGOXIN)
ELIXIR
PEDIATRIC
Each mL contains
50 μg (0.05 mg)
PLEASANTLY FLAVORED
GlaxoWellcome
Glaxo Wellcome Inc.
Research Triangle Park, NC 27709
Made in U.S.A. Rev. 2/96 542404
Alcohol 10%, Methylparaben 0.1% (added as a preservative)
For indications, dosage, precautions, etc., see accompanying package insert.
Store at 15° to 25°C (59° to 77°F) and protect from light.
CAUTION: Federal law prohibits dispensing without prescription.
LOT
EXP

65. Mr. Ceney, admitted for contact dermatitis, receives elixir of Benadryl 10 mL po q 6 h prn for relief of itching. The drug is supplied as 12.5 mg/5 mL. This dose delivers _______ mg.

66. The licensed prescriber orders Indocin 50 mg po twice a day. How many capsules will the nurse administer per dose? _______

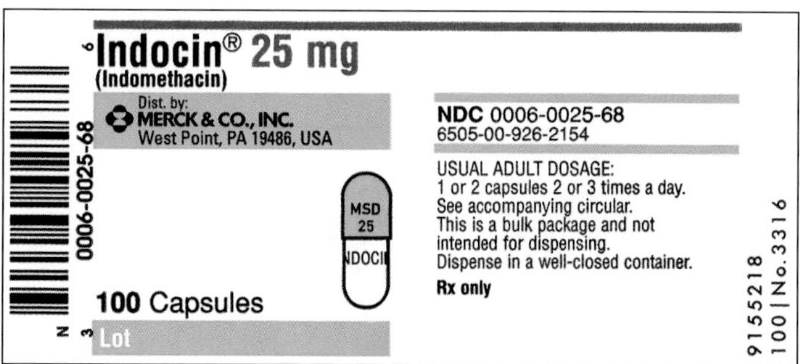
Indocin® 25 mg
(Indomethacin)
Dist. by:
MERCK & CO., INC.
West Point, PA 19486, USA
0006-0025-68
NDC 0006-0025-68
6505-00-926-2154
USUAL ADULT DOSAGE:
1 or 2 capsules 2 or 3 times a day.
See accompanying circular.
This is a bulk package and not intended for dispensing.
Dispense in a well-closed container.
Rx only
MSD
25
100 Capsules
Lot
9155218
100 | No. 3316

67. Your patient receives Dilantin 90 mg po three times a day for past seizure activity. How many capsules will you administer per dose? _______

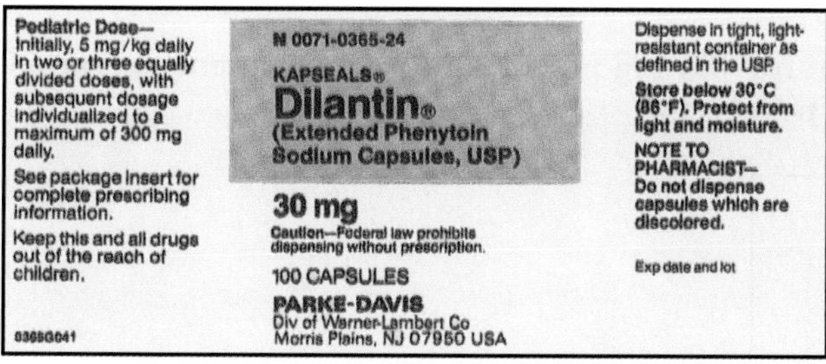
Pediatric Dose—Initially, 5 mg/kg daily in two or three equally divided doses, with subsequent dosage individualized to a maximum of 300 mg daily.
See package insert for complete prescribing information.
Keep this and all drugs out of the reach of children.
N 0071-0365-24
KAPSEALS®
Dilantin®
(Extended Phenytoin Sodium Capsules, USP)
30 mg
Caution—Federal law prohibits dispensing without prescription.
100 CAPSULES
PARKE-DAVIS
Div of Warner-Lambert Co
Morris Plains, NJ 07950 USA
Dispense in tight, light-resistant container as defined in the USP.
Store below 30°C (86°F). Protect from light and moisture.
NOTE TO PHARMACIST—Do not dispense capsules which are discolored.
Exp date and lot

68. The licensed prescriber orders Lipitor 40 mg po daily. You have available 10-mg, 20-mg, and 40-mg tablets. Which tablet would be most appropriate? _______ How many tablets will you administer per dose? _______

69. Your patient, admitted with a small-bowel obstruction, has KCl 10 mEq po daily ordered for his low potassium level. The drug is available as a liquid in KCl 20 mEq/15 mL. How many milliliters will you administer per dose? _______

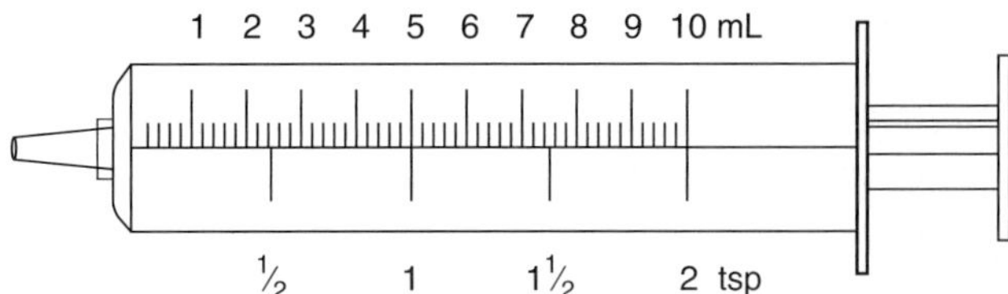

70. Mr. Brown receives dexamethasone 1.5 mg po q 12 h for inflammation. How many tablets will the nurse administer per dose? _______

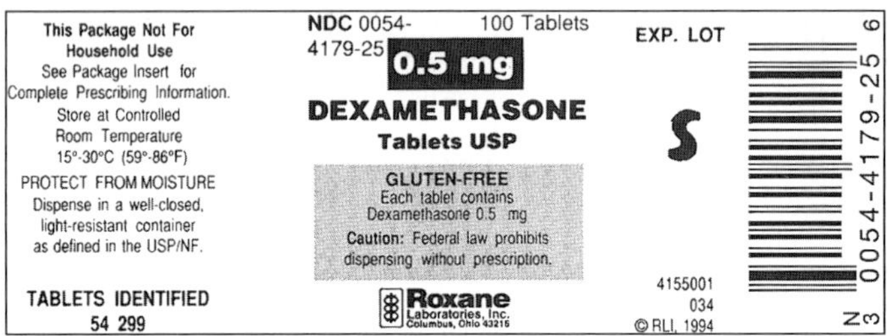

71. Mrs. Roget has been receiving digoxin 0.5 mg po daily for her cardiac dysrhythmia. The drug is available in 0.25-mg tablets. How many tablets will the nurse administer per dose? _______

72. Acetaminophen 650 mg po q 4 h is prescribed for a temperature of more than 38.5° C × 24 h. How many tablets will the nurse administer every 4 hours? _______

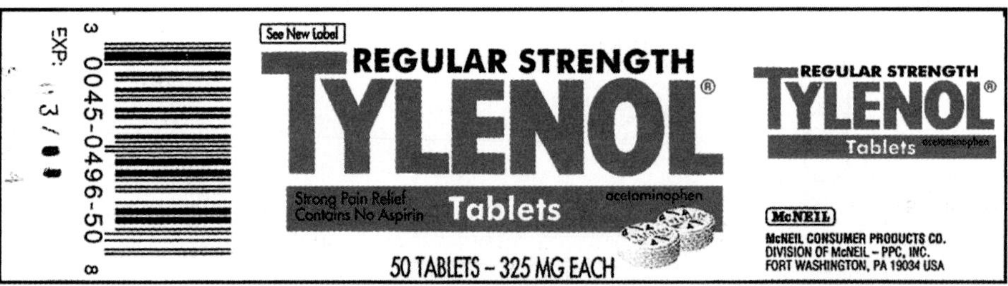

73. The licensed prescriber prescribes Decadron 0.5 mg po q 12 h for your patient's keratitis. How many tablets will you administer per dose? _______

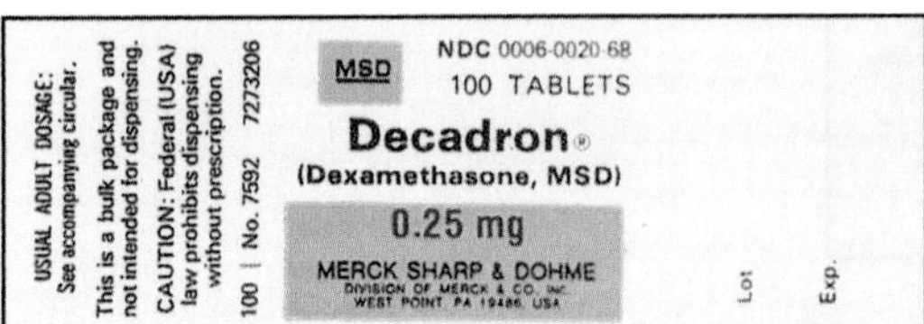

74. The licensed prescriber orders Keflex 375 mg po q 6 h for Mr. Pein for cellulitis. How many milliliters will the nurse administer per dose? _______

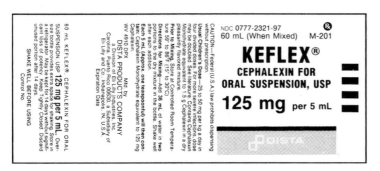

75. Mrs. Fare receives codeine 30 mg po q 3 h prn for pain relief after knee replacement surgery. How many tablets will you administer? _______

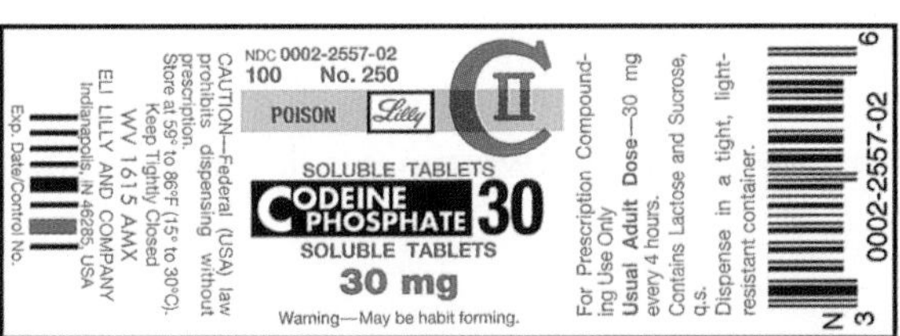

76. The licensed prescriber orders Crystodigin 0.3 mg po daily. You have Crystodigin in 0.05-mg, 0.15-mg, and 0.2-mg tablets. The best way to administer this drug is to give _______ tablets of _______ mg each.

77. Mr. Zeman has prednisone 7.5 mg po daily ordered for exfoliative dermatitis. Prednisone is supplied in 5-mg scored tablets. How many tablets will the nurse administer per dose? _______

78. Your patient who has had a partial craniotomy has Ceclor suspension 250 mg po four times a day ordered. How many milliliters will you administer per dose? _______

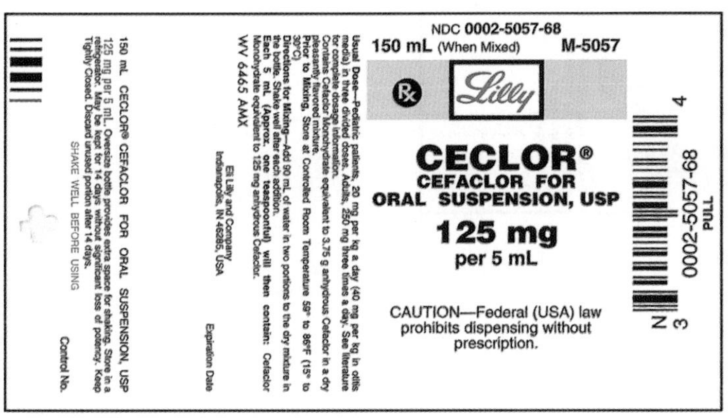

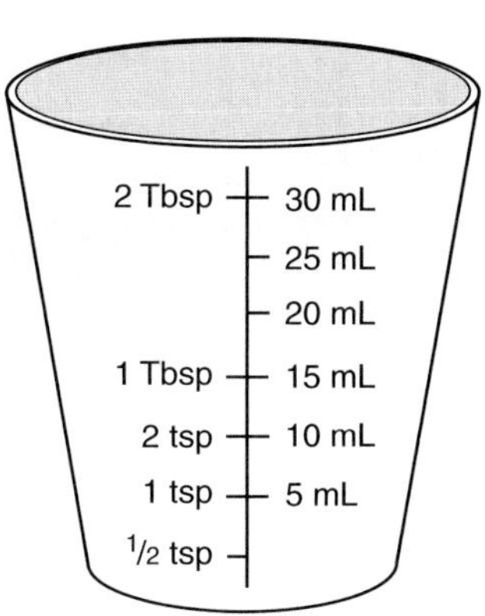

79. Your patient, who has undergone a coronary artery bypass graft, receives Surfak 250 mg po daily as a stool softener. How many capsules will you administer per dose? _______

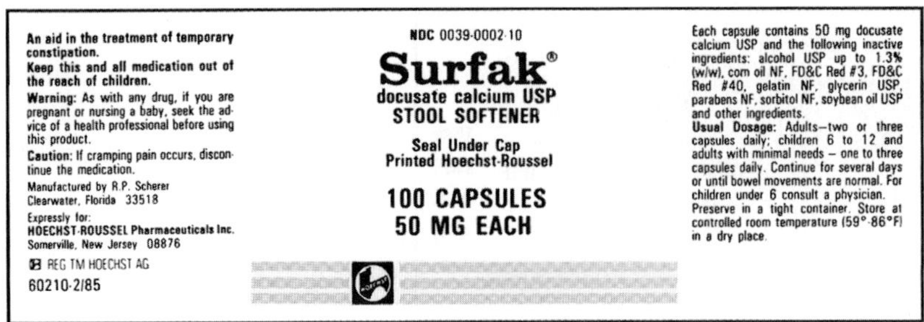

80. The licensed prescriber orders 20 mEq KCl elixir po three times a day. Elixir of KCl 15 mEq/11.25 mL is available. How many milliliters will you administer per dose? _______

81. Your patient with epilepsy receives phenobarbital 55 mg po two times a day. How many milliliters will you administer per dose? _______

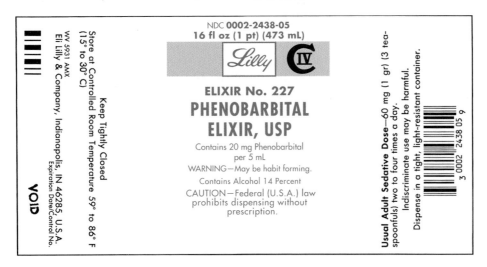

82. The licensed prescriber orders Aldomet 250 mg po two times a day. How many tablets will the nurse administer per dose? _______

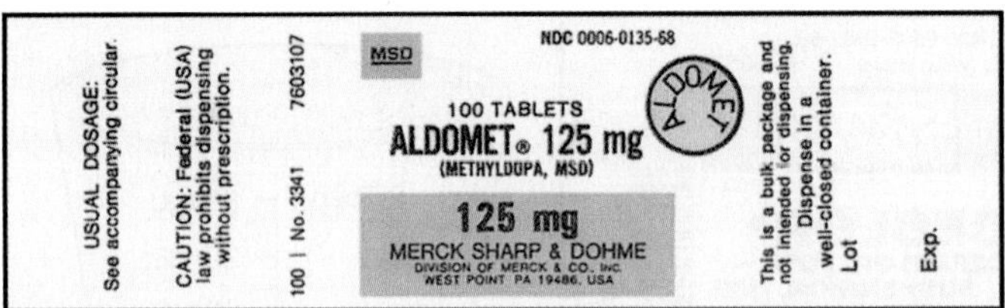

83. Mrs. Richardson, a patient who had a thyroidectomy, receives Synthroid 0.05 mg po daily in the morning. How many tablets will the nurse administer per dose? _______

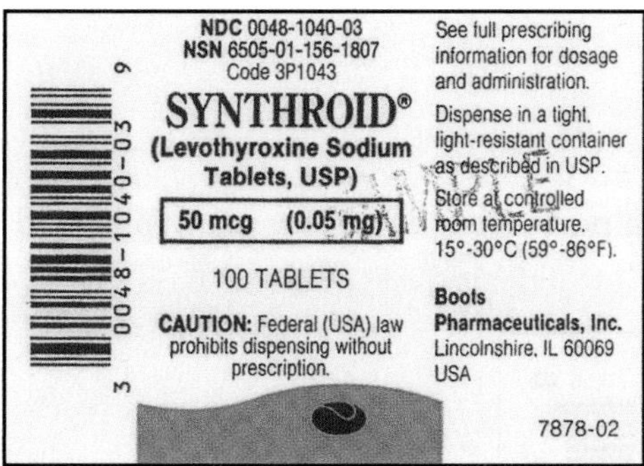

84. The licensed prescriber orders Theo-Dur 0.2 g po q 8 h. Theo-Dur is supplied in 100-mg, 200-mg, and 300-mg sustained-action tablets. Give _______ tablets of _______ mg. How many milligrams will be given per day? _______

85. Your patient who had a valve repair begins receiving Coumadin 15 mg po STAT. Coumadin 5-mg scored tablets are available. How many tablets will you administer per dose? _______

86. Your patient, who has an ulcer, receives cimetidine 800 mg po at bedtime. How many tablets will you administer each night? _______

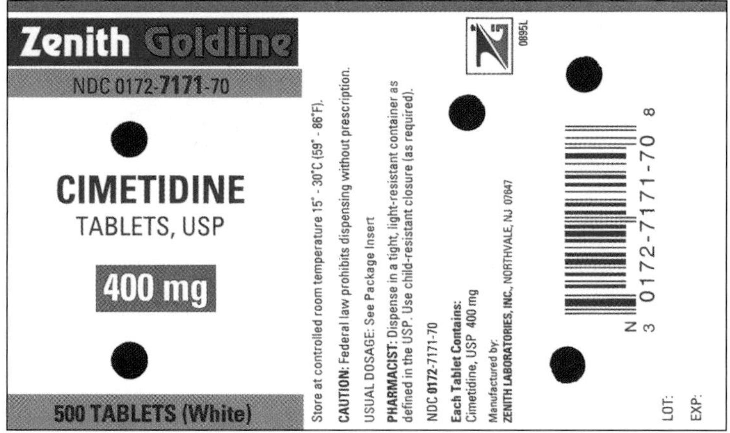

87. Your patient receives Keflex 0.5 g po four times a day. You have Keflex 250-mg capsules available. How many capsules will you administer? _______

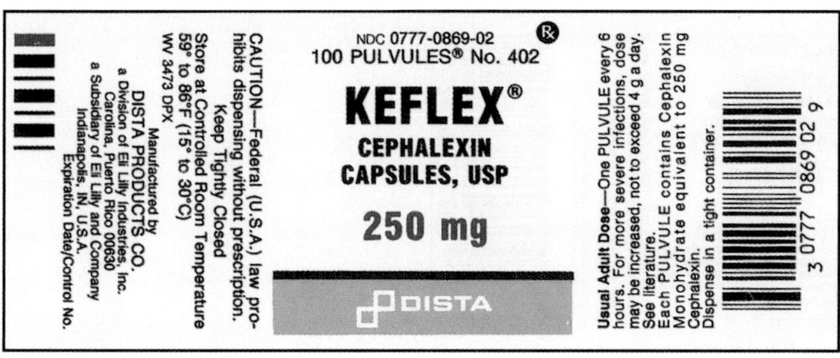

88. The licensed prescriber orders imipramine 50 mg po once in the morning and once at bedtime. The drug is supplied in 25-mg tablets. How many tablets will the nurse administer per dose? _______

89. Your patient with depression receives Prozac 30 mg po twice a day. How many pills will you administer per dose? _______

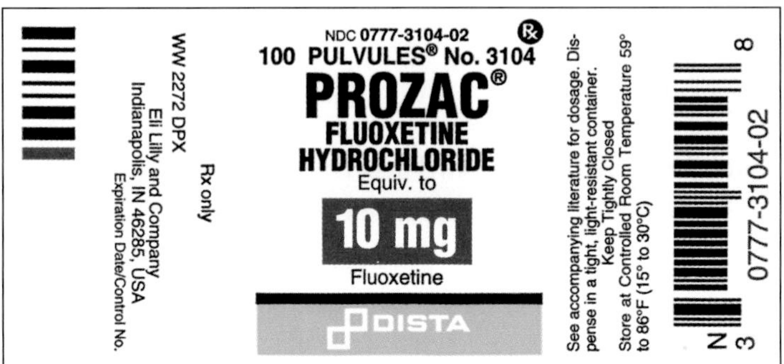

90. A patient receives Furosemide 6 mg po twice a day with meals. How many milliliters will be given per dose? _______

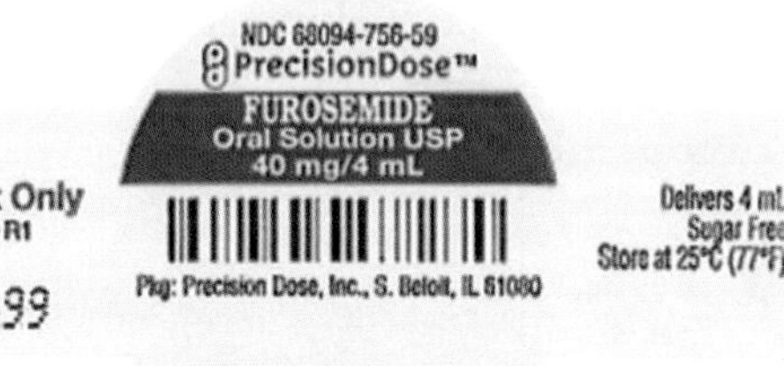

91. Mrs. Adams receives Cleocin 150 mg po q 6 h for her upper respiratory tract infection. Cleocin is supplied in 75-mg capsules. How many capsules will the nurse administer per dose? _______

92. Your patient receives Dilantin 200 mg po three times a day for seizures. How many capsules will you administer per dose? _______

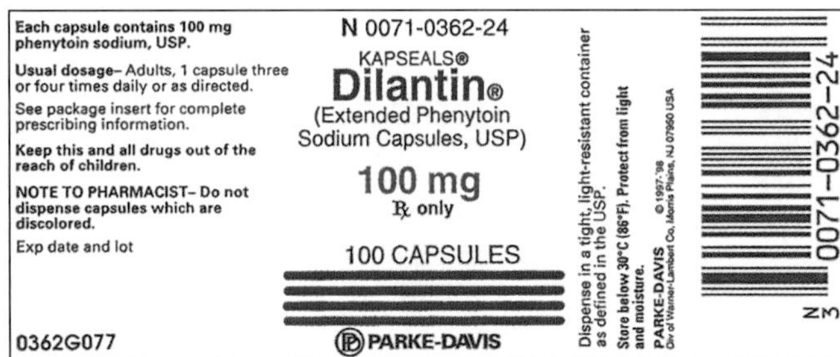

93. The licensed prescriber orders Coumadin 10 mg po at 1800 today. How many tablets will the nurse administer per dose? _______

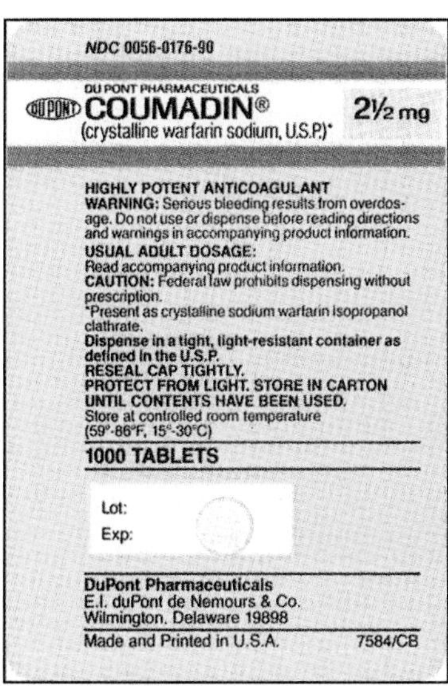

94. Your patient with diabetes receives Diabinese 0.25 g po daily in the morning. How many tablets will you administer per dose? _______

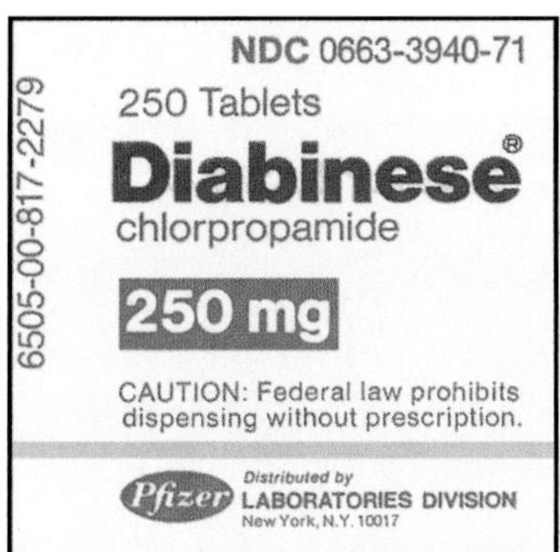

95. The licensed prescriber prescribes Apresoline 25 mg po two times a day for Mr. Yu's hypertension. You have Apresoline scored tablets 10 mg available. How many tablets will you administer per dose? _______

96. The licensed prescriber orders Flexeril 30 mg po at bedtime. Flexeril 10-mg tablets are available. How many tablets will the nurse administer per dose? _______

97. Your patient has begun receiving prednisone 15 mg po daily for asthma. Prednisone is available in 5-mg tablets. How many tablets will you administer per dose? _______

98. Mr. Gray, who has undergone cervical diskectomy, receives Restoril 0.015 g po at bedtime for insomnia. How many capsules will the nurse administer per dose? _______

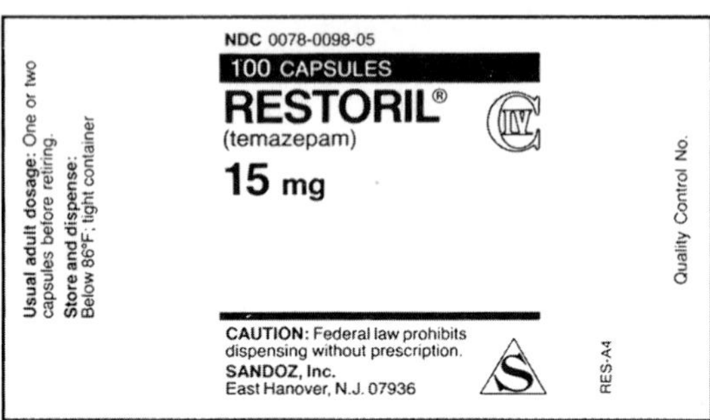

99. A patient receives KCl elixir 30 mEq po three times a day with juice. KCl 6.7 mEq/5 mL is available. How many milliliters will the nurse administer per dose? _______

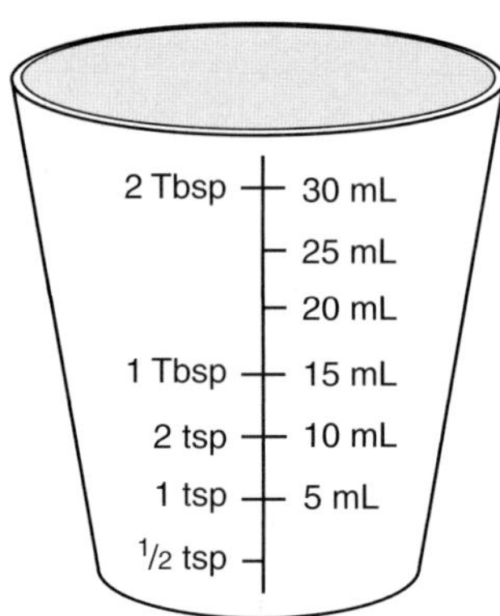

100. Mrs. Endres receives furosemide 20 mg po q 8 h for congestive heart failure. How many tablets will the nurse administer per dose? _______

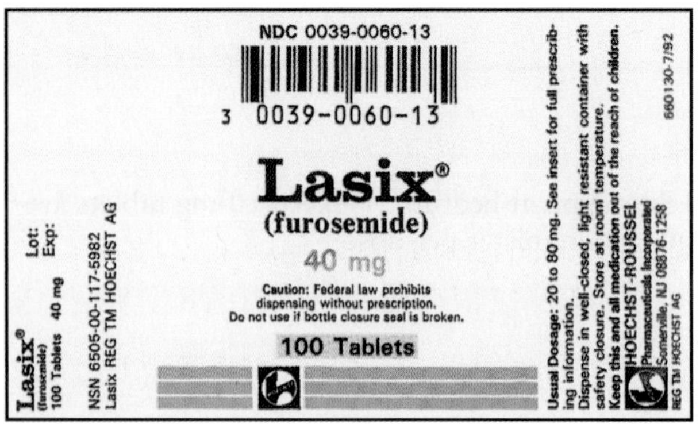

ANSWERS ON PP. 252–256 AND 258–274.

NAME ______________________

DATE ______________________

ACCEPTABLE SCORE **24**

YOUR SCORE ______

CHAPTER 11
Oral Dosages

POSTTEST 1

DIRECTIONS: The medication order is listed at the beginning of each problem. Calculate the oral doses. Show your work. Shade each medicine cup or oral syringe when provided to indicate the correct dose.

1. The licensed prescriber orders Cymbalta 60 mg po once a day for a patient with an anxiety disorder. How many tablets will the nurse administer per dose? _______

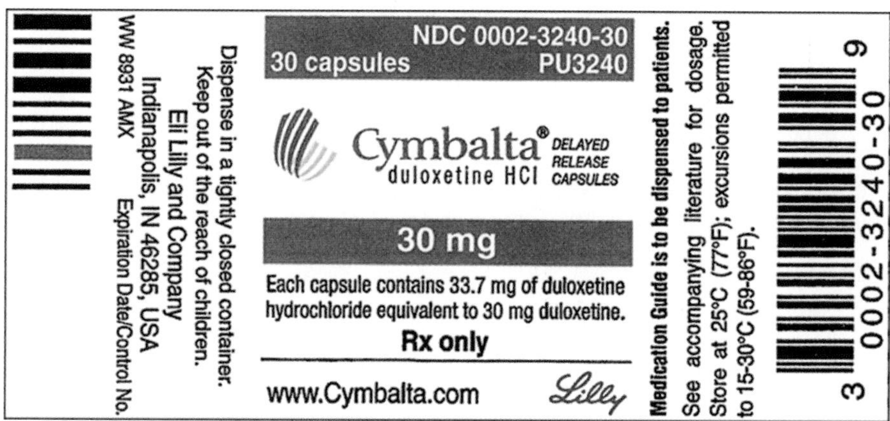

2. Mr. Clay receives tetracycline 0.5 g po four times a day for a gastrointestinal infection. How many capsules will the nurse administer per dose? _______

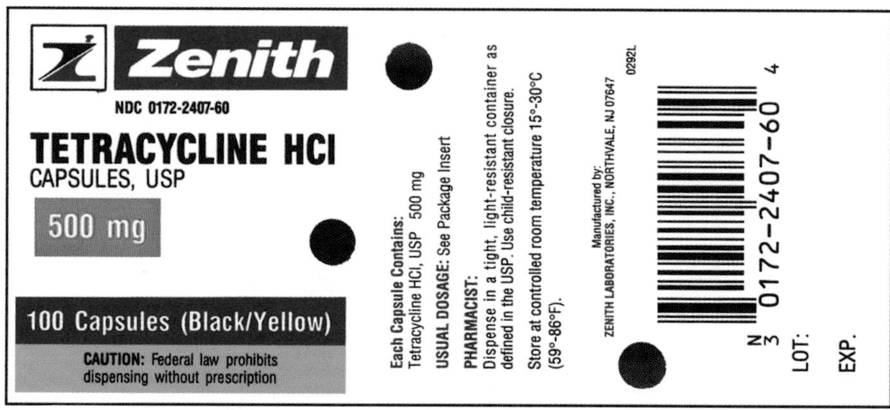

3. The licensed prescriber orders ampicillin 1 g po q 6 h for treatment of shigellosis. How many capsules will the nurse administer per dose? _______

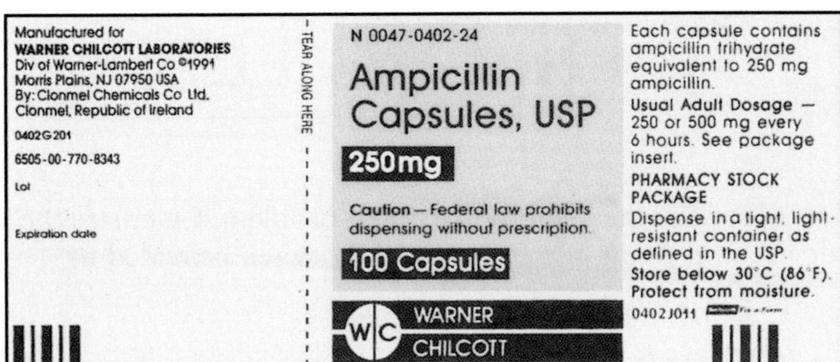

4. The licensed prescriber prescribes Allegra 60 mg two times a day for your patient's complaints of allergic rhinitis. You have 0.03-g tablets available. How many tablets will you administer per dose? _______

5. The licensed prescriber orders levothyroxine 100 mcg po daily. You have 0.05-mg tablets available. How many tablets will you administer per dose? _______

6. Mr. Shen, admitted with a psychoneurotic disorder, receives Atarax 25 mg po daily in the morning. You have Atarax 10 mg/5 mL. How many milliliters will you administer per dose? _______

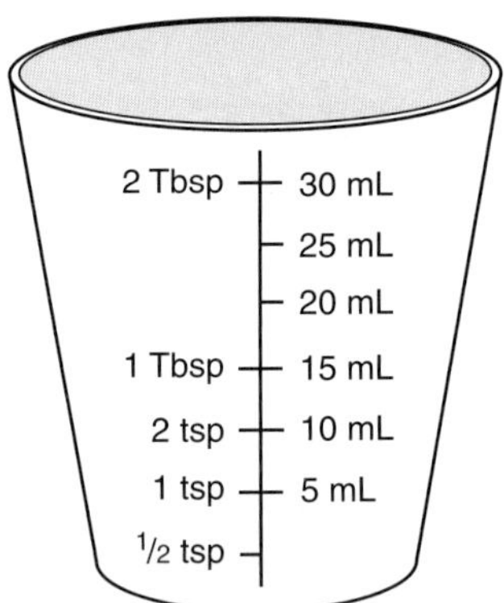

7. Your cardiac patient has Cardizem 60 mg four times a day ordered. How many tablets will you administer per dose? ____

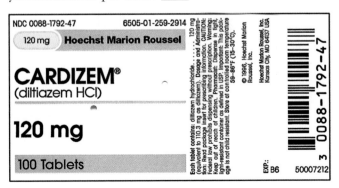

8. The licensed prescriber prescribes codeine 30 mg po q 3 h prn for pain relief for your patient with a total hip replacement. How many tablets will you administer per dose? _______

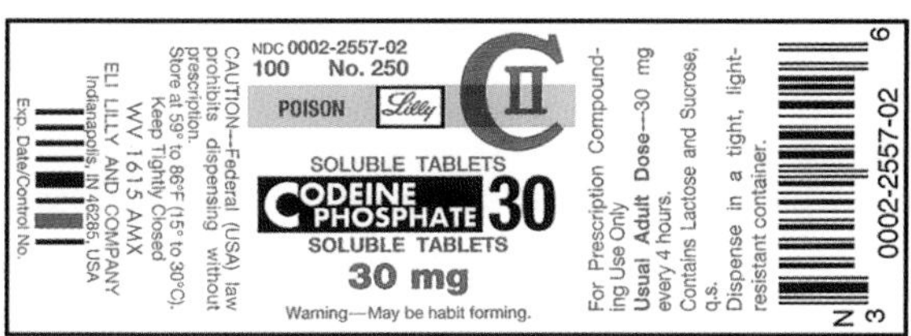

9. Your patient receives Vistaril 50 mg po three times a day for preoperative anxiety. Vistaril oral suspension 25 mg/5 mL is available. How many milliliters will you administer per dose? _______

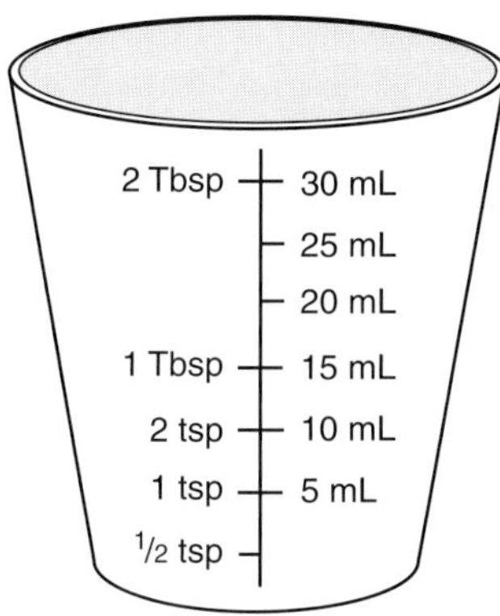

10. The licensed prescriber orders Prozac liquid 30 mg po twice a day. How many milliliters will you administer per dose? _______

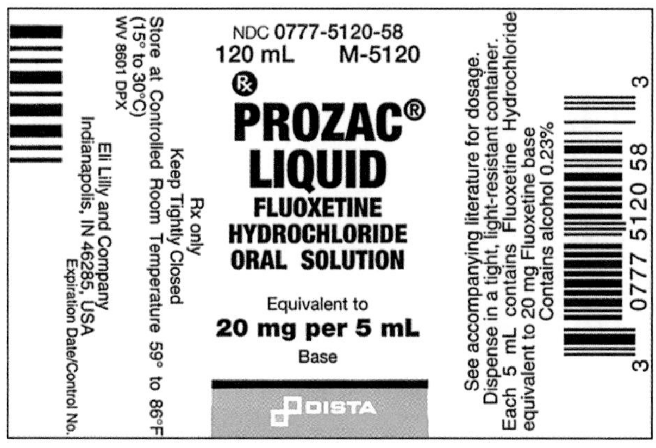

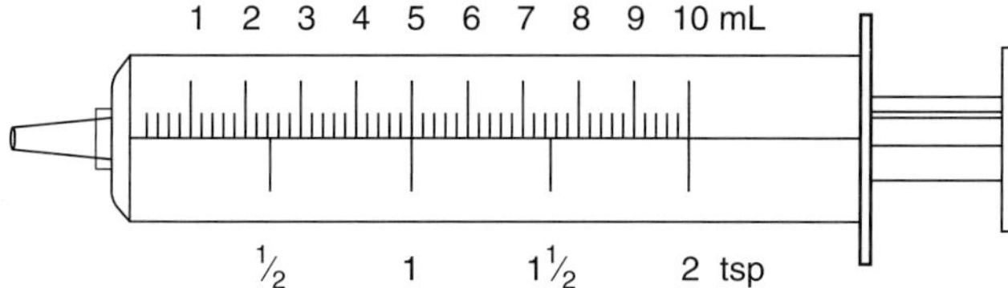

11. Your patient receives Crystodigin 0.1 mg po daily for an atrial arrhythmia. Crystodigin tablets 0.2 mg are available. How many tablets will you administer per dose? _______

12. The licensed prescriber prescribes KCl 20 mEq po twice a day for hypokalemia. KCl liquid is supplied 30 mEq/22.5 mL. How many milliliters will the nurse administer per dose? _______

13. The licensed prescriber orders Lipitor 40 mg po daily. How many tablets will you give per dose? _______

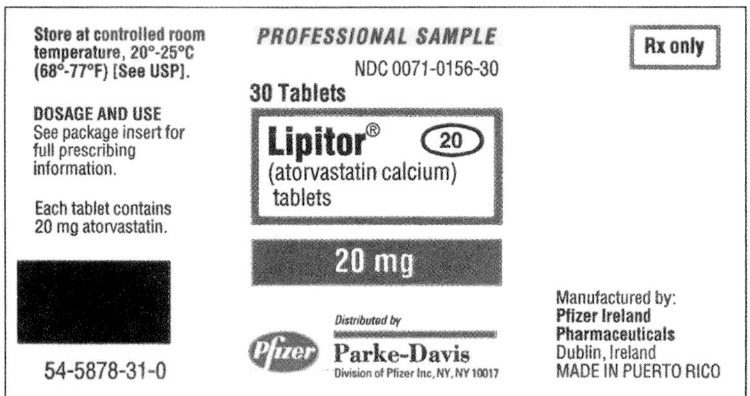

14. Your patient with a lumbar laminectomy has Benadryl 100 mg po at bedtime prn ordered for insomnia. How many capsules will you administer per dose? _______

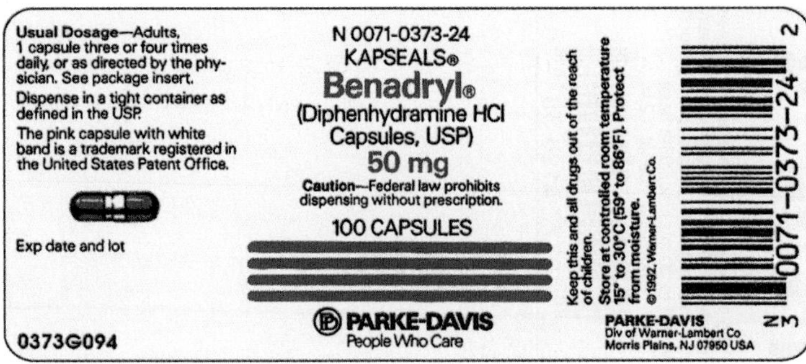

15. Your patient has Lasix 38 mg po q 12 h ordered for hypercalcemia. You have Lasix 10 mg/mL. How many milliliters will you administer per dose? _______

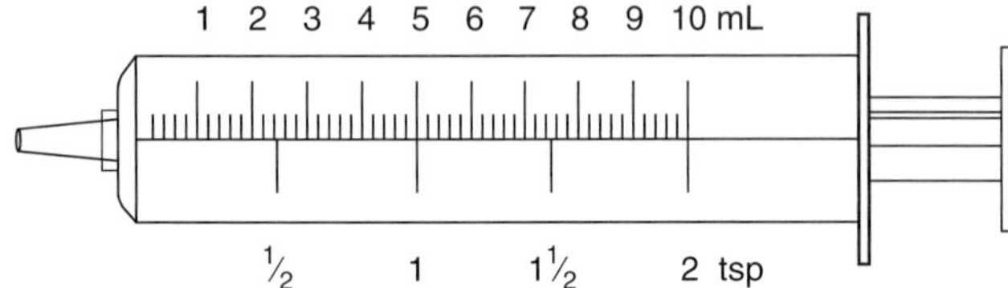

16. Mrs. Cook receives Keflex 100 mg po q 6 h for a sinus infection. How many milliliters will the nurse administer per dose? _______

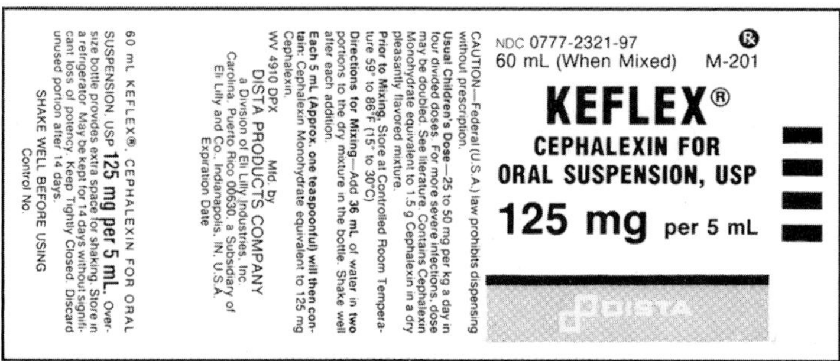

17. The licensed prescriber orders Mevacor 30 mg po daily to be given with the evening meal. You have 10-mg tablets available. How many tablets will you administer per dose? _______

18. Mr. Jones receives Inderal 80 mg po two times a day for a dysrhythmia. You have Inderal 40-mg scored tablets. How many tablets will you administer per dose? _______

19. The licensed prescriber prescribes Apresoline 20 mg po three times a day for your patient's hypertension. You have 10-mg tablets available. How many tablets will you administer per dose? _______

20. Your patient with epilepsy receives phenobarbital 90 mg po three times a day. How many tablets will you administer in each dose? _______ How many tablets will you administer in 1 day? _______

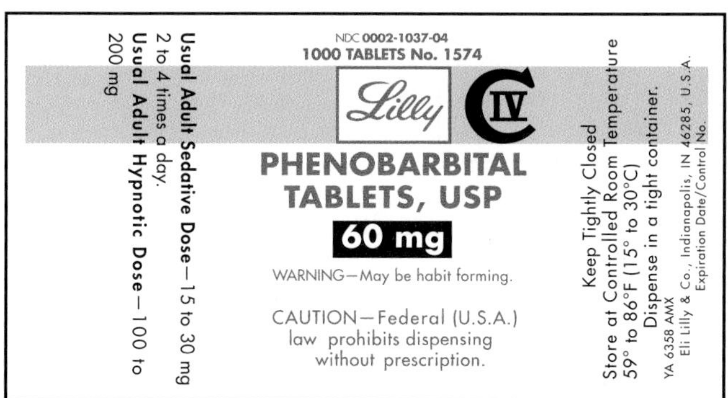

21. Mrs. Luther has alprazolam 0.5 mg po three times a day prescribed for her panic disorder. You have 0.25-mg tablets available. How many tablets will you administer per dose? _______

22. Mr. Barry has Ambien 10 mg po at bedtime ordered for insomnia. How many tablets will the nurse administer per dose? _______

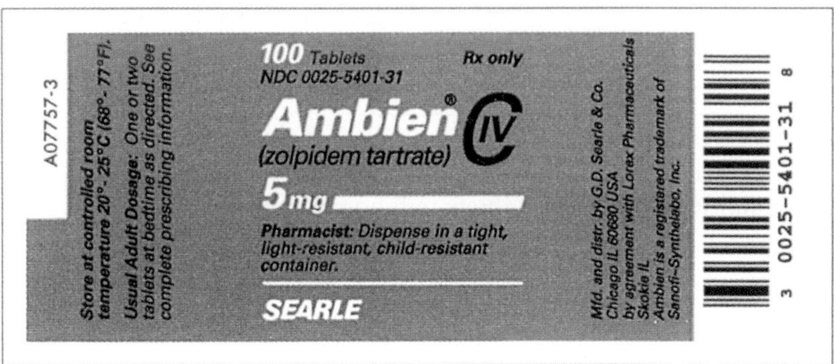

23. Mrs. Torres has metoprolol 150 mg po twice daily ordered for hypertension. You have metoprolol 100-mg scored tablets available. How many tablets will you administer per dose? _______

24. The licensed prescriber orders Zocor 30 mg po daily in the evening. How many tablets will you administer per dose? _______

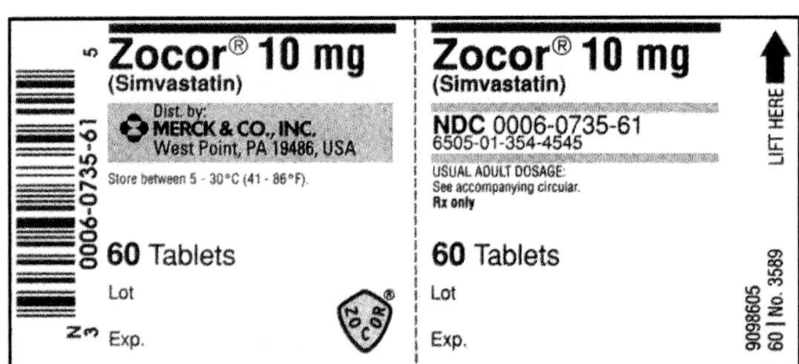

25. Mr. Bond has Allegra 60 mg po twice a day ordered. Allegra 30-mg tablets are available. How many tablets will you administer per dose? _______

ANSWERS ON PP. 256–257 AND 274–278.

NAME ______________________

DATE ______________________

ACCEPTABLE SCORE **24**

YOUR SCORE ______

CHAPTER 11
Oral Dosages

POSTTEST 2

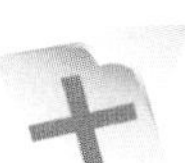

DIRECTIONS: The medication order is listed at the beginning of each problem. Calculate the oral doses. Show your work. Shade each medicine cup or oral syringe when provided to indicate correct dose.

1. Your patient receives Feldene 20 mg po daily for gouty arthritis. Feldene 10-mg capsules are available. How many capsules will you administer per dose? ______

2. The licensed prescriber orders Zofran 8 mg po before chemotherapy. How many milliliters will the nurse administer per dose? ______

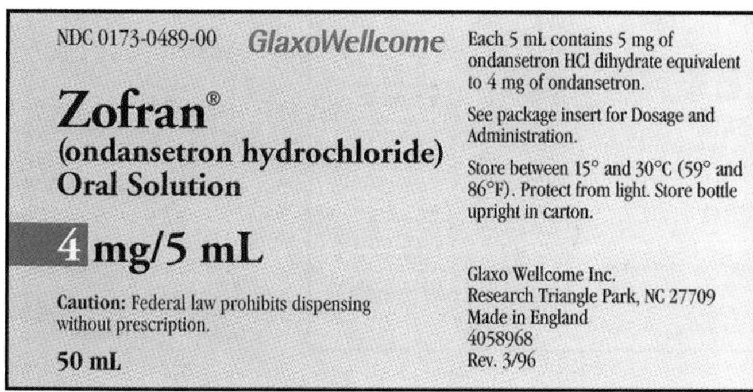
NDC 0173-0489-00 GlaxoWellcome
Zofran®
(ondansetron hydrochloride)
Oral Solution
4 mg/5 mL
Caution: Federal law prohibits dispensing without prescription.
50 mL
Each 5 mL contains 5 mg of ondansetron HCl dihydrate equivalent to 4 mg of ondansetron.
See package insert for Dosage and Administration.
Store between 15° and 30°C (59° and 86°F). Protect from light. Store bottle upright in carton.
Glaxo Wellcome Inc.
Research Triangle Park, NC 27709
Made in England
4058968
Rev. 3/96

3. Mr. Theson receives Vistaril 60 mg po q 6 h for relief of nausea after his acoustic neuroma revision. Vistaril oral suspension, 25 mg/5 mL, is supplied. How many milliliters will the nurse administer? ______

4. The licensed prescriber orders Glucotrol 15 mg daily. Glucotrol 10-mg scored tablets are available. How many tablets will the nurse administer per dose? ______

5. Your patient who is being treated for congestive heart failure requires KCl 5 mEq po two times a day for hypokalemia. KCl 20 mEq/30 mL is available. How many milliliters will you administer per dose? _______

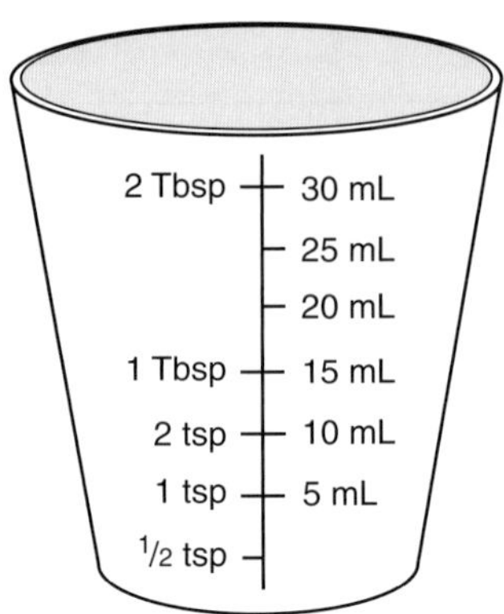

6. Your patient who has an upper and lower respiratory infection receives Keflex 250 mg po four times a day. How many capsules will you administer per dose? _______

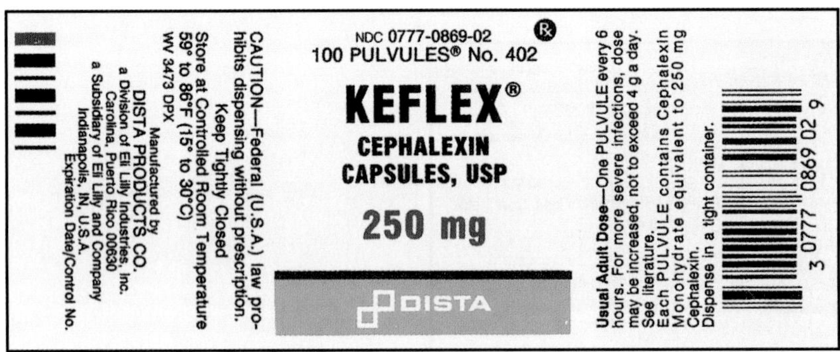

7. Mrs. Pace receives prednisone 7.5 mg po four times a day for asthma. How many tablets will the nurse administer per dose? _______

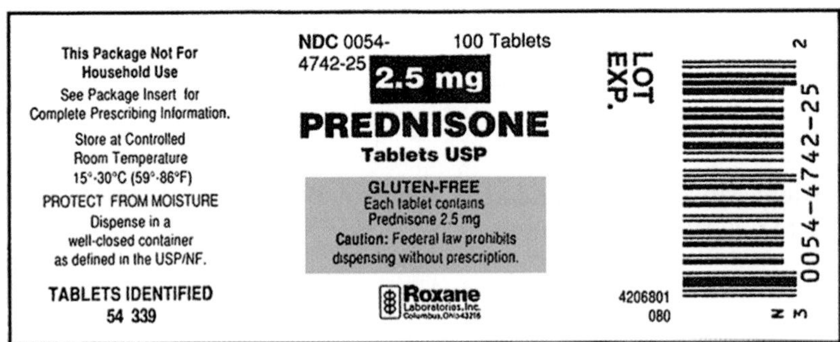

8. Your patient receives Lanoxin 0.05 mg po daily for cardiac arrhythmia. How many milliliters will you administer per dose? _______

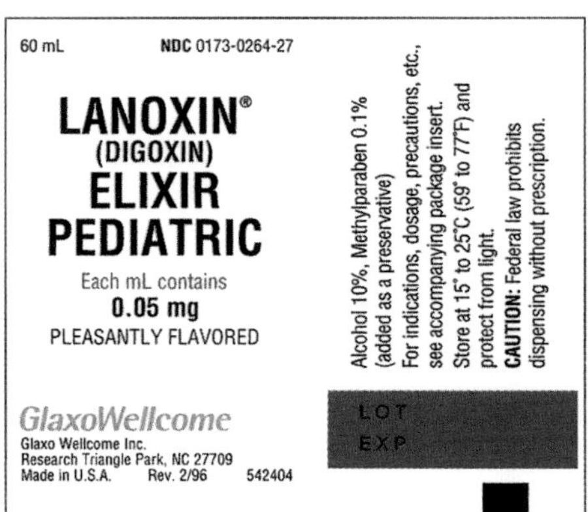
60 mL
NDC 0173-0264-27
LANOXIN®
(DIGOXIN)
ELIXIR
PEDIATRIC
Each mL contains
0.05 mg
PLEASANTLY FLAVORED
Alcohol 10%, Methylparaben 0.1%
(added as a preservative)
For indications, dosage, precautions, etc.,
see accompanying package insert.
Store at 15° to 25°C (59° to 77°F) and
protect from light.
CAUTION: Federal law prohibits
dispensing without prescription.
GlaxoWellcome
Glaxo Wellcome Inc.
Research Triangle Park, NC 27709
Made in U.S.A. Rev. 2/96 542404
LOT
EXP

9. The licensed prescriber orders Macrodantin 0.1 g po four times a day. How many capsules will the nurse administer per dose? _______

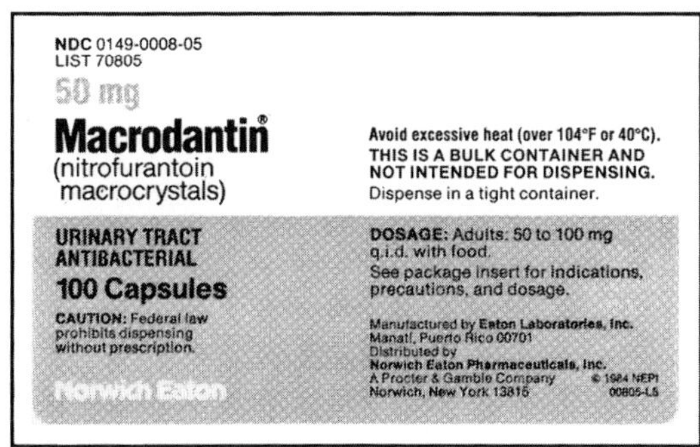
NDC 0149-0008-05
LIST 70805
50 mg
Macrodantin®
(nitrofurantoin
macrocrystals)
URINARY TRACT
ANTIBACTERIAL
100 Capsules
CAUTION: Federal law prohibits dispensing without prescription.
Norwich Eaton
Avoid excessive heat (over 104°F or 40°C).
THIS IS A BULK CONTAINER AND NOT INTENDED FOR DISPENSING.
Dispense in a tight container.
DOSAGE: Adults: 50 to 100 mg q.i.d. with food.
See package insert for indications, precautions, and dosage.
Manufactured by Eaton Laboratories, Inc.
Manatí, Puerto Rico 00701
Distributed by
Norwich Eaton Pharmaceuticals, Inc.
A Procter & Gamble Company
Norwich, New York 13815

10. Your patient who had a bilateral turbinate reduction receives acetaminophen 650 mg po q 4 h for pain relief. Acetaminophen is supplied in 325-mg tablets. How many tablets will you administer per dose? _______

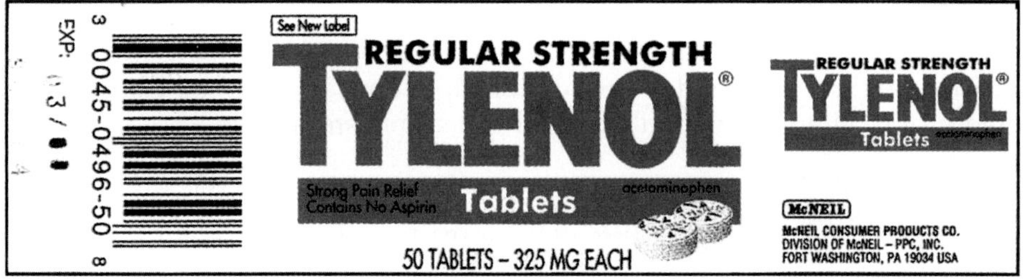
3 00045-0496-50 8
EXP:
See New Label
REGULAR STRENGTH
TYLENOL®
Strong Pain Relief
Contains No Aspirin
Tablets
acetaminophen
50 TABLETS – 325 MG EACH
REGULAR STRENGTH
TYLENOL®
Tablets
McNEIL
McNEIL CONSUMER PRODUCTS CO.
DIVISION OF McNEIL – PPC, INC.
FORT WASHINGTON, PA 19034 USA

11. The licensed prescriber prescribes Dilantin 100 mg po twice a day for seizure activity in your patient with epilepsy. Dilantin 50-mg Infatabs are available. How many tablets will you administer per dose? _______

12. Mr. Bales requires Pen-V K 250 mg po q 6 h for bacterial endocarditis. Pen-V K solution 125 mg/5 mL is available. How many milliliters will the nurse administer per dose? _______

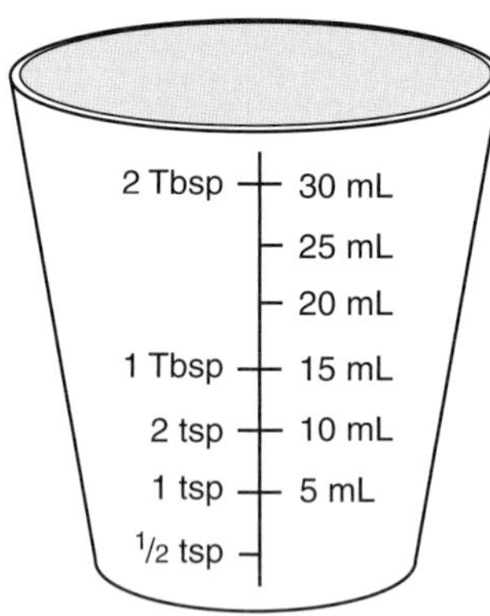

13. The licensed prescriber orders Deltasone 20 mg po four times a day. Deltasone is supplied in 2.5-mg, 5-mg, and 50-mg tablets. The nurse will give _______ tablets of _______ mg.

14. Mr. Cy, who has had mitral valve repair, receives Lanoxin 0.25 mg po daily. How many tablets will the nurse administer per dose? _______

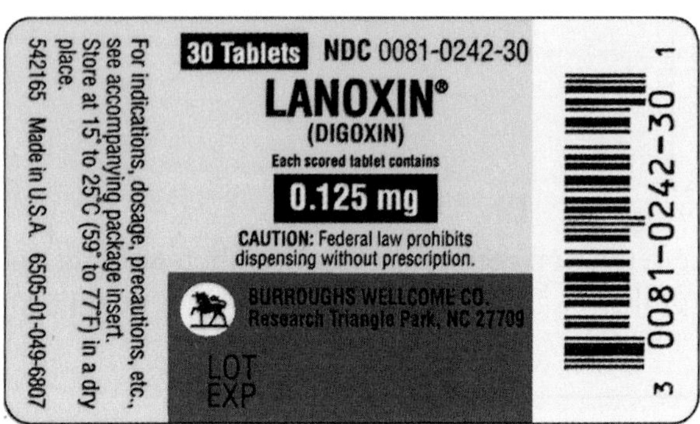

15. Colace syrup 25 mg po three times a day prn for constipation is ordered for your patient after an ethmoidectomy. How many milliliters will you administer per dose? _______

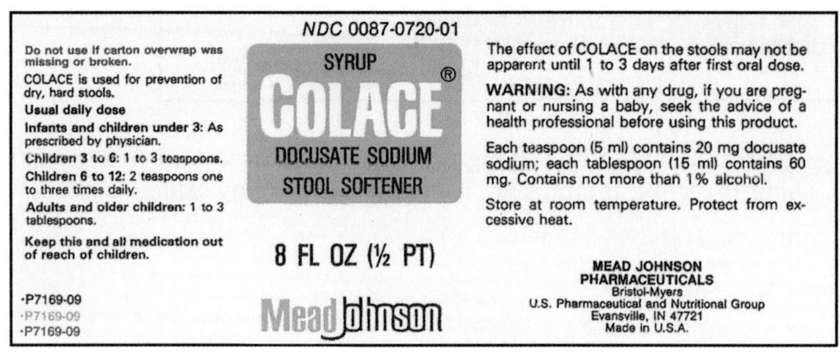

16. Mr. Tate, who suffers from chronic gout, has Zyloprim 0.15 g po daily in the mornings. How many tablets will he receive per dose? _______

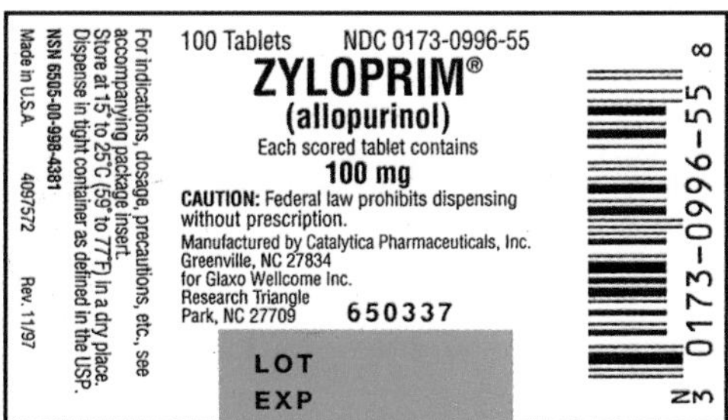

17. Your patient with hypertension has verapamil 80 mg po three times a day ordered. You have 40-mg tablets. How many tablets will you administer per dose? _______

18. The licensed prescriber orders Zyprexa 15 mg po daily for bipolar mania. How many tablets will the nurse administer per dose? _______

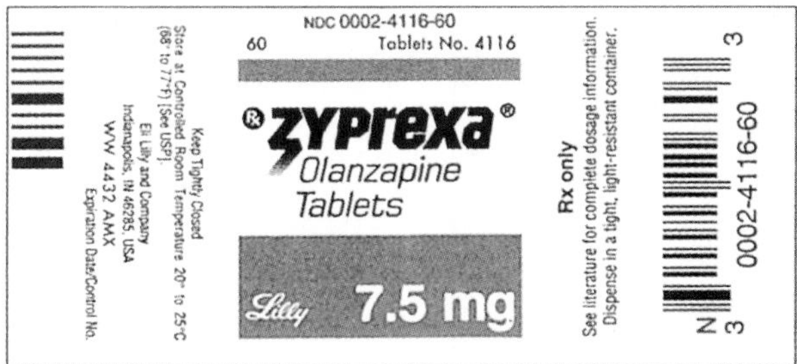

19. Your patient was admitted with seizure activity. The licensed prescriber orders phenobarbital 30 mg po q 8 h. How many tablets will you administer per dose?

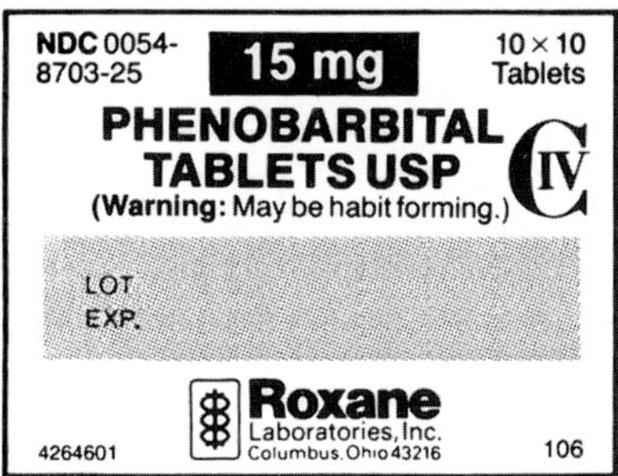

20. The licensed prescriber orders Flagyl 750 mg po three times a day for 5 days for a yeast infection. Flagyl is supplied in 250-mg tablets. How many tablets will the nurse administer per dose? _______

21. Mr. Luke's licensed prescriber has ordered Norvasc 10 mg po daily for hypertension. Norvasc 5-mg tablets are available. How many tablets will you administer per dose? _______

22. Mrs. Martin is prescribed Tofranil-PM 0.225 g po at bedtime for depression. How many capsules will you administer per dose? _______

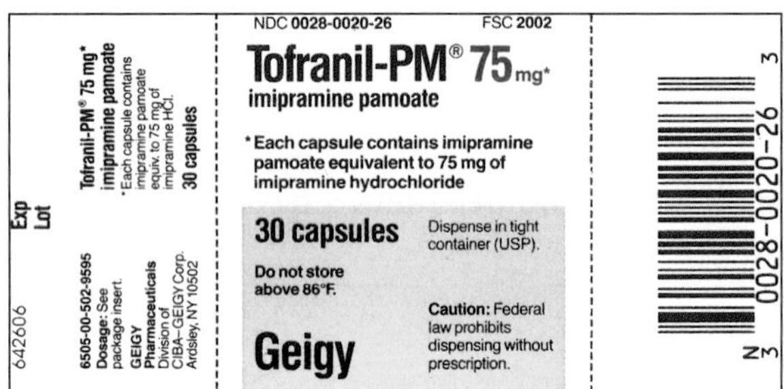

23. The licensed prescriber orders Vibramycin 100 mg po daily. You have Vibramycin syrup 50 mg/5 mL. How many milliliters will you administer per dose? _______

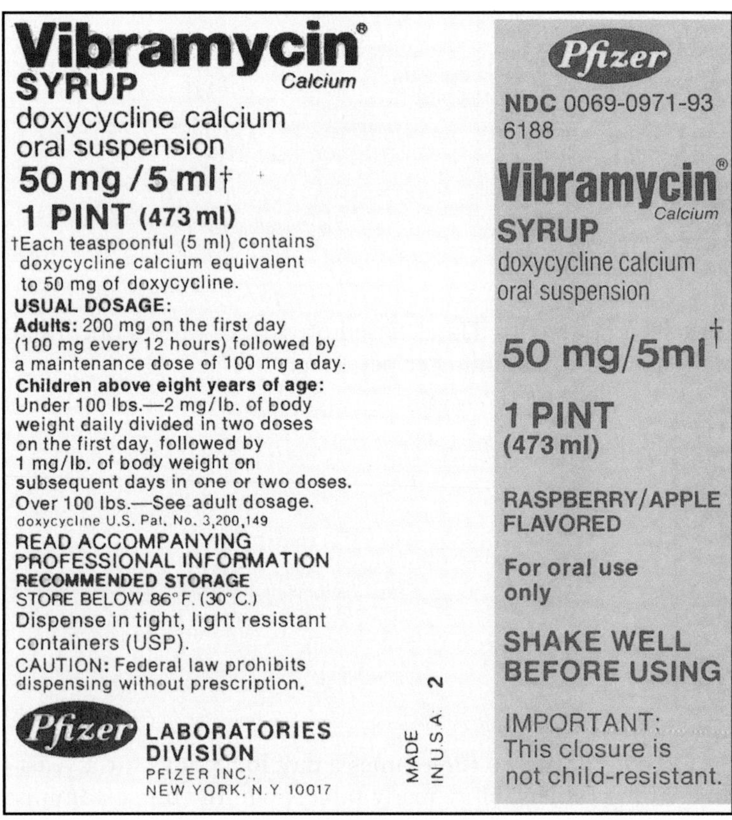

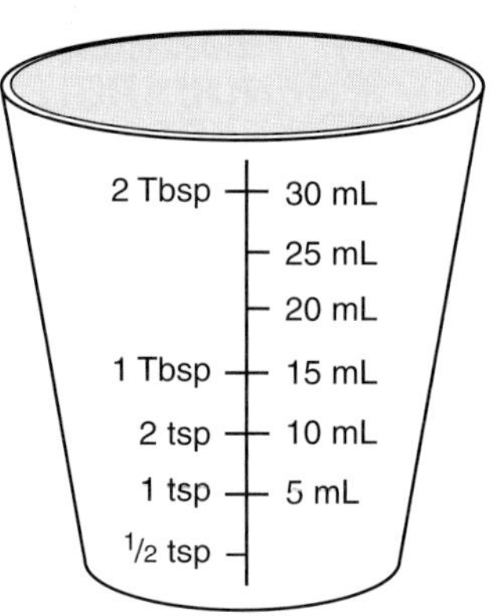

24. Vasotec 5 mg po twice a day is ordered for Mr. Butter's congestive heart failure. How many tablets will the nurse administer per dose? _______

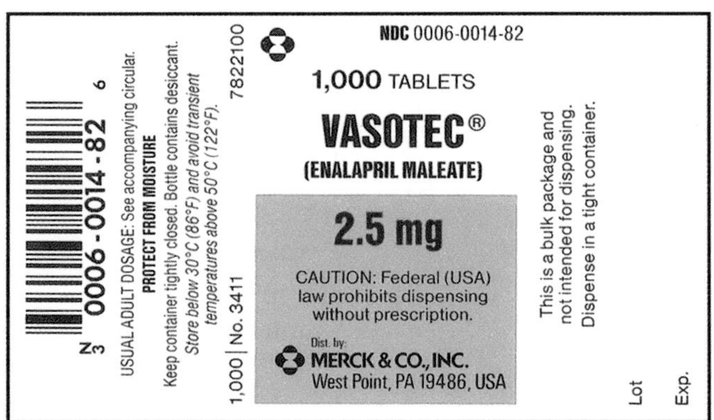

25. Ms. Wang is to receive Zithromax oral suspension 1 g po now. How many milliliters will you administer per dose? _______

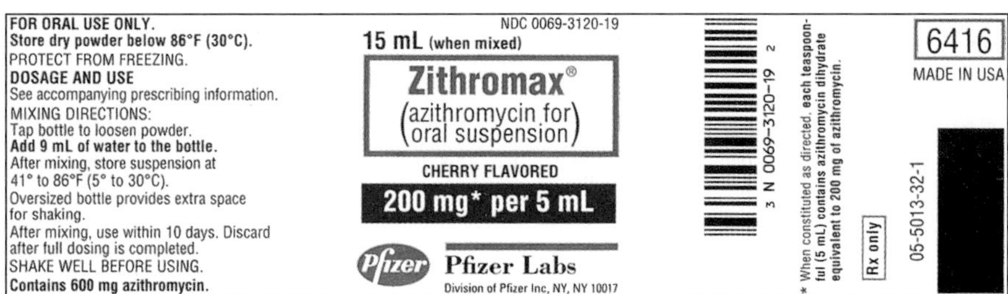

ANSWERS ON PP. 257–258 AND 279–282.

evolve For additional practice problems, refer to the Oral Dosages section of *Elsevier's Interactive Drug Calculation Application*, version 1.

ANSWERS

CHAPTER 11 Dimensional Analysis—Worksheet, pp. 215–238

1. $x \text{ capsules} = \dfrac{1 \text{ capsule}}{1 \text{ mg}} \times \dfrac{2 \text{ mg}}{1}$
   $= 2 \text{ capsules}$

2. $x \text{ mL} = \dfrac{5 \text{ mL}}{20 \text{ mg}} \times \dfrac{30 \text{ mg}}{1} = 7.5 \text{ mL}$

3. $x \text{ tablets} = \dfrac{1 \text{ tablet}}{0.05 \text{ mg}} \times \dfrac{0.2 \text{ mg}}{1}$
   $= 4 \text{ tablets}$
   $x \text{ tablets} = \dfrac{1 \text{ tablet}}{0.05 \text{ mg}} \times \dfrac{0.15 \text{ mg}}{1}$
   $= 3 \text{ tablets}$

4. $x \text{ tablets} = \dfrac{1 \text{ tablet}}{250 \text{ mg}} \times \dfrac{500 \text{ mg}}{1} = 2 \text{ tablets}$

5. $x \text{ mL} = \dfrac{5 \text{ mL}}{5 \text{ mg}} \times \dfrac{2.5 \text{ mg}}{1} = 2.5 \text{ mL}$

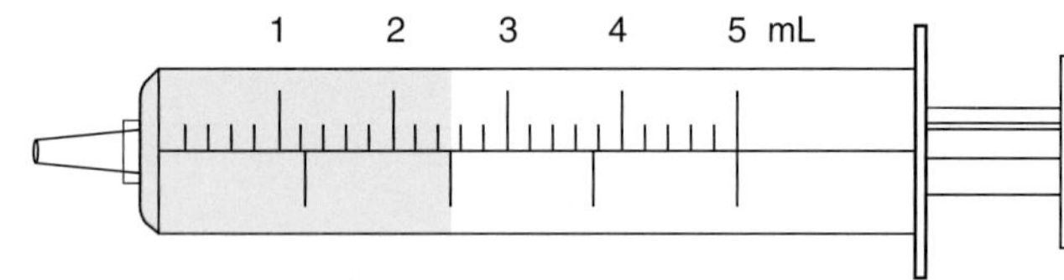

6. $x \text{ tablets} = \dfrac{1 \text{ tablet}}{1 \text{ mg}} \times \dfrac{2 \text{ mg}}{1} = 2 \text{ tablets}$

7. $x \text{ tablets} = \dfrac{1 \text{ tablet}}{10 \text{ mg}} \times \dfrac{20 \text{ mg}}{1} = 2 \text{ tablets}$

8. $x \text{ tablets} = \dfrac{1 \text{ tablet}}{0.5 \text{ g}} \times \dfrac{1 \text{ g}}{1} = 2 \text{ tablets}$

9. $x \text{ mL} = \dfrac{5 \text{ mL}}{20 \text{ mg}} \times \dfrac{40 \text{ mg}}{1} = 10 \text{ mL}$

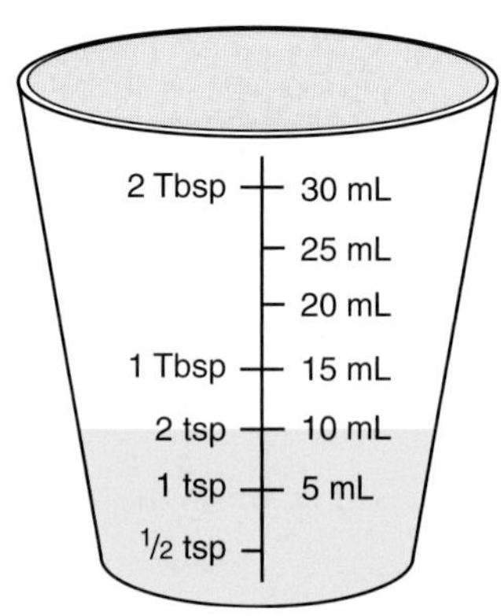

10. $x \text{ tablets} = \dfrac{1 \text{ tablet}}{0.5 \text{ mg}} \times \dfrac{1 \text{ mg}}{1} = 2 \text{ tablets}$

11. $x \text{ tablets} = \dfrac{1 \text{ tablet}}{400 \text{ mg}} \times \dfrac{800 \text{ mg}}{1} = 2 \text{ tablets}$

12. $x \text{ tablets} = \dfrac{1 \text{ tablet}}{300 \text{ mg}} \times \dfrac{1000 \text{ mg}}{1 \text{ g}} \times \dfrac{0.6 \text{ g}}{1}$
    $= 2 \text{ tablets}$
    $x \text{ mg} = \dfrac{300 \text{ mg}}{1 \text{ tablet}} \times \dfrac{2 \text{ tablets}}{1 \text{ dose}} \times \dfrac{2 \text{ doses}}{1 \text{ day}}$
    $= 1200 \text{ mg}$

13. $x \text{ tablets} = \dfrac{1 \text{ tablet}}{10 \text{ mg}} \times \dfrac{30 \text{ mg}}{1} = 3 \text{ tablets}$

14. $x \text{ tablets} = \dfrac{1 \text{ tablet}}{750 \text{ mg}} \times \dfrac{1000 \text{ mg}}{1 \text{ g}} \times \dfrac{0.75 \text{ g}}{1}$
    $= 1 \text{ tablet}$

15. $x \text{ capsules} = \dfrac{1 \text{ capsule}}{40 \text{ mg}} \times \dfrac{80 \text{ mg}}{1}$
    $= 2 \text{ capsules}$

16. $x \text{ tablets} = \dfrac{1 \text{ tablet}}{0.5 \text{ g}} \times \dfrac{4 \text{ g}}{1} = 8 \text{ tablets}$
    $x \text{ tablets} = \dfrac{1 \text{ tablet}}{0.5 \text{ g}} \times \dfrac{2 \text{ g}}{1} = 4 \text{ tablets}$

17. $x \text{ tablets} = \dfrac{1 \text{ tablet}}{400 \text{ mg}} \times \dfrac{800 \text{ mg}}{1} = 2 \text{ tablets}$

18. $x = \dfrac{30 \text{ mL}}{\text{Dose}} \times \dfrac{4 \text{ doses}}{1} = 120 \text{ mL}$

19. $x \text{ mL} = \dfrac{5 \text{ mL}}{12.5 \text{ mg}} \times \dfrac{30 \text{ mg}}{1} = 12 \text{ mL}$

20. $x \text{ tablets} = \dfrac{1 \text{ tablet}}{30 \text{ mg}} \times \dfrac{60 \text{ mg}}{1}$
    $= 2 \text{ tablets}$

21. $x \text{ mg} = \dfrac{125 \text{ mg}}{5 \text{ mL}} \times \dfrac{5.5 \text{ mL}}{1} = 137.5 \text{ mg}$

22. $x \text{ tablets} - \dfrac{1 \text{ tablet}}{40 \text{ mg}} \times \dfrac{80 \text{ mg}}{1} = 2 \text{ tablets}$

23. $x \text{ mg} = \dfrac{0.4 \text{ mg}}{1 \text{ tablet}} \times \dfrac{2 \text{ tablets}}{1} = 0.8 \text{ mg}$

24. $x \text{ mL} = \dfrac{5 \text{ mL}}{0.5 \text{ mg}} \times \dfrac{1.5 \text{ mg}}{1} = 15 \text{ mL}$

$x \text{ oz} = \dfrac{1 \text{ oz}}{30 \text{ mL}} \times \dfrac{15 \text{ mL}}{1} = 0.5 \text{ oz}$

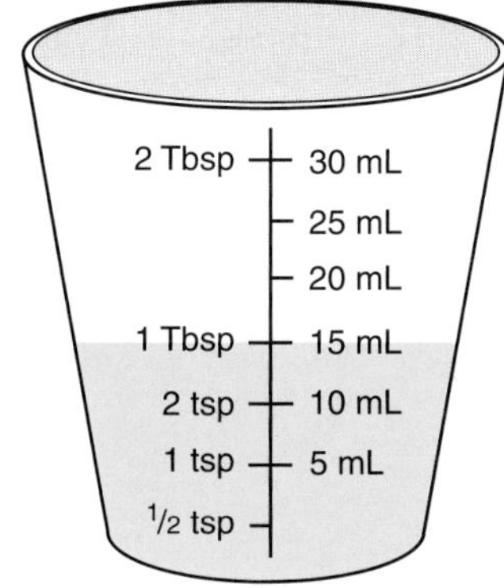

25. $x \text{ mL} = \dfrac{5 \text{ mL}}{375 \text{ mg}} \times \dfrac{500 \text{ mg}}{1} = 6.7 \text{ mL}$

26. $x \text{ tablets} = \dfrac{1 \text{ tablet}}{50 \text{ mg}} \times \dfrac{25 \text{ mg}}{1} = 0.5 \text{ tablet}$

27. $x \text{ doses} = \dfrac{1 \text{ dose}}{30 \text{ mL}} \times \dfrac{360 \text{ mL}}{1} = 12 \text{ doses}$

28. $x \text{ tablets} = \dfrac{1 \text{ tablet}}{0.125 \text{ mg}} \times \dfrac{0.25 \text{ mg}}{1} = 2 \text{ tablets}$

29. $x \text{ tablets} = \dfrac{1 \text{ tablet}}{30 \text{ mg}} \times \dfrac{15 \text{ mg}}{1} = 0.5 \text{ tablet}$

30. $x \text{ mL} = \dfrac{5 \text{ mL}}{250 \text{ mg}} \times \dfrac{125 \text{ mg}}{1} = 2.5 \text{ mL}$

31. $x \text{ tablets} = \dfrac{1 \text{ tablet}}{50 \text{ mg}} \times \dfrac{25 \text{ mg}}{1} = 0.5 \text{ tablet}$

32. $x \text{ tablets} = \dfrac{1 \text{ tablet}}{200 \text{ mg}} \times \dfrac{1000 \text{ mg}}{1 \text{ g}} \times \dfrac{0.6 \text{ g}}{1} = 3 \text{ tablets}$

$x \text{ tablets} = \dfrac{3 \text{ tablets}}{1 \text{ dose}} \times \dfrac{6 \text{ doses}}{1} = 18 \text{ tablets}$

33. $x \text{ mL} = \dfrac{5 \text{ mL}}{4 \text{ mg}} \times \dfrac{8 \text{ mg}}{1} = 10 \text{ mL}$

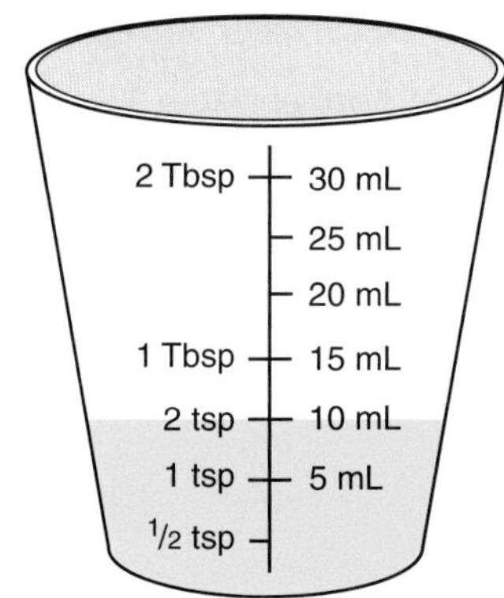

34. $x \text{ mL} = \dfrac{5 \text{ mL}}{500 \text{ mg}} \times \dfrac{750 \text{ mg}}{1} = 7.5 \text{ mL}$

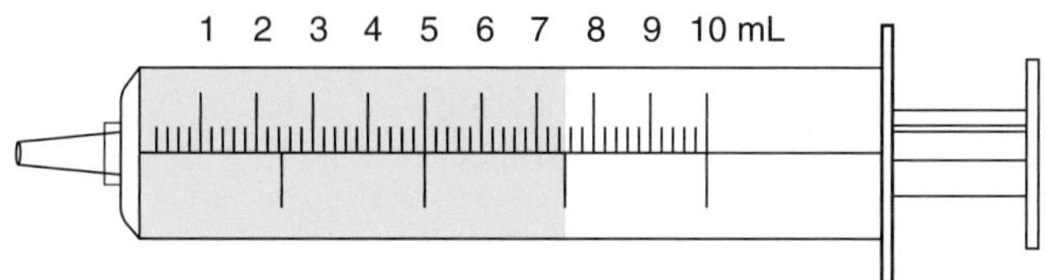

35. $x \text{ mL} = \dfrac{5 \text{ mL}}{20 \text{ mg}} \times \dfrac{100 \text{ mg}}{1} = 25 \text{ mL}$

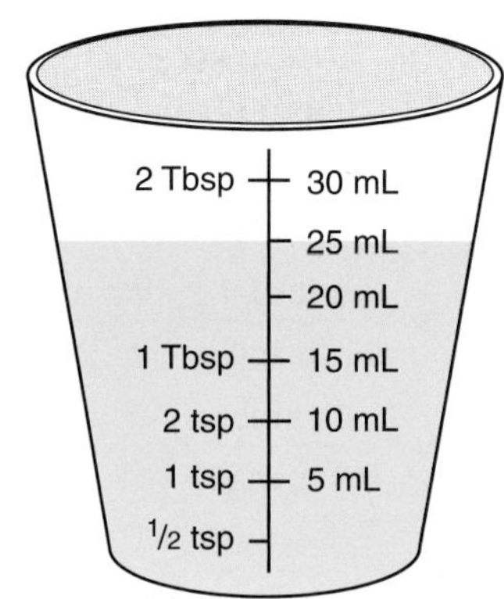

36. $x \text{ tablets} = \dfrac{1 \text{ tablet}}{500 \text{ mg}} \times \dfrac{1000 \text{ mg}}{1 \text{ g}} \times \dfrac{1 \text{ g}}{1} = 2 \text{ tablets}$

37. $x \text{ tablets} = \dfrac{1 \text{ tablet}}{2.5 \text{ mg}} \times \dfrac{7.5 \text{ mg}}{1} = 3 \text{ tablets}$

38. $x \text{ tablets} = \dfrac{1 \text{ tablet}}{100 \text{ mg}} \times \dfrac{1000 \text{ mg}}{1 \text{ g}} \times \dfrac{0.2 \text{ g}}{1} = 2 \text{ tablets}$

39. $x \text{ tablets} = \frac{1 \text{ tablet}}{5 \text{ mg}/500 \text{ mg}} \times \frac{5 \text{ mg}/500 \text{ mg}}{1} = 1 \text{ tablet}$

$x \text{ acetaminophen} = \frac{500 \text{ mg}}{1 \text{ tablet}} \times \frac{1 \text{ tablet}}{1} = 500 \text{ mg acetaminophen}$

40. $x \text{ tablets} = \frac{1 \text{ tablet}}{0.25 \text{ mg}} \times \frac{0.5 \text{ mg}}{1} = 2 \text{ tablets}$

41. $x \text{ tablets} = \frac{1 \text{ tablet}}{5 \text{ mg}} \times \frac{10 \text{ mg}}{1} = 2 \text{ tablets}$

42. $x \text{ tablets} = \frac{1 \text{ tablet}}{50 \text{ mg}} \times \frac{100 \text{ mg}}{1} = 2 \text{ tablets}$

43. $x \text{ capsules} = \frac{1 \text{ capsule}}{300 \text{ mg}} \times \frac{600 \text{ mg}}{1} = 2 \text{ capsules}$

44. $x \text{ tablets} = \frac{1 \text{ tablet}}{0.125 \text{ mg}} \times \frac{0.25 \text{ mg}}{1} = 2 \text{ tablets}$

45. $x \text{ capsules} = \frac{1 \text{ capsule}}{250 \text{ mg}} \times \frac{500 \text{ mg}}{1} = 2 \text{ capsules}$

$x \text{ capsules} = \frac{2 \text{ capsules}}{1 \text{ dose}} \times \frac{4 \text{ doses}}{1} = 8 \text{ capsules}$

46. $x \text{ capsules} = \frac{1 \text{ capsule}}{20 \text{ mg}} \times \frac{40 \text{ mg}}{1} = 2 \text{ capsules}$

47. $x \text{ tablets} = \frac{1 \text{ tablet}}{30 \text{ mg}} \times \frac{90 \text{ mg}}{1} = 3 \text{ tablets}$

48. $x \text{ tablets} = \frac{1 \text{ tablet}}{75 \text{ mg}} \times \frac{150 \text{ mg}}{1} = 2 \text{ tablets}$

49. $x \text{ tablets} = \frac{1 \text{ tablet}}{12.5 \text{ mg}} \times \frac{25 \text{ mg}}{1} = 2 \text{ tablets}$

50. $x \text{ mL} = \frac{1 \text{ mL}}{15 \text{ mg}} \times \frac{150 \text{ mg}}{1} = 10 \text{ mL}$

51. $x \text{ tablets} = \frac{1 \text{ tablet}}{250 \text{ mg}} \times \frac{500 \text{ mg}}{1} = 2 \text{ tablets}$

52. $x \text{ tablets} = \frac{1 \text{ tablet}}{0.1 \text{ mg}} \times \frac{0.2 \text{ mg}}{1} = 2 \text{ tablets}$

53. $x \text{ capsules} = \frac{1 \text{ capsule}}{10 \text{ mg}} \times \frac{20 \text{ mg}}{1} = 2 \text{ capsules}$

54. $x \text{ mL} = \frac{5 \text{ mL}}{10 \text{ mg}} \times \frac{30 \text{ mg}}{1} = 15 \text{ mL}$

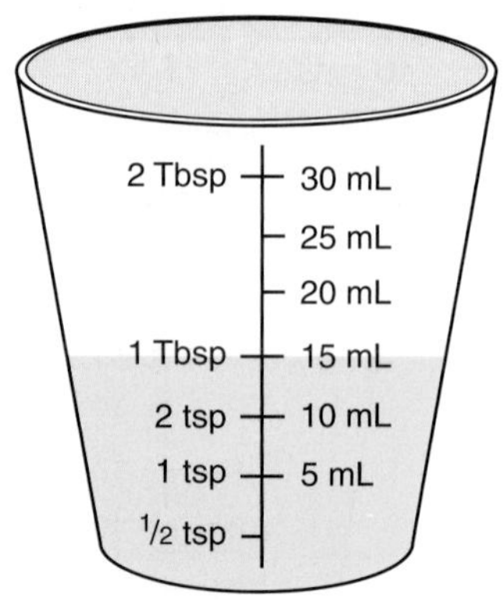

55. $x \text{ tablets} = \frac{1 \text{ tablet}}{250 \text{ mg}} \times \frac{1000 \text{ mg}}{1 \text{ g}} \times \frac{0.75 \text{ g}}{1} = 3 \text{ tablets}$

56. $x \text{ mL} = \frac{5 \text{ mL}}{4 \text{ mg}} \times \frac{8 \text{ mg}}{1} = \frac{40}{4} = 10 \text{ mL}$

57. $x \text{ mL} = \frac{5 \text{ mL}}{25 \text{ mg}} \times \frac{15 \text{ mg}}{1} = 3 \text{ mL}$

58. $x \text{ tablets} = \frac{1 \text{ tablet}}{50 \text{ mg}} \times \frac{100 \text{ mg}}{1} = 2 \text{ tablets}$

59. $x \text{ tablets} = \frac{1 \text{ tablet}}{500 \text{ mg}} \times \frac{1000 \text{ mg}}{1 \text{ g}} \times \frac{1 \text{ g}}{1} = 2 \text{ tablets}$

60. $x \text{ mL} = \frac{5 \text{ mL}}{150 \text{ mg}} \times \frac{250 \text{ mg}}{1} = 8.3 \text{ mL}$

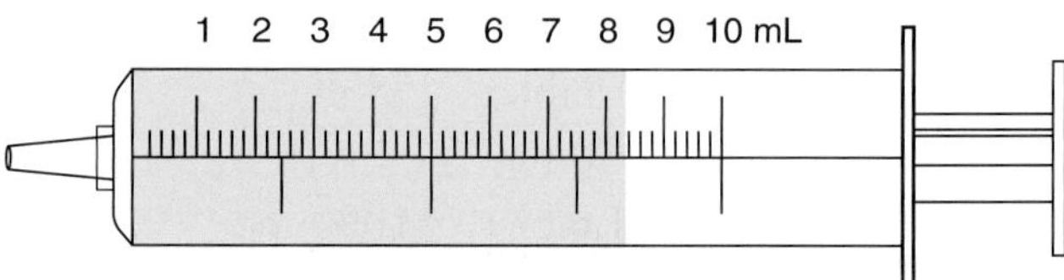

61. $x \text{ mL} = \frac{5 \text{ mL}}{50 \text{ mg}} \times \frac{100 \text{ mg}}{1} = 10 \text{ mL}$

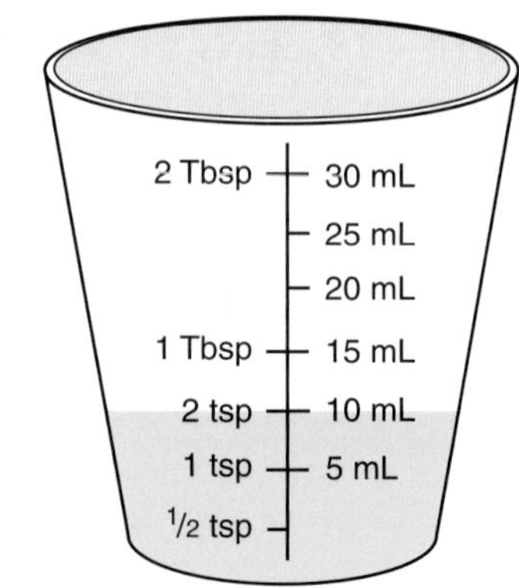

62. $x \text{ tablets} = \frac{1 \text{ tablet}}{50 \text{ mg}} \times \frac{25 \text{ mg}}{1} = 0.5 \text{ tablet}$

63. $x \text{ tablets} = \frac{1 \text{ tablet}}{80 \text{ mg}} \times \frac{240 \text{ mg}}{1} = 3 \text{ tablets}$

64. $x \text{ mL} = \frac{1 \text{ mL}}{0.05 \text{ mg}} \times \frac{1 \text{ mg}}{1000 \text{ mcg}} \times \frac{90 \text{ mcg}}{1}$
$= 1.8 \text{ mL}$

65. $x \text{ mg} = \frac{12.5 \text{ mg}}{5 \text{ mL}} \times \frac{10 \text{ mL}}{1} = 25 \text{ mg}$

66. $x \text{ capsules} = \frac{1 \text{ capsule}}{25 \text{ mg}} \times \frac{50 \text{ mg}}{1}$
$= 2 \text{ capsules}$

67. $x \text{ capsules} = \frac{1 \text{ capsule}}{30 \text{ mg}} \times \frac{90 \text{ mg}}{1}$
$= 3 \text{ capsules}$

68. 40-mg tablet
$x \text{ tablets} = \frac{1 \text{ tablet}}{40 \text{ mg}} \times \frac{40 \text{ mg}}{1} = 1 \text{ tablet}$

69. $x \text{ mL} = \frac{15 \text{ mL}}{20 \text{ mEq}} \times \frac{10 \text{ mEq}}{1} = 7.5 \text{ mL}$

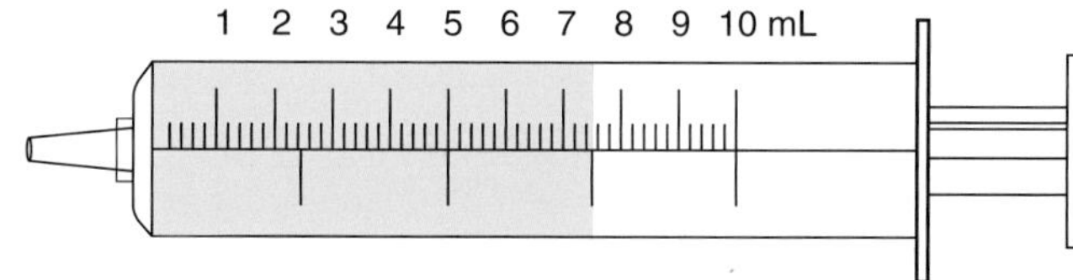

70. $x \text{ tablets} = \frac{1 \text{ tablet}}{0.5 \text{ mg}} \times \frac{1.5 \text{ mg}}{1} = 3 \text{ tablets}$

71. $x \text{ tablets} = \frac{1 \text{ tablet}}{0.25 \text{ mg}} \times \frac{0.5 \text{ mg}}{1} = 2 \text{ tablets}$

72. $x \text{ tablets} = \frac{1 \text{ tablet}}{325 \text{ mg}} \times \frac{650 \text{ mg}}{1} = 2 \text{ tablets}$

73. $x \text{ tablets} = \frac{1 \text{ tablet}}{0.25 \text{ mg}} \times \frac{0.5 \text{ mg}}{1} = 2 \text{ tablets}$

74. $x \text{ mL} = \frac{5 \text{ mL}}{125 \text{ mg}} \times \frac{375 \text{ mg}}{1} = 15 \text{ mL}$

75. $x \text{ tablets} = \frac{1 \text{ tablet}}{30 \text{ mg}} \times \frac{30 \text{ mg}}{1} = 1 \text{ tablet}$

76. $x \text{ tablets} = \frac{1 \text{ tablet}}{0.15 \text{ mg}} \times \frac{0.3 \text{ mg}}{1}$
$= 2 \text{ tablets of } 0.15 \text{ mg}$

77. $x \text{ tablets} = \frac{1 \text{ tablet}}{5 \text{ mg}} \times \frac{7.5 \text{ mg}}{1}$
$= 1.5 \text{ tablets}$

78. $x \text{ mL} = \frac{5 \text{ mL}}{125 \text{ mg}} \times \frac{250 \text{ mg}}{1} = 10 \text{ mL}$

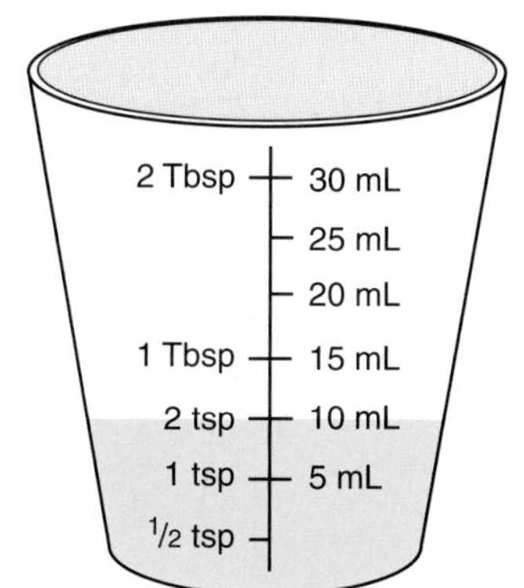

79. $x \text{ capsules} = \frac{1 \text{ capsule}}{50 \text{ mg}} \times \frac{250 \text{ mg}}{1}$
$= 5 \text{ capsules}$

80. $x \text{ mL} = \frac{11.25 \text{ mL}}{15 \text{ mEq}} \times \frac{20 \text{ mEq}}{1} = 15 \text{ mL}$

81. $x \text{ mL} = \frac{5 \text{ mL}}{20 \text{ mg}} \times \frac{55 \text{ mg}}{1} = 13.75 \text{ mL}$

82. $x \text{ tablets} = \frac{1 \text{ tablet}}{125 \text{ mg}} \times \frac{250 \text{ mg}}{1} = 2 \text{ tablets}$

83. $x \text{ tablets} = \frac{1 \text{ tablet}}{0.05 \text{ mg}} \times \frac{0.05 \text{ mg}}{1} = 1 \text{ tablet}$

84. $x \text{ mg} = \frac{1000 \text{ mg}}{1 \text{ g}} \times \frac{0.2 \text{ g}}{1}$
$= 1 \text{ tablet of } 200 \text{ mg}$
$x \text{ mg} = \frac{200 \text{ mg}}{1 \text{ dose}} \times \frac{3 \text{ doses}}{1} = 600 \text{ mg}$

85. $x \text{ tablets} = \frac{1 \text{ tablet}}{5 \text{ mg}} \times \frac{15 \text{ mg}}{1} = 3 \text{ tablets}$

86. $x \text{ tablets} = \frac{1 \text{ tablet}}{400 \text{ mg}} \times \frac{800 \text{ mg}}{1} = 2 \text{ tablets}$

87. $x \text{ capsules} = \frac{1 \text{ capsule}}{250 \text{ mg}} \times \frac{500 \text{ mg}}{1}$
$= 2 \text{ capsules}$

88. $x \text{ tablets} = \frac{1 \text{ tablet}}{25 \text{ mg}} \times \frac{50 \text{ mg}}{1} = 2 \text{ tablets}$

89. $x \text{ pills} = \frac{1 \text{ pill}}{10 \text{ mg}} \times \frac{30 \text{ mg}}{1} = 3 \text{ pills}$

90. $x \text{ mL} = \frac{4 \text{ mL}}{40 \text{ mg}} \times \frac{6 \text{ mg}}{1} = 0.6 \text{ mL}$

91. $x \text{ capsules} = \frac{1 \text{ capsule}}{75 \text{ mg}} \times \frac{150 \text{ mg}}{1}$
$= 2 \text{ capsules}$

92. $x \text{ capsules} = \frac{1 \text{ capsule}}{100 \text{ mg}} \times \frac{200 \text{ mg}}{1}$
$= 2 \text{ capsules}$

93. $x \text{ tablets} = \frac{1 \text{ tablet}}{2.5 \text{ mg}} \times \frac{10 \text{ mg}}{1} = 4 \text{ tablets}$

94. $x \text{ tablets} = \frac{1 \text{ tablet}}{250 \text{ mg}} \times \frac{1000 \text{ mg}}{1 \text{ g}} \times \frac{0.25 \text{ g}}{1}$
$= 1 \text{ tablet}$

95. $x \text{ tablets} = \frac{1 \text{ tablet}}{10 \text{ mg}} \times \frac{25 \text{ mg}}{1} = 2.5 \text{ tablets}$

96. $x \text{ tablets} = \frac{1 \text{ tablet}}{10 \text{ mg}} \times \frac{30 \text{ mg}}{1} = 3 \text{ tablets}$

97. $x \text{ tablets} = \frac{1 \text{ tablet}}{5 \text{ mg}} \times \frac{15 \text{ mg}}{1} = 3 \text{ tablets}$

98. $x \text{ capsules} = \frac{1 \text{ capsule}}{15 \text{ mg}} \times \frac{1000 \text{ mg}}{1 \text{ g}} \times \frac{0.015 \text{ g}}{1}$
$= 1 \text{ capsule}$

99. $x \text{ mL} = \frac{5 \text{ mL}}{6.7 \text{ mEq}} \times \frac{30 \text{ mEq}}{1} = 22.4 \text{ mL}$

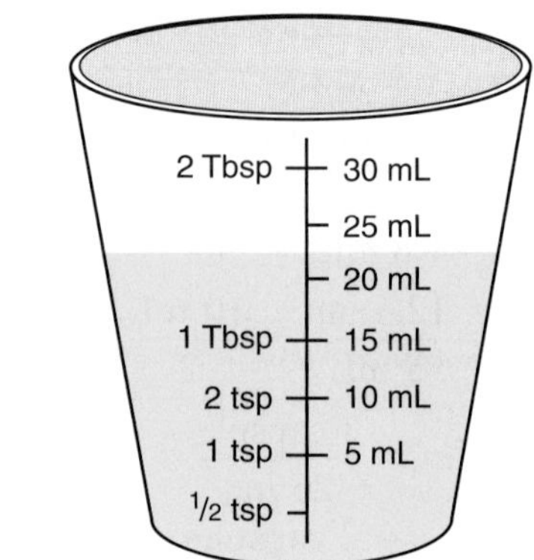

100. $x \text{ tablets} = \frac{1 \text{ tablet}}{40 \text{ mg}} \times \frac{20 \text{ mg}}{1} = 0.5 \text{ tablet}$

CHAPTER 11 Dimensional Analysis—Posttest 1, pp. 239–244

1. $x \text{ tablets} = \frac{1 \text{ tablet}}{30 \text{ mg}} \times \frac{60 \text{ mg}}{1} = 2 \text{ tablets}$

2. $x \text{ capsules} = \frac{1 \text{ capsule}}{500 \text{ mg}} \times \frac{1000 \text{ mg}}{1 \text{ g}} \times \frac{0.5 \text{g}}{1}$
$= 1 \text{ capsule}$

3. $x \text{ capsules} = \frac{1 \text{ capsule}}{250 \text{ mg}} \times \frac{1000 \text{ mg}}{1} \times \frac{1 \text{ g}}{1}$
$= 4 \text{ capsules}$

4. $x \text{ tablets} = \frac{1 \text{ tablet}}{0.03 \text{ g}} \times \frac{1 \text{ g}}{1000 \text{ mg}} \times \frac{60 \text{ mg}}{1}$
$= 2 \text{ tablets}$

5. $x \text{ tablets} = \frac{1 \text{ tablet}}{0.05 \text{ mg}} \times \frac{1 \text{ mg}}{1000 \text{ mcg}} \times \frac{100 \text{ mcg}}{1}$
$= 2 \text{ tablets}$

6. $x \text{ mL} = \frac{5 \text{ mL}}{10 \text{ mg}} \times \frac{25 \text{ mg}}{1} = 12.5 \text{ mL}$

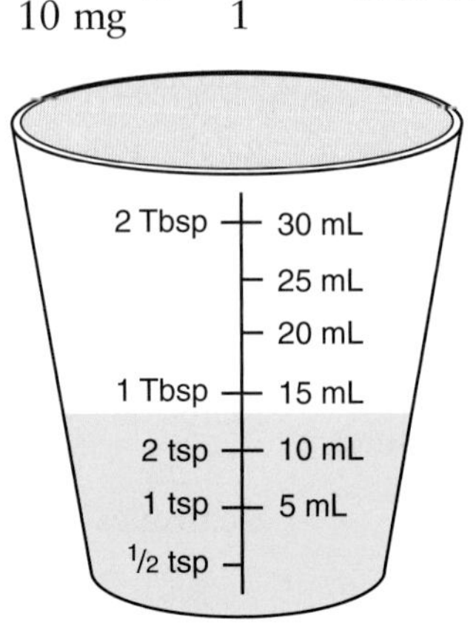

7. $x \text{ tablets} = \frac{1 \text{ tablet}}{120 \text{ mg}} \times \frac{60 \text{ mg}}{1} = 0.5 \text{ tablet}$

8. $x \text{ tablets} = \frac{1 \text{ tablet}}{30 \text{ mg}} \times \frac{30 \text{ mg}}{1} = 1 \text{ tablet}$

9. $x \text{ mL} = \frac{5 \text{ mL}}{25 \text{ mg}} \times \frac{50 \text{ mg}}{1} = 10 \text{ mL}$

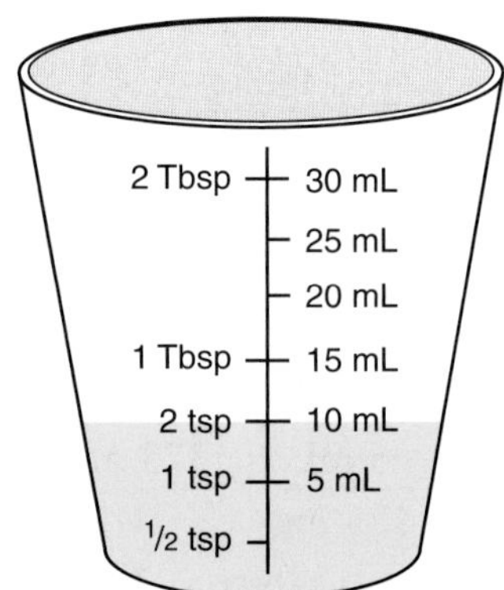

10. $x \text{ mL} = \frac{5 \text{ mL}}{20 \text{ mg}} \times \frac{30 \text{ mg}}{1} = 7.5 \text{ mL}$

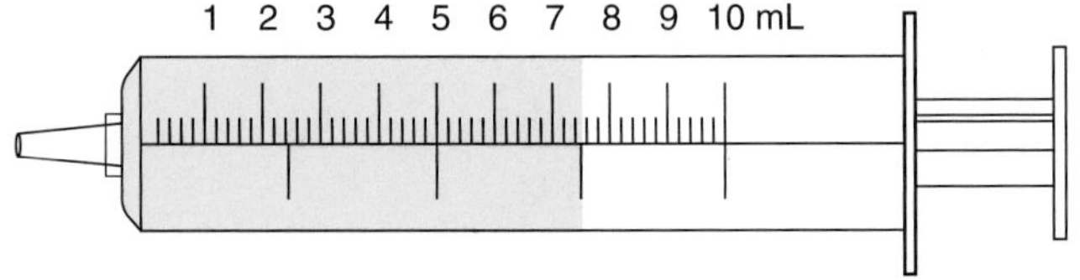

ANSWERS

11. $x \text{ tablets} = \frac{1 \text{ tablet}}{0.2 \text{ mg}} \times \frac{0.1 \text{ mg}}{1} = 0.5 \text{ tablet}$

12. $x \text{ mL} = \frac{22.5 \text{ mL}}{30 \text{ mEq}} \times \frac{20 \text{ mEq}}{1} = 15 \text{ mL}$

13. $x \text{ tablets} = \frac{1 \text{ tablet}}{20 \text{ mg}} \times \frac{40 \text{ mg}}{1} = 2 \text{ tablets}$

14. $x \text{ capsules} = \frac{1 \text{ capsule}}{50 \text{ mg}} \times \frac{100 \text{ mg}}{1}$
$= 2 \text{ capsules}$

15. $x \text{ mL} = \frac{1 \text{ mL}}{10 \text{ mg}} \times \frac{38 \text{ mg}}{1} = 3.8 \text{ mL}$

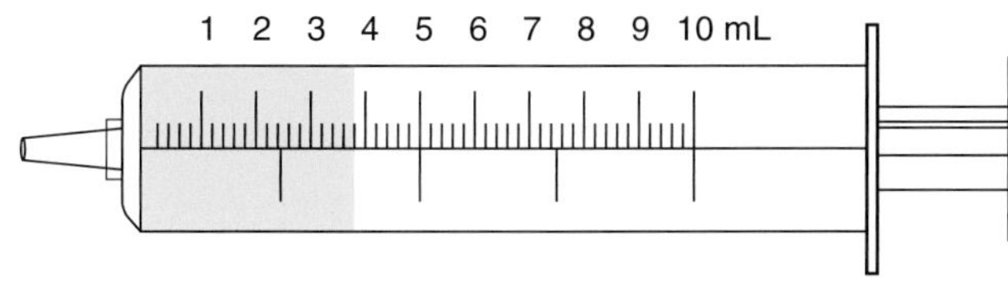

16. $x \text{ mL} = \frac{5 \text{ mL}}{125 \text{ mg}} \times \frac{100 \text{ mg}}{1} = 4 \text{ mL}$

17. $x \text{ tablets} = \frac{1 \text{ tablet}}{10 \text{ mg}} \times \frac{30 \text{ mg}}{1} = 3 \text{ tablets}$

18. $x \text{ tablets} = \frac{1 \text{ tablet}}{40 \text{ mg}} \times \frac{80 \text{ mg}}{1} = 2 \text{ tablets}$

19. $x \text{ tablets} = \frac{1 \text{ tablet}}{10 \text{ mg}} \times \frac{20 \text{ mg}}{1} = 2 \text{ tablets}$

20. $x \text{ tablets} = \frac{1 \text{ tablet}}{60 \text{ mg}} \times \frac{90 \text{ mg}}{1} = 1.5 \text{ tablets}$

$x \frac{\text{tablets}}{\text{day}} = \frac{1.5 \text{ tablets}}{1 \text{ dose}} \times \frac{3 \text{ doses}}{1 \text{ day}}$
$= 4.5 \text{ tablets/day}$

21. $x \text{ tablets} = \frac{1 \text{ tablet}}{0.25 \text{ mg}} \times \frac{0.5 \text{ mg}}{1} = 2 \text{ tablets}$

22. $x \text{ tablets} = \frac{1 \text{ tablet}}{5 \text{ mg}} \times \frac{10 \text{ mg}}{1} = 2 \text{ tablets}$

23. $x \text{ tablets} = \frac{1 \text{ tablet}}{100 \text{ mg}} \times \frac{150 \text{ mg}}{1} = 1.5 \text{ tablets}$

24. $x \text{ tablets} = \frac{1 \text{ tablet}}{10 \text{ mg}} \times \frac{30 \text{ mg}}{1} = 3 \text{ tablets}$

25. $x \text{ tablets} = \frac{1 \text{ tablet}}{30 \text{ mg}} \times \frac{60 \text{ mg}}{1} = 2 \text{ tablets}$

CHAPTER 11 Dimensional Analysis—Posttest 2, pp. 245–251

1. $x \text{ capsules} = \frac{1 \text{ capsule}}{10 \text{ mg}} \times \frac{20 \text{ mg}}{1}$
$= 2 \text{ capsules}$

2. $x \text{ mL} = \frac{5 \text{ mL}}{4 \text{ mg}} \times \frac{8 \text{ mg}}{1} = 10 \text{ mL}$

3. $x \text{ mL} = \frac{5 \text{ mL}}{25 \text{ mg}} \times \frac{60 \text{ mg}}{1} = 12 \text{ mL}$

4. $x \text{ tablets} = \frac{1 \text{ tablet}}{10 \text{ mg}} \times \frac{15 \text{ mg}}{1} = 1.5 \text{ tablets}$

5. $x \text{ mL} = \frac{30 \text{ mL}}{20 \text{ mEq}} \times \frac{5 \text{ mEq}}{1} = 7.5 \text{ mL}$

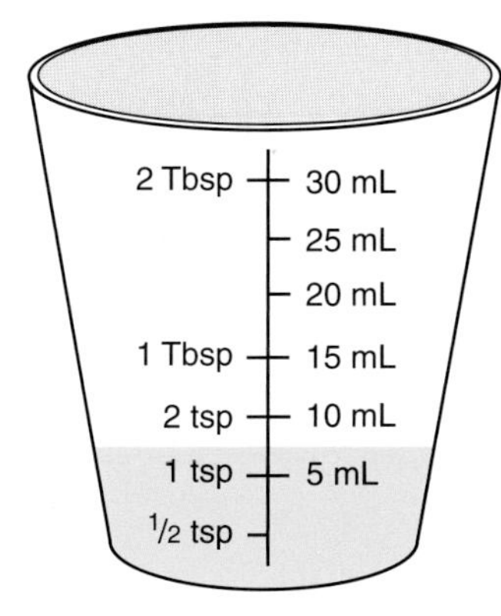

6. $x \text{ capsules} = \frac{1 \text{ capsule}}{250 \text{ mg}} \times \frac{250 \text{ mg}}{1}$
$= 1 \text{ capsule}$

7. $x \text{ tablets} = \frac{1 \text{ tablet}}{2.5 \text{ mg}} \times \frac{7.5 \text{ mg}}{1} = 3 \text{ tablets}$

8. $x \text{ mL} = \frac{1 \text{ mL}}{0.05 \text{ mg}} \times \frac{0.05 \text{ mg}}{1} = 1 \text{ mL}$

9. $x \text{ capsules} = \frac{1 \text{ capsule}}{50 \text{ mg}} \times \frac{1000 \text{ mg}}{1 \text{ g}} \times \frac{0.1 \text{ g}}{1}$
$= 2 \text{ capsules}$

10. $x \text{ tablets} = \frac{1 \text{ tablet}}{325 \text{ mg}} \times \frac{650 \text{ mg}}{1} = 2 \text{ tablets}$

11. $x \text{ tablets} = \frac{1 \text{ tablet}}{50 \text{ mg}} \times \frac{100 \text{ mg}}{1} = 2 \text{ tablets}$

12. $x \text{ mL} = \frac{5 \text{ mL}}{125 \text{ mg}} \times \frac{250 \text{ mg}}{1} = 10 \text{ mL}$

13. $x \text{ tablets} = \frac{1 \text{ tablet}}{5 \text{ mg}} \times \frac{20 \text{ mg}}{1}$
$= 4 \text{ tablets of } 5 \text{ mg}$

14. $x \text{ tablets} = \frac{1 \text{ tablet}}{0.125 \text{ mg}} \times \frac{0.25 \text{ mg}}{1}$
$= 2 \text{ tablets}$

15. $x \text{ mL} = \frac{5 \text{ mL}}{20 \text{ mg}} \times \frac{25 \text{ mg}}{1} = 6.25 \text{ mL}$

16. $x \text{ tablets} = \frac{1 \text{ tablet}}{100 \text{ mg}} \times \frac{1000 \text{ mg}}{1 \text{ g}} \times \frac{0.15 \text{ g}}{1}$
$= 1.5 \text{ tablets}$

17. $x \text{ tablets} = \frac{1 \text{ tablet}}{40 \text{ mg}} \times \frac{80 \text{ mg}}{1} = 2 \text{ tablets}$

18. $x \text{ tablets} = \frac{1 \text{ tablet}}{7.5 \text{ mg}} \times \frac{15 \text{ mg}}{1} = 2 \text{ tablets}$

19. $x \text{ tablets} = \frac{1 \text{ tablet}}{15 \text{ mg}} \times \frac{30 \text{ mg}}{1} = 2 \text{ tablets}$

20. $x \text{ tablets} = \frac{1 \text{ tablet}}{250 \text{ mg}} \times \frac{750 \text{ mg}}{1} = 3 \text{ tablets}$

21. $x \text{ tablets} = \frac{1 \text{ tablet}}{5 \text{ mg}} \times \frac{10 \text{ mg}}{1} = 2 \text{ tablets}$

22. $x \text{ capsules} = \frac{1 \text{ capsule}}{75 \text{ mg}} \times \frac{1000 \text{ mg}}{1 \text{ g}} \times \frac{0.225 \text{ g}}{1}$
$= 3 \text{ capsules}$

23. $x \text{ mL} = \frac{5 \text{ mL}}{50 \text{ mg}} \times \frac{100 \text{ mg}}{1} = 10 \text{ mL}$

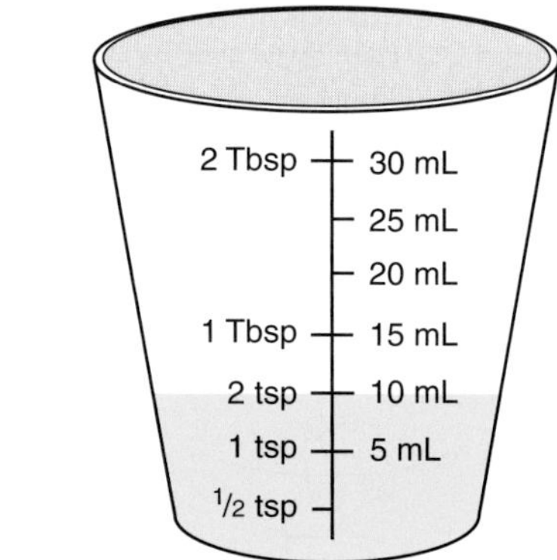

24. $x \text{ tablets} = \frac{1 \text{ tablet}}{2.5 \text{ mg}} \times \frac{5 \text{ mg}}{1} = 2 \text{ tablets}$

25. $x \text{ mL} = \frac{5 \text{ mL}}{200 \text{ mg}} \times \frac{1000 \text{ mg}}{1 \text{ g}} \times \frac{1 \text{ g}}{1}$
$= 25 \text{ mL}$

CHAPTER 11 Proportion/Formula Method—Worksheet, pp. 215–238

Proportion	Formula
1. 1 mg : 1 cap :: 2 mg : x cap 1 : 1 :: 2 : x $x = 2$ capsules	$\frac{2 \text{ mg}}{1 \text{ mg}} \times 1 \text{ cap} = 2 \text{ capsules}$
2. 20 mg : 5 mL :: 30 mg : x mL 20 : 5 :: 30 : x $20x = 150$ $x = \frac{150}{20}$ $x = 7.5$ mL	$\frac{30 \text{ mg}}{20 \text{ mg}} \times 5 \text{ mL} =$ $\frac{30}{\cancel{20}_4} \times \frac{\cancel{5}^1}{1} = \frac{30}{4}$ $\frac{30}{4} = 7.5 \text{ mL}$

ANSWERS

Proportion	Formula
3. 0.05 mg : 1 tab :: 0.2 mg : x tab 0.05 : 1 :: 0.2 : x $0.05x = 0.2$ $x = \frac{0.2}{0.05}$ $x = 4$ tablets 0.05 mg : 1 tab :: 0.15 mg : x tab 0.05 : 1 :: 0.15 : x $0.05x = 0.15$ $x = \frac{0.15}{0.05}$ $x = 3$ tablets	$\frac{0.2 \text{ mg}}{0.05 \text{ mg}} \times 1 \text{ tab} =$ $\frac{0.2}{0.05} = 4$ tablets $\frac{0.15 \text{ mg}}{0.05 \text{ mg}} \times 1 \text{ tab} =$ $\frac{0.15}{0.05} = 3$ tablets
4. 250 mg : 1 tab :: 500 mg : x tab 250 : 1 :: 500 : x $250x = 500$ $x = \frac{500}{250}$ $x = 2$ tablets	$\frac{500}{250} \times 1 \text{ tab} =$ $\frac{\overset{2}{\cancel{500}}}{\underset{1}{\cancel{250}}} =$ $\frac{2}{1} = 2$ tablets
5. 5 mg : 5 mL :: 2.5 mg : x mL 5 : 5 :: 2.5 : x $5x = 12.5$ $x = \frac{12.5}{5}$ $x = 2.5$ mL	$\frac{2.5 \text{ mg}}{5 \text{ mg}} \times 5 \text{ mL} =$ $\frac{2.5}{\underset{1}{\cancel{5}}} \times \frac{\overset{1}{\cancel{5}}}{1} = \frac{2.5}{1} = 2.5$ mL

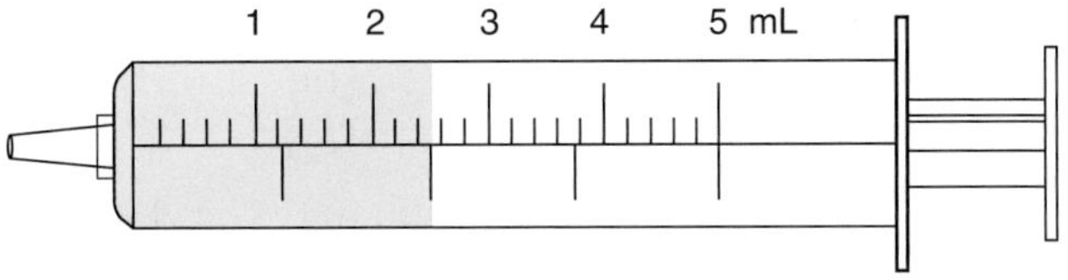

1 2 3 4 5 mL

Proportion	Formula
6. 1 mg : 1 tab :: 2 mg : x tab 1 : 1 :: 2 : x $x = 2$ tablets	$\frac{2 \text{ mg}}{1 \text{ mg}} \times 1 \text{ tab} =$ $\frac{2}{1} = 2$ tablets
7. 10 mg : 1 tab :: 20 mg : x tab 10 : 1 :: 20 : x $10x = 20$ $x = \frac{20}{10}$ $x = 2$ tablets	$\frac{20}{10} \times 1 \text{ tab} =$ $\frac{\overset{2}{\cancel{20}}}{\underset{1}{\cancel{10}}} = 2$ tablets
8. 0.5 g : 1 tab :: 1 g : x tab 0.5 : 1 :: 1 : x $0.5x = 1$ $x = \frac{1}{0.5}$ $x = 2$ tablets	$\frac{1 \text{ g}}{0.5 \text{ g}} \times 1 \text{ tab} =$ $\frac{1}{0.5} = 2$ tablets

Proportion	Formula
9. $20 \text{ mg} : 5 \text{ mL} :: 40 \text{ mg} : x \text{ mL}$ $20 : 5 :: 40 : x$ $20x = 200$ $x = \frac{200}{20}$ $x = 10 \text{ mL}$	$\frac{40}{20} \times 5 \text{ mL} =$ $\frac{\overset{10}{\cancel{40}}}{\underset{\underset{1}{\cancel{4}}}{\cancel{20}}} \times \frac{5}{1} =$ $\frac{10}{1} = 10 \text{ mL}$
10. $0.5 \text{ mg} : 1 \text{ tab} :: 1 \text{ mg} : x \text{ tab}$ $0.5 : 1 :: 1 : x$ $0.5x = 1$ $x = \frac{1}{0.5}$ $x = 2$ tablets	$\frac{1 \text{ mg}}{0.5 \text{ mg}} \times 1 \text{ tab} =$ $\frac{1}{0.5} = 2$ tablets
11. $400 \text{ mg} : 1 \text{ tab} :: 800 : x \text{ tab}$ $400 : 1 :: 800 : x$ $400x = 800$ $x = \frac{800}{400}$ $x = 2$ tablets	$\frac{800 \text{ mg}}{400 \text{ mg}} \times 1 \text{ tab} =$ $\frac{800}{400} = 2$ tablets
12. $1000 \text{ mg} : 1 \text{ g} : x \text{ mg} : 0.6 \text{ g}$ $1000 : 1 :: x : 0.6$ $x = 600 \text{ mg}$ $300 \text{ mg} : 1 \text{ tab} :: 600 \text{ mg} : x \text{ tab}$ $300 : 1 :: 600 : x$ $300x = 600$ $x = \frac{600}{300}$ $x = 2$ tablets $600 \text{ mg} : 1 \text{ dose} :: x \text{ mg} : 2 \text{ dose}$ $600 : 1 :: x : 2$ $x = 1200 \text{ mg}$	$\frac{600 \text{ mg}}{300 \text{ mg}} \times 1 \text{ tab} =$ $\frac{600}{300} = 2$ tablets $\frac{600 \text{ mg}}{1 \text{ dose}} \times \frac{2 \text{ doses}}{1 \text{ day}} = 1200 \text{ mg}$
13. $10 \text{ mg} : 1 \text{ tablet} :: 30 \text{ mg} : x \text{ tablets}$ $10x = 30$ $x = \frac{30}{10}$ $x = 3$ tablets	$\frac{30 \text{ mg}}{10 \text{ mg}} \times 1 \text{ tab} =$ $\frac{30}{10} = 3$ tablets
14. $1 \text{ g} : 1000 \text{ mg} :: 0.75 \text{ g} : x \text{ mg}$ $1 : 1000 :: 0.75 : x$ $x = 750 \text{ mg}$ $750 \text{ mg} : 1 \text{ tab} :: 750 \text{ mg} : x \text{ tab}$ $750 : 1 :: 750 : x$ $750x = 750$ $x = \frac{750}{750}$ $x = 1$ tablet	$\frac{750 \text{ mg}}{750 \text{ mg}} \times 1 \text{ tab} =$ $\frac{750}{750} = 1$ tablet

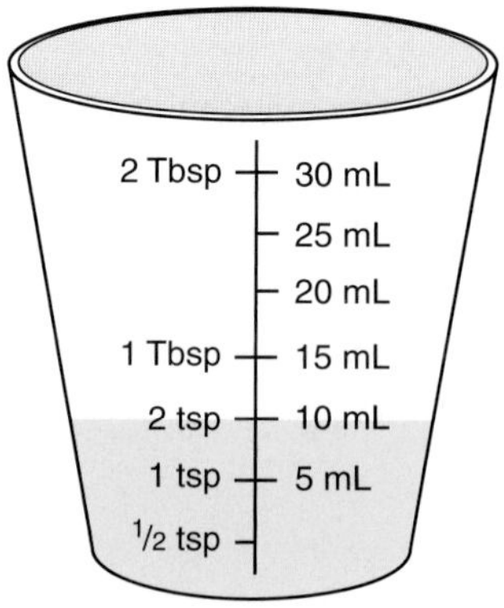

Proportion	Formula
15. 40 mg : 1 cap :: 80 mg : x cap 40 : 1 :: 80 : x $40x = 80$ $x = 2$ capsules	$\frac{80 \text{ mg}}{40 \text{ mg}} \times 1 \text{ cap} =$ $\frac{80}{40} = 2$ capsules
16. 0.5 g : 1 tab :: 4 g : x tab 0.5 : 1 :: 4 : x $0.5x = 4$ $x = \frac{4}{0.5}$ $x = 8$ tablets 0.5 g : 1 tab :: 2 g : x tab 0.5 : 1 :: 2 : x $0.5x = 2$ $x = \frac{2}{0.5}$ $x = 4$ tablets	$\frac{4 \text{ g}}{0.5 \text{ g}} \times 1 \text{ tab} =$ $\frac{4}{0.5} = 8$ tablets $\frac{2 \text{ g}}{0.5 \text{ g}} \times 1 \text{ tab} =$ $\frac{2}{0.5} = 4$ tablets
17. 400 mg : 1 tab :: 800 mg : x tab 400 : 1 :: 800 : x $400x = 800$ $x = \frac{800}{400}$ $x = 2$ tablets	$\frac{800 \text{ mg}}{400 \text{ mg}} \times 1 \text{ tab} =$ $\frac{\overset{2}{\cancel{800}}}{\underset{1}{\cancel{400}}} = 2$ tablets
18. 30 mL : 1 dose :: x mL : 4 doses 120 mL $= x$ 120 mL given each day	
19. 12.5 mg : 5 mL :: 30 mg : x mL 12.5 : 5 :: 30 : x $12.5x = 150$ $x = \frac{150}{12.5}$ $x = 12$ mL	$\frac{30 \text{ mg}}{12.5 \text{ mg}} \times \frac{5 \text{ mL}}{1} =$ $\frac{30}{12.5} \times \frac{5}{1} =$ $\frac{150}{12.5} = 12$ mL
20. 30 mg : 1 tab :: 60 mg : x tab 30 : 1 :: 60 : x $30x = 60$ $x = \frac{60}{30}$ $x = 2$ tablets	$\frac{60 \text{ mg}}{30 \text{ mg}} \times 1 \text{ tab} =$ $\frac{60}{30} = 2$ tablets
21. 125 mg : 5 mL :: x mg : 5.5 mL 125 : 5 :: x : 5.5 $5x = 687.5$ $x = \frac{687.5}{5}$ $x = 137.5$ mg	$\frac{x \text{ mg}}{125 \text{ mg}} \times 5 \text{ mL} = 5.5 \text{ mL}$ $\frac{x}{\underset{25}{\cancel{125}}} \times \frac{\overset{1}{\cancel{5}}}{1} = 5.5$ $\frac{x}{25} = 5.5$ $\frac{\overset{1}{\cancel{25}}}{1} \times \frac{x}{\underset{1}{\cancel{25}}} = 5.5 \times 25$ $x = 137.5$ mg

ANSWERS

Proportion / **Formula**

22\. Proportion:

$40 \text{ mg} : 1 \text{ tab} :: 80 \text{ mg} : x \text{ tab}$

$40 : 1 :: 80 : x$

$40x = 80$

$x = \dfrac{80}{40}$

$x = 2 \text{ tablets}$

Formula:

$\dfrac{80 \text{ mg}}{40 \text{ mg}} \times 1 \text{ tab} =$

$\dfrac{80}{40} = 2 \text{ tablets}$

23\. Proportion:

$0.4 \text{ mg} : 1 \text{ tab} :: x \text{ mg} : 2 \text{ tab}$

$0.4 : 1 :: x : 2$

$x = 0.8 \text{ mg}$

Formula:

$\dfrac{x \text{ mg}}{0.4 \text{ mg}} \times 1 \text{ tab} = 2 \text{ tablets}$

$\dfrac{x}{0.4} = 2$

$x = 2 \times 0.4$

$x = 0.8 \text{ mg}$

24\. Proportion:

$0.5 \text{ mg} : 5 \text{ mL} :: 1.5 \text{ mg} : x \text{ mL}$

$0.5 : 5 :: 1.5 : x$

$0.5x = 7.5$

$x = \dfrac{7.5}{0.5}$

$x = 15 \text{ mL}$

$30 \text{ mL} : 1 \text{ fl oz} :: 15 \text{ mL} : x \text{ fl oz}$

$30 : 1 :: 15 : x$

$30x = 15$

$x = \dfrac{15}{30}$

$x = ½ \text{ fl oz}$

Formula:

$\dfrac{1.5 \text{ mg}}{0.5 \text{ mg}} \times \dfrac{5 \text{ mL}}{1} =$

$\dfrac{1.5}{0.5} \times \dfrac{5}{1} = \dfrac{7.5}{0.5}$

$\dfrac{7.5}{0.5} = 15 \text{ mL}$

$15 \text{ mL} \times \dfrac{1 \text{ oz}}{30 \text{ mL}} = \dfrac{1}{2} \text{ fl oz}$

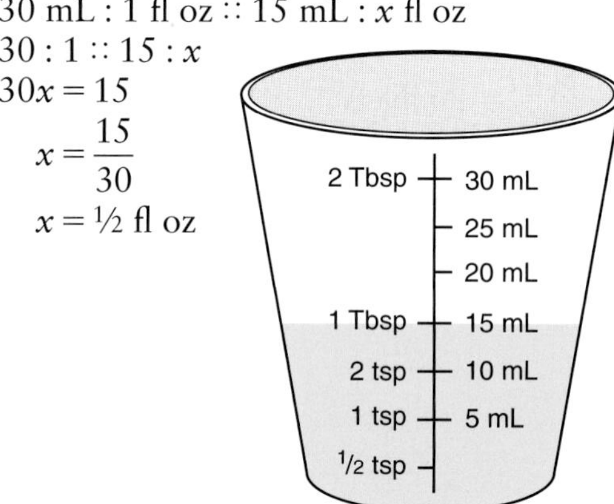

25\. Proportion:

$375 \text{ mg} : 5 \text{ mL} :: 500 \text{ mg} : x \text{ mL}$

$375 : 5 :: 500 : x$

$375x = 2500$

$x = \dfrac{2500}{375}$

$x = 6.6666 \text{ mL or } 6.7 \text{ mL}$

Formula:

$\dfrac{500 \text{ mg}}{375 \text{ mg}} \times 5 \text{ mL} =$

$\dfrac{500}{\cancel{375}_{75}} \times \dfrac{\cancel{5}^{1}}{1} =$

$\dfrac{500}{75} = 6.7 \text{ mL}$

26\. Proportion:

$50 \text{ mg} : 1 \text{ tab} :: 25 \text{ mg} : x \text{ tab}$

$50 : 1 :: 25 : x$

$50x = 25$

$x = \dfrac{25}{50}$

$x = ½ \text{ tablet}$

Formula:

$\dfrac{25 \text{ mg}}{50 \text{ mg}} \times 1 \text{ tab} =$

$\dfrac{25}{50} = ½ \text{ tablet}$

27\. Proportion:

Supplied in 12-oz bottle

$1 \text{ fl oz} : 1 \text{ dose} :: 12 \text{ fl oz} : x \text{ dose}$

$1 : 1 :: 12 : x$

$x = 12 \text{ doses}$

Formula:

$\dfrac{1 \text{ dose}}{1 \text{ oz}} \times 12 \text{ oz} = 12 \text{ doses}$

$30 \text{ mL} = 1 \text{ fl oz}$

Order is for 1 fl oz

Proportion

28. $0.125 \text{ mg} : 1 \text{ tab} :: 0.25 \text{ mg} : x \text{ tab}$

$0.125 : 1 :: 0.25 : x$

$0.125x = 0.25$

$x = \dfrac{0.25}{0.125}$

$x = 2 \text{ tablets}$

29. $30 \text{ mg} : 1 \text{ tab} :: 15 \text{ mg} : x \text{ tab}$

$30 : 1 :: 15 : x$

$30x = 15$

$x = \dfrac{15}{30}$

$x = \frac{1}{2} \text{ tablet}$

30. $250 \text{ mg} : 5 \text{ mL} :: 125 \text{ mg} : x \text{ mL}$

$250 : 5 :: 125 : x$

$250x = 625$

$x = \dfrac{625}{250}$

$x = 2.5 \text{ mL}$

31. $50 \text{ mg} : 1 \text{ tab} :: 25 \text{ mg} : x \text{ tab}$

$50 : 1 :: 25 : x$

$50x = 25$

$x = \dfrac{25}{50}$

$x = \frac{1}{2} \text{ tablet}$

32. $1000 \text{ mg} : 1 \text{ g} :: x \text{ mg} : 0.6 \text{ g}$

$1000 : 1 :: x : 0.6$

$x = 600 \text{ mg}$

$200 \text{ mg} : 1 \text{ tab} :: 600 \text{ mg} : x \text{ tab}$

$200 : 1 :: 600 : x$

$200x = 600$

$x = \dfrac{600}{200}$

$x = 3 \text{ tablets}$

$3 \text{ tablets} : 1 \text{ dose} :: x \text{ tab} : 6 \text{ doses}$

$3 : 1 :: x : 6$

$x = 18 \text{ tablets}$

33. $4 \text{ mg} : 5 \text{ mL} :: 8 \text{ mg} : x \text{ mL}$

$4 : 5 :: 8 : x$

$4x = 40$

$x = \dfrac{40}{4}$

$x = 10 \text{ mL}$

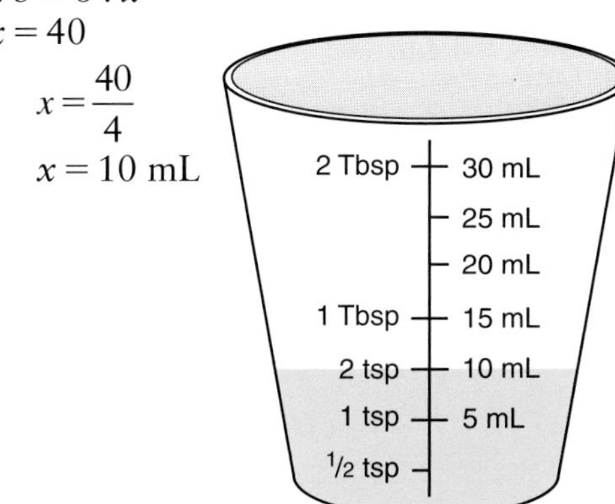

Formula

28. $\dfrac{0.25 \text{ mg}}{0.125 \text{ mg}} \times 1 \text{ tab} =$

$\dfrac{0.25}{0.125} = 2 \text{ tablets}$

29. $\dfrac{15 \text{ mg}}{30 \text{ mg}} \times 1 \text{ tab} =$

$\dfrac{15}{30} = \frac{1}{2} \text{ tablet}$

30. $\dfrac{125 \text{ mg}}{250 \text{ mg}} \times 5 \text{ mL} =$

$\dfrac{\overset{1}{\cancel{125}}}{\underset{2}{\cancel{250}}} \times \dfrac{5}{1} = \dfrac{5}{2}$

$\dfrac{5}{2} = 2.5 \text{ mL}$

31. $\dfrac{25 \text{ mg}}{50 \text{ mg}} \times 1 \text{ tab} =$

$\dfrac{25}{50} = \frac{1}{2} \text{ tablet}$

32. $\dfrac{600 \text{ mg}}{200 \text{ mg}} = 1 \text{ tab} =$

$\dfrac{600}{200} = 3 \text{ tablets}$

$6 \text{ doses} \times \dfrac{3 \text{ tab}}{1 \text{ dose}} = 18 \text{ tablets}$

33. $\dfrac{8 \text{ mg}}{4 \text{ mg}} \times 5 \text{ mL} =$

$\dfrac{\overset{2}{\cancel{8}}}{\underset{1}{\cancel{4}}} \times \dfrac{5}{1} =$

$\dfrac{2 \times 5}{1} = 10 \text{ mL}$

Proportion	**Formula**

34. 500 mg : 5 mL :: 750 mg : x mL
500 : 5 :: 750 : x
$500x = 3750$
$x = \frac{3750}{500}$
$x = 7.5$ mL

$$\frac{750 \text{ mg}}{500 \text{ mg}} \times 5 \text{ mL} =$$
$$\frac{\overset{15}{\cancel{750}}}{\underset{2}{\cancel{\underset{100}{\cancel{500}}}}} \times \frac{\overset{1}{\cancel{5}}}{1} =$$
$$\frac{15}{2} = 7.5 \text{ mL}$$

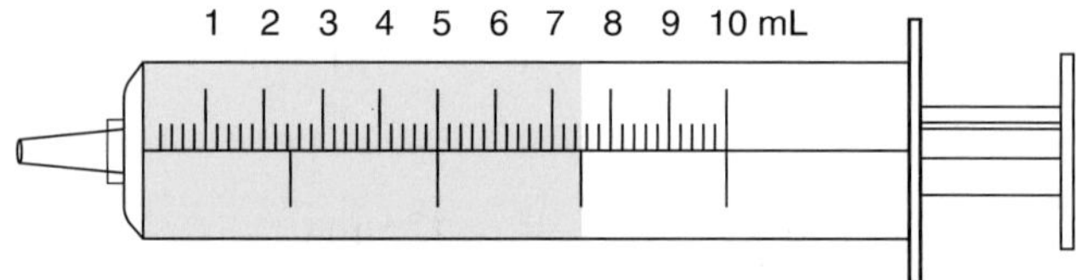

35. 20 mg : 5 mL :: 100 mg : x mL
20 : 5 :: 100 : x
$20x = 500$
$x = \frac{500}{20}$
$x = 25$ mL

$$\frac{100 \text{ mg}}{20 \text{ mg}} \times 5 \text{ mL} =$$
$$\frac{100}{\underset{4}{\cancel{20}}} \times \frac{\overset{1}{\cancel{5}}}{1} =$$
$$\frac{100}{4} = 25 \text{ mL}$$

36. 500 mg : 1 tab :: 1000 mg : x tab
500 : 1 :: 1000 : x
$500x = 1000$
$x = \frac{1000}{500}$
$x = 2$ tablets

$$\frac{1000 \text{ mg}}{500 \text{ mg}} \times 1 \text{ tab} =$$
$$\frac{1000}{500} = 2 \text{ tablets}$$

37. 2.5 mg : 1 tab :: 7.5 mg : x tab
2.5 : 1 :: 7.5 : x
$2.5x = 7.5$
$x = \frac{7.5}{2.5}$
$x = 3$ tablets

$$\frac{7.5 \text{ mg}}{2.5 \text{ mg}} \times 1 \text{ tab} =$$
$$\frac{7.5}{2.5} = 3 \text{ tablets}$$

38. 1000 mg : 1 g :: x mg : 0.2 g
1000 : 1 :: x : 0.2
$x = 200$ mg
100 mg : 1 tab :: 200 mg : x tab
100 : 1 :: 200 : x
$100x = 200$
$x = \frac{200}{100}$
$x = 2$ tablets

$$\frac{200 \text{ mg}}{100 \text{ mg}} \times 1 \text{ tab} =$$
$$\frac{200}{100} = 2 \text{ tablets}$$

Proportion	Formula
39. 1 tablet 500 mg acetaminophen in each tablet	
40. 0.25 mg : 1 tab :: 0.5 mg : x tab 0.25 : 1 :: 0.5 : x $0.25x = 0.5$ $x = \frac{0.5}{0.25}$ $x = 2$ tablets	$\frac{0.5 \text{ mg}}{0.25 \text{ mg}} \times 1 \text{ tab} =$ $\frac{0.5}{0.25} = 2$ tablets
41. 5 mg : 1 tab :: 10 mg : x tab 5 : 1 :: 10 : x $5x = 10$ $x = \frac{10}{5}$ $x = 2$ tablets	$\frac{10 \text{ mg}}{5 \text{ mg}} \times 1 \text{ tab} =$ $\frac{10}{5} = 2$ tablets
42. 50 mg : 1 tab :: 100 mg : x tab 50 : 1 :: 100 : x $50x = 100$ $x = \frac{100}{50}$ $x = 2$ tablets	$\frac{100 \text{ mg}}{50 \text{ mg}} \times 1 \text{ tab} =$ $\frac{100}{50} = 2$ tablets
43. 300 mg : 1 cap :: 600 mg : x cap 300 : 1 :: 600 : x $300x = 600$ $x = \frac{600}{300}$ $x = 2$ capsules	$\frac{600 \text{ mg}}{300 \text{ mg}} \times 1 \text{ cap} =$ $\frac{600}{300} = 2$ capsules
44. 0.125 mg : 1 tab :: 0.25 mg : x tab 0.125 : 1 :: 0.25 : x $0.125x = 0.25$ $x = \frac{0.25}{0.125}$ $x = 2$ tablets	$\frac{0.25 \text{ mg}}{0.125 \text{ mg}} \times 1 \text{ tab} =$ $\frac{0.25}{0.125} = 2$ tablets
45. 250 mg : 1 cap :: 500 mg : x cap 250 : 1 :: 500 : x $250x = 500$ $x = \frac{500}{250}$ $x = 2$ capsules 2 cap : 1 dose :: x cap : 4 doses 2 : 1 :: x : 4 $x = 8$ capsules	$\frac{500 \text{ mg}}{250 \text{ mg}} \times 1 \text{ cap} =$ $\frac{500}{250} = 2$ capsules $\frac{2 \text{ cap}}{1 \text{ dose}} \times 4 \text{ doses} = 8$ capsules
46. 20 mg : 1 cap :: 40 mg : x cap 20 : 1 :: 40 : x $20x = 40$ $x = \frac{40}{20}$ $x = 2$ capsules	$\frac{40 \text{ mg}}{20 \text{ mg}} \times 1 \text{ cap} =$ $\frac{40}{20} = 2$ capsules

Proportion	Formula
47. 30 mg : 1 tab :: 90 mg : x tab 30 : 1 :: 90 : x $30x = 90$ $x = \frac{90}{30}$ $x = 3$ tablets	$\frac{90\text{ mg}}{30\text{ mg}} \times 1\text{ tab} =$ $\frac{90}{30} = 3$ tablets
48. 75 mg : 1 tab :: 150 mg : x tab 75 : 1 :: 150 : x $75x = 150$ $x = \frac{150}{75}$ $x = 2$ tablets	$\frac{150\text{ mg}}{75\text{ mg}} \times 1\text{ tab} =$ $\frac{150}{75} = 2$ tablets
49. 12.5 mg : 1 tab :: 25 mg : x tab 12.5 : 1 :: 25 : x $12.5x = 25$ $x = \frac{25}{12.5}$ $x = 2$ tablets	$\frac{25\text{ mg}}{12.5\text{ mg}} \times 1\text{ tab} =$ $\frac{25}{12.5} = 2$ tablets
50. 15 mg : 1 mL :: 150 mg : x mL 15 : 1 :: 150 : x $15x = 150$ $x = \frac{150}{15}$ $x = 10$ mL	$\frac{150\text{ mg}}{15\text{ mg}} \times 1\text{ mL} =$ $\frac{\overset{10}{\cancel{150}}}{\underset{1}{\cancel{15}}} = 10$ mL
51. 250 mg : 1 tab :: 500 mg : x tab 250 : 1 :: 500 : x $250x = 500$ $x = \frac{500}{250}$ $x = 2$ tablets	$\frac{500\text{ mg}}{250\text{ mg}} \times 1\text{ tab} =$ $\frac{500}{250} = 2$ tablets
52. 1000 mcg : 1 mg :: x mcg : 0.2 mg 1000 : 1 :: x : 0.2 $x = 200$ mcg 100 mcg : 1 tablet :: 200 mcg : x tab 100 : 1 :: 200 : x $100x = 200$ $x = \frac{200}{100}$ $x = 2$ tablets	$\frac{200\text{ mcg}}{100\text{ mcg}} \times 1\text{ tab} =$ $\frac{200}{100} = 2$ tablets
53. 10 mg : 1 cap :: 20 mg : x cap 10 : 1 :: 20 : x $10x = 20$ $x = \frac{20}{10}$ $x = 2$ capsules	$\frac{20\text{ mg}}{10\text{ mg}} \times 1\text{ cap} =$ $\frac{20}{10} = 2$ capsules

Proportion	**Formula**
54. $10\text{ mg} : 5\text{ mL} :: 30\text{ mg} : x\text{ mL}$ $10 : 5 :: 30 : x$ $10x = 150$ $x = \frac{150}{10}$ $x = 15\text{ mL}$	$\frac{30\text{ mg}}{10\text{ mg}} \times 5\text{ mL} =$ $\frac{\overset{15}{\cancel{30}}}{\underset{1}{\cancel{\underset{2}{\cancel{10}}}}} \times \frac{\overset{1}{\cancel{5}}}{1} =$ $\frac{15}{1} = 15\text{ mL}$
55. $1000\text{ mg} : 1\text{ g} :: x\text{ mg} : 0.75\text{ g}$ $1000 : 1 :: x : 0.75$ $x = 1000 \times 0.75$ $x = 750\text{ mg}$ $250\text{ mg} : 1\text{ tab} :: 750\text{ mg} : x\text{ tab}$ $250 : 1 :: 750 : x$ $250x = 750$ $x = \frac{750}{250}$ $x = 3\text{ tablets}$	$\frac{750\text{ mg}}{250\text{ mg}} \times 1\text{ tab} =$ $\frac{750}{250} = 3\text{ tablets}$
56. $4\text{ mg} : 5\text{ mL} :: 8\text{ mg} : x\text{ mL}$ $4 : 5 :: 8 : x$ $4x = 40$ $x = \frac{40}{4}$ $x = 10\text{ mL}$	$\frac{8\text{ mg}}{4\text{ mg}} \times 5\text{ mL} =$ $\frac{8}{4} \times \frac{5}{1} = \frac{40}{4}$ $\frac{40}{4} = 10\text{ mL}$
57. $25\text{ mg} : 5\text{ mL} :: 15\text{ mg} : x\text{ mL}$ $25 : 5 :: 15 : x$ $25x = 75$ $x = \frac{75}{25}$ $x = 3\text{ mL}$	$\frac{15\text{ mg}}{25\text{ mg}} \times 5\text{ mL} =$ $\frac{15}{\underset{5}{\cancel{25}}} \times \frac{\overset{1}{\cancel{5}}}{1} = \frac{15}{5}$ $\frac{15}{5} = 3\text{ mL}$
58. $50\text{ mg} : 1\text{ tab} :: 100\text{ mg} : x\text{ tab}$ $50 : 1 :: 100 : x$ $50x = 100$ $x = \frac{100}{50}$ $x = 2\text{ tablets}$	$\frac{100\text{ mg}}{50\text{ mg}} \times 1\text{ tab} =$ $\frac{\overset{2}{\cancel{100}}}{\underset{1}{\cancel{50}}} = \frac{2}{1}$ $\frac{2}{1} = 2\text{ tablets}$

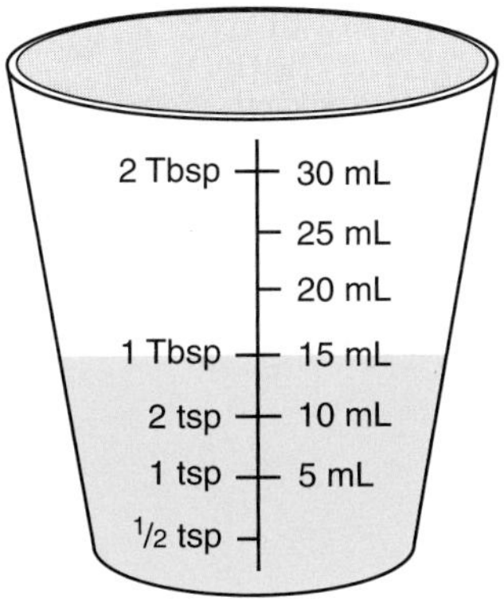

Proportion	Formula
59. 500 mg : 1 tab :: 1000 mg : x tab 500 : 1 :: 1000 : x $500x = 1000$ $x = \frac{1000}{500}$ $x = 2$ tablets	$\frac{1000 \text{ mg}}{500 \text{ mg}} \times 1 \text{ tab} =$ $\frac{1000}{500} = 2$ tablets
60. 150 mg : 5 mL :: 250 mg : x mL 150 : 5 :: 250 : x $150x = 1250$ $x = \frac{1250}{150}$ $x = 8.33$ mL or 8.3 mL	$\frac{250 \text{ mg}}{150 \text{ mg}} \times 5 \text{ mL} =$ $\frac{250}{\cancel{150}_{30}} \times \frac{\cancel{5}^{1}}{1} = \frac{250}{30}$ $\frac{250}{30} = 8.33$ mL or 8.3 mL

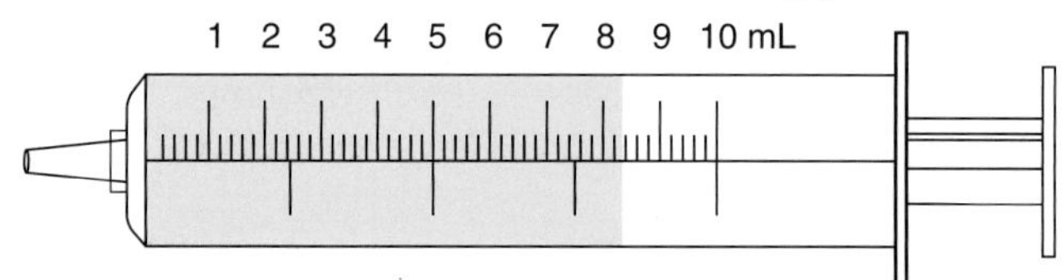

Proportion	Formula
61. 50 mg : 5 mL :: 100 mg : x mL 50 : 5 :: 100 : x $50x = 500$ $x = \frac{500}{50}$ $x = 10$ mL	$\frac{100 \text{ mg}}{50 \text{ mg}} \times 5 \text{ mL} =$ $\frac{100}{\cancel{50}_{10}} \times \frac{\cancel{5}^{1}}{1} =$ $\frac{100}{10} = 10$ mL

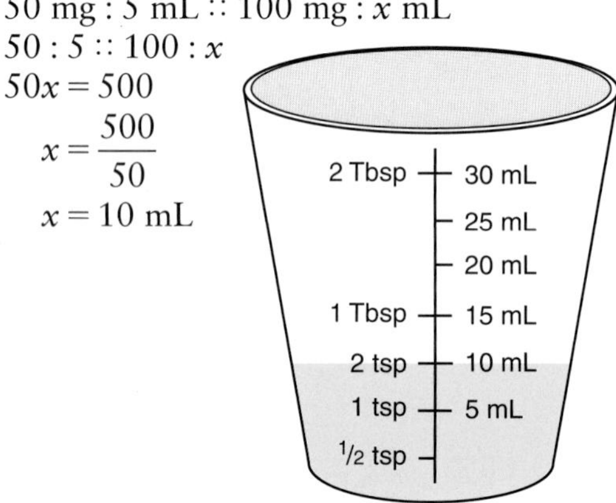

Proportion	Formula
62. 50 mg : 1 tab :: 25 mg : x tab 50 : 1 :: 25 : x $50x = 25$ $x = \frac{25}{50}$ $x = ½$ tablet	$\frac{25 \text{ mg}}{50 \text{ mg}} \times 1 \text{ tab} =$ $\frac{25}{50} = ½$ tablet
63. 80 mg : 1 tab :: 240 mg : x tab 80 : 1 :: 240 : x $80x = 240$ $x = \frac{240}{80}$ $x = 3$ tablets	$\frac{240 \text{ mg}}{80 \text{ mg}} \times 1 \text{ tab} =$ $\frac{240}{80} = 3$ tablets
64. 1000 mcg : 1 mg :: x mcg : 0.05 mg 1000 : 1 :: x : 0.05 $x = 50$ mcg 50 mcg : 1 mL :: 90 mcg : x mL 50 : 1 :: 90 : x $50x = 90$ $x = \frac{90}{50}$ $x = 1.8$ mL	$\frac{90 \text{ mcg}}{50 \text{ mcg}} \times 1 \text{ mL} =$ $\frac{90}{50} = 1.8$ mL

Proportion | **Formula**

65. $12.5\text{ mg} : 5\text{ mL} :: x\text{ mg} : 10\text{ mL}$

$12.5 : 5 :: x : 10$

$5x = 125$

$x = \frac{125}{5}$

$x = 25\text{ mg}$

$\frac{x\text{ mg}}{12.5\text{ mg}} \times 5\text{ mL} = 10\text{ mL}$

$\frac{x}{12.5} \times \frac{5}{1} = 10$

$\frac{\overset{1}{\cancel{12.5}}}{1} \times \frac{x}{\underset{1}{\cancel{12.5}}} \times \frac{5}{1} = \frac{10}{1} \times 12.5$

$5x = 125$

$x = \frac{125}{5}$

$x = 25\text{ mg}$

66. $25\text{ mg} : 1\text{ cap} :: 50\text{ mg} : x\text{ cap}$

$25 : 1 :: 50 : x$

$25x = 50$

$x = \frac{50}{25}$

$x = 2$ capsules

$\frac{50\text{ mg}}{25\text{ mg}} \times 1\text{ cap} =$

$\frac{50}{25} = 2$ capsules

67. $30\text{ mg} : 1\text{ cap} :: 90\text{ mg} : x\text{ cap}$

$30 : 1 :: 90 : x$

$30x = 90$

$x = \frac{90}{30}$

$x = 3$ capsules

$\frac{90\text{ mg}}{30\text{ mg}} \times 1\text{ cap} =$

$\frac{90}{30} = 3$ capsules

68. 40-mg tablet

$40\text{ mg} : 1\text{ tab} :: 40\text{ mg} : x\text{ tab}$

$40 : 1 :: 40 : x$

$40x = 40$

$x = \frac{40}{40}$

$x = 1$ tablet

40-mg tablets. The other strengths of the medication would require swallowing more pills.

$40\text{ mg} \times \frac{1\text{ tab}}{40\text{ mg}} = 1$ tablet

69. $20\text{ mEq} : 15\text{ mL} :: 10\text{ mEq} : x\text{ mL}$

$20 : 15 :: 10 : x$

$20x = 150$

$x = \frac{150}{20}$

$x = 7.5\text{ mL}$

$\frac{10\text{ mEq}}{20\text{ mEq}} \times \frac{15\text{mL}}{1} =$

$\frac{10}{\underset{4}{\cancel{20}}} \times \frac{\overset{3}{\cancel{15}}}{1} = \frac{30}{4}$

$\frac{30}{4} = 7.5\text{ mL}$

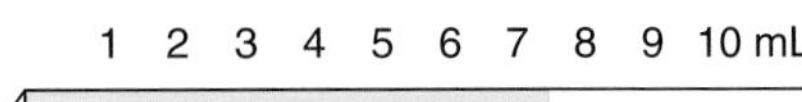

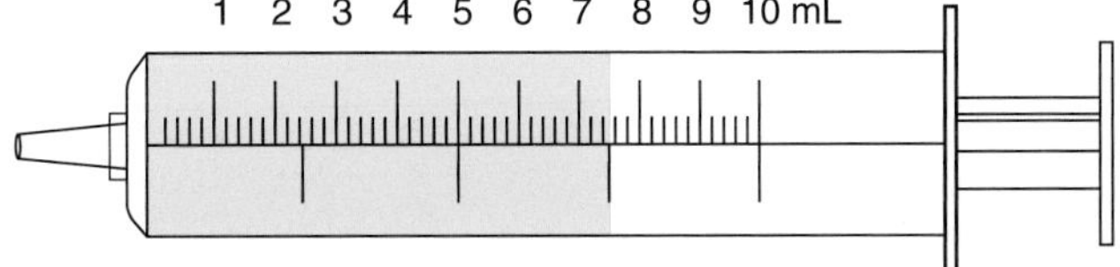

70. $0.5\text{ mg} : 1\text{ tab} :: 1.5\text{ mg} : x\text{ tab}$

$0.5 : 1 :: 1.5 : x$

$0.5x = 1.5$

$x = \frac{1.5}{0.5}$

$x = 3$ tablets

$\frac{1.5\text{ mg}}{0.5\text{ mg}} \times 1\text{ tab} =$

$\frac{1.5}{0.5} = 3$ tablets

Proportion	Formula
71. $0.25\text{ mg} : 1\text{ tab} :: 0.5\text{ mg} : x\text{ tab}$ $0.25 : 1 :: 0.5 : x$ $0.25x = 0.5$ $x = \frac{0.5}{0.25}$ $x = 2$ tablets	$\frac{0.5\text{ mg}}{0.25\text{ mg}} \times 1\text{ tab} =$ $\frac{0.5}{0.25} = 2$ tablets
72. $325\text{ mg} : 1\text{ tab} :: 650\text{ mg} : x\text{ tab}$ $325 : 1 :: 650 : x$ $325x = 650$ $x = \frac{650}{325}$ $x = 2$ tablets	$\frac{\overset{2}{\cancel{650}}\text{ mg}}{\underset{1}{\cancel{325}}\text{ mg}} \times 1\text{ tab} =$ $\frac{2}{1} = 2$ tablets
73. $0.25\text{ mg} : 1\text{ tab} :: 0.5\text{ mg} : x\text{ tab}$ $0.25 : 1 :: 0.5 : x$ $0.25x = 0.5$ $x = \frac{0.5}{0.25}$ $x = 2$ tablets	$\frac{0.5\text{ mg}}{0.25\text{ mg}} \times 1\text{ tab} =$ $\frac{0.5}{0.25} = 2$ tablets
74. $375\text{ mg} : x\text{ mL} :: 125\text{ mg} : 5\text{ mL}$ $375 : x :: 125 : 5$ $125x = 1875$ $x = 15\text{ mL}$	$\frac{375\text{ mg}}{125\text{ mg}} \times 5\text{ mL} = 15\text{ mL}$
75. $30\text{ mg} : 1\text{ tab} :: 30\text{ mg} : x\text{ tab}$ $30 : 1 :: 30 : x$ $30x = 30$ $x = \frac{30}{30}$ $x = 1$ tab	$\frac{30\text{ mg}}{30\text{ mg}} \times 1\text{ tab} =$ $\frac{30}{30} = 1$ tablet
76. $0.15\text{ mg} : 1\text{ tab} :: 0.3\text{ mg} : x\text{ tab}$ $0.15 : 1 :: 0.3 : x$ $0.15x = 0.3$ $x = \frac{0.3}{0.15}$ $x = 2$ tablets of 0.15 mg	$\frac{0.3\text{ mg}}{0.15\text{ mg}} \times 1\text{ tab} =$ $\frac{0.3}{0.15} = 2$ tablets of 0.15 mg
77. $5\text{ mg} : 1\text{ tab} :: 7.5\text{ mg} : x\text{ tab}$ $5 : 1 :: 7.5 : x$ $5x = 7.5$ $x = \frac{7.5}{5}$ $x = 1.5$ tablets	$\frac{7.5\text{ mg}}{5\text{ mg}} \times 1\text{ tab} =$ $\frac{7.5}{5} = 1.5$ tablets

Proportion | **Formula**

78. 125 mg : 5 mL :: 250 mg : x mL
125 : 5 :: 250 : x
$125x = 1250$
$$x = \frac{1250}{125}$$
$x = 10$ mL

$$\frac{250 \text{ mg}}{125 \text{ mg}} \times 5 \text{ mL} =$$
$$\frac{\overset{2}{\cancel{250}}}{\underset{1}{\cancel{125}}} \times \frac{5}{1} = \frac{10}{1}$$
$$\frac{10}{1} = 10 \text{ mL}$$

79. 50 mg : 1 cap :: 250 mg : x cap
50 : 1 :: 250 : x
$50x = 250$
$$x = \frac{250}{50}$$
$x = 5$ capsules

$$\frac{250 \text{ mg}}{50 \text{ mg}} \times 1 \text{ cap} =$$
$$\frac{250}{50} = 5 \text{ capsules}$$

80. 15 mEq : 11.25 mL :: 20 mEq : x mL
15 : 11.25 :: 20 : x
$15x = 225$
$$x = \frac{225}{15}$$
$x = 15$ mL

$$\frac{20 \text{ mEq}}{15 \text{ mEq}} \times 11.25 \text{ mL} =$$
$$x = \frac{20 \times 11.25}{15}$$
$$x = \frac{225}{15}$$
$x = 15$ mL

81. 20 mg : 5 mL :: 55 mg : x mL
20 : 5 :: 55 : x
$20x = 275$
$$x = \frac{275}{20}$$
$x = 13.75$ mL or 13.8 mL

$$\frac{55 \text{ mg}}{20 \text{ mg}} \times 5 \text{ mL} =$$
$$\frac{55}{\underset{4}{\cancel{20}}} \times \frac{\overset{1}{\cancel{5}}}{1} = \frac{55}{4}$$
$$\frac{55}{4} = 13.75 \text{ mL or } 13.8 \text{ mL}$$

82. 125 mg : 1 tab :: 250 mg : x tab
125 : 1 :: 250 : x
$125x = 250$
$$x = \frac{250}{125}$$
$x = 2$ tablets

$$\frac{250 \text{ mg}}{125 \text{ mg}} \times 1 \text{ tab} =$$
$$\frac{250}{125} = 2 \text{ tablets}$$

83. 0.05 mg : 1 tab :: 0.05 mg : x tab
0.05 : 1 :: 0.05 : x
$0.05x = 0.05$
$$x = \frac{0.05}{0.05}$$
$x = 1$ tablet

$$\frac{0.05 \text{ mg}}{0.05 \text{ mg}} \times 1 \text{ tab} =$$
$$\frac{0.05}{0.05} = 1 \text{ tablet}$$

Proportion	Formula
84. 1000 mg : 1 g :: x mg : 0.2 g 1000 : 1 :: x : 0.2 $x = 200$ mg Give 1 tablet of 200 mg 200 mg : 1 dose :: x mg : 3 doses $x = 600$ mg will be given per day	$\frac{200\text{ mg}}{200\text{ mg}} \times 1\text{ tab} =$ $\frac{200}{200} = 1\text{ tablet}$ $\frac{200\text{ mg}}{1\text{ dose}} \times 3\text{ doses} = 600\text{ mg}$
85. 5 mg : 1 tab :: 15 mg : x tab 5 : 1 :: 15 : x $5x = 15$ $x = \frac{15}{5}$ $x = 3$ tablets	$\frac{15\text{ mg}}{5\text{ mg}} \times 1\text{ tab} =$ $\frac{15}{5} = 3\text{ tablets}$
86. 400 mg : 1 tab :: 800 mg : x tab 400 : 1 :: 800 : x $400x = 800$ $x = \frac{800}{400}$ $x = 2$ tablets	$\frac{800\text{ mg}}{400\text{ mg}} \times 1\text{ tab} =$ $\frac{800}{400} = 2\text{ tablets}$
87. 250 mg : 1 cap :: 500 mg : x cap 250 : 1 :: 500 : x $250x = 500$ $x = \frac{500}{250}$ $x = 2$ capsules	$\frac{500\text{ mg}}{250\text{ mg}} \times 1\text{ cap} =$ $\frac{500}{250} = 2\text{ capsules}$
88. 25 mg : 1 tab :: 50 mg : x tab 25 : 1 :: 50 : x $25x = 50$ $x = \frac{50}{25}$ $x = 2$ tablets	$\frac{50\text{ mg}}{25\text{ mg}} \times 1\text{ tab} =$ $\frac{50}{25} = 2\text{ tablets}$
89. 10 mg : 1 pill :: 30 mg : x pills 10 : 1 :: 30 : x $10x = 30$ $x = \frac{30}{10}$ $x = 3$ pills	$\frac{30\text{ mg}}{10\text{ mg}} \times 1\text{ pill} =$ $\frac{30}{10} = 3\text{ pills}$
90. 40 mg : 4 mL : 6 mg : x mL 40 : 4 :: 6 : x $40x = 24$ $x = \frac{24}{40}$ $x = 0.6$ mL	$\frac{6\text{ mg}}{40\text{ mg}} \times 4\text{ mL} = \frac{24}{40} = 0.6\text{ mL}$
91. 75 mg : 1 cap :: 150 mg : x cap 75 : 1 :: 150 : x $75x = 150$ $x = \frac{150}{75}$ $x = 2$ capsules	$\frac{150\text{ mg}}{75\text{ mg}} \times 1\text{ cap} =$ $\frac{150}{75} = 2\text{ capsules}$

Proportion	Formula
92. 100 mg : 1 cap :: 200 mg : x cap 100 : 1 :: 200 : x $100x = 200$ $x = \frac{200}{100}$ $x = 2$ capsules	$\frac{200\text{ mg}}{100\text{ mg}} \times 1\text{ cap} =$ $\frac{200}{100} = 2$ capsules
93. 2.5 mg : 1 tab :: 10 mg : x tab 2.5 : 1 :: 10 : x $2.5x = 10$ $x = \frac{10}{2.5}$ $x = 4$ tablets	$\frac{10\text{ mg}}{2.5\text{ mg}} \times 1\text{ tab} =$ $\frac{10}{2.5} = 4$ tablets
94. 1000 mg : 1 g :: x mg : 0.25 g 1000 : 1 :: x : 0.25 $x = 250$ mg 250 mg : 1 tab :: 250 mg : x tab 250 : 1 :: 250 : x $250x = 250$ $x = 1$ tablet	$\frac{250\text{ mg}}{250\text{ mg}} \times 1\text{ tab} =$ $\frac{250}{250} = 1$ tablet
95. 10 mg : 1 tab :: 25 mg : x tab 10 : 1 :: 25 : x $10x = 25$ $x = \frac{25}{10}$ $x = 2.5$ tablets	$\frac{25\text{ mg}}{10\text{ mg}} \times 1\text{ tab} =$ $\frac{25}{10} = 2.5$ tablets
96. 10 mg : 1 tab :: 30 mg : x tab 10 : 1 :: 30 : x $10x = 30$ $x = \frac{30}{10}$ $x = 3$ tablets	$\frac{30\text{ mg}}{10\text{ mg}} \times 1\text{ tab} =$ $\frac{\cancel{30}^{3}}{\cancel{10}_{1}} = 3$ tablets
97. 5 mg : 1 tab :: 15 mg : x tab 5 : 1 :: 15 : x $5x = 15$ $x = \frac{15}{5}$ $x = 3$ tablets	$\frac{15\text{ mg}}{5\text{ mg}} \times 1\text{ tab} =$ $\frac{15}{5} = 3$ tablets
98. 1000 mg : 1 g :: x mg : 0.015 g 1000 : 1 :: x : 0.015 $x = 15$ mg 15 mg : 1 cap :: 15 mg : x cap 15 : 1 :: 15 : x $15x = 15$ $x = \frac{15}{15}$ $x = 1$ capsule	$\frac{15\text{ mg}}{15\text{ mg}} \times 1\text{ cap} =$ $\frac{15}{15} = 1$ capsule

Proportion	Formula
99. 6.7 mEq : 5 mL :: 30 mEq : x mL 6.7 : 5 :: 30 : x $6.7x = 150$ $x = \dfrac{150}{6.7}$ $x = 22.4$ mL	$\dfrac{30 \text{ mEq}}{6.7 \text{ mEq}} \times 5 \text{ mL} =$ $\dfrac{30}{6.7} \times \dfrac{5}{1} = \dfrac{150}{6.7}$ $\dfrac{150}{6.7} = 22.4$ mL
100. 40 mg : 1 tab :: 20 mg : x tab 40 : 1 :: 20 : x $40x = 20$ $x = \dfrac{20}{40}$ $x = ½$ tablet	$\dfrac{20 \text{ mg}}{40 \text{ mg}} \times 1 \text{ tab} =$ $\dfrac{20}{40} = ½$ tablet

CHAPTER 11 Proportion/Formula Method—Posttest 1, pp. 239–244

Proportion	Formula
1. 30 : 1 tab :: 60 : x tab 30 : 1 :: 60 : x $30x = 60$ $x = \dfrac{60}{30}$ $x = 2$ tablets	$\dfrac{60 \text{ mg}}{30 \text{ mg}} \times 1 \text{ tab} =$ $\dfrac{60}{30} = 2$ tablets
2. 1000 mg : 1 g :: x mg : 0.5 g 1000 : 1 :: x : 0.5 $x = 500$ mg 500 mg : 1 cap :: 500 mg : x cap 500 : 1 :: 500 : x $500x = 500$ $x = \dfrac{500}{500}$ $x = 1$ capsule	$\dfrac{500 \text{ mg}}{500 \text{ mg}} \times 1 \text{ cap} =$ $\dfrac{500}{500} = 1$ capsule
3. 250 mg : 1 cap :: 1000 mg : x cap 250 : 1 :: 1000 : x $250x = 1000$ $x = \dfrac{1000}{250}$ $x = 4$ capsules	$\dfrac{1000 \text{ mg}}{250 \text{ mg}} \times 1 \text{ cap} =$ $\dfrac{1000}{250} = 4$ capsules

Proportion	**Formula**
4. 30 mg : 1 tab :: 60 mg : x tab 30 : 1 :: 60 : x $30x = 60$ $x = \frac{\overset{2}{\cancel{60}}}{\underset{1}{\cancel{30}}}$ $x = 2$ tablets	$\frac{60 \text{ mg}}{30 \text{ mg}} \times 1 \text{ tab} =$ $\frac{\overset{2}{\cancel{60}}}{\underset{1}{\cancel{30}}} = 2$ tablets
5. 100 mcg = 0.1 mg 0.05 mg : 1 tab :: 0.1 : x tab 0.05 : 1 :: 0.1 : x $0.05x = 0.1$ $x = \frac{0.1}{0.05}$ $x = 2$ tablets	$\frac{0.1 \text{ mg}}{0.05 \text{ mg}} \times 1 \text{ tab} =$ $\frac{0.1}{0.05} = 2$ tablets
6. 10 mg : 5 mL :: 25 mg : x mL 10 : 5 :: 25 : x $10x = 125$ $x = \frac{125}{10}$ $x = 12.5$ mL	$\frac{25 \text{ mg}}{10 \text{ mg}} \times 5 \text{ mL} =$ $\frac{25}{\underset{2}{\cancel{10}}} \times \frac{\overset{1}{\cancel{5}}}{1} = \frac{25}{2}$ $\frac{25}{2} = 12.5$ mL

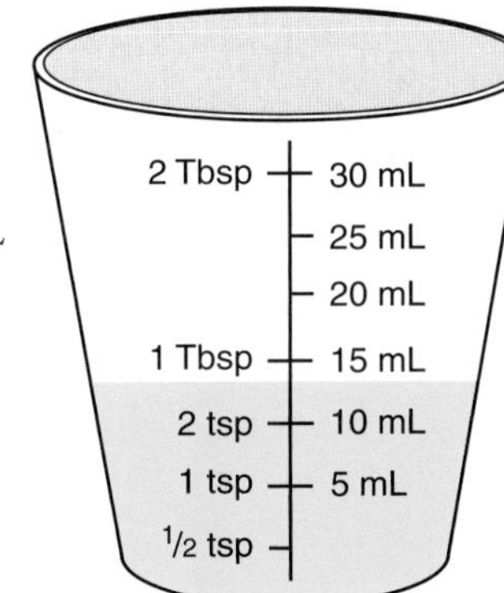

Proportion	**Formula**
7. 120 mg : 1 tab :: 60 mg : x tab 120 : 1 :: 60 : x $120x = 60$ $x = \frac{60}{120}$ $x = \frac{1}{2}$ tablet	$\frac{60 \text{ mg}}{120 \text{ mg}} \times 1 \text{ tab} =$ $\frac{\overset{1}{\cancel{60}}}{\underset{2}{\cancel{120}}} = \frac{1}{2}$ tablet
8. 30 mg : 1 tab :: 30 mg : x tab 30 : 1 :: 30 : x $30x = 30$ $x = \frac{30}{30}$ $x = 1$ tablet	$\frac{30 \text{ mg}}{30 \text{ mg}} \times 1 \text{ tab} =$ $\frac{30}{30} = 1$ tablet

Proportion	Formula
9. 25 mg : 5 mL :: 50 mg : x mL 25 : 5 :: 50 : x $25x = 250$ $x = \frac{250}{25}$ $x = 10$ mL	$\frac{50 \text{ mg}}{25 \text{ mg}} \times 5 \text{ mL} =$ $\frac{\overset{5}{\cancel{50}}}{\underset{1}{\cancel{25}}} \times \frac{\overset{1}{\cancel{5}}}{1} =$ (25 cancelled to 5, then to 1) $\frac{10}{1} = 10$ mL

Proportion	Formula
10. 20 mg : 5 mL :: 30 mg : x mL 20 : 5 :: 30 : x $20x = 150$ $x = \frac{150}{20}$ $x = 7.5$ mL	$\frac{30 \text{ mg}}{20 \text{ mg}} \times 5 \text{ mL} =$ $\frac{30}{\underset{4}{\cancel{20}}} \times \frac{\overset{1}{\cancel{5}}}{1} =$ $\frac{30}{4} = 7.5$ mL

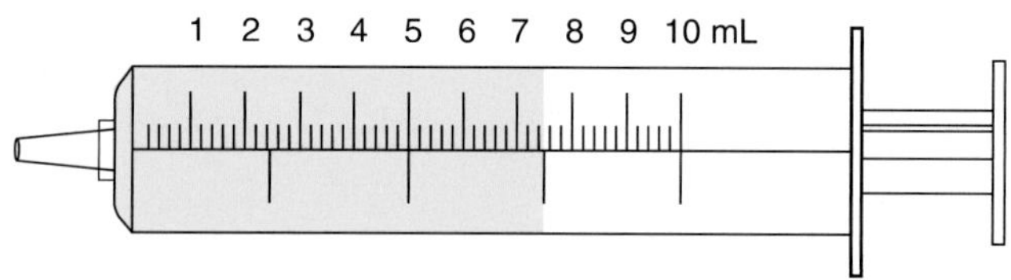

Proportion	Formula
11. 0.2 mg : 1 tab :: 0.1 mg : x tab 0.2 : 1 :: 0.1 : x $0.2x = 0.1$ $x = \frac{0.1}{0.2}$ $x = \frac{1}{2}$ tablet	$\frac{0.1 \text{ mg}}{0.2 \text{ mg}} \times 1 \text{ tab} =$ $\frac{0.1}{0.2} = \frac{1}{2}$ tablet
12. 30 mEq : 22.5 mL :: 20 mEq : x mL 30 : 22.5 :: 20 : x $30x = 450$ $x = \frac{450}{30}$ $x = 15$ mL	$\frac{20 \text{ mEq}}{30 \text{ mEq}} \times 22.5 \text{ mL} =$ $\frac{\overset{2}{\cancel{20}}}{\underset{3}{\cancel{30}}} \times \frac{22.5}{1} = \frac{45}{3}$ $\frac{\overset{15}{\cancel{45}}}{\underset{1}{\cancel{3}}} = 15$ mL

Proportion	Formula
13. 20 mg : 1 tab :: 40 mg : x tab 20 : 1 :: 40 : x $20x = 40$ $x = \frac{40}{20}$ $x = 2$ tablets	$\frac{40\text{ mg}}{20\text{ mg}} \times 1\text{ tab} =$ $\frac{40}{20} = 2$ tablets
14. 50 mg : 1 cap :: 100 mg : x cap 50 : 1 :: 100 : x $50x = 100$ $x = \frac{100}{50}$ $x = 2$ capsules	$\frac{100\text{ mg}}{50\text{ mg}} \times 1\text{ cap} =$ $\frac{100}{50} = 2$ capsules
15. 10 mg : 1 mL :: 38 mg : x mL 10 : 1 :: 38 : x $10x = 38$ $x = \frac{38}{10}$ $x = 3.8$ mL	$\frac{38\text{ mg}}{10\text{ mg}} \times 1\text{ mL} =$ $\frac{38}{10} = 3.8$ mL

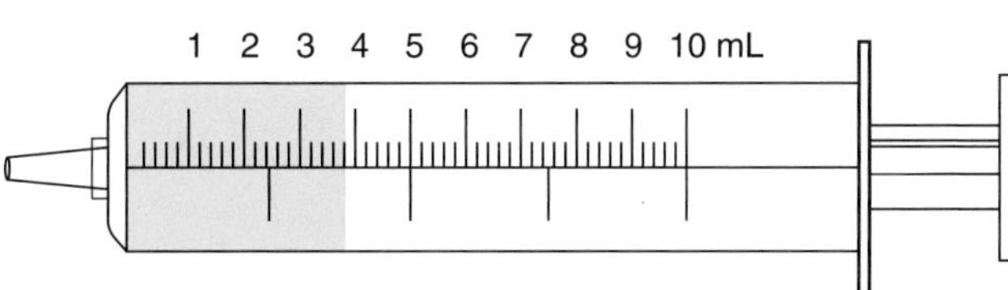

Proportion	Formula
16. 125 mg : 5 mL :: 100 mg : x mL 125 : 5 :: 100 : x $125x = 500$ $x = \frac{500}{125}$ $x = 4$ mL	$\frac{100\text{ mg}}{125\text{ mg}} \times 5\text{ mL} =$ $\frac{100}{\cancel{125}_{25}} \times \frac{\cancel{5}^{1}}{1} = \frac{100}{25}$ $\frac{100}{25} = 4$ mL
17. 10 mg : 1 tab :: 30 mg : x tab 10 : 1 :: 30 : x $10x = 30$ $x = \frac{30}{10}$ $x = 3$ tablets	$\frac{30\text{ mg}}{10\text{ mg}} \times 1\text{ tab} =$ $\frac{30}{10} = 3$ tablets
18. 40 mg : 1 tab :: 80 mg : x tab 40 : 1 :: 80 : x $40x = 80$ $x = \frac{80}{40}$ $x = 2$ tablets	$\frac{80\text{ mg}}{40\text{ mg}} \times 1\text{ tab} =$ $\frac{80}{40} = 2$ tablets
19. 10 mg : 1 tab :: 20 mg : x tab 10 : 1 :: 20 : x $10x = 20$ $x = \frac{20}{10}$ $x = 2$ tablets	$\frac{20\text{ mg}}{10\text{ mg}} \times 1\text{ tab} =$ $\frac{20}{10} = 2$ tablets

Proportion	Formula
20. $60 \text{ mg} : 1 \text{ tab} :: 90 \text{ mg} : x \text{ tab}$ $60 : 1 :: 90 : x$ $60x = 90$ $x = \frac{90}{60}$ $x = 1\frac{1}{2}$ tablets per dose $1\frac{1}{2} \text{ tab} : 1 \text{ dose} :: x \text{ tab} : 3 \text{ doses}$ $\frac{3}{2} : 1 :: x : 3$ $x = \frac{3}{2} \times \frac{3}{1}$ $x = \frac{9}{2}$ $x = 4\frac{1}{2}$ tablets/day	$\frac{90 \text{ mg}}{60 \text{ mg}} \times 1 \text{ tab} =$ $\frac{90}{60} = 1\frac{1}{2}$ tablets per dose
21. $0.25 \text{ mg} : 1 \text{ tab} :: 0.5 \text{ mg} : x \text{ tab}$ $0.25 : 1 :: 0.5 : x$ $0.25x = 0.5$ $x = \frac{0.5}{0.25}$ $x = 2$ tablets	$\frac{0.5 \text{ mg}}{0.25 \text{ mg}} \times 1 \text{ tab} =$ $\frac{0.5}{0.25} = 2$ tablets
22. $5 \text{ mg} : 1 \text{ tab} :: 10 \text{ mg} : x \text{ tab}$ $5 : 1 :: 10 : x$ $5x = 10$ $x = \frac{10}{5}$ $x = 2$ tablets	$\frac{10 \text{ mg}}{5 \text{ mg}} \times 1 \text{ tab} =$ $\frac{10}{5} = 2$ tablets
23. $100 \text{ mg} : 1 \text{ tab} :: 150 \text{ mg} : x \text{ tab}$ $100 : 1 :: 150 : x$ $100x = 150$ $x = \frac{150}{100}$ $x = 1\frac{1}{2}$ tablets	$\frac{150 \text{ mg}}{100 \text{ mg}} \times 1 \text{ tab} =$ $\frac{150}{100} = 1\frac{1}{2}$ tablets
24. $10 \text{ mg} : 1 \text{ tab} :: 30 \text{ mg} : x \text{ tab}$ $10 : 1 :: 30 : x$ $10x = 30$ $x = \frac{30}{10}$ $x = 3$ tablets	$\frac{30 \text{ mg}}{10 \text{ mg}} \times 1 \text{ tab} =$ $\frac{30}{10} = 3$ tablets
25. $30 \text{ mg} : 1 \text{ tab} :: 60 \text{ mg} : x \text{ tab}$ $30 : 1 :: 60 : x$ $30x = 60$ $x = \frac{60}{30}$ $x = 2$ tablets	$\frac{60 \text{ mg}}{30 \text{ mg}} \times 1 \text{ tab} =$ $\frac{60}{30} = 2$ tablets

CHAPTER 11 Proportion/Formula Method—Posttest 2, pp. 245–251

Proportion

1. 10 mg : 1 cap :: 20 mg : x cap
   10 : 1 :: 20 : x
   $10x = 20$
   $x = \frac{20}{10}$
   $x = 2$ capsules

2. 4 mg : 5 mL :: 8 mg : x mL
   4 : 5 :: 8 : x
   $4x = 40$
   $x = \frac{40}{4}$
   $x = 10$ mL

3. 25 mg : 5 mL :: 60 mg : x mL
   25 : 5 :: 60 : x
   $25x = 300$
   $x = \frac{300}{25}$
   $x = 12$ mL

4. 10 mg : 1 tab :: 15 mg : x tab
   10 : 1 :: 15 : x
   $10x = 15$
   $x = \frac{15}{10}$
   $x = 1\frac{1}{2}$ tablets

5. 20 mEq : 30 mL :: 5 mEq : x mL
   20 : 30 :: 5 : x
   $20x = 150$
   $x = \frac{150}{20}$
   $x = 7.5$ mL

6. 1000 mg : 1 g :: x mg : 0.25 g
   1000 : 1 :: x : 0.25
   $x = 250$ mg
   250 mg : 1 cap :: 250 mg : x cap
   250 : 1 :: 250 : x
   $250x = 250$
   $x = \frac{250}{250}$
   $x = 1$ capsule

Formula

1. $\frac{20 \text{ mg}}{10 \text{ mg}} \times 1 \text{ cap} =$
   $\frac{20}{10} = 2$ capsules

2. $\frac{8 \text{ mg}}{4 \text{ mg}} \times 5 \text{ mL} =$
   $\frac{\overset{2}{\cancel{8}}}{\underset{1}{\cancel{4}}} \times \frac{5}{1} = \frac{10}{1} = 10 \text{ mL}$

3. $\frac{60 \text{ mg}}{25 \text{ mg}} \times 5 \text{ mL} =$
   $\frac{60}{\underset{5}{\cancel{25}}} \times \frac{\overset{1}{\cancel{5}}}{1} = \frac{60}{5}$
   $\frac{60}{5} = 12 \text{ mL}$

4. $\frac{15 \text{ mg}}{10 \text{ mg}} \times 1 \text{ tab} =$
   $\frac{15}{10} = 1\frac{1}{2}$ tablets

5. $\frac{5 \text{ mEq}}{20 \text{ mEq}} \times 30 \text{ mL} =$
   $\frac{5}{\underset{2}{\cancel{20}}} \times \frac{\overset{3}{\cancel{30}}}{1} = \frac{15}{2}$
   $\frac{15}{2} = 7.5 \text{ mL}$

6. $\frac{250 \text{ mg}}{250 \text{ mg}} \times 1 \text{ cap} =$
   $\frac{250}{250} = 1$ capsule

Proportion	Formula
7. $2.5 \text{ mg} : 1 \text{ tab} :: 7.5 \text{ mg} : x \text{ tab}$ $2.5 : 1 :: 7.5 : x$ $2.5x = 7.5$ $x = \frac{7.5}{2.5}$ $x = 3 \text{ tablets}$	$\frac{7.5 \text{ mg}}{2.5 \text{ mg}} \times 1 \text{ cap} =$ $\frac{7.5}{2.5} = 3 \text{ tablets}$
8. $0.05 \text{ mg} : 1 \text{ mL} :: 0.05 \text{ mg} : x \text{ mL}$ $0.05 : 1 :: 0.05 : x$ $0.05x = 0.05$ $x = \frac{0.05}{0.05}$ $x = 1 \text{ mL}$	$\frac{0.05 \text{ mg}}{0.05 \text{ mg}} \times 1 \text{ mL} =$ $\frac{0.05}{0.05} = 1 \text{ mL}$
9. $1000 \text{ mg} : 1 \text{ g} :: x \text{ mg} : 0.1 \text{ g}$ $1000 : 1 :: x : 0.1$ $x = 100 \text{ mg}$ $50 \text{ mg} : 1 \text{ cap} :: 100 \text{ mg} : x \text{ cap}$ $50 : 1 :: 100 : x$ $50x = 100$ $x = \frac{100}{50}$ $x = 2 \text{ capsules}$	$\frac{100 \text{ mg}}{50 \text{ mg}} \times 1 \text{ cap} =$ $\frac{100}{50} = 2 \text{ capsules}$
10. $325 \text{ mg} : 1 \text{ tab} :: 650 \text{ mg} : x \text{ tab}$ $325 : 1 :: 650 : x$ $325x = 650$ $x = \frac{650}{325}$ $x = 2 \text{ tablets}$	$\frac{650 \text{ mg}}{325 \text{ mg}} \times 1 \text{ tab} =$ $\frac{650}{325} = 2 \text{ tablets}$
11. $50 \text{ mg} : 1 \text{ tab} :: 100 \text{ mg} : x \text{ tab}$ $50 : 1 :: 100 : x$ $50x = 100$ $x = \frac{100}{50}$ $x = 2 \text{ tablets}$	$\frac{100 \text{ mg}}{50 \text{ mg}} \times 1 \text{ tab} =$ $\frac{100}{50} = 2 \text{ tablets}$
12. $125 \text{ mg} : 5 \text{ mL} :: 250 \text{ mg} : x \text{ mL}$ $125 : 5 :: 250 : x$ $125x = 1250$ $x = \frac{1250}{125}$ $x = 10 \text{ mL}$	$\frac{250 \text{ mg}}{125 \text{ mg}} \times 5 \text{ mL} =$ $\frac{250}{\cancel{125}_{25}} \times \frac{\cancel{5}^{1}}{1} = \frac{250}{25}$ $\frac{250}{25} = 10 \text{ mL}$

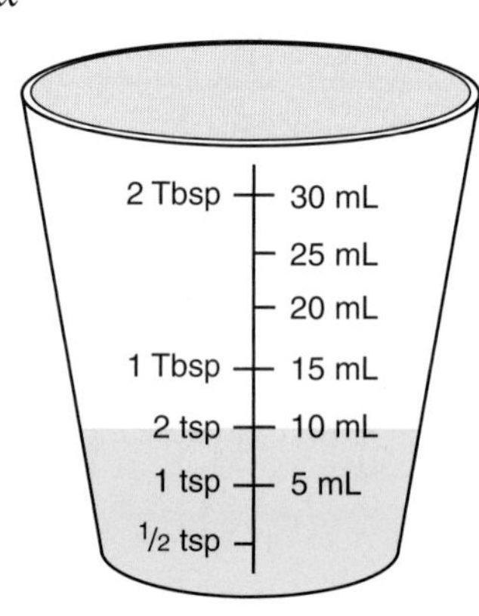

Proportion	Formula
13. 5 mg : 1 tab :: 20 mg : x tab $5 : 1 :: 20 : x$ $5x = 20$ $x = \frac{20}{5}$ $x = 4$ tablets of 5 mg/tab	$\frac{20\text{ mg}}{5\text{ mg}} \times 1\text{ tab} =$ $\frac{20}{5} = 4$ tablets of 5 mg/tab
14. 0.125 mg : 1 tab :: 0.25 mg : x tab $0.125 : 1 :: 0.25 : x$ $0.125x = 0.25$ $x = \frac{0.25}{0.125}$ $x = 2$ tablets	$\frac{0.25\text{ mg}}{0.125\text{ mg}} \times 1\text{ tab} =$ $\frac{0.25}{0.125} = 2$ tablets
15. 20 mg : 5 mL :: 25 mg : x mL $20 : 5 :: 25 : x$ $20x = 125$ $x = \frac{125}{20}$ $x = 6.25$ mL or 6.3 mL	$\frac{25\text{ mg}}{20\text{ mg}} \times 5\text{ mL} =$ $\frac{25}{\cancel{20}_{4}} \times \frac{\cancel{5}^{1}}{1} = \frac{25}{4}$ $\frac{25}{4} = 6.25$ mL or 6.3 mL
16. 1000 mg : 1 g :: x mg : 0.15 g $x = 150$ mg 100 mg : 1 tab :: 150 mg : x tab $100 : 1 :: 150 : x$ $100x = 150$ $x = \frac{150}{100}$ $x = 1.5$ tablets	$\frac{150\text{ mg}}{100\text{ mg}} \times 1\text{ tab}$ $\frac{150}{100} = 1.5$ tablets
17. 40 mg : 1 tab :: 80 mg : x tab $40 : 1 :: 80 : x$ $40x = 80$ $x = \frac{80}{40}$ $x = 2$ tablets	$\frac{80\text{ mg}}{40\text{ mg}} \times 1\text{ tab} =$ $\frac{\cancel{80}^{2}}{\cancel{40}_{1}} = 2$ tablets
18. 7.5 mg : 1 tab :: 15 mg : x tab $7.5 : 1 :: 15 : x$ $7.5x = 15$ $x = \frac{15}{7.5}$ $x = 2$ tablets	$\frac{15\text{ mg}}{7.5\text{ mg}} \times 1\text{ tab} =$ $\frac{15}{7.5} = 2$ tablets
19. 15 mg : 1 tab :: 30 mg : x tab $15 : 1 :: 30 : x$ $15x = 30$ $x = \frac{30}{15}$ $x = 2$ tablets	$\frac{30\text{ mg}}{15\text{ mg}} \times 1\text{ tab} =$ $\frac{30}{15} = 2$ tablets

Proportion / **Formula**

20. Proportion:

$250 \text{ mg} : 1 \text{ tab} :: 750 \text{ mg} : x \text{ tab}$
$250 : 1 :: 750 : x$
$250x = 750$
$x = \dfrac{750}{250}$
$x = 3 \text{ tablets}$

Formula:

$\dfrac{750 \text{ mg}}{250 \text{ mg}} \times 1 \text{ tab} =$
$\dfrac{750}{250} = 3 \text{ tablets}$

21. Proportion:

$5 \text{ mg} : 1 \text{ tab} :: 10 \text{ mg} : x \text{ tab}$
$5 : 1 :: 10 : x$
$5x = 10$
$x = \dfrac{10}{5}$
$x = 2 \text{ tablets}$

Formula:

$\dfrac{10 \text{ mg}}{5 \text{ mg}} \times 1 \text{ tab} =$
$\dfrac{10}{5} = 2 \text{ tablets}$

22. Proportion:

$75 \text{ mg} : 1 \text{ capsule} :: 225 \text{ mg} : x \text{ tab}$
$75 : 1 :: 225 : x$
$75x = 225$
$x = \dfrac{225}{75}$
$x = 3 \text{ capsules}$

Formula:

$\dfrac{225 \text{ mg}}{75 \text{ mg}} \times 1 \text{ capsule} =$
$\dfrac{225}{75} = 3 \text{ capsules}$

23. Proportion:

$50 \text{ mg} : 5 \text{ mL} :: 100 \text{ mg} : x \text{ mL}$
$50 : 5 :: 100 : x$
$50x = 500$
$x = \dfrac{500}{50}$
$x = 10 \text{ mL}$

Formula:

$\dfrac{100 \text{ mg}}{50 \text{ mg}} \times 5 \text{ mL} =$
$\dfrac{100}{\underset{10}{\cancel{50}}} \times \dfrac{\overset{1}{\cancel{5}}}{1} =$
$\dfrac{100}{10} = 10 \text{ mL}$

24. Proportion:

$2.5 \text{ mg} : 1 \text{ tab} :: 5 \text{ mg} : x \text{ tab}$
$2.5 : 1 :: 5 : x$
$2.5x = 5$
$x = \dfrac{5}{2.5}$
$x = 2 \text{ tablets}$

Formula:

$\dfrac{5 \text{ mg}}{2.5 \text{ mg}} \times 1 \text{ tab} =$
$\dfrac{5}{2.5} = 2 \text{ tablets}$

25. Proportion:

$200 \text{ mg} : 5 \text{ mL} :: 1000 \text{ mg} : x \text{ mL}$
$200 : 5 :: 1000 : x$
$200x = 5000$
$x = \dfrac{5000}{200}$
$x = 25 \text{ mL}$

Formula:

$\dfrac{1000 \text{ mg}}{200 \text{ mg}} \times 5 \text{ mL} =$
$\dfrac{1000}{\underset{40}{\cancel{200}}} \times \dfrac{\overset{1}{\cancel{5}}}{1} =$
$\dfrac{1000}{40} = 25 \text{ mL}$

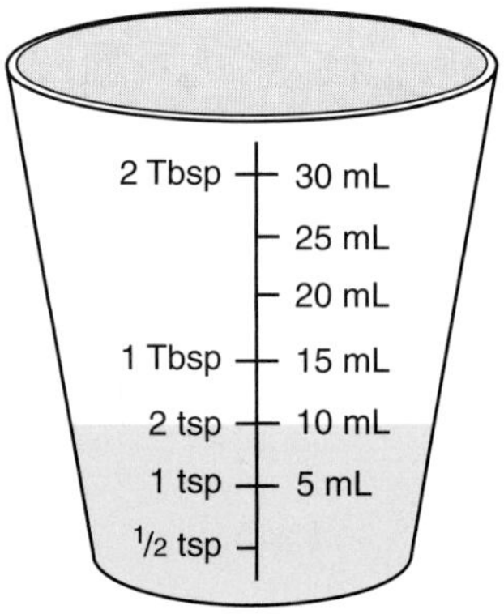

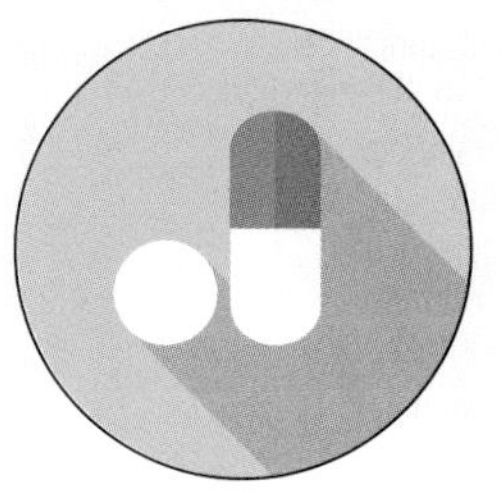

Parenteral Dosages

LEARNING OBJECTIVES

Upon completion of the materials provided in this chapter, you will be able to perform computations accurately by mastering the following mathematical concepts:

1. Using the dimensional analysis method to solve parenteral dosage problems
2. Converting all measures within the problem to equivalent measures in one system of measurement if required
3. Using a proportion to solve parenteral dosage problems
4. Using the stated formula as an alternative method of solving parenteral dosage problems

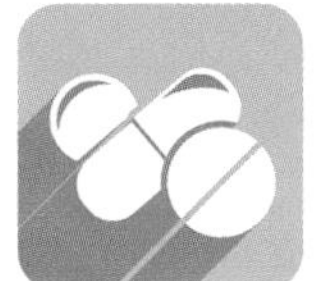

Parenteral refers to outside the alimentary canal or gastrointestinal tract. Medications may be given parenterally when they cannot be taken by mouth or when rapid action is desired. Some medications are not available by any other method of administration. Parenteral medications are absorbed directly into the bloodstream; therefore the amount of drug needed can be determined more accurately. This type of administration of medications is necessary for the uncooperative or unconscious patient, or for a patient who has been designated *NPO*. An advantage of intravenous (IV) parenteral medications is that the patient does not have to endure the discomfort of multiple injections, especially when the medications are used for pain control.

Parenteral medications are administered by (1) subcutaneous injection—beneath the skin, in fat; (2) intramuscular (IM) injection—within the muscle; or (3) intradermal injection—within the skin (Figure 12-1). Parenteral medications may also be given intravenously (IV)—within the vein. IV drugs may be diluted and administered by themselves, in conjunction with existing IV fluids,

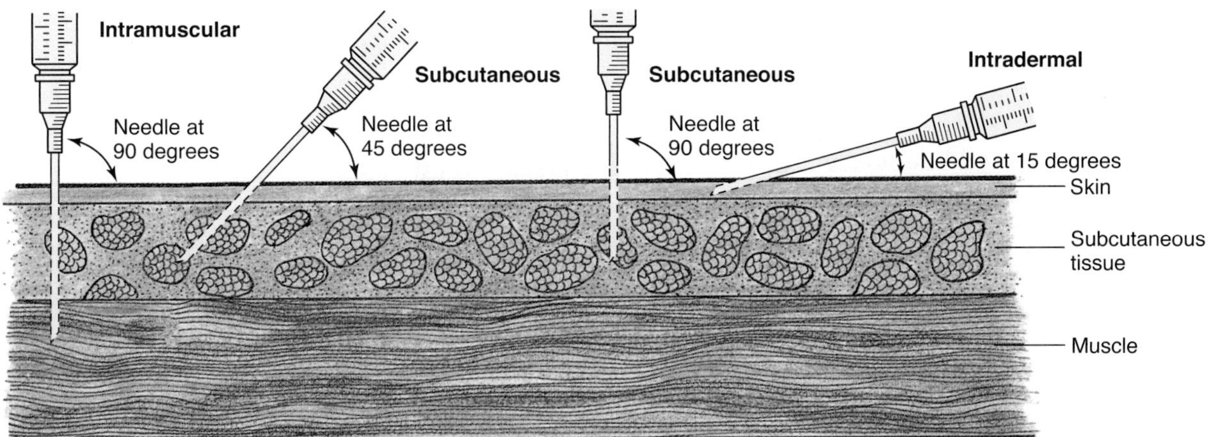

FIGURE 12-1 Intramuscular, subcutaneous, and intradermal injections, with comparison of the angles of insertion. (From Perry AG, Potter PA, Ostendorf WR: *Clinical nursing skills and techniques,* ed 9, St Louis, 2018, Elsevier.)

or in addition to IV fluids. Any time that the integrity of the skin—the body's prime defense against microorganisms—is threatened, infection may occur. Thus the nurse must use sterile technique when preparing and administering parenteral medications.

Drugs for parenteral use are supplied as liquids or powders. The medications are packaged in a variety of forms. A liquid may be contained in an ampule, which is a single-dose container that must be broken at the neck to withdraw the drug (Figures 12-2 and 12-3).

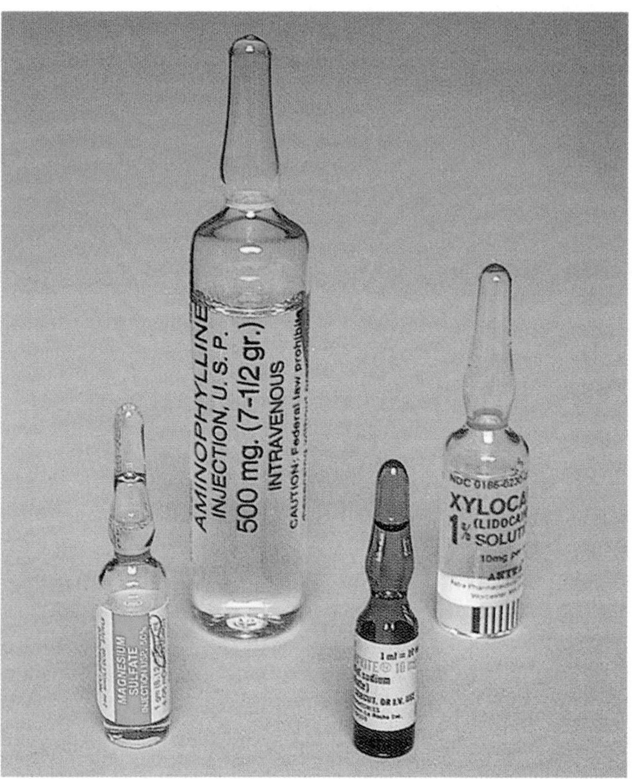

FIGURE 12-2 Examples of ampules. (From Perry AG, Potter PA, Ostendorf WR: *Clinical nursing skills and techniques,* ed 9, St Louis, 2018, Elsevier.)

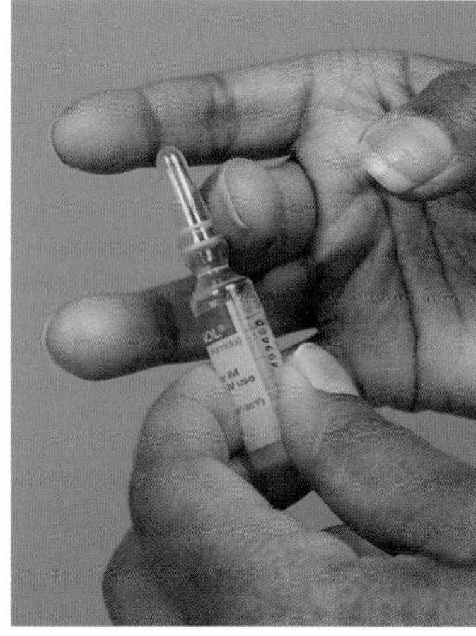

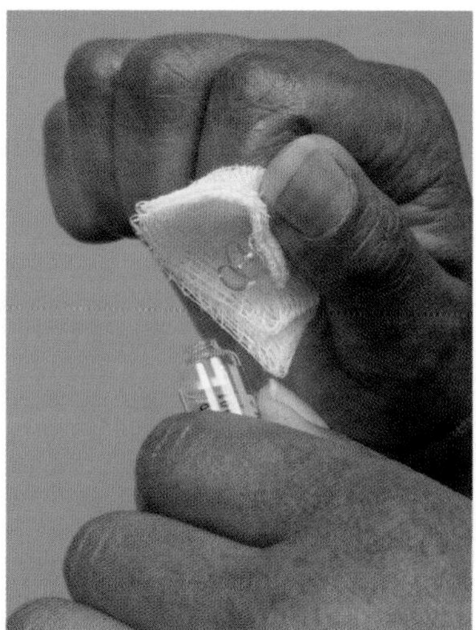

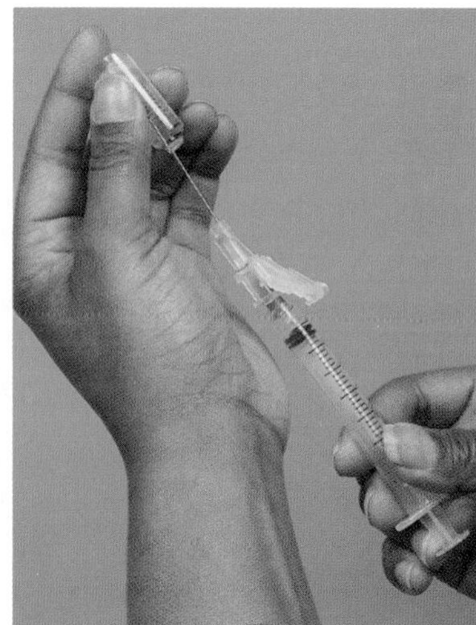

FIGURE 12-3 Breaking the ampule to withdraw the medication. (From Perry AG, Potter PA, Ostendorf WR: *Clinical nursing skills and techniques,* ed 9, St Louis, 2018, Elsevier.)

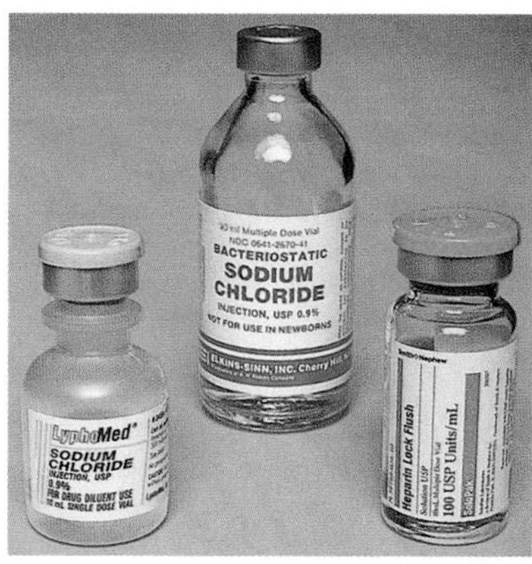

FIGURE 12-4 Examples of vials. (From Perry AG, Potter PA, Ostendorf WR: *Clinical nursing skills and techniques,* ed 9, St Louis, 2018, Elsevier.)

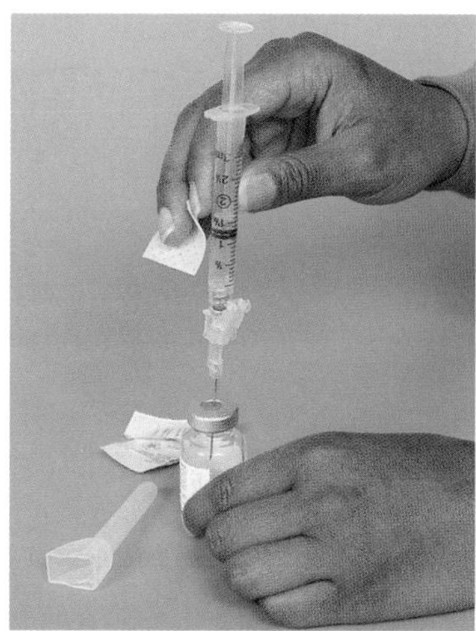

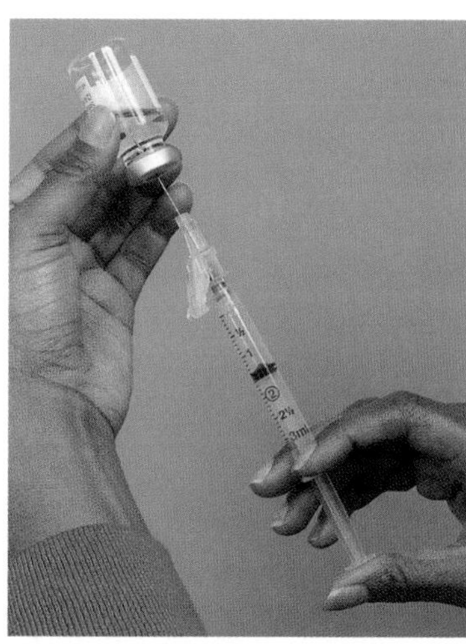

FIGURE 12-5 Withdrawing medication from a vial through the rubber stopper. (From Perry AG, Potter PA, Ostendorf WR: *Clinical nursing skills and techniques,* ed 9, St Louis, 2018, Elsevier.)

Vials are also used to package parenteral medications in liquid or powder form. A vial is a glass or plastic container that is sealed with a rubber stopper (Figure 12-4). Because vials usually contain more than one dose of a medication, the amount desired is withdrawn by inserting a needle through the rubber stopper and removing the required amount (Figure 12-5).

Some of the more unstable drugs may be supplied in vials that have a compartment containing the liquid diluent. Pressure applied to the top of the vial releases the stopper between the compartments and allows the drug to be dissolved. These are called *Mix-O-Vials* (Figure 12-6).

Medications may also be supplied in either prefilled disposable syringes or a plastic reusable syringe with a disposable cartridge and a needle unit. Such units contain a specific amount of medication. If the medication order is less than the amount supplied, discard the unneeded portion before administering the medication to the patient. If the discard is a narcotic, follow your institution's rules for documentation.

Syringes

For accurate measurement of medications that are to be administered by the parenteral route, a syringe must be used. Each syringe is supplied in a sterile package. Although syringes may be

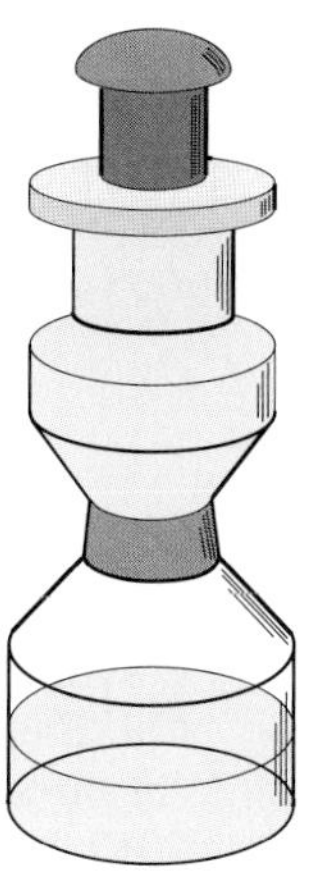

FIGURE 12-6 A Mix-O-Vial or Act-O-Vial. This vial works by pushing the top down. This allows the powder to drop into the liquid for mixing. Shake to thoroughly mix. (From Clayton BD, Willihnganz MJ: *Basic pharmacology for nurses,* ed 16, St Louis, 2013, Mosby.)

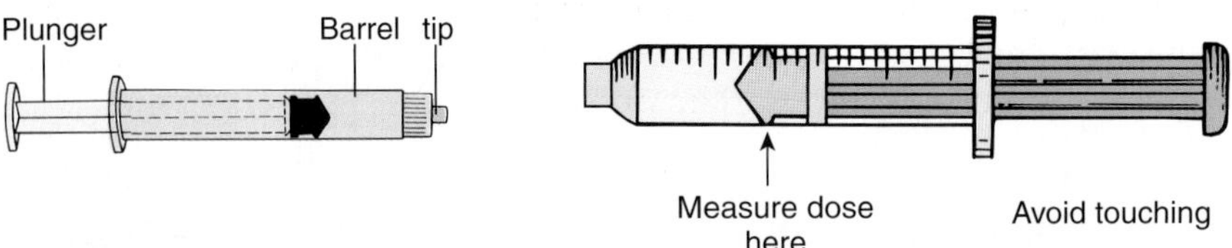

FIGURE 12-7 Parts of a syringe. (From Perry AG, Potter PA, Ostendorf WR: *Clinical nursing skills and techniques,* ed 9, St Louis, 2018, Elsevier.)

made of glass or plastic, plastic syringes are more commonly used. All are designed to be used only once and then discarded. Figure 12-7 shows the parts of a syringe.

1. TIP. The tip is located at the end of the syringe. This is the part that holds the needle.
2. BARREL. This is the outer part of the syringe and the part that holds the medication. The various calibrations are printed on the outside of the barrel.
3. PLUNGER. This is the interior part of the syringe, which slides within the barrel. The plunger is moved backward to withdraw and measure the medication. Then it is pushed forward to inject the medication into the patient.

Syringes come in a variety of sizes. The size used depends on the amount and type of medication to be administered. There are three types of syringes: hypodermic, tuberculin, and insulin syringes (Figure 12-8).

Syringes vary in size as to the amount of fluid they can measure. The most commonly used sizes are 2-, 2½-, 3-, and 5-mL syringes (Figure 12-9). Syringes are also available in 10-, 20-, 30-, and 50-mL sizes.

Syringes that are smaller in capacity can easily be used to measure decimal fractions of a milliliter. Longer lines mark the half- and whole-number milliliters, and shorter lines mark the decimal fractions. Each line indicates one tenth of

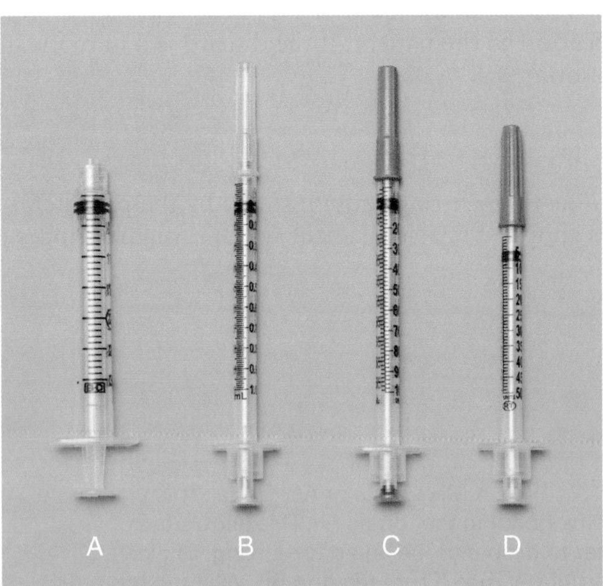

FIGURE 12-8 Examples of types of syringes. **A,** 5-mL syringe. **B,** 3-mL syringe. **C,** Tuberculin syringe marked in 0.01 (hundredths) increments of less than 1 mL. **D,** Insulin syringe marked in units (50). (From Perry AG, Potter PA, Ostendorf WR: *Clinical nursing skills and techniques,* ed 9, St Louis, 2018, Elsevier.)

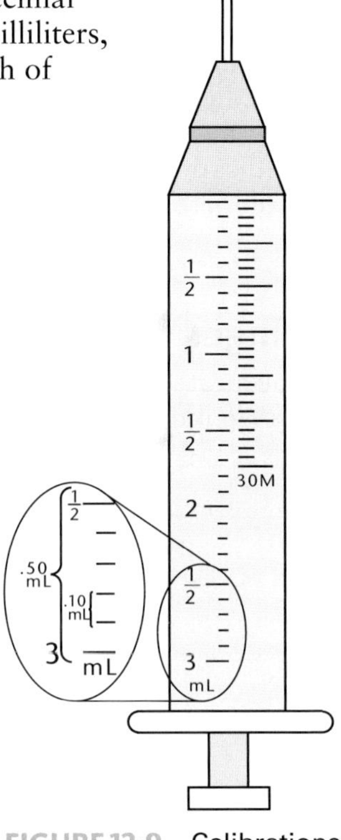

FIGURE 12-9 Calibrations on a 3-mL syringe. (From Clayton BD, Willihnganz MJ: *Basic pharmacology for nurses,* ed 16, St Louis, 2013, Mosby.)

a milliliter. With larger-capacity syringes, each mark may represent a 0.2-mL increment or whole milliliter increments. The larger-capacity syringes are not appropriate for measuring smaller quantities of medication for administration. The nurse must select the proper size of syringe for the calculated volume of medication.

Tuberculin Syringes. A tuberculin syringe is a thin, 1-mL syringe (Figure 12-10). The mL side of the syringe includes markings for hundredths of a milliliter. These syringes are commonly used in pediatrics and also to measure medications given in very small amounts, such as heparin. Tuberculin syringes should not be confused with insulin syringes.

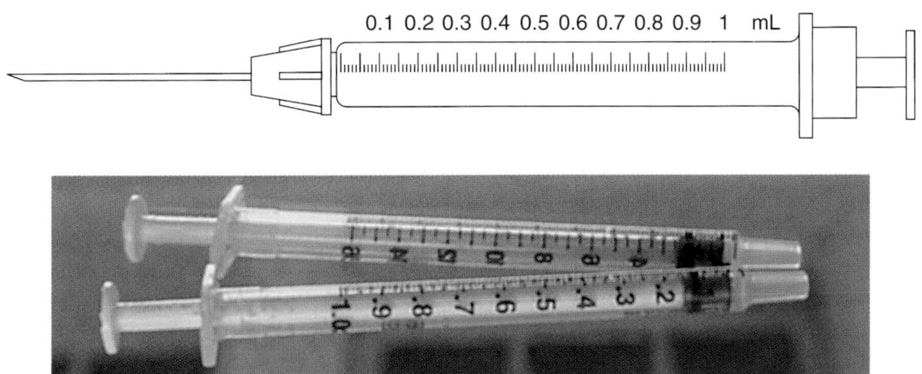

FIGURE 12-10 BD tuberculin syringes. (From Becton, Dickinson and Company, Franklin Lakes, NJ.)

Needleless System. The Occupational Safety and Health Administration has recommended administration of parenteral medications with the use of a needleless system. This recommendation is for the protection of both patients and nurses from needlesticks. Needleless systems provide a shield that protects the needle device and are only for IV use (Figure 12-10).

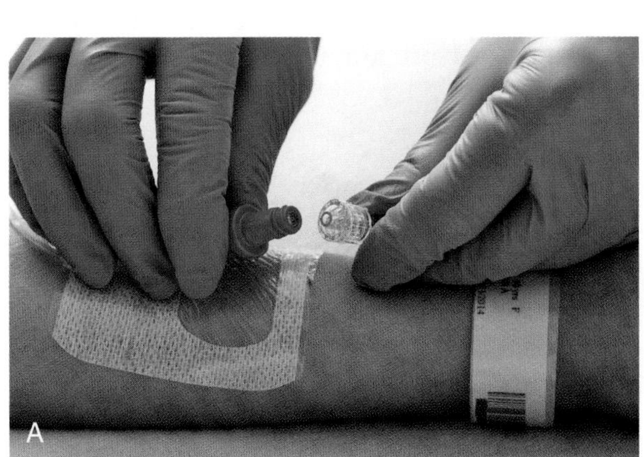

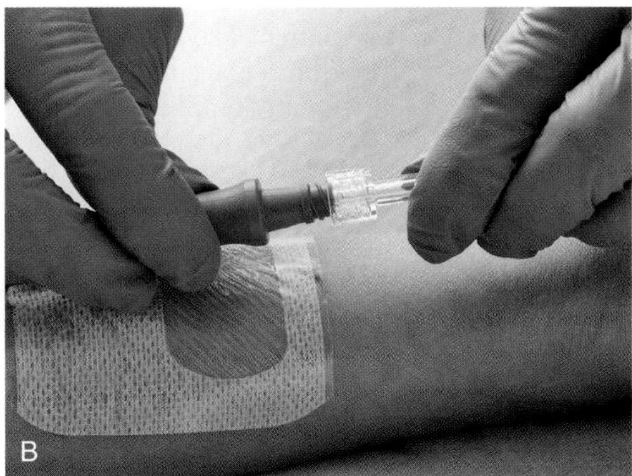

FIGURE 12-11 **A,** Needleless lock cannula system. **B,** Blunt-ended cannula inserts into port and locks. (From Perry AG, Potter PA, Ostendorf WR: *Clinical nursing skills and techniques,* ed 9, St Louis, 2018, Elsevier.)

Calculation of Parenteral Drug Dosages: Dimensional Analysis Method

EXAMPLE 1: The licensed prescriber orders Apresoline 30 mg IM. Apresoline 20 mg/mL is available. How many milliliters will the nurse administer?

Step 1. On the left side of the equation, place the name or abbreviation of the drug form of x, or what you are solving for.

$$x \text{ mL} =$$

Step 2. On the right side of the equation, place the available information related to the measurement or abbreviation that was placed on the left side. In this example that is *mL*. This information is placed in the equation as part of a fraction; match the appropriate abbreviation. Thus the abbreviation that matches the x quantity must be placed in the numerator. We also know that each mL contains 20 mg of Apresoline. 20 mg is the denominator of our fraction.

$$x \text{ mL} = \frac{1 \text{ mL}}{20 \text{ mg}}$$

Step 3. Next, find the information that matches the measurement or abbreviation used in the denominator of the fraction you created. In this example *mg* is in the denominator and our desired dosage is 30 mg. Therefore the full equation is

$$x \text{ mL} = \frac{1 \text{ mL}}{20 \text{ mg}} \times \frac{30 \text{ mg}}{1}$$

Step 4. Now cancel out the like abbreviations on the right side of the equation. If you have set up the problem correctly, the remaining measurement or abbreviation should match that used on the left side of the equation. You are now ready to solve for x.

$$x \text{ mL} = \frac{1 \text{ mL}}{\underset{2}{\cancel{20}} \ \cancel{\text{mg}}} \times \frac{\overset{3}{\cancel{30}} \ \cancel{\text{mg}}}{1}$$

$$x = \frac{1 \times 3}{2 \times 1} = \frac{3}{2}$$

$$x = 1.5 \text{ mL}$$

The answer to the problem is 1.5 mL.

EXAMPLE 2: The patient may receive Dilaudid 3 mg IM q 3 h for relief of pain caused by a total hip replacement. Dilaudid is supplied in 1-mL ampules containing 4 mg. How many milliliters will you administer?

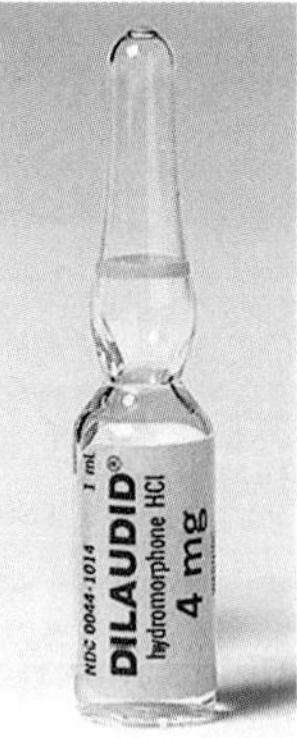

Step 1. On the left side of the equation, place the name or abbreviation of the drug form of x, or what you are solving for.

$$x \text{ mL} =$$

Step 2. On the right side of the equation, place the available information related to the measurement or abbreviation that was placed on the left side. In this example that is *mL*. This information is placed in the equation as part of a fraction; match the appropriate abbreviation. Thus the abbreviation that matches the x

quantity must be placed in the numerator. We also know that each mL contains 4 mg of Dilaudid. 4 mg is the denominator of our fraction.

$$x \text{ mL} = \frac{1 \text{ mL}}{4 \text{ mg}}$$

Step 3. Next, find the information that matches the measurement or abbreviation used in the denominator of the fraction you created. In this example *mg* is in the denominator and our desired dosage is 3 mg. Therefore the full equation is

$$x \text{ mL} = \frac{1 \text{ mL}}{4 \text{ mg}} \times \frac{3 \text{ mg}}{1}$$

Step 4. Now cancel out the like abbreviations on the right side of the equation. If you have set up the problem correctly, the remaining measurement or abbreviation should match that used on the left side of the equation. You are now ready to solve for x.

$$x \text{ mL} = \frac{1 \text{ mL}}{4 \cancel{\text{mg}}} \times \frac{3 \cancel{\text{mg}}}{1}$$

$$x = \frac{1 \times 3}{4 \times 1} = \frac{3}{4}$$

$$x = 0.75 \text{ mL}$$

The answer to the problem is 0.75 mL.

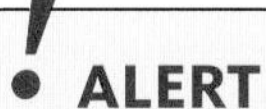

ALERT

Remember to use a leading zero for all dosages less than a whole number (e.g., 0.2 mL, NOT .2 mL). The decimal point might not be noticed and could be read as 2 mL, resulting in a grave medication error.

EXAMPLE 3: The licensed prescriber orders Cleocin phosphate 450 mg IV q 6 h. Cleocin 150 mg/mL is available. How many milliliters will the nurse administer?

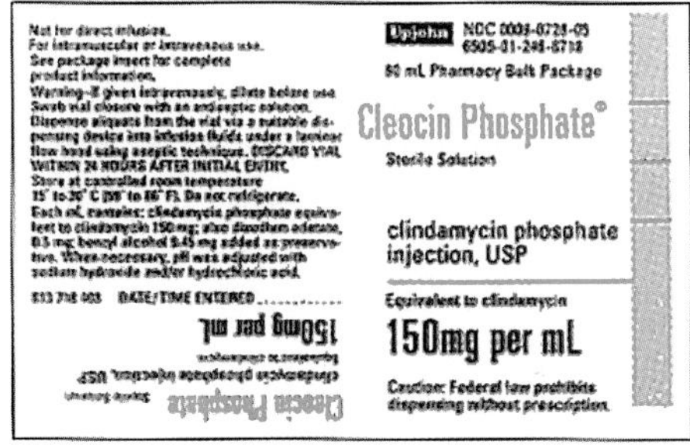

Step 1. On the left side of the equation, place the name or abbreviation of the drug form of x, or what you are solving for.

$$x \text{ mL} =$$

Step 2. On the right side of the equation, place the available information related to the measurement or abbreviation that was placed on the left side. In this example that is *mL*. This information is placed in the equation as part of a fraction; match the appropriate abbreviation. Thus the abbreviation that matches the x quantity must be placed in the numerator. We also know that each mL contains 150 mg of Cleocin. 150 mg is the denominator of our fraction.

$$x \text{ mL} = \frac{1 \text{ mL}}{150 \text{ mg}}$$

Step 3. Next, find the information that matches the measurement or abbreviation used in the denominator of the fraction you created. In this example *mg* is in the denominator and our desired dosage is 450 mg. Therefore the full equation is

$$x \text{ mL} = \frac{1 \text{ mL}}{150 \text{ mg}} \times \frac{450 \text{ mg}}{1}$$

Step 4. Now cancel out the like abbreviations on the right side of the equation. If you have set up the problem correctly, the remaining measurement or abbreviation should match that used on the left side of the equation. You are now ready to solve for x.

$$x \text{ mL} = \frac{1 \text{ mL}}{\underset{1}{\cancel{150}} \ \cancel{\text{mg}}} \times \frac{\overset{3}{\cancel{450}} \ \cancel{\text{mg}}}{1}$$

$$x = \frac{1 \times 3}{1 \times 1} = \frac{3}{1}$$

$$x = 3 \text{ mL}$$

The answer to the problem is 3 mL.

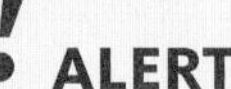

ALERT

Remember, do NOT use a trailing zero after a whole number (e.g., 4 mL, NOT 4.0 mL). The decimal point might not be noticed and could be read as 40 mL, resulting in a grave medical error.

EXAMPLE 4: The order states Kantrex 400 mg IM q 12 h. The drug is supplied as 0.5 g/2 mL. How many milliliters will the nurse administer?

Step 1. On the left side of the equation, place the name or abbreviation of the drug form of x, or what you are solving for.

$$x \text{ mL} =$$

Step 2. On the right side of the equation, place the available information related to the measurement or abbreviation that was placed on the left side. In this example that is *mL*. This information is placed in the equation as part of a fraction; match the appropriate abbreviation. Remember that the abbreviation that matches the x quantity must be placed in the numerator. We know from the problem that each 2 mL contains 0.5 g of Kantrex.

$$x \text{ mL} = \frac{2 \text{ mL}}{0.5 \text{ g}}$$

Step 3. Because the order is for 400 mg and the medication is supplied to us as 0.5 g/2 mL, a conversion would normally be required. However, with the dimensional analysis method, an additional fraction is added on the right side of the equation. From information supplied in earlier chapters, we know that 1 g equals 1000 mg. This information is then placed in the equation next in the form of the fraction $\frac{1 \text{ g}}{1000 \text{ mg}}$. Note that the abbreviation or measurement in the *numerator* of this fraction must match the abbreviation or measurement in the *denominator* of the immediate previous fraction. The equation now looks like

$$x \text{ mL} = \frac{2 \text{ mL}}{0.5 \text{ g}} \times \frac{1 \text{ g}}{1000 \text{ mg}}$$

Step 4. Next, place the amount of drug ordered in the equation. Note that this will once again match the measurement or abbreviation of the denominator of the fraction immediately before. In this example, that is 400 mg. Therefore the full equation is

$$x \text{ mL} = \frac{2 \text{ mL}}{0.5 \text{ g}} \times \frac{1 \text{ g}}{1000 \textbf{ mg}} \times \frac{400 \textbf{ mg}}{1}$$

Step 5. For the final step, cancel out the like abbreviations on the right side of the equation. If the equation has been set up correctly, the remaining abbreviation should match that used on the left side. Now solve for x.

$$x \text{ mL} = \frac{2 \text{ mL}}{0.5 \not{\text{g}}} \times \frac{1 \not{\text{g}}}{1000 \not{\text{mg}}} \times \frac{400 \not{\text{mg}}}{1}$$

$$x = \frac{2 \times 400}{0.5 \times 1000}$$

$$x = \frac{800}{500}$$

$$x = 1.6 \text{ mL}$$

The answer to the problem is 1.6 mL.

Calculation of Parenteral Drug Dosages: Proportion Method

Parenteral drug dosages may also be calculated by using a proportion. The licensed prescriber order and the available medication must be in the same system of measurement to write a proportion for the actual amount of medication to be administered. Examples of parenteral drug dosage problems follow.

EXAMPLE 1: The licensed prescriber orders Apresoline 30 mg IM. Apresoline 20 mg/mL is available. How many milliliters will the nurse administer?

Step 1. On the left side of the proportion, place what you know or have available. In this example, each milliliter contains 20 mg. Therefore the left side of the proportion would be

$$20 \text{ mg} : 1 \text{ mL} ::$$

Step 2. The right side of the proportion is determined by the licensed prescriber's order and the abbreviations placed on the left side of the proportion. Remember, only *two* different abbreviations may be used in a single proportion. The abbreviations must be placed in the same position on the right side as they are on the left.

$$20 \text{ mg} : 1 \text{ mL} :: \_\_\_\_\_\_ \text{ mg} : \_\_\_\_\_\_ \text{ mL}$$

The licensed prescriber ordered 30 mg.

$$20 \text{ mg} : 1 \text{ mL} :: 30 \text{ mg} : \_\_\_\_\_\_ \text{ mL}$$

The symbol x is used to represent the unknown number of milliliters.

$$20 \text{ mg} : 1 \text{ mL} :: 30 \text{ mg} : x \text{ mL}$$

Step 3. Rewrite the proportion without the abbreviations.

$$20 : 1 :: 30 : x$$

Step 4. Solve for x.

$$20x = 30$$

$$x = \frac{30}{20}$$

$$x = 1.5$$

Step 5. Label your answer as determined by the abbreviation placed next to x in the original proportion.

$$1.5 \text{ mL}$$

The patient would receive 1.5 mL of Apresoline containing 30 mg.

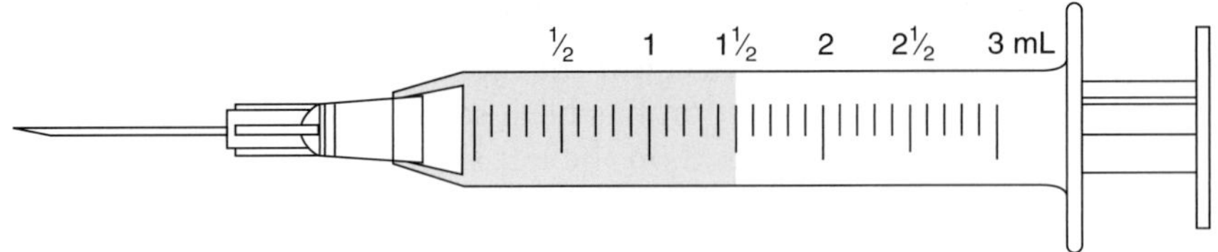

EXAMPLE 2: The licensed prescriber orders meperidine 30 mg IM q 4 h prn. Meperidine 25 mg/mL is available. How many milliliters will the nurse administer?

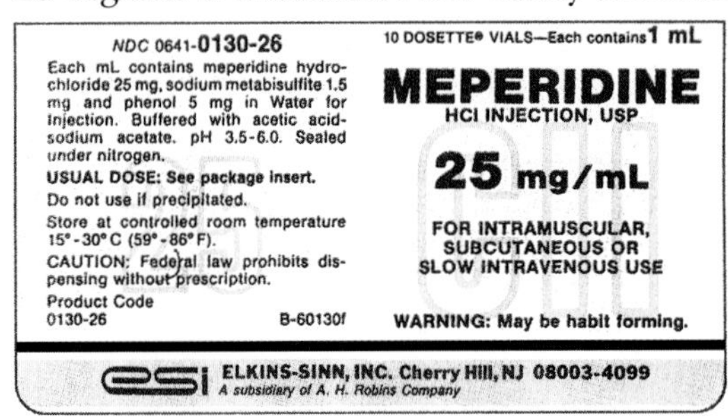

Step 1. On the left side of the proportion, place what you know or have available. In this example, each milliliter contains 25 mg. So the left side of the proportion would be

$$25 \text{ mg} : 1 \text{ mL} ::$$

Step 2. The right side of the proportion is determined by the licensed prescriber's order and the abbreviations on the left side of the proportion. Only *two* different abbreviations may be used in a single proportion. The abbreviations must be in the same position on the right side as they are on the left.

$$25 \text{ mg} : 1 \text{ mL} :: \_\_\_\_\_\_ \text{ mg} : \_\_\_\_\_\_ \text{ mL}$$

In this example, the licensed prescriber ordered 30 mg.

$$25 \text{ mg} : 1 \text{ mL} :: 30 \text{ mg} : \_\_\_\_\_\_ \text{ mL}$$

We need to find the number of milliliters to be given, so we use the symbol x to represent the unknown.

$$25 \text{ mg} : 1 \text{ mL} :: 30 \text{ mg} : x \text{ mL}$$

Step 3. Rewrite the proportion without the abbreviations.

$$25 : 1 :: 30 : x$$

Step 4. Solve for x.

$$25x = 1 \times 30$$

$$25x = 30$$

$$x = \frac{30}{25}$$

$$x = 1.2$$

Step 5. Label your answer as determined by the abbreviation placed next to x in the original proportion.

The nurse would measure 1.2 mL to administer 30 mg of Demerol.

EXAMPLE 3: The licensed prescriber orders Cleocin phosphate 450 mg IV q 6 h. Cleocin 150 mg/mL is available. How many milliliters will the nurse administer?

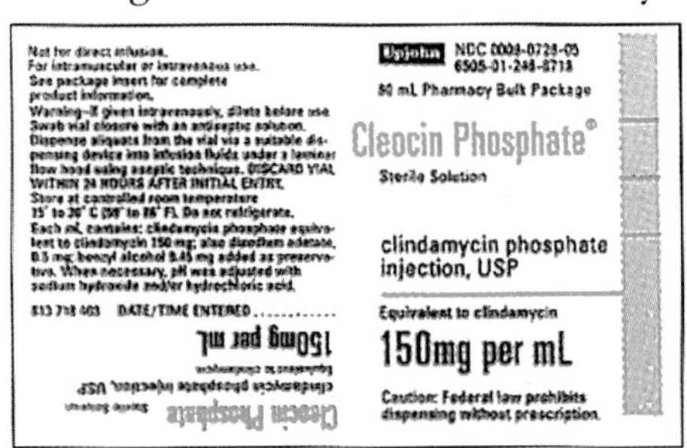

Step 1. 150 mg : 1 mL ::

Step 2. 150 mg : 1 mL :: _______ mg : _______ mL

150 mg : 1 mL :: 450 mg : x mL

Step 3. $150 : 1 :: 450 : x$

Step 4. $150x = 450$

$$x = \frac{450}{150}$$

$$x = 3$$

Step 5. Label your answer as determined by the abbreviation placed next to x in the original proportion.

$x = 3$ mL

The nurse would measure 3 mL to administer 450 mg of Cleocin.

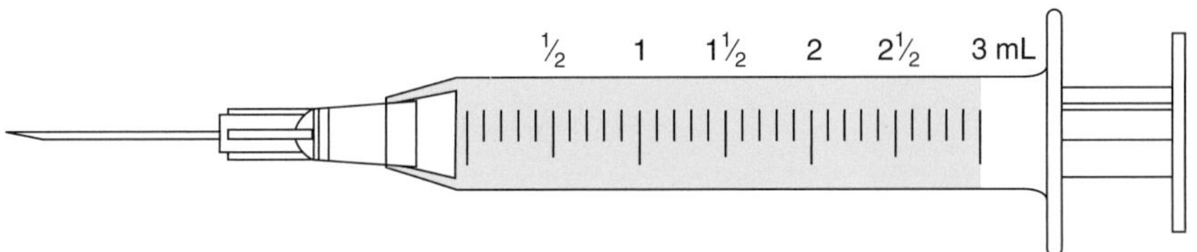

Parenteral Drug Dosage Calculation: Alternative Formula Method

In Chapter 11, the alternative formula was introduced as another method of calculating drug dosages. This formula also may be used when parenteral drug dosages are calculated.

Remember, the formula is

$$\frac{D}{A} \times Q = x$$

or

$$\frac{\text{Desired}}{\text{Available}} \times \text{Quantity available} = x \text{ (unknown)}$$

EXAMPLE 1: The licensed prescriber orders Amikin 150 mg IM q 8 h. Amikin 500 mg/2 mL is available. How many milliliters will the nurse administer?

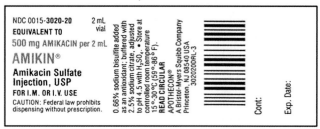

Step 1. The desired amount of Amikin is 150 mg.

$$\underline{150 \text{ mg}}$$

Step 2. The available amount of Amikin is 500 mg.

$$\frac{150 \text{ mg}}{500 \text{ mg}}$$

Step 3. The quantity of the medication for 500 mg is 2 mL.

$$\frac{150 \text{ mg}}{500 \text{ mg}} \times \frac{2 \text{ mL}}{1}$$

Step 4. We can now solve for x.

$$x = \frac{150 \text{ mg}}{500 \text{ mg}} \times \frac{2 \text{ mL}}{1}$$

$$x = \frac{150 \cancel{\text{mg}}}{\underset{250}{\cancel{500}} \cancel{\text{mg}}} \times \frac{\overset{1}{\cancel{2}} \text{ mL}}{1} = \frac{150}{250}$$

$$x = \frac{150}{250}$$

$$x = \frac{3}{5} \text{ or } 0.6$$

Step 5. Label your answer as determined by the quantity.

$$150 \text{ mg} = 0.6 \text{ mL of Amikin}$$

EXAMPLE 2: Mr. Davis is to receive atropine 0.4 mg IM STAT. Atropine 0.4 mg/mL is available. How many milliliters will the nurse administer?

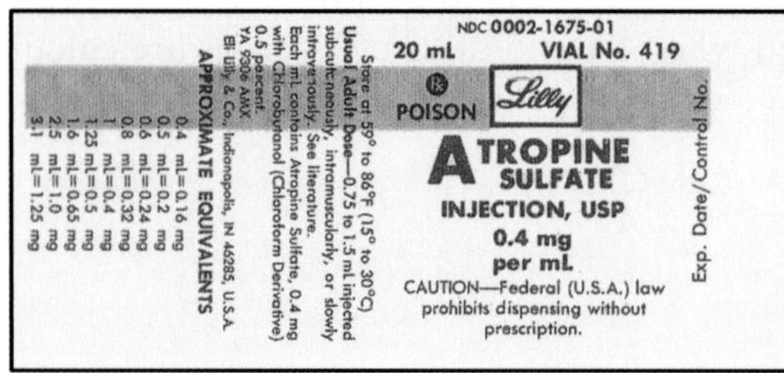

Step 1. The desired amount is 0.4 mg.

$$\underline{0.4 \text{ mg}}$$

Step 2. The available amount or strength of atropine is 0.4 mg.

$$\frac{0.4 \text{ mg}}{0.4 \text{ mg}}$$

Step 3. The quantity available is in 1 mL.

$$\frac{0.4 \cancel{\text{mg}}}{0.4 \cancel{\text{mg}}} \times \frac{1 \text{ mL}}{1}$$

Step 4. Solve for x

$$x = \frac{0.4 \times 1}{0.4 \times 1}$$

$$x = 1$$

Step 5. Label your answer as determined by the quantity.

$$0.4 \text{ mg} = 1 \text{ mL of atropine}$$

EXAMPLE 3: Mr. Lewis's licensed prescriber has ordered 200 mg of Tigan IM for treatment of nausea. Tigan 100 mg/mL is available. How many milliliters will the nurse administer?

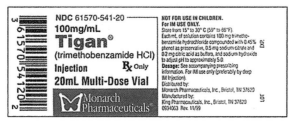

Step 1. The desired amount of Tigan is 200 mg.

$$\underline{200 \text{ mg}}$$

Step 2. The available amount or strength is 100 mg.

$$\frac{200 \text{ mg}}{100 \text{ mg}}$$

Step 3. The quantity available is 1 mL.

$$\frac{200 \text{ mg}}{100 \text{ mg}} \times 1 \text{ mL}$$

Step 4. Solve for x.

$$x = \frac{200 \text{ mg}}{100 \text{ mg}} \times \frac{1 \text{ mL}}{1}$$

$$x = \frac{200 \cancel{\text{mg}} \times 1 \text{ mL}}{100 \cancel{\text{mg}} \times 1}$$

$$x = \frac{200}{100}$$

$$x = 2$$

Step 5. Label your answer as determined by the quantity.

$$200 \text{ mg} = 2 \text{ mL of Tigan}$$

Complete the following work sheet, which provides for extensive practice in the calculation of parenteral drug dosages. Check your answers. If you have difficulties, go back and review the necessary material. When you feel ready to evaluate your learning, take the first posttest. Check your answers. An acceptable score as indicated on the posttest signifies that you have successfully completed this chapter. An unacceptable score signifies a need for further study before taking the second posttest.

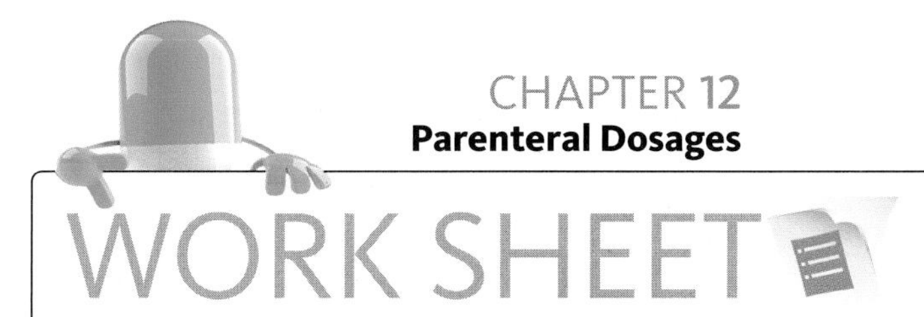

DIRECTIONS: The medication order is listed at the beginning of each problem. Calculate the parenteral doses. Show your work. Shade the syringe when provided to indicate the correct dose.

1. The licensed prescriber orders streptomycin 500 mg IM q 12 h for your patient with an infection. How many milliliters will you administer? _______

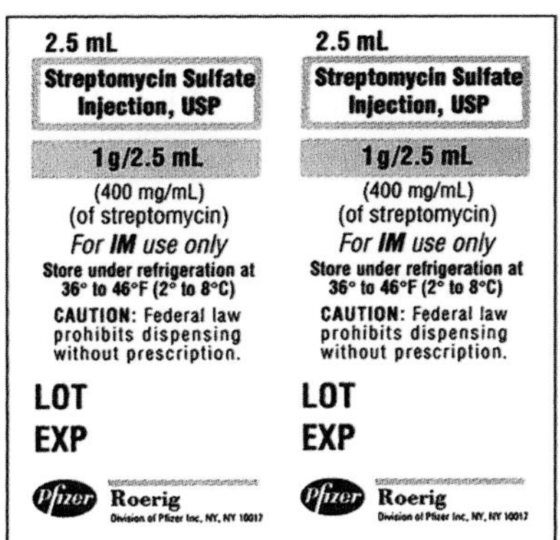

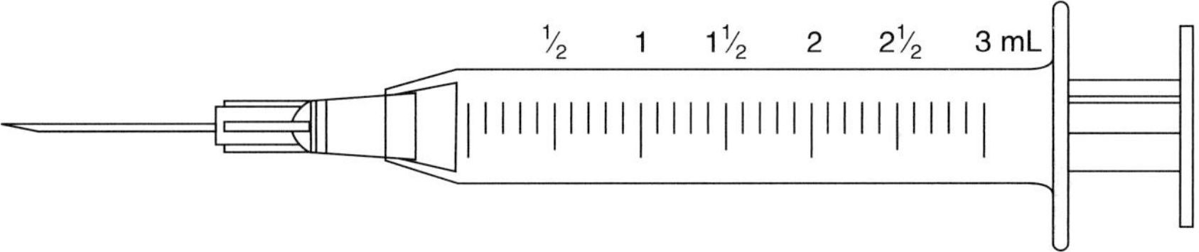

2. Your patient with an atrial valve repair has Digoxin 110 mcg IV q 12 h ordered. How many milliliters will you prepare? _______

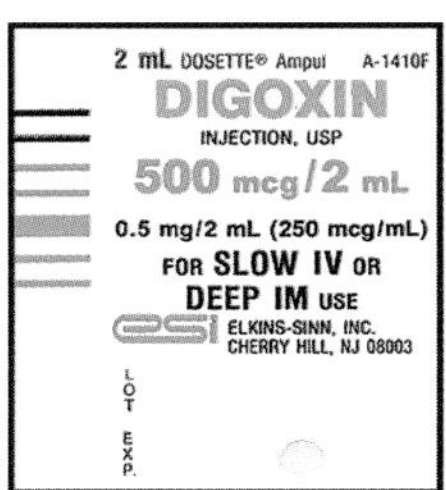

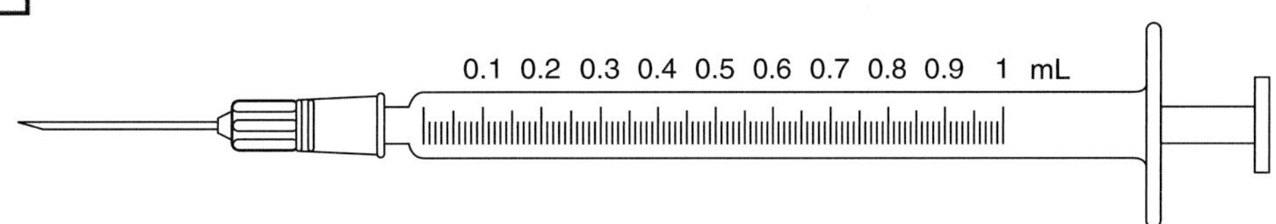

3. The licensed prescriber orders atropine 0.3 mg IM at 0615. How many milliliters will the nurse administer? _______

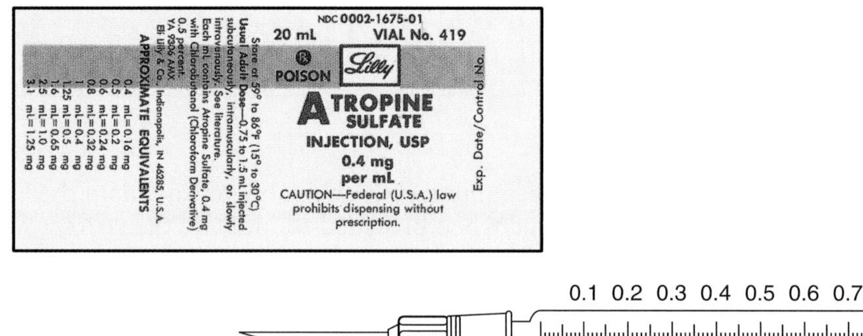

4. Your patient who has undergone pacemaker placement complains of nausea and has Compazine 10 mg IM q 6 h ordered. How many milliliters will you administer? _______

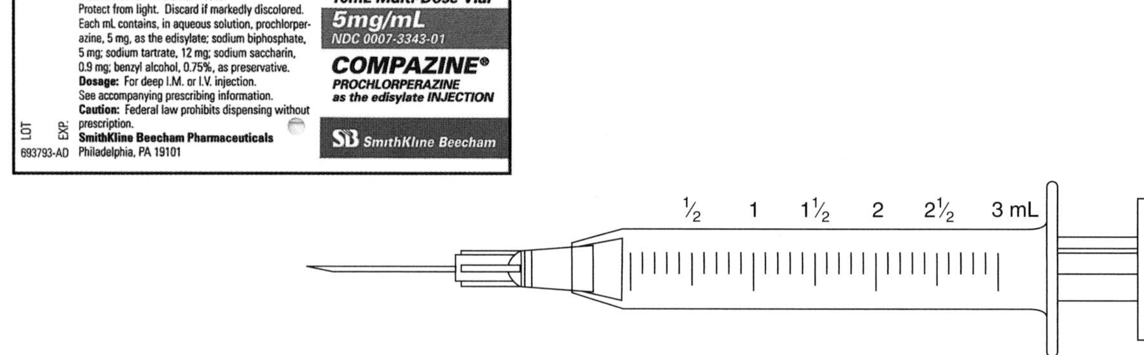

5. The licensed prescriber orders ranitidine hydrochloride 50 mg IM q 6 h. How many milliliters will the nurse administer? _______

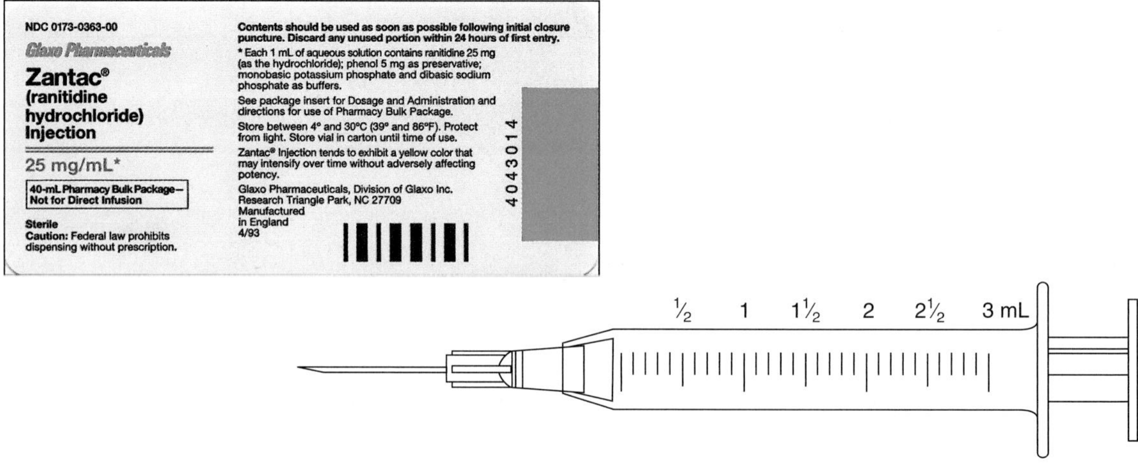

6. The licensed prescriber orders piperacillin 3 g IV q 8 h for your patient with sepsis. You have piperacillin 1 g/2.5 mL available. How many milliliters will you prepare? _______

7. The licensed prescriber orders morphine 5 mg subcutaneous q 4 h. How many milliliters will the nurse administer? _______

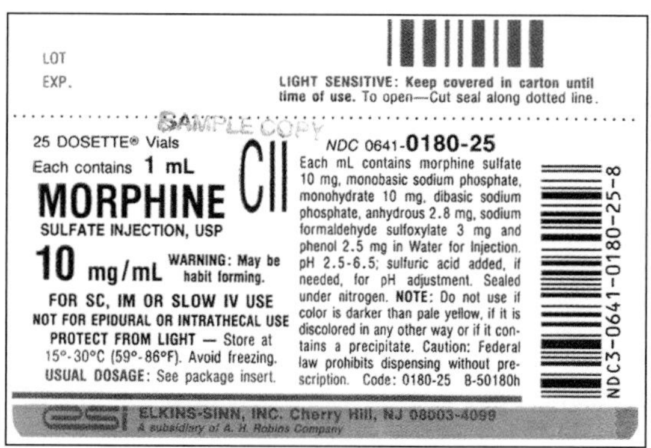

8. The licensed prescriber orders diazepam 4 mg IV q 12 h for your patient with anxiety. How many milliliters will you prepare? _______

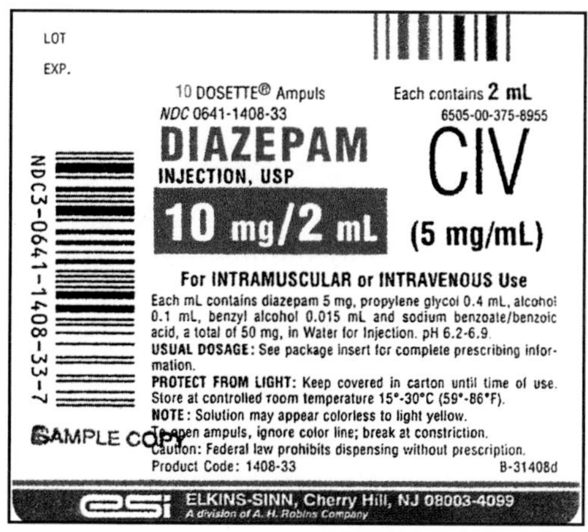

9. Your patient with congestive heart failure requires furosemide 30 mg IV STAT. How many milliliters will you administer? _______

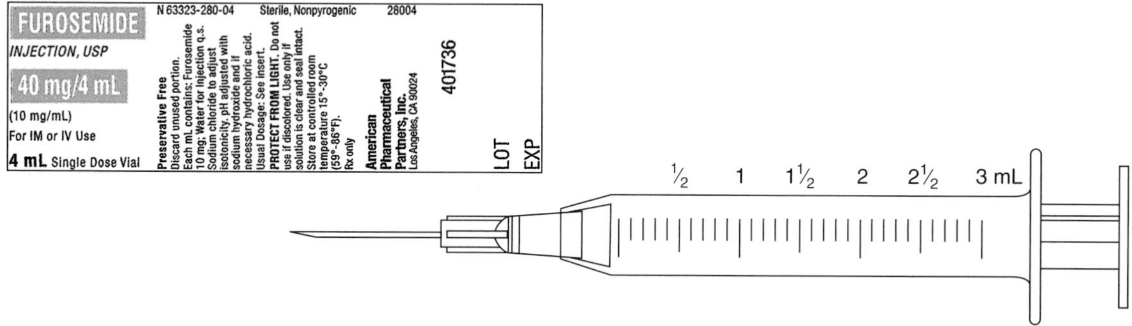

10. Your postoperative patient has Toradol 15 mg IM q 6 h for 3 days ordered. You have 30 mg/mL prefilled syringes. How many milliliters will you administer? _______

11. The licensed prescriber orders D_5W 1000 mL plus sodium bicarbonate ($NaHCO_3$) 25.8 mEq at 12 mL/h IV. $NaHCO_3$ is supplied in a 50-mL ampule containing 44.6 mEq. How many milliliters of $NaHCO_3$ will be added to the 1000 mL of D_5W? _______

12. Your patient with asthma requires aminophylline 100 mg IV q 6 h. How many milliliters will you prepare? _______

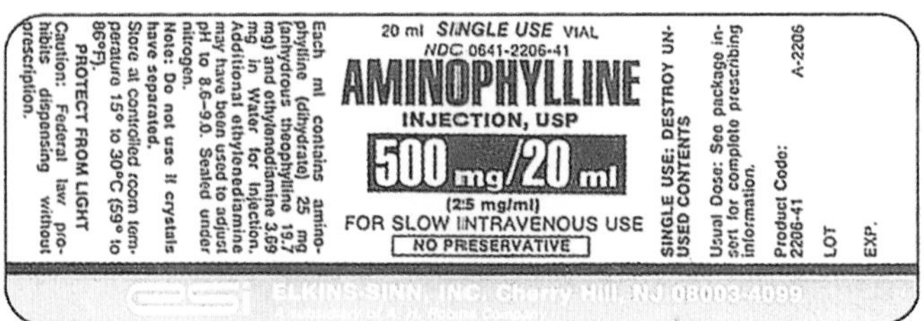

13. The licensed prescriber orders amphotericin B 350 mg IV every day. You have a 100-mg/20-mL vial. How many milliliters will you prepare? _______

14. The licensed prescriber orders Cipro 300 mg q 12 h IV. How many milliliters will you prepare? _______

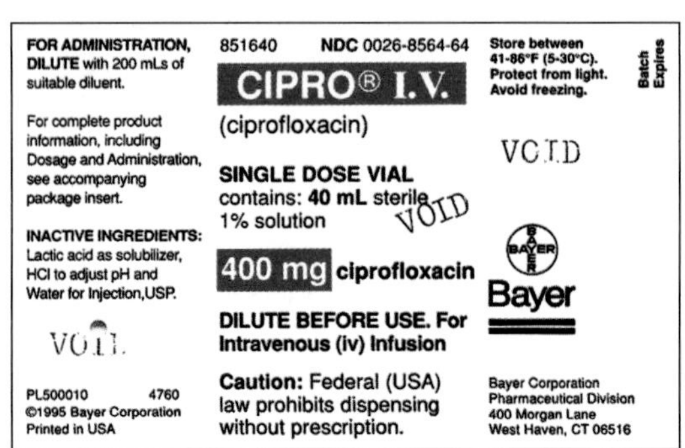

15. The licensed prescriber orders Solu-Cortef 0.05 g IM q 6 h for your patient with scleroderma. How many milliliters will you administer? _______

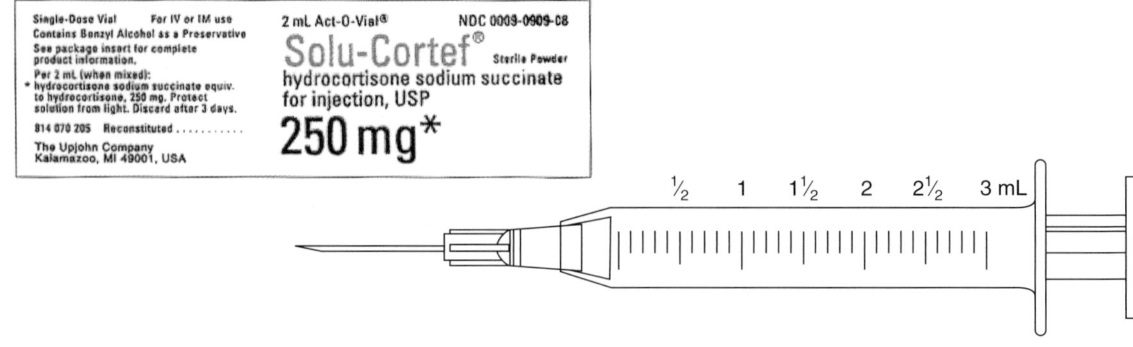

16. The licensed prescriber orders naloxone 0.6 mg IV STAT. How many milliliters will you administer? _______

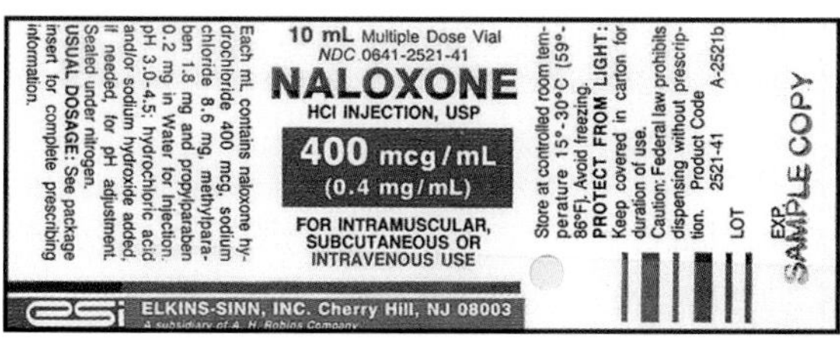

17. The licensed prescriber orders Tagamet 300 mg IV q 6 h. How many milliliters will the nurse prepare? _______

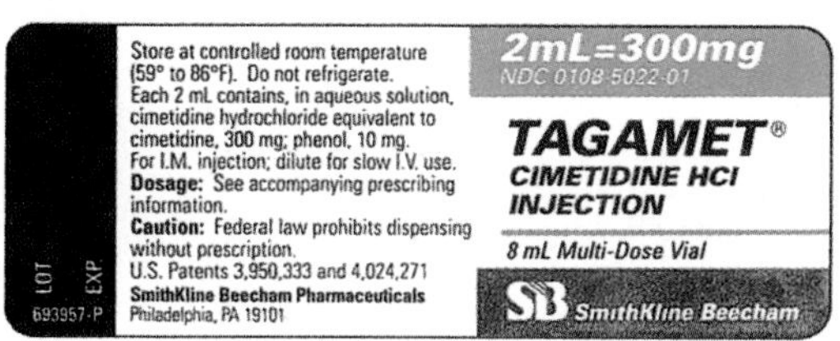

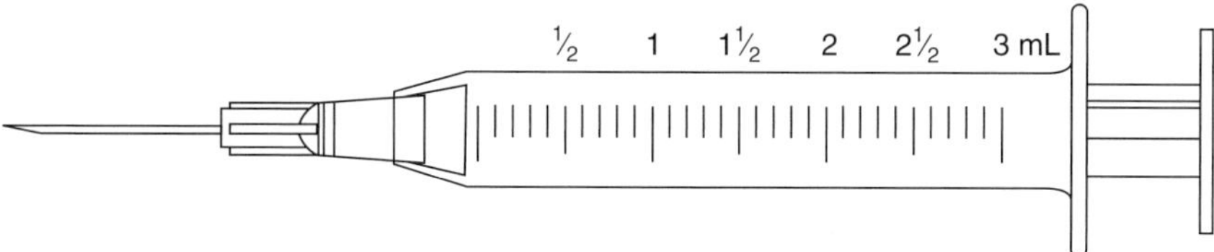

18. Mrs. Andis requires Duramorph 6 mg IV q 4 h for pain. How many milliliters will the nurse administer? _______

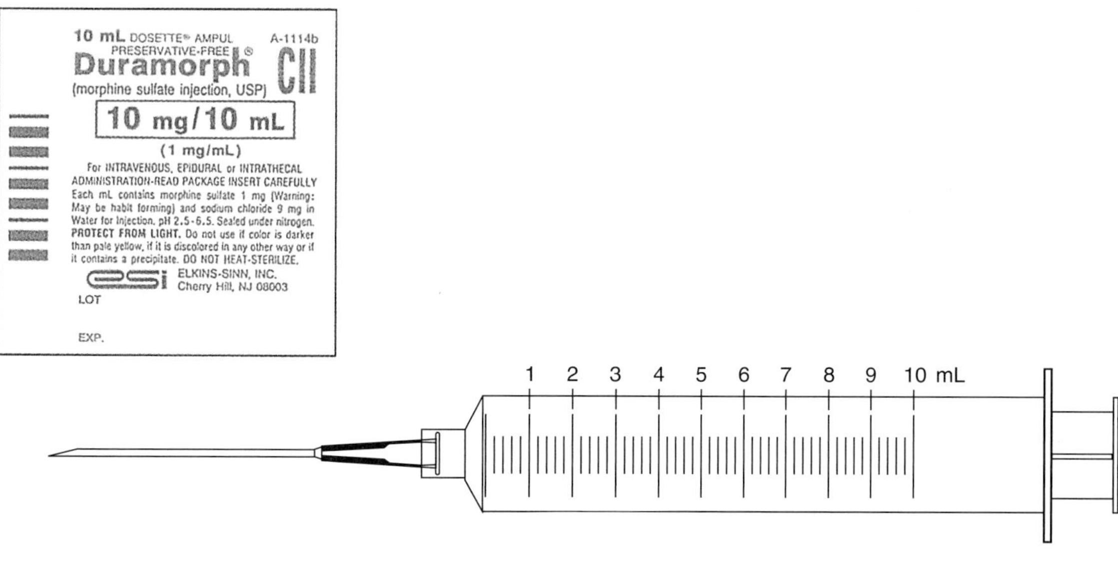

19. Loxapine 25 mg IM now is ordered for Mrs. Switzer, who has been diagnosed with a psychotic disorder. Loxapine 50 mg/mL is available. How many milliliters will the nurse administer? _______

20. Mr. Lewis requires Ativan 1 mg IM STAT for severe agitation. How many milliliters will the nurse administer? _______

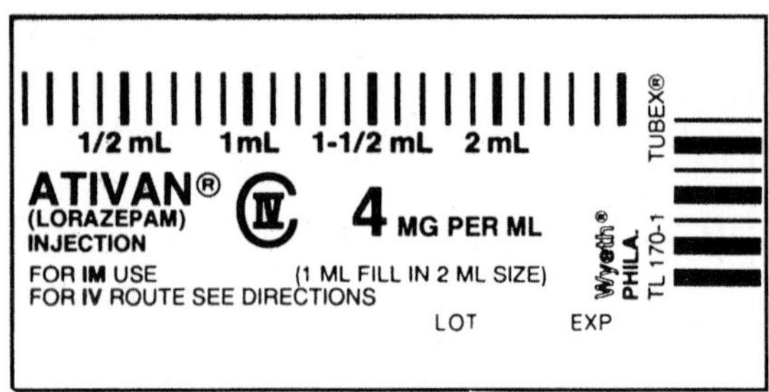

21. Mrs. Carroll requires Apresoline 10 mg IM q 6 h for high blood pressure. Apresoline is supplied in 1-mL ampules containing 20 mg. How many milliliters will the nurse prepare? _______

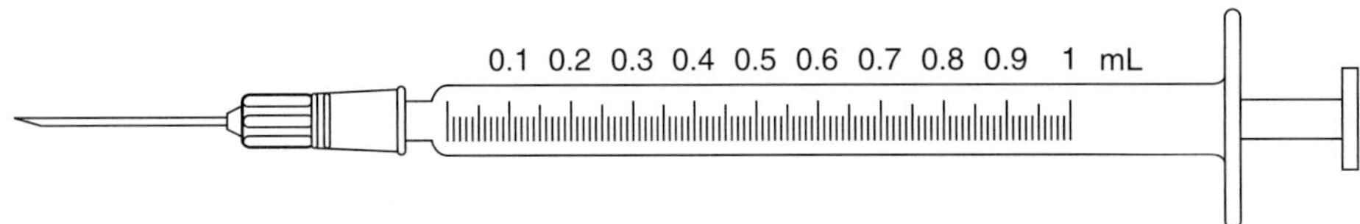

22. Mr. Fry has amikacin sulfate 400 mg IV q 8 h ordered. You have amikacin sulfate for injection 500 mg/2 mL. How many milliliters will you administer? _______

23. The licensed prescriber orders diazepam 7.5 mg IM q 6 h for your anxious patient. How many milliliters will you administer? _______

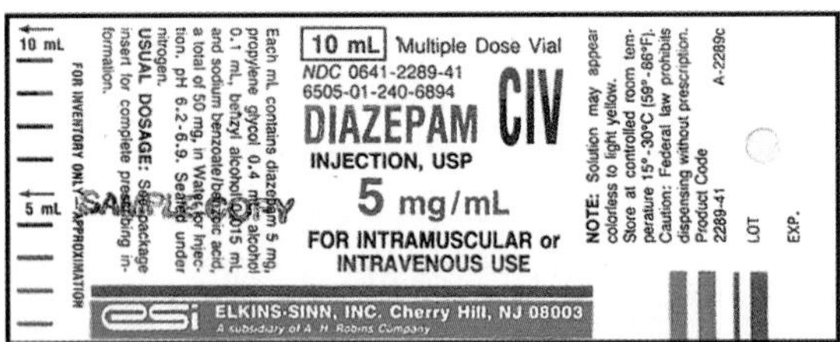

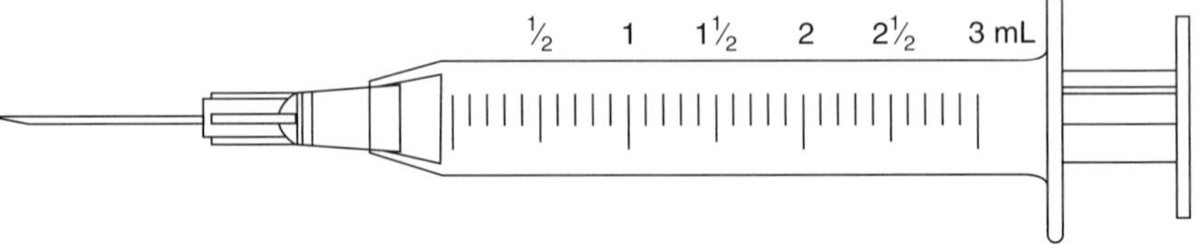

24. Mr. Keesling is diagnosed with an acoustic neuroma and complains of pain. He has codeine 15 mg IM q 3 h prn ordered. How many milliliters will the nurse administer? _______

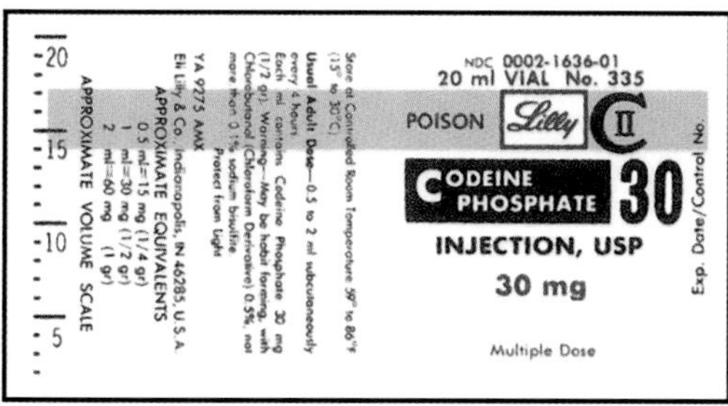

25. The licensed prescriber orders AquaMEPHYTON 0.01 g IM every morning. How many milliliters will the nurse administer? _______

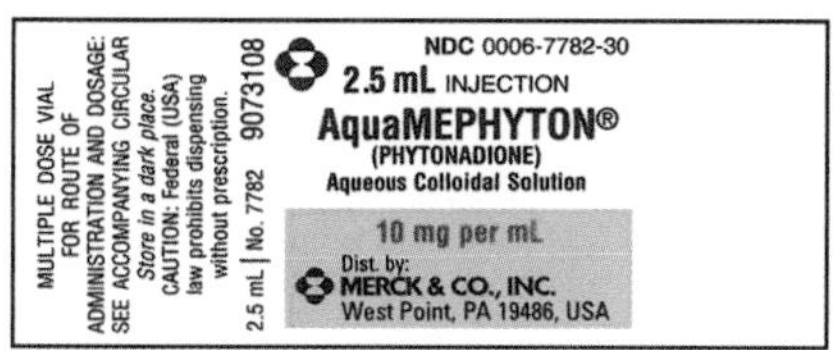

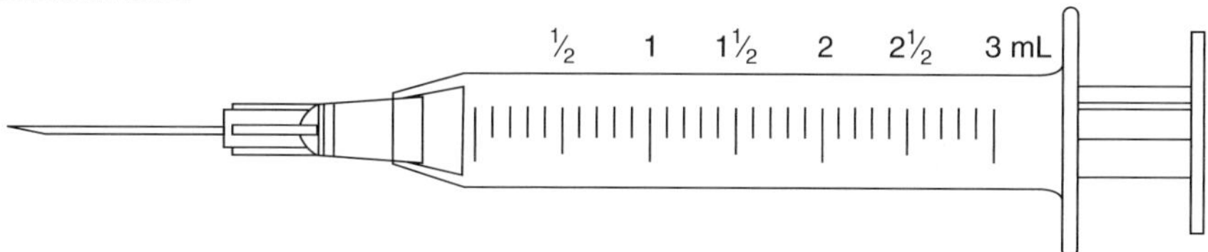

26. The licensed prescriber orders Cipro 0.2 g IV q 12 h. How many milliliters will the nurse prepare? _______

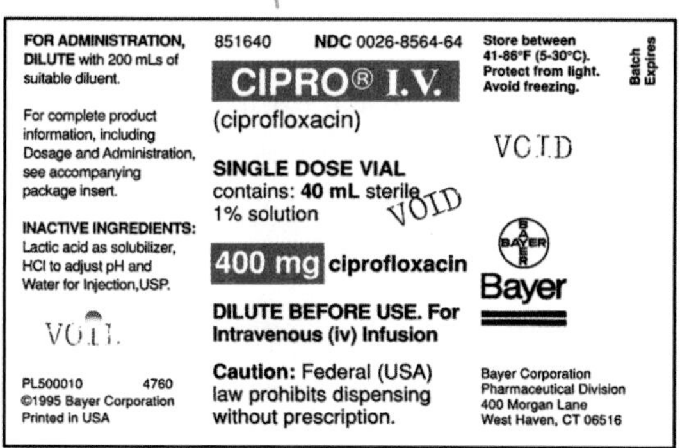

27. Mrs. Ring, who has undergone a hysterectomy, has morphine 6 mg IV q 4 h prn ordered for pain relief. How many milliliters will the nurse administer? _______

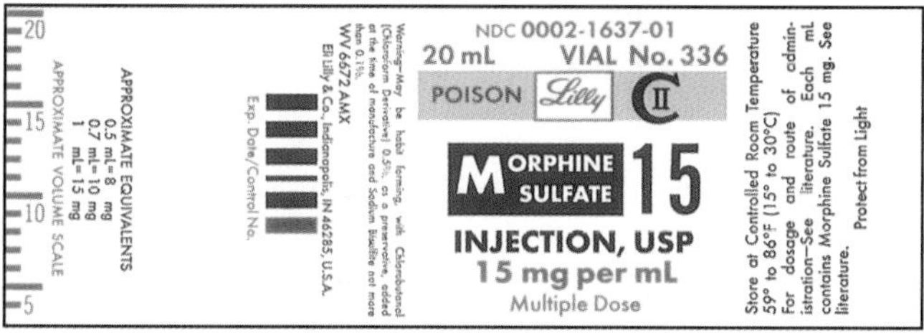

28. The licensed prescriber orders Benadryl 100 mg IM four times a day. How many milliliters will the nurse administer? _______

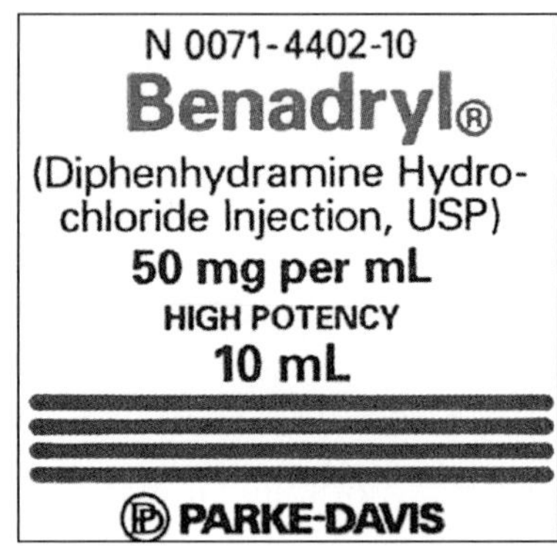

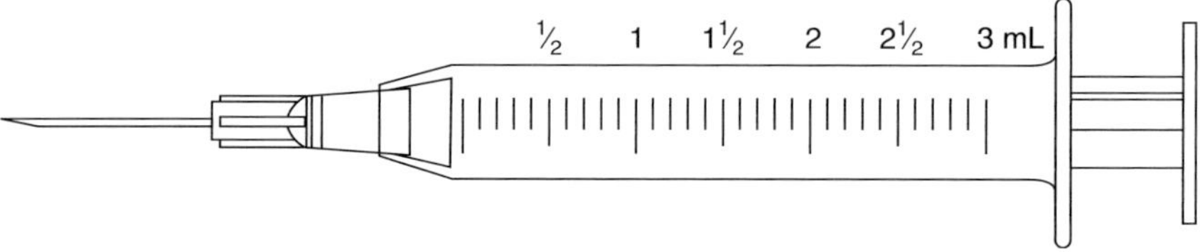

29. Mr. Fields requires digoxin 100 mcg IM daily for his cardiac dysrhythmia. How many milliliters will the nurse administer? _______

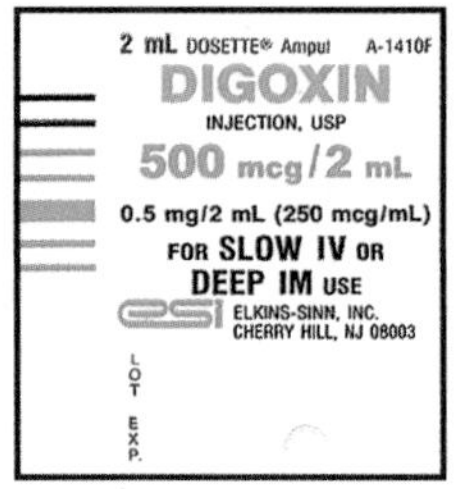

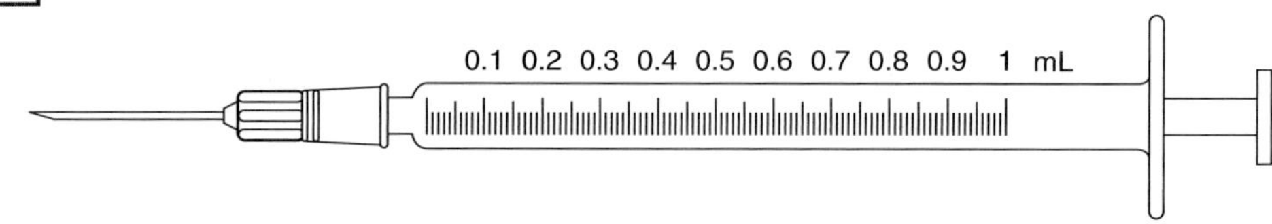

30. The licensed prescriber orders Amikin 700 mg IV q 12 h. How many milliliters will the nurse prepare? _______

31. The licensed prescriber orders Stadol 1.5 mg IV q 4 h for pain. How many milliliters will the nurse administer? _______

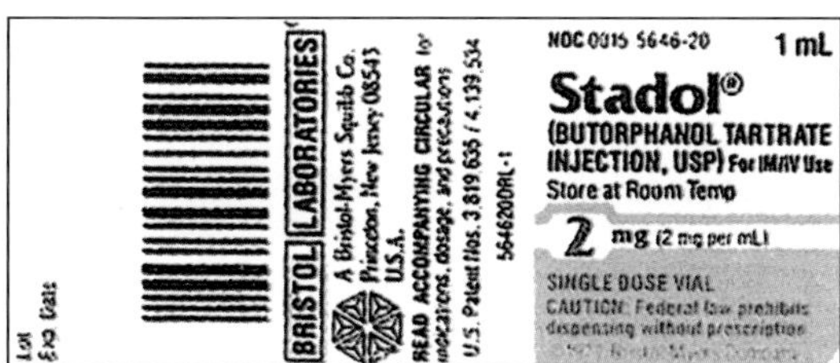

32. The licensed prescriber orders Solu-Cortef 100 mg IV q 8 h for your patient with severe contact dermatitis. How many milliliters will you administer? _______

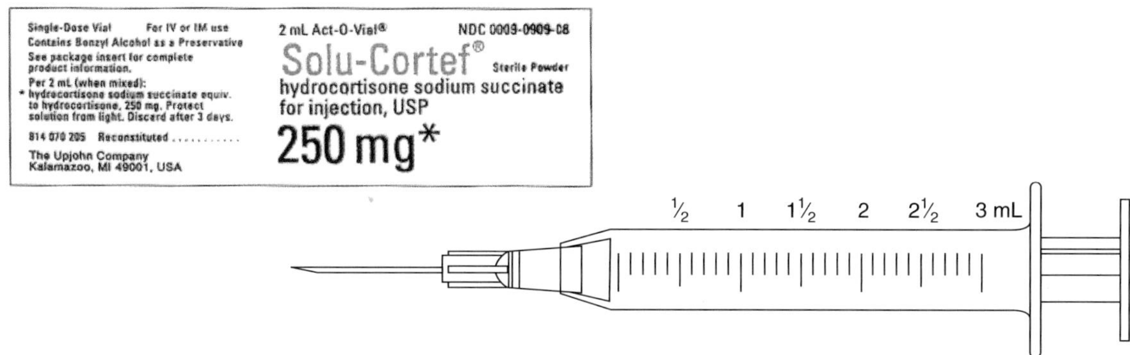

33. The licensed prescriber orders D_5W 250 mL plus NaCl 7.5 mEq at 2 mL IV per hour. NaCl is supplied in a 40-mL vial containing 2.5 mEq/mL. How many milliliters of NaCl will be added to the 250 mL of D_5W? _______

34. Your patient with a lumbar laminectomy receives Vistaril 25 mg IM three times a day. How many milliliters does this patient receive in each dose? _______

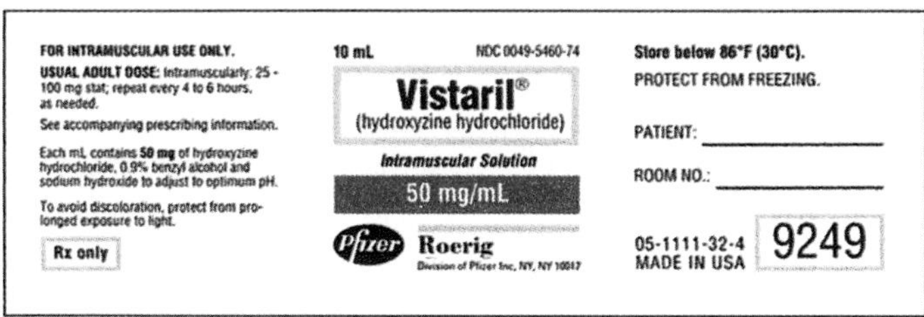

35. The licensed prescriber orders atropine 0.6 mg IM STAT for your preoperative patient. How many milliliters will you administer? _______

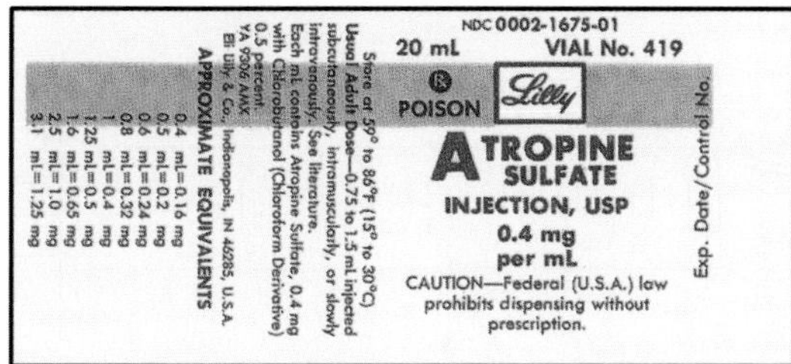

36. Your patient admitted with neuroleptic disorder has Valproate 150 mg IM at bedtime prn ordered. The drug is available for injection at 100 mg/mL. How many milliliters will you administer? _______

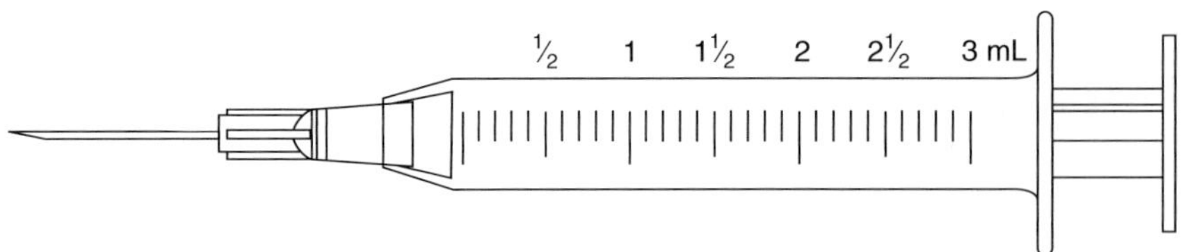

37. Ms. Barry has orders for bumetanide 0.5 mg IV q 3 h for edema caused by congestive heart failure. How many milliliters will the nurse administer? _______

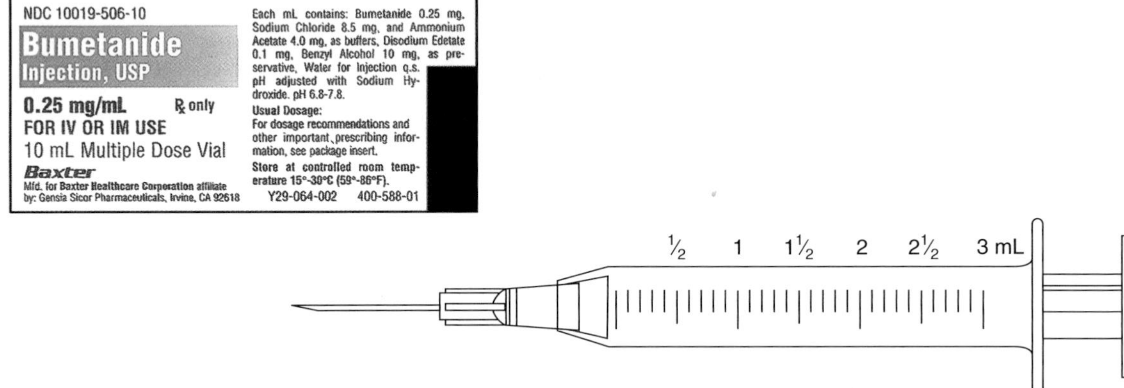

38. Your patient with chronic obstructive pulmonary disease receives aminophylline 75 mg IV q 6 h. How many milliliters will you prepare? _______

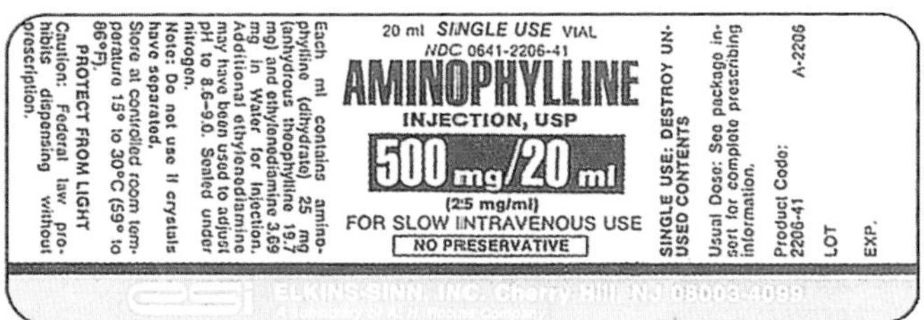

39. The licensed prescriber orders naloxone 0.6 mg IM STAT. How many milliliters will the nurse prepare? _______

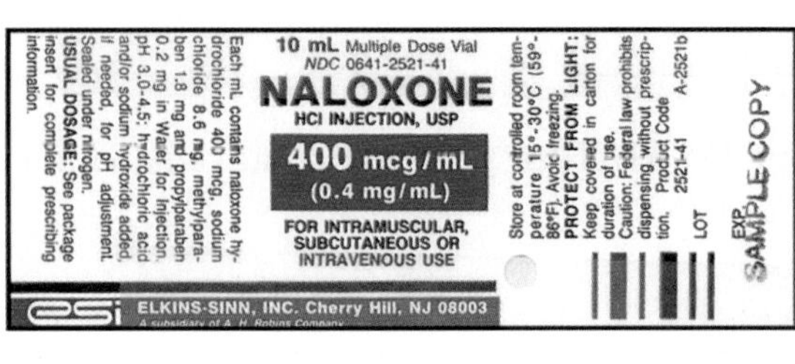

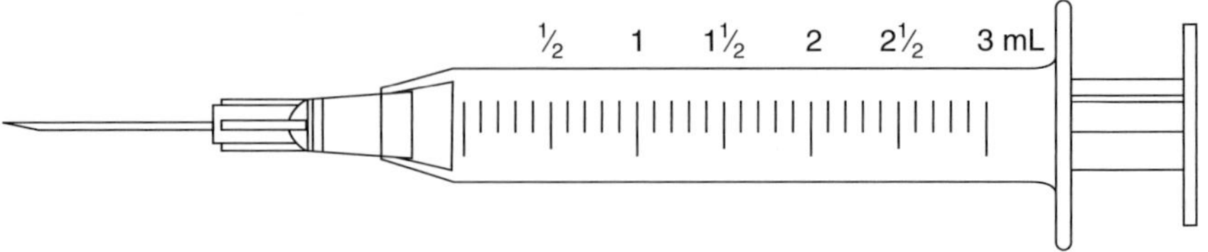

40. The licensed prescriber orders diazepam 10 mg IV STAT. How many milliliters will the nurse prepare? _______

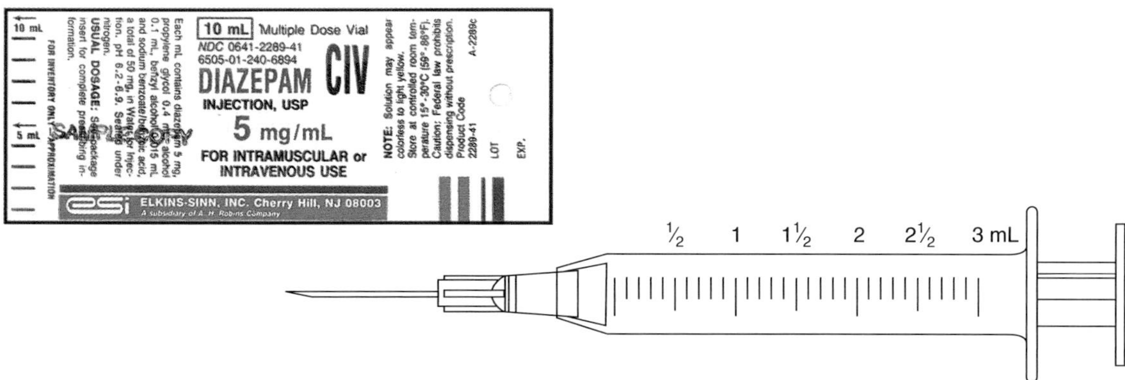

41. Mr. Ortiz has psoriasis and requires hydrocortisone 25 mg IM daily. The drug is available at a concentration of 100 mg/2 mL. How many milliliters will the nurse administer? _______

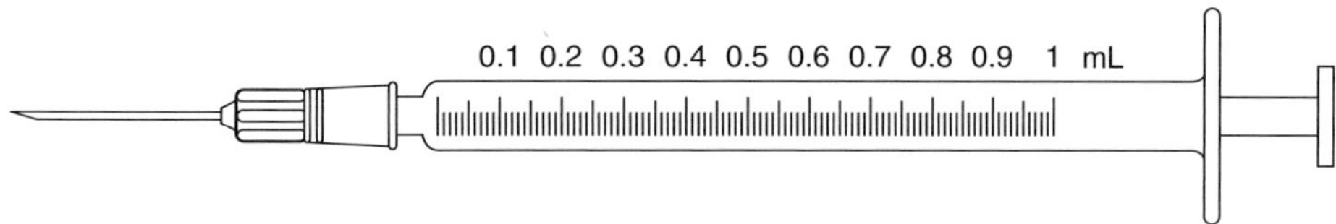

42. Mrs. Kite has ciprofloxacin 200 mg IV q 12 h ordered for a urinary tract infection. How many milliliters will the nurse administer? _______

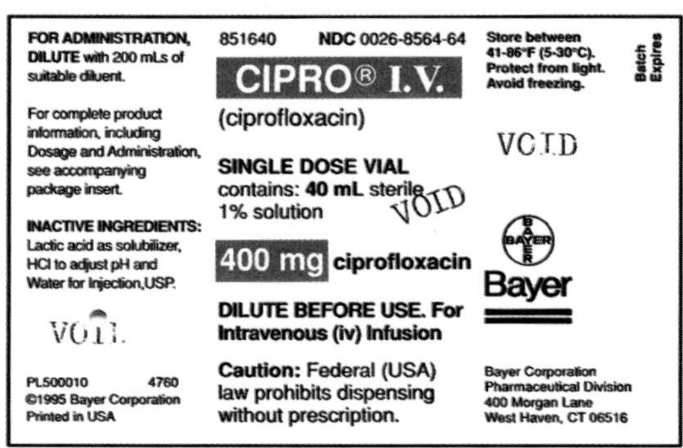

43. The licensed prescriber orders ascorbic acid 0.25 g IM daily for your patient admitted with an alcohol abuse problem. You have ascorbic acid 500 mg/mL. How many milliliters will you administer? _______

44. The licensed prescriber orders D_5W 250 mL plus calcium chloride ($CaCl_2$) 5 mEq at 2 mL/h IV. $CaCl_2$ is supplied in a 10-mL ampule containing 13.6 mEq. How many milliliters of $CaCl_2$ will be added to the 250 mL of D_5W? _______

45. The licensed prescriber orders phenobarbital sodium 70 mg IV q 8 h for your patient with epilepsy. The drug is supplied in a 1-mL ampule containing 130 mg. How many milliliters will you administer? _______

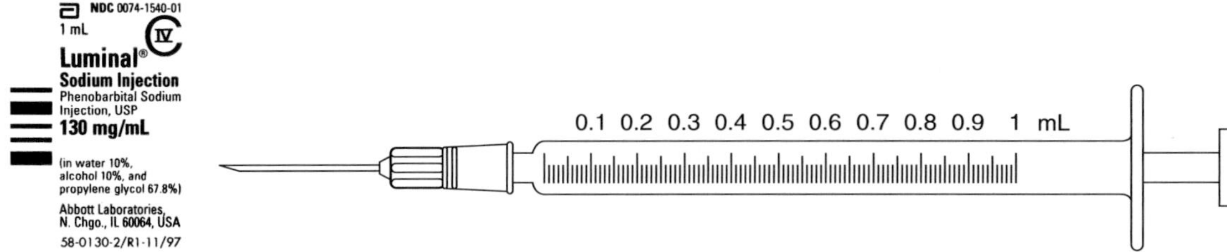

46. The licensed prescriber orders Vibramycin 200 mg IV daily. You have Vibramycin 10 mg/mL after reconstitution. How many milliliters will you prepare? _______

47. The licensed prescriber orders Dilaudid 2 mg IV q 4 h prn for pain. How many milliliters will the nurse administer? _______

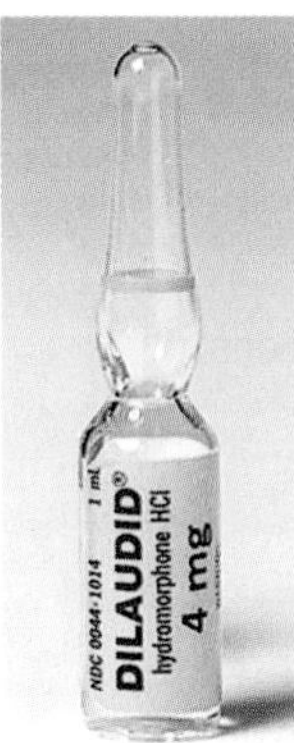

48. Your patient with atrial fibrillation has digoxin 0.2 mg IM daily ordered. How many milliliters will you administer? _______

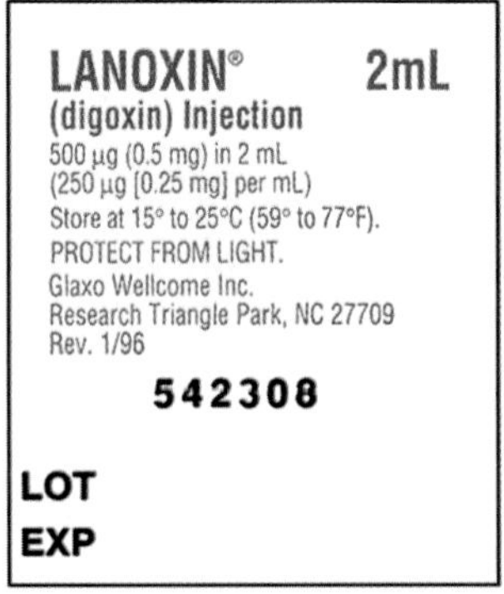

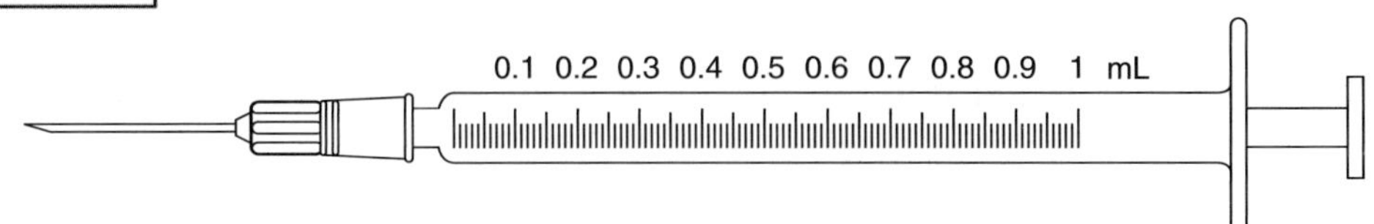

49. The licensed prescriber orders morphine 10 mg subcutaneous q 3 h. How many milliliters will the nurse administer? _______

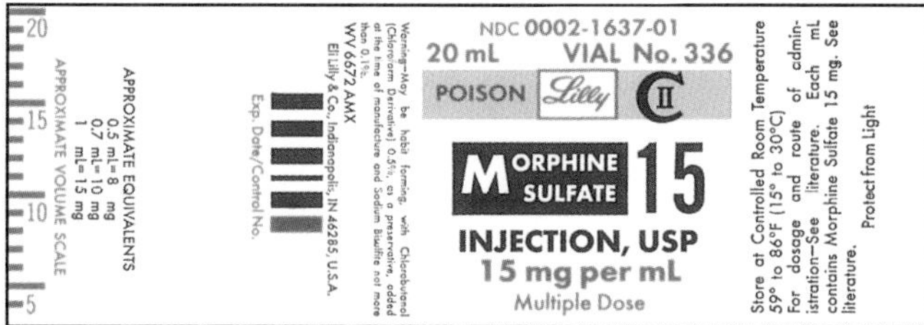

50. Mr. Lee is receiving Benadryl 25 mg IV q 6 h for severe itching. How many milliliters will the nurse administer? _______

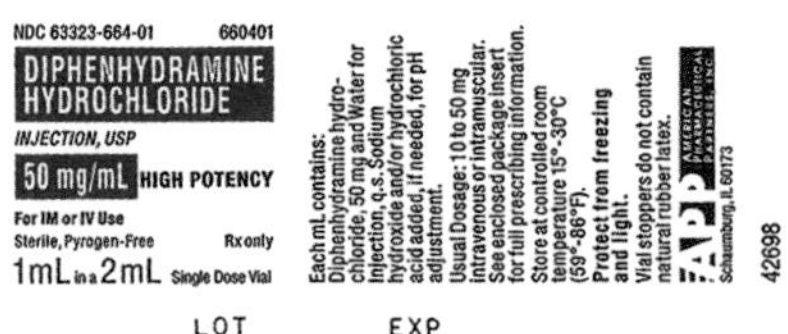

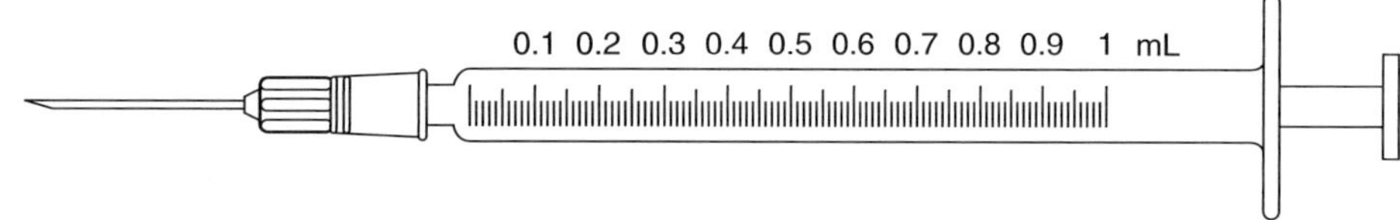

51. The licensed prescriber orders Cefadyl 600 mg IM q 6 h. How many milliliters will the nurse administer? _______

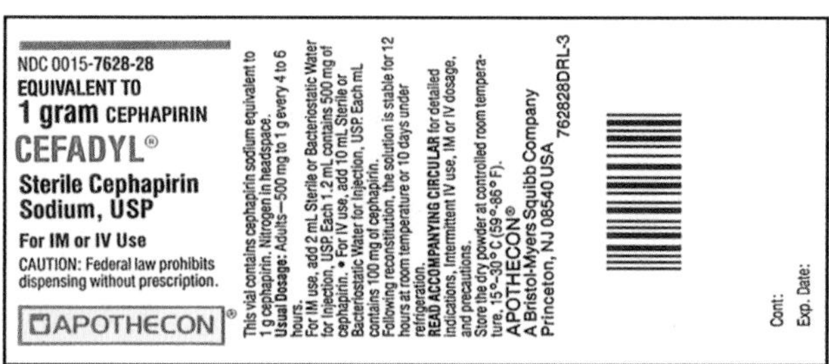

52. Your preoperative patient needs atropine 0.9 mg IM at 0615. How many milliliters will you administer? _______

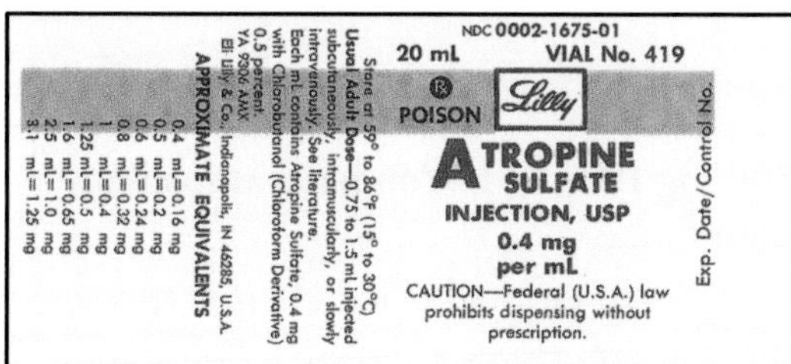

53. The licensed prescriber orders codeine 30 mg subcutaneous q 4 h for your patient after a lumbar laminectomy for pain relief. How many milliliters will you administer? _______

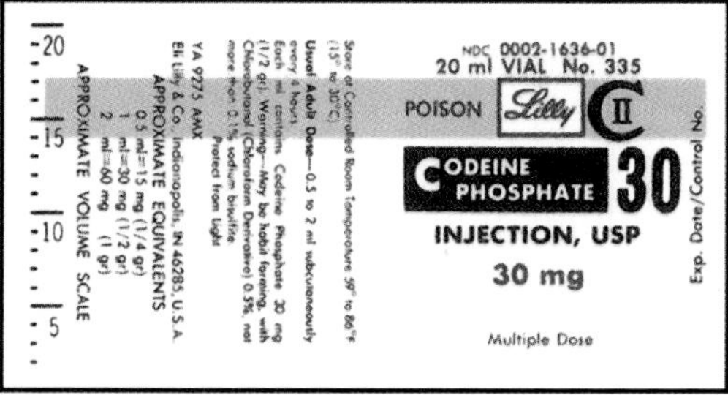

54. Mrs. Das has Ativan 3 mg IM now ordered for anxiety. How many milliliters will the nurse administer? _______

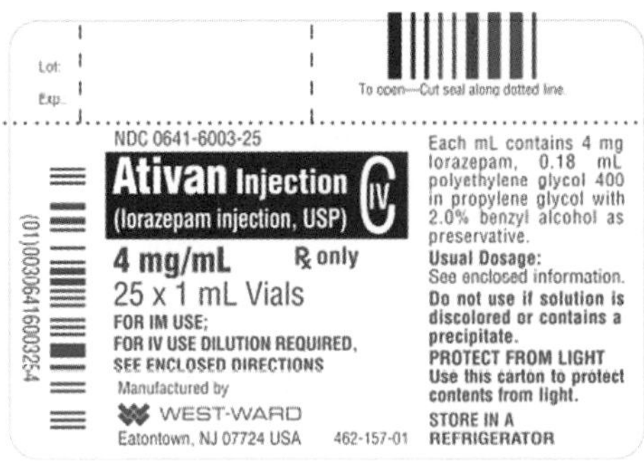

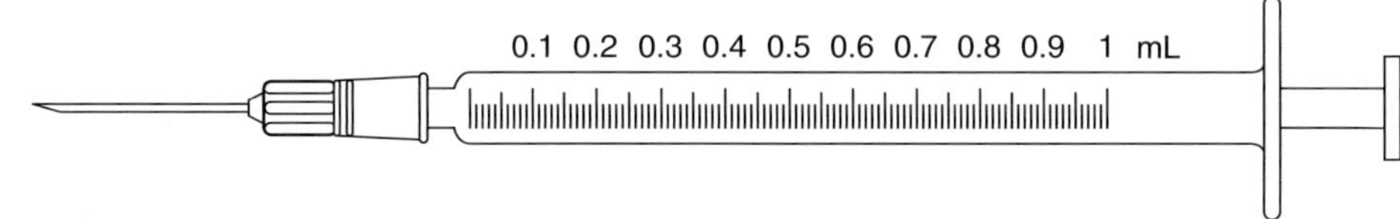

55. The licensed prescriber orders D_5W 500 mL plus 6 mEq of $NaHCO_3$ at 42 mL/h IV. $NaHCO_3$ is available in a 10-mL ampule containing 0.89 mEq/mL. How many milliliters of $NaHCO_3$ will be added to the 500 mL of D_5W? _______

56. Mrs. Luther has Decadron 10 mg IV now ordered for cerebral edema. Decadron 20 mg/mL is available. How many milliliters will the nurse administer? _______

57. Mr. Ali receives Thorazine 5 mg q 4 h for severe hiccups. How many milliliters does Mr. Ali receive in each dose? _______

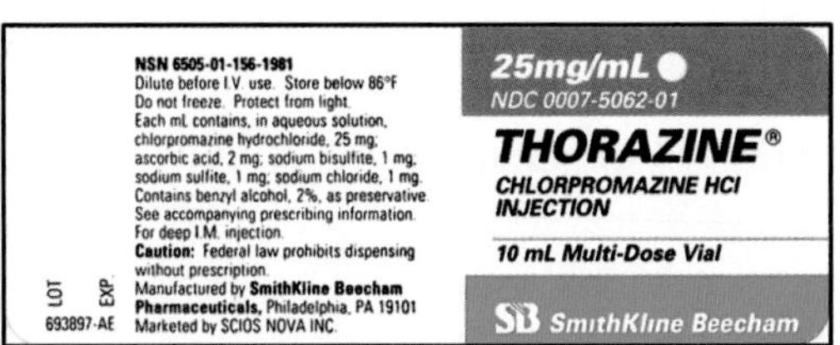

58. Your patient with sinusitis receives ampicillin 500 mg IV q 12 h. You have ampicillin 125 mg/mL. How many milliliters will you prepare? _______

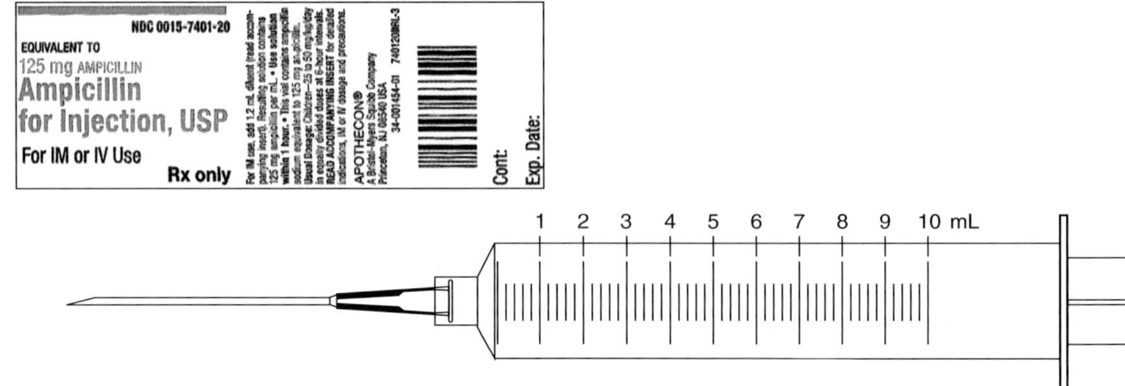

59. Mrs. Calhoun has ergonovine 0.2 mg IM STAT. Ergonovine 0.25 mg/mL is available. How many milliliters will the nurse administer? _______

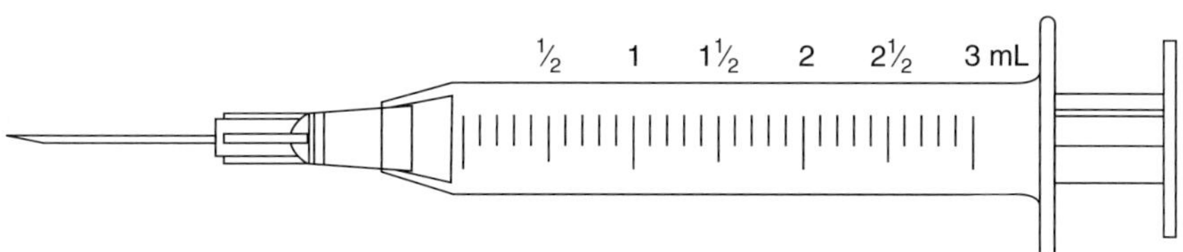

60. The licensed prescriber orders Ativan 0.5 mg IM STAT for your patient with severe anxiety. The drug is supplied in a 1-mL vial containing 2 mg/mL. How many milliliters will you administer? _______

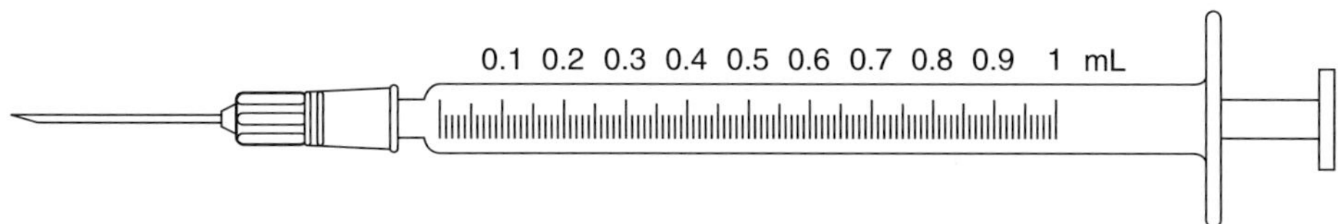

61. Aminophylline 0.2 g IV three times a day is ordered. Aminophylline is supplied in a 20-mL single-use vial containing 500 mg/20 mL. How many milliliters will the nurse prepare? _______

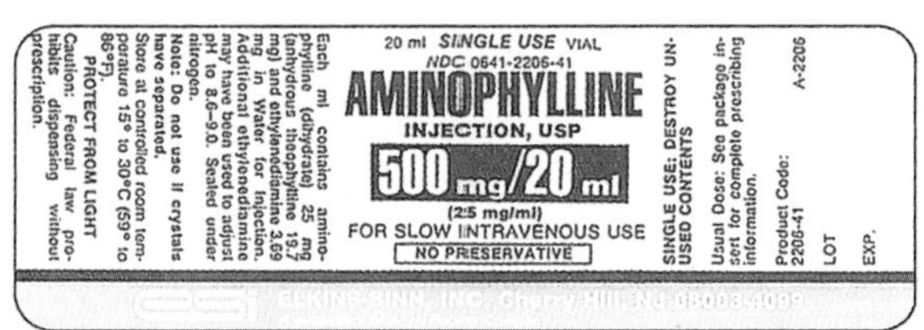

62. Codeine 15 mg IM q 4 h is ordered. Codeine is available in a vial containing 30 mg/mL. How many milliliters will the nurse administer? _______

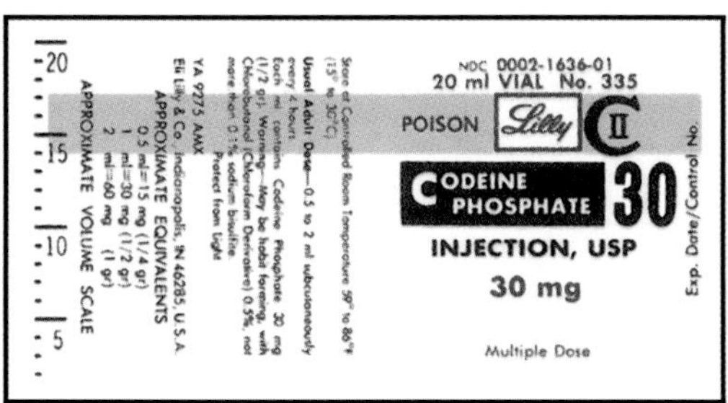

63. Mr. Ciele, who has undergone partial craniotomy, receives Dilantin 100 mg IV q 8 h. How many milliliters will you prepare? _______

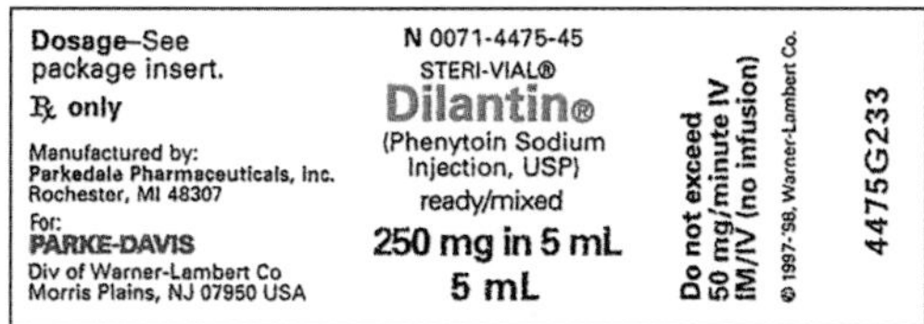

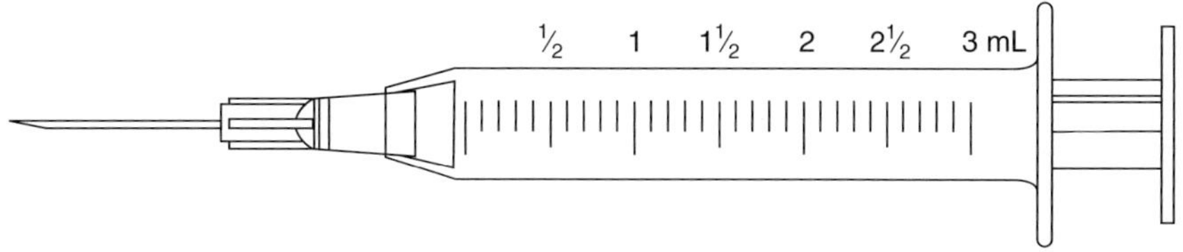

64. The licensed prescriber orders digoxin 0.25 mg IV daily for your patient with atrial flutter. Digoxin is supplied in a 2-mL ampule containing 0.5 mg. How many milliliters will you prepare? _______

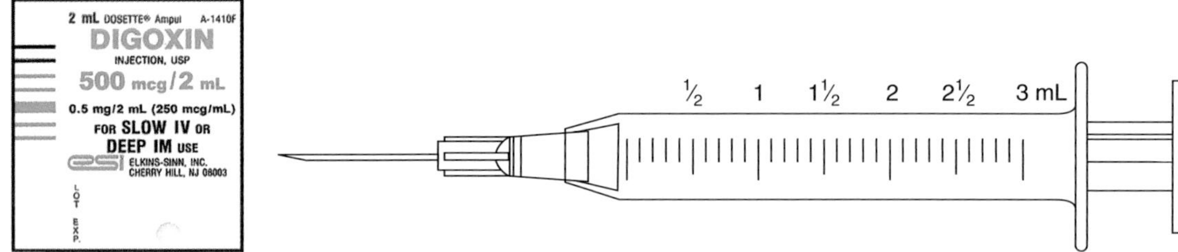

65. Mrs. Snow has Kytril 500 mcg IV ordered 30 minutes before beginning her chemotherapy. Kytril is available in 1 mg/mL. How many milliliters will the nurse administer? _______

66. The licensed prescriber orders D_5W 250 mL plus calcium gluconate 5 mEq at 2 mL IV per hour. Calcium gluconate is supplied in a 10-mL ampule containing 4.8 mEq. How many milliliters of calcium gluconate will be added to the 250 mL of D_5W? _______

67. Mr. Thompson, admitted with erythrasma, receives Cleocin 50 mg IV q 8 h. How many milliliters will the nurse prepare? _______

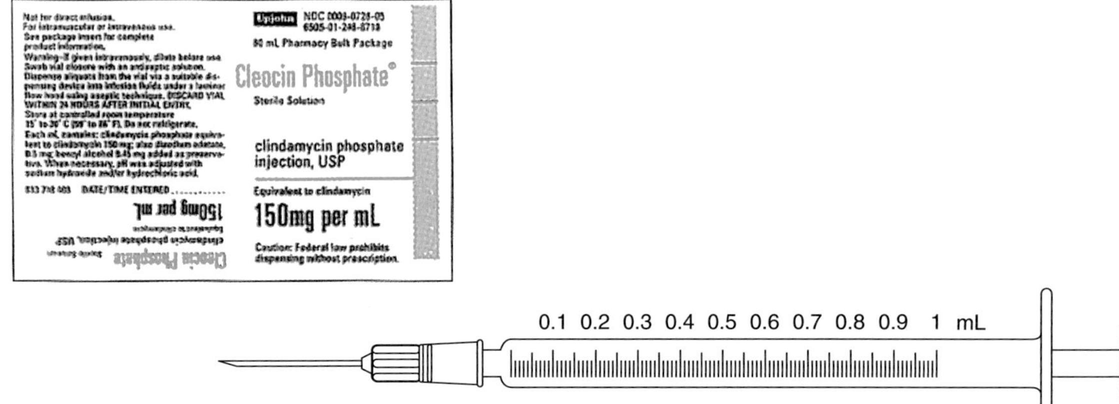

68. Atropine 0.2 mg IM at 0730 is ordered. How many milliliters will the nurse administer? _______

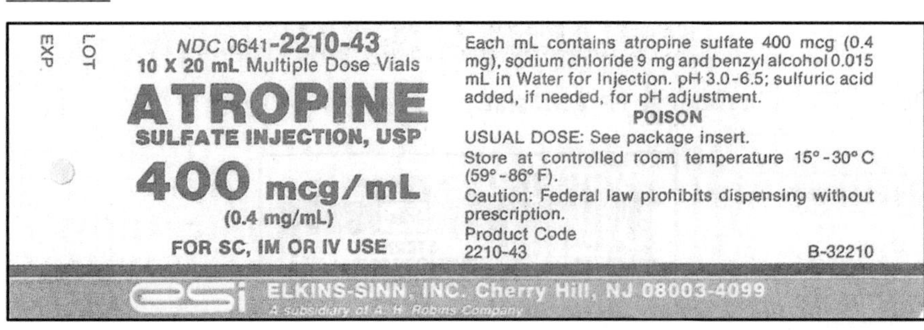

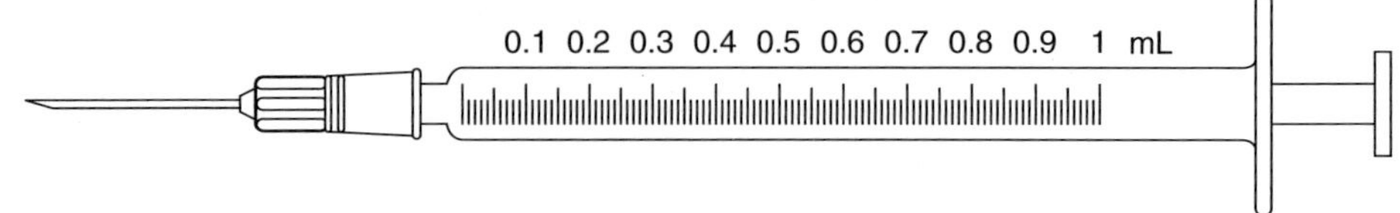

69. Mr. Riley receives tobramycin sulfate 55 mg IV q 8 h for sepsis. How many milliliters will the nurse prepare? _______

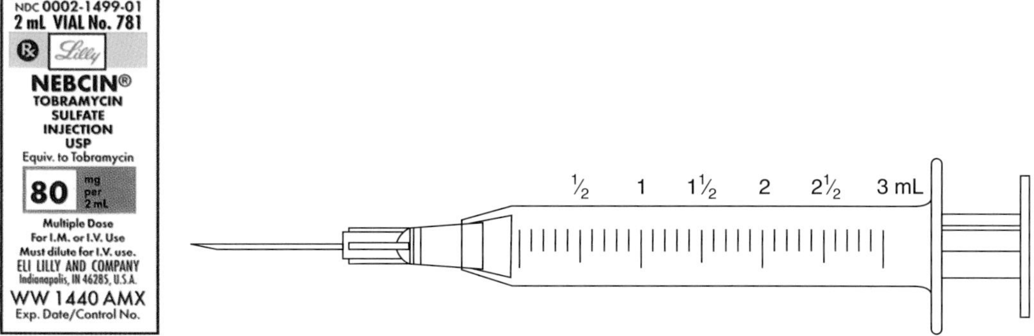

70. Mr. Russo has amikacin sulfate 600 mg IV q 8 h ordered. You have amikacin sulfate for injection 500 mg/2 mL. How many milliliters will you administer? _______

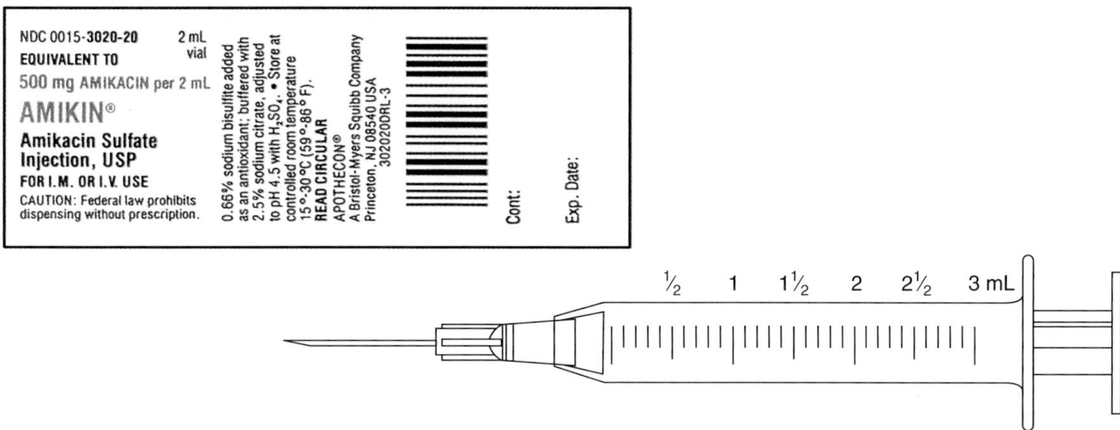

71. Your patient needs morphine 6 mg subcutaneous STAT for myocardial infarction. How many milliliters will you administer? _______

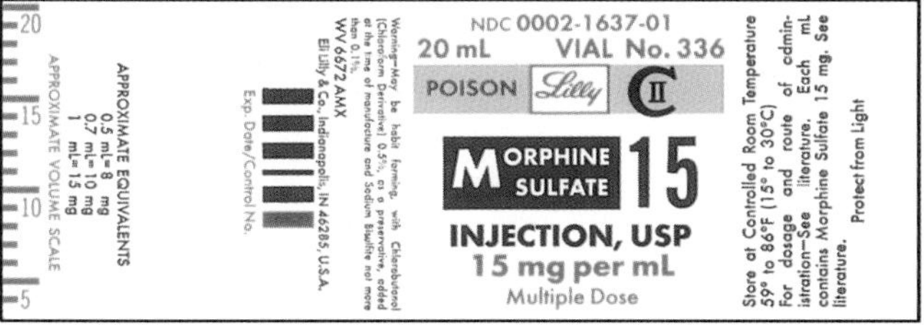

72. The licensed prescriber orders vitamin B_{12} 1000 mcg IM every Monday. How many milliliters will the nurse administer? _______

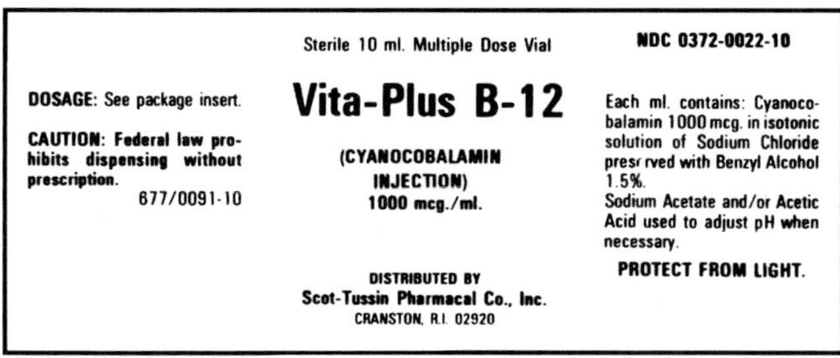

73. The licensed prescriber orders Monocid 800 mg IM daily. How many milliliters will the nurse administer? ______

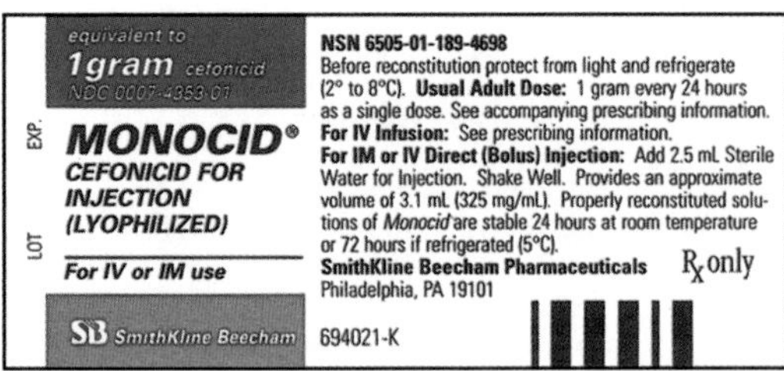

74. Mr. Paley receives promethazine 30 mg IM at 0930 for relief of nausea after a colonoscopy. How many milliliters will the nurse administer? ______

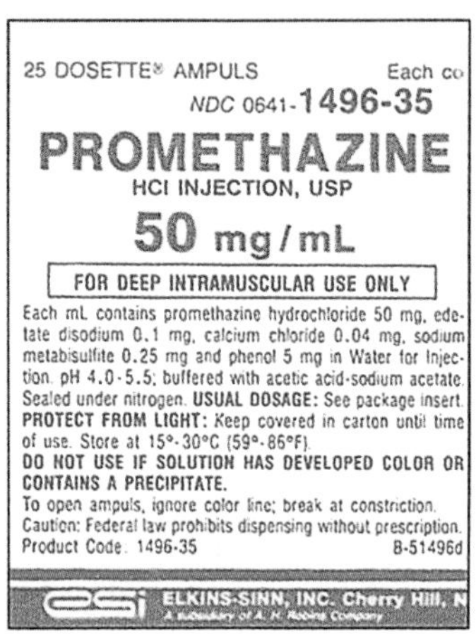

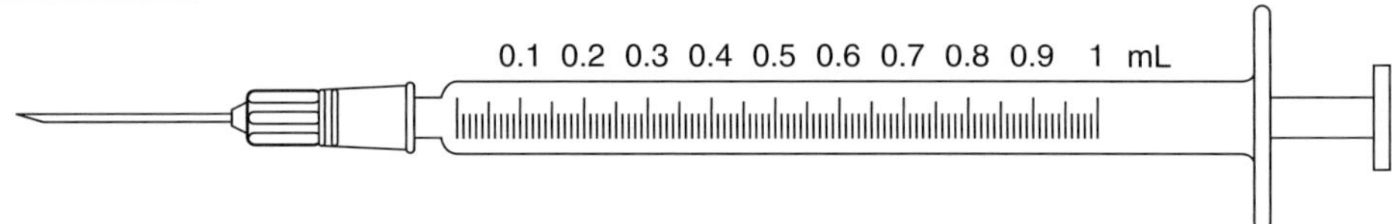

75. Your patient receives Robinul 0.28 mg IM at 0600. How many milliliters will you administer? ______

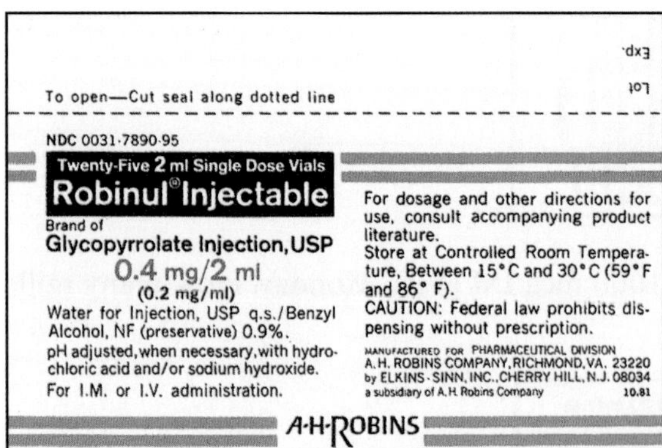

76. Mrs. Lopez has Ativan 3 mg IM ordered at bedtime for insomnia. Ativan is supplied in a 4 mg/mL prefilled syringe. How many milliliters will the nurse administer? ______

77. The licensed prescriber orders D_5W 1000 mL plus NaCl 15 mEq at 30 mL IV per hour. NaCl is supplied in a 40-mL vial containing 100 mEq. How many milliliters of NaCl will be added to the 1000 mL of D_5W? ______

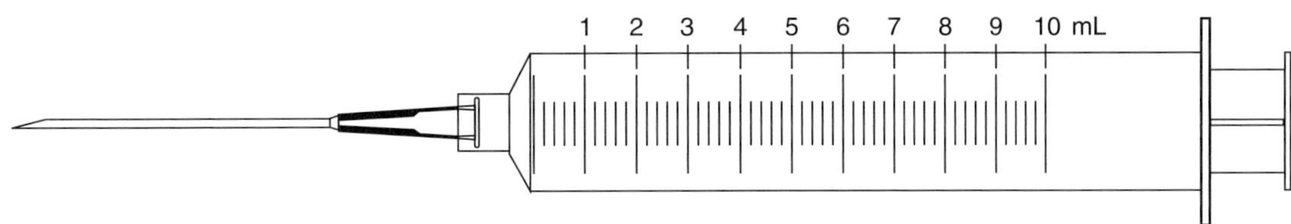

78. Mr. Neal receives Kefzol 250 mg IV q 6 h for 12 doses after an ethmoidectomy. How many milliliters will the nurse prepare? ______

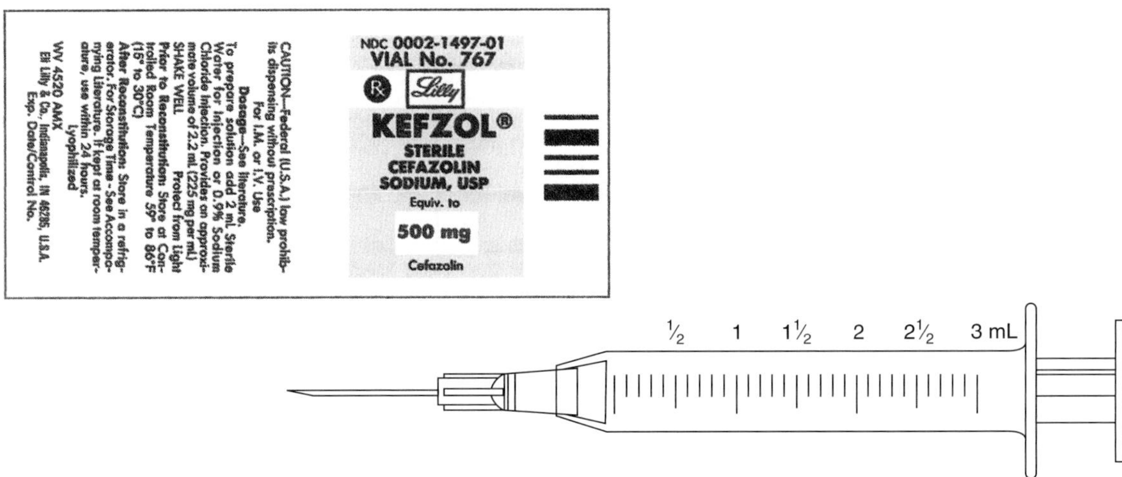

79. Your patient receives the antibiotic Cleocin phosphate 300 mg IV q 6 h for treatment of diphtheria. How many milliliters will you prepare? ______

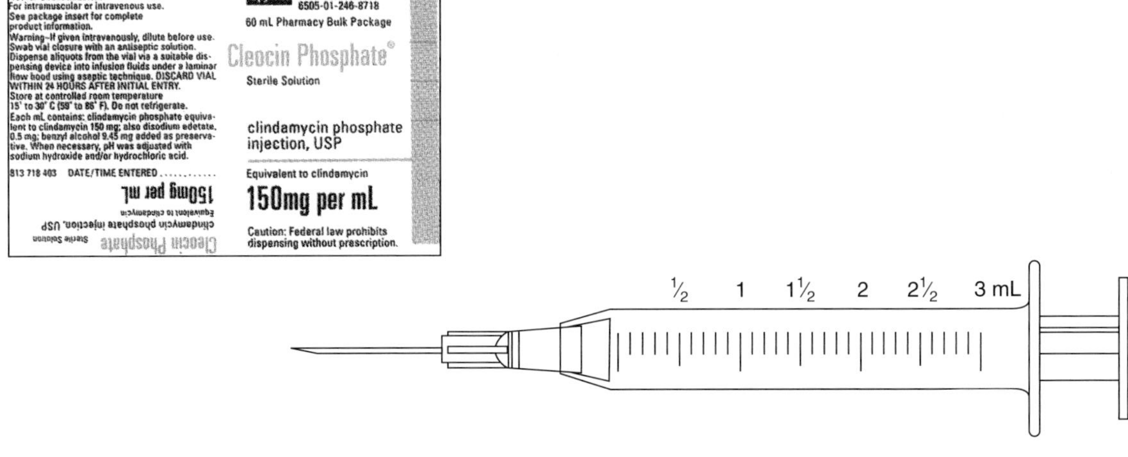

80. The licensed prescriber orders lidocaine 75 mg IV STAT. Lidocaine is available in a 5-mL vial containing 100 mg/5 mL. How many milliliters will the nurse prepare? ______

81. The licensed prescriber orders Ticar 0.8 g IM q 6 h. How many milliliters will the nurse prepare? _______

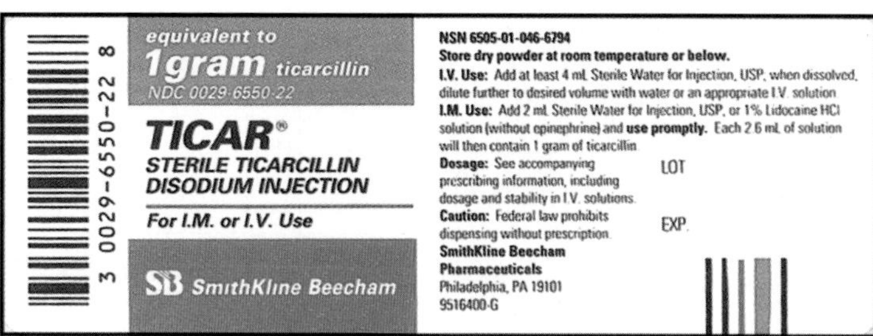

82. The licensed prescriber orders Solu-Medrol 100 mg IV STAT. How many milliliters will the nurse prepare? _______

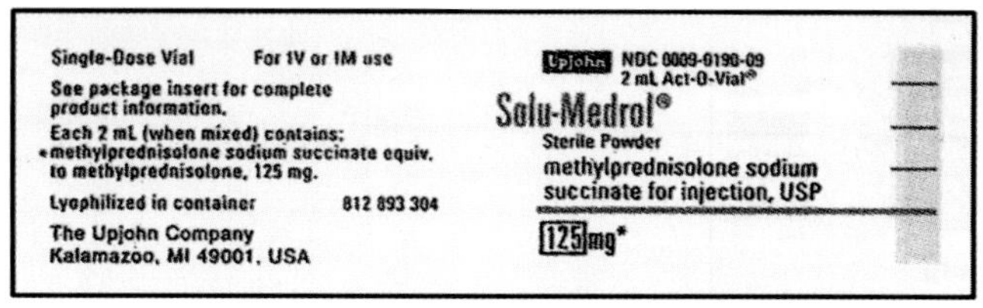
Single-Dose Vial For IV or IM use
See package insert for complete product information.
Each 2 mL (when mixed) contains:
*methylprednisolone sodium succinate equiv. to methylprednisolone, 125 mg.
Lyophilized in container 812 893 304
The Upjohn Company
Kalamazoo, MI 49001, USA
Upjohn NDC 0009-0190-09
2 mL Act-O-Vial®
Solu-Medrol®
Sterile Powder
methylprednisolone sodium succinate for injection, USP
125 mg*

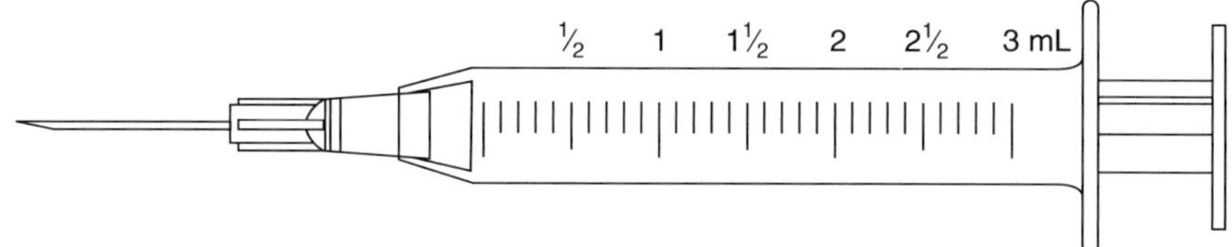

83. Mr. Scott takes Cerebyx 300 mg IV STAT for grand mal seizures. Cerebyx 75 mg/mL in a 10-mL vial is available. How many milliliters will the patient receive? _______

84. The licensed prescriber orders scopolamine 0.4 mg subcutaneous at 0700. How many milliliters will the nurse administer? _______

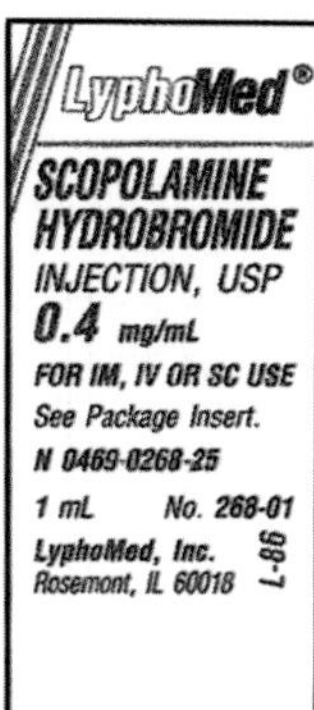

85. The licensed prescriber orders for your patient promethazine 10 mg IM STAT for relief of nausea and vomiting. How many milliliters will the patient receive? _______

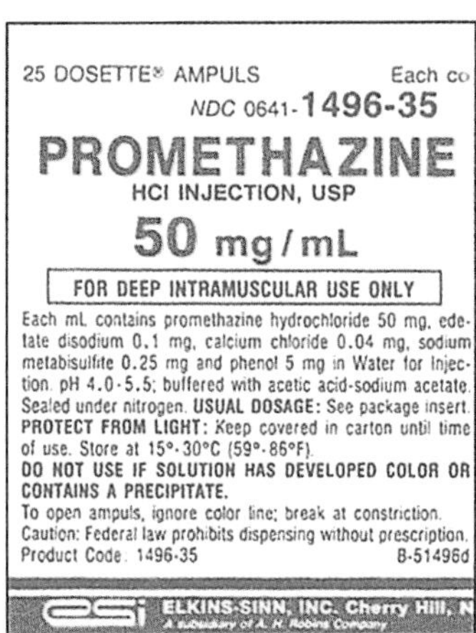

86. The licensed prescriber orders Dilaudid 1 mg IV q 4 h prn. How many milliliters will the nurse administer? _______

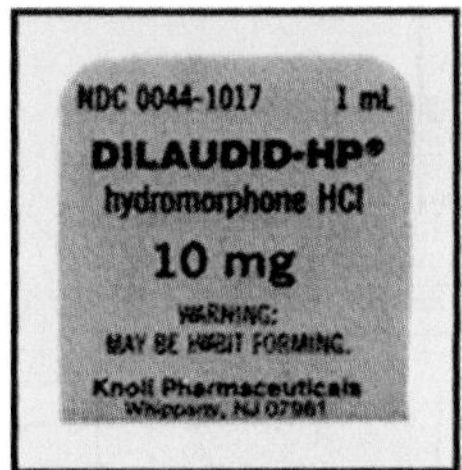

87. Your patient requires Vistaril 50 mg IM q 4 h prn for severe agitation. How many milliliters will you administer? _______

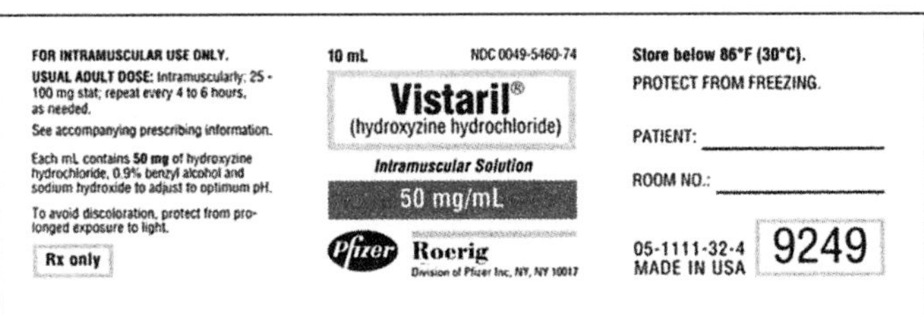

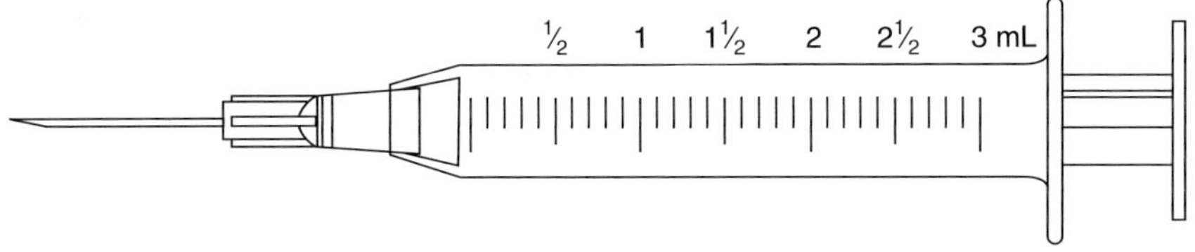

88. Ms. Jones has fentanyl citrate 60 mcg IM ordered q 2 h prn for pain. How many milliliters will the nurse administer? _______

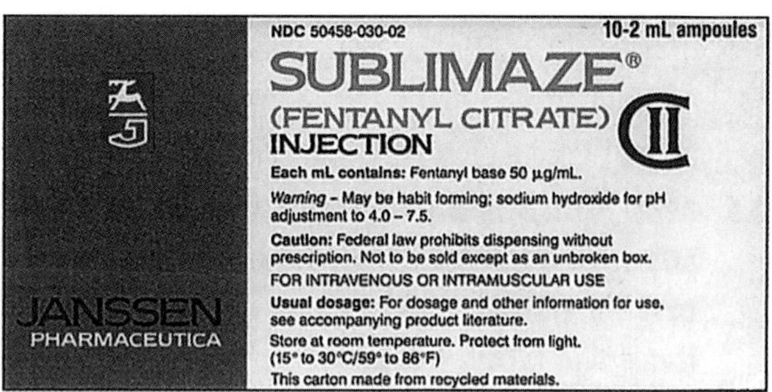

89. Atropine 0.5 mg IM STAT is ordered. How many milliliters will the nurse administer? _______

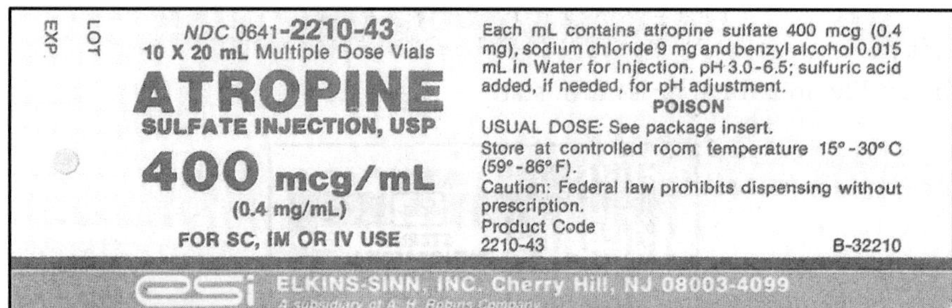

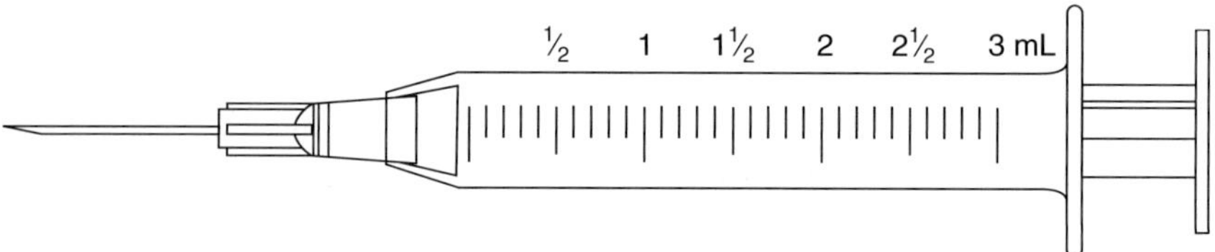

90. Your patient has Thorazine 15 mg IM q 6 h ordered for severe agitation. How many milliliters will you administer? _______

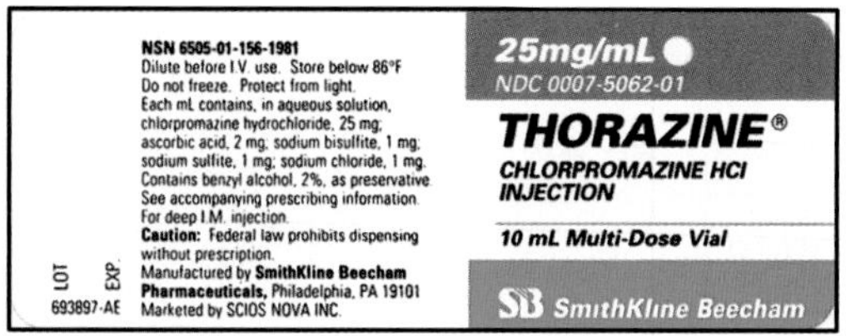

91. The licensed prescriber orders Tigan 150 mg IM for treatment of nausea. How many milliliters will the nurse prepare? _______

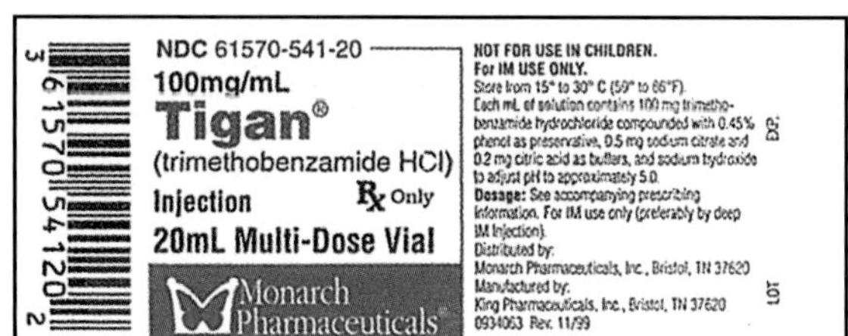

92. Mr. Garcia has Robinul 75 mcg IM ordered 30 minutes before surgery. Robinul 0.2 mg/mL is available. How many milliliters will the nurse administer? _______

93. Your patient with a seizure disorder receives diazepam 2 mg IM q 4 h. How many milliliters will you administer? _______

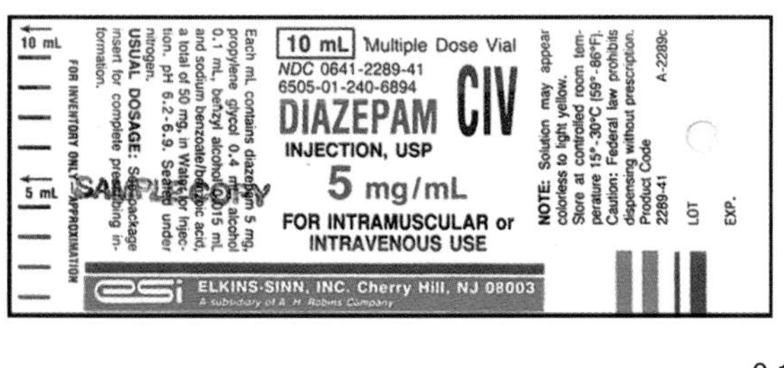

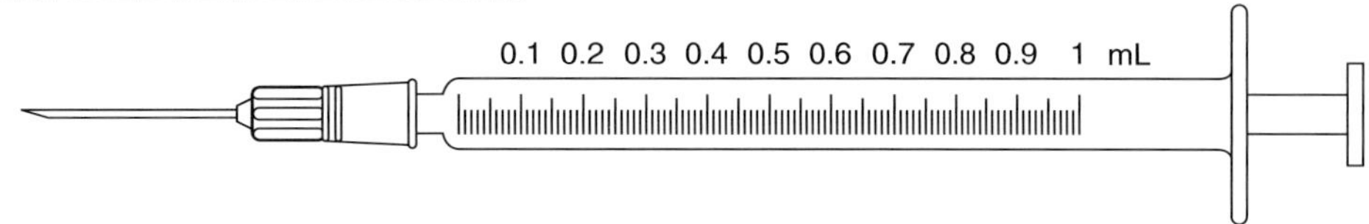

94. The licensed prescriber orders Flagyl 500 mg IV q 6 h to treat Ms. King's yeast infection. After reconstitution you have Flagyl 100 mg/mL. How many milliliters will you prepare? _______

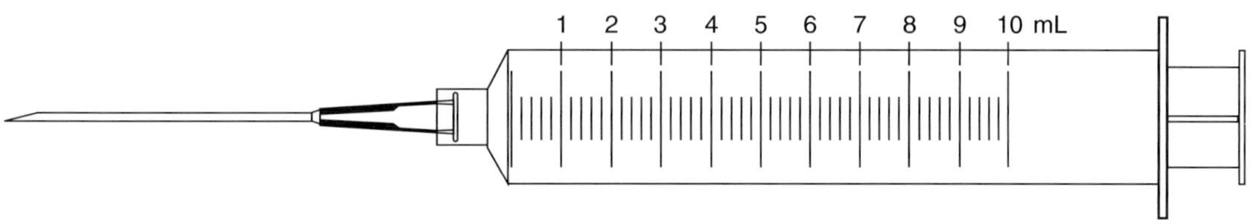

95. The licensed prescriber orders streptomycin 0.64 g IM daily. After reconstitution you have streptomycin 400 mg/mL. How many milliliters will you administer? _______

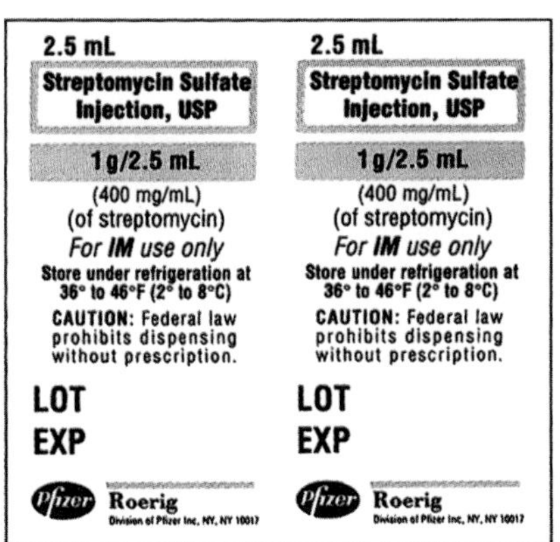

96. Your patient receives nafcillin 500 mg IM q 6 h for treatment of a *Staphylococcus aureus* infection. You have nafcillin 250 mg/mL. How many milliliters will you administer? _______

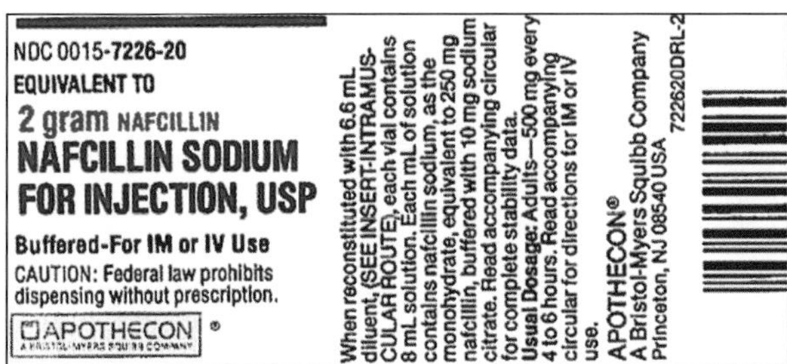

97. The licensed prescriber orders Stadol 0.5 mg IV q 4 h for pain. How many milliliters will the nurse administer? _______

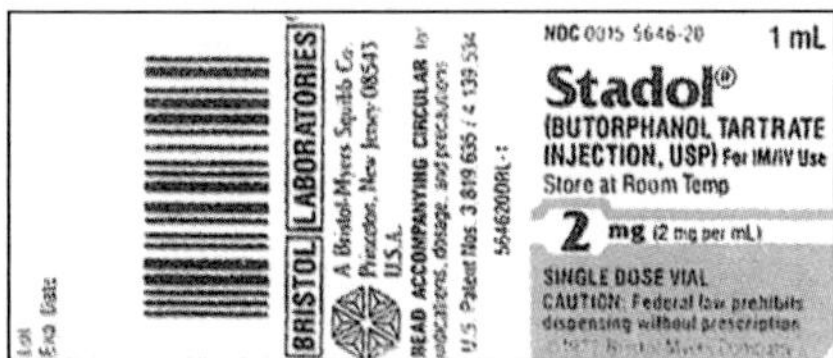

98. The licensed prescriber orders Imferon 100 mg IM every other day for your patient with pernicious anemia. The drug is supplied in ampules containing 25 mg/0.5 mL. How many milliliters will you administer? _______

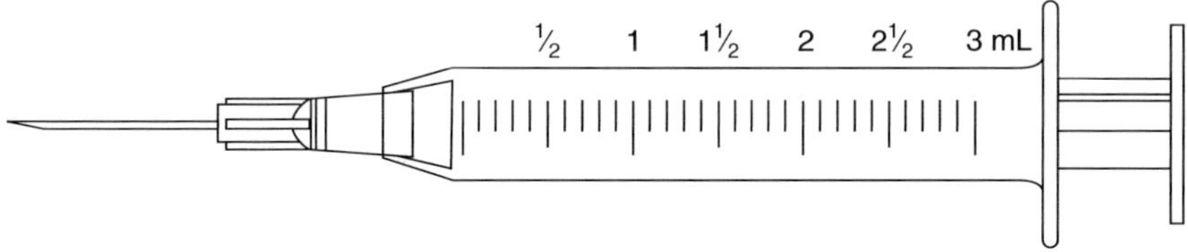

99. Your patient with arthritis receives Solganal 10 mg IM. Solganal is supplied as 50 mg/mL. How many milliliters will you administer? _______

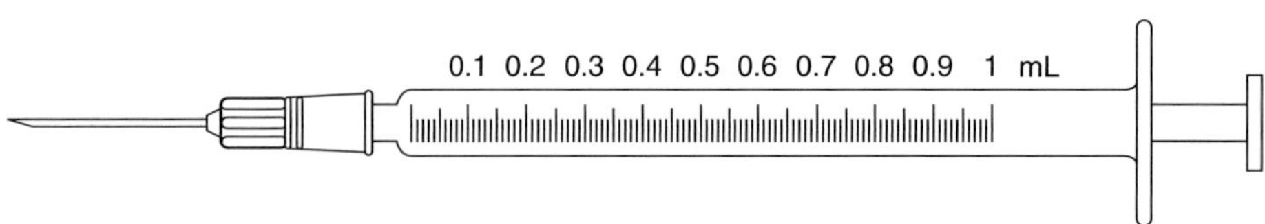

100. Mrs. Sutter has midazolam 3.5 mg IV ordered 1 hour before her surgery. How many milliliters will you administer? _______

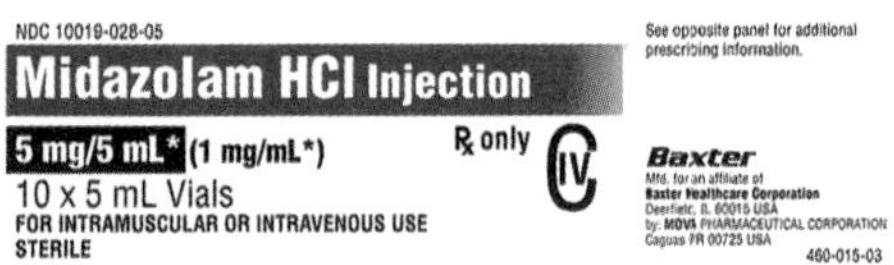

ANSWERS ON PP. 333–342 AND 346–363.

NAME ______________________

DATE ______________________

ACCEPTABLE SCORE **19**

YOUR SCORE ______

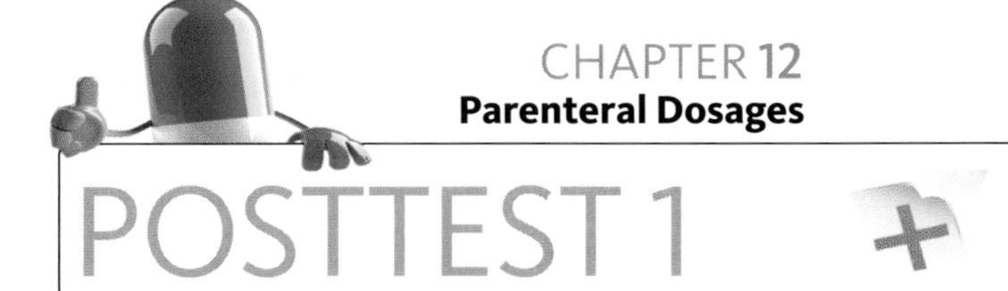

CHAPTER 12
Parental Dosages

POSTTEST 1

DIRECTIONS: The medication order is listed at the beginning of each problem. Calculate the parenteral doses. Show your work. Shade the syringe when provided to indicate the correct dose.

1. The licensed prescriber orders Vistaril 25 mg IM three times a day q 6 h prn to enhance the effects of pain medication for your patient with a thyroidectomy. How many milliliters will you administer? _______

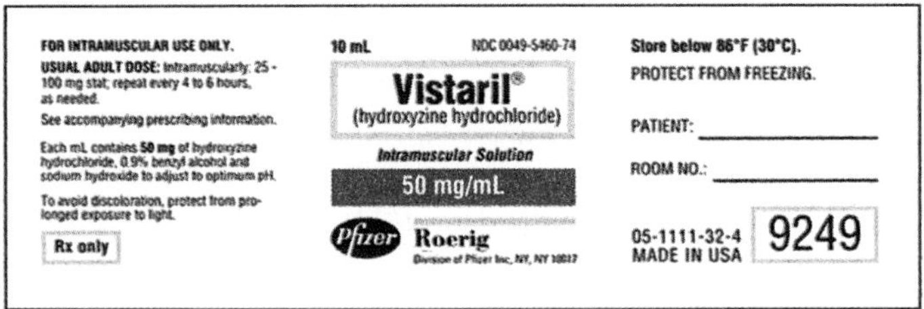

2. Your patient with a septoplasty complains of nausea and has promethazine 25 mg IM four times a day ordered. How many milliliters will you administer? _______

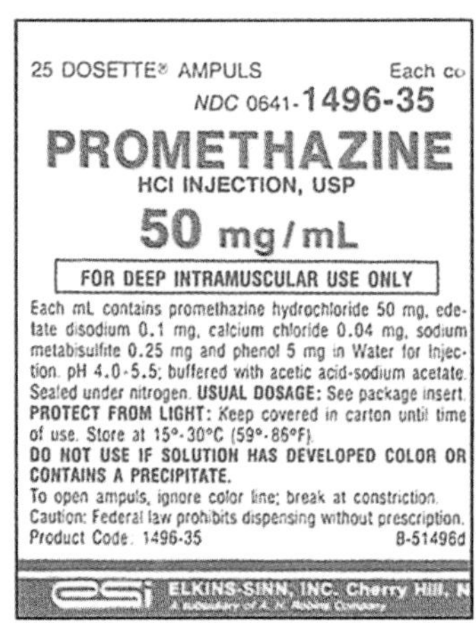

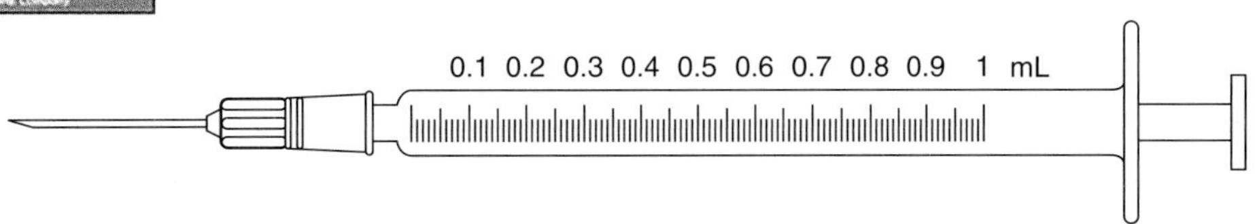

3. Your patient who has undergone tympanomastoidectomy complains of pain and has codeine 30 mg IM q 2 h prn ordered. Codeine is supplied in a 1-mL ampule containing 15 mg. How many milliliters will you administer? _______

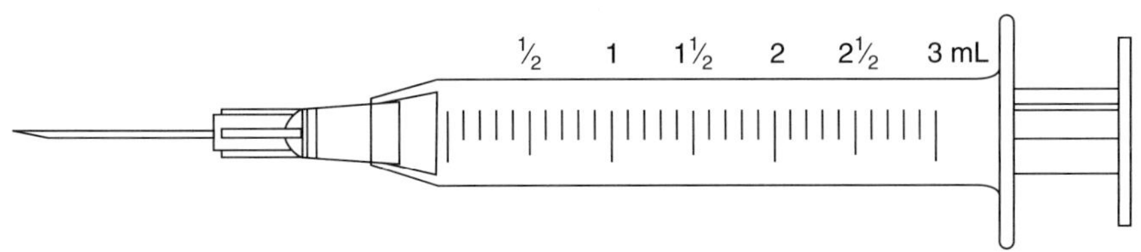

4. The licensed prescriber orders Keflin 500 mg IM q 6 h for your patient with a *Klebsiella* infection. Keflin 1 g/10 mL is available. How many milliliters will you administer? _______

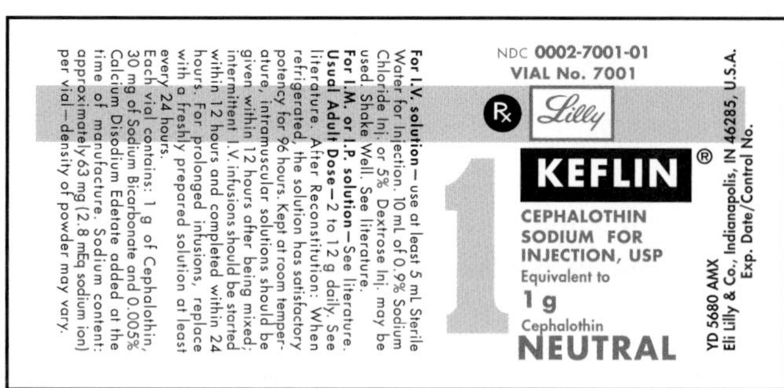

5. Your patient, who has undergone medullary carcinoma excision, has hydrocortisone 50 mg IM twice a day ordered. You have hydrocortisone 100 mg/2 mL available. How many milliliters will you administer? _______

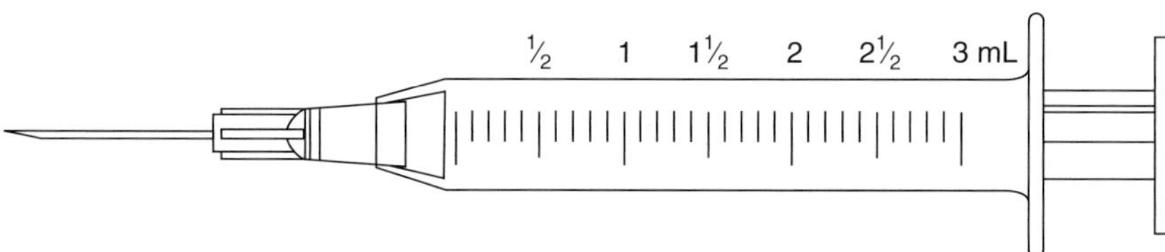

6. The licensed prescriber orders Dilaudid 0.5 mg IM q 4 h prn for pain. How many milliliters will the nurse administer? _______

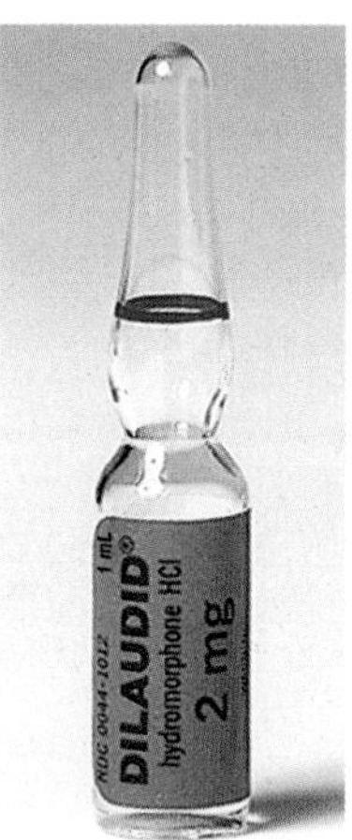

7. Mr. Harrison has Toradol 15 mg IM ordered q 6 h for pain after a hip replacement. A prefilled syringe with Toradol 30 mg/mL is available. How many milliliters will the nurse administer? _______

8. The licensed prescriber orders scopolamine 0.2 mg IM at 0600 before surgery. How many milliliters will the nurse administer? _______

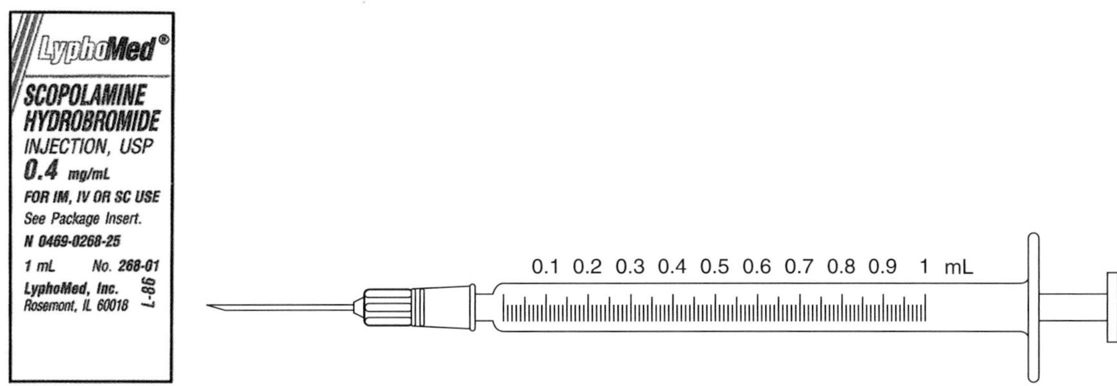

9. The licensed prescriber orders Thorazine 100 mg IM STAT. Thorazine is supplied in a 10-mL vial containing 25 mg/mL. How many milliliters will the nurse administer? _______

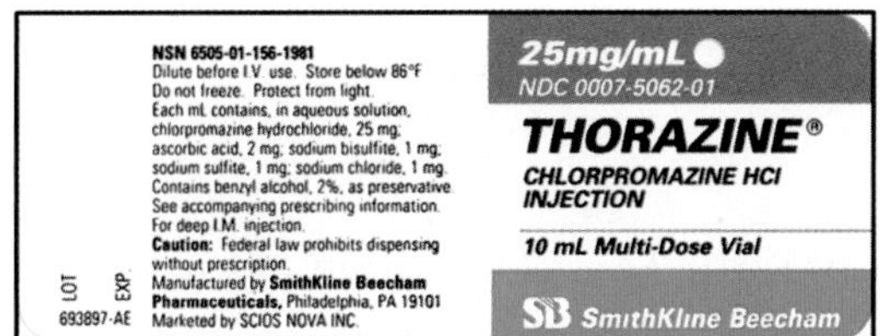

10. Your severely agitated patient has diazepam 2 mg IM q 6 h prn ordered. How many milliliters will you administer? _______

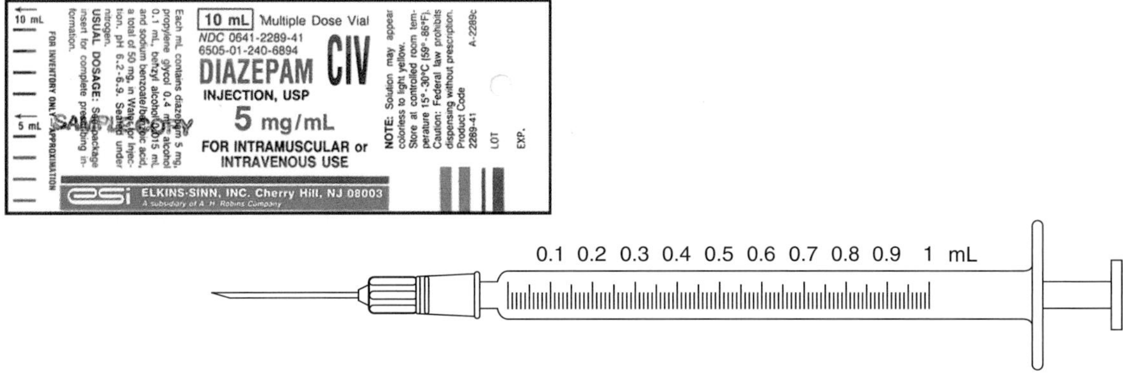

11. Atropine 0.7 mg IM STAT is ordered for your patient before surgery. You have atropine 0.5 mg/mL. How many milliliters will you administer? _______

12. Your patient with a medication reaction complains of pruritus and has Benadryl 25 mg IM prn ordered. You have Benadryl 50 mg/mL available. How many milliliters will you administer? _______

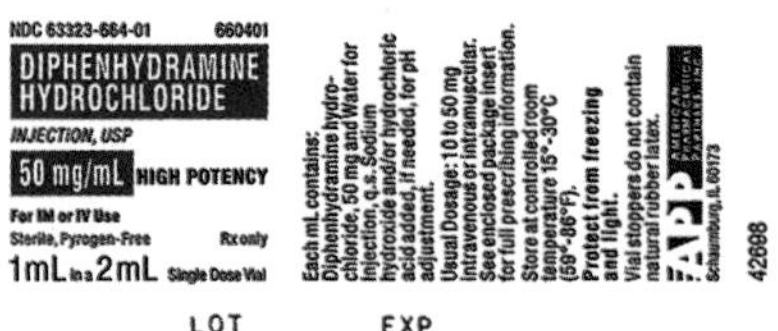

13. The licensed prescriber orders Depo-Medrol 50 mg IM twice a day. How many milliliters will the nurse administer? _______

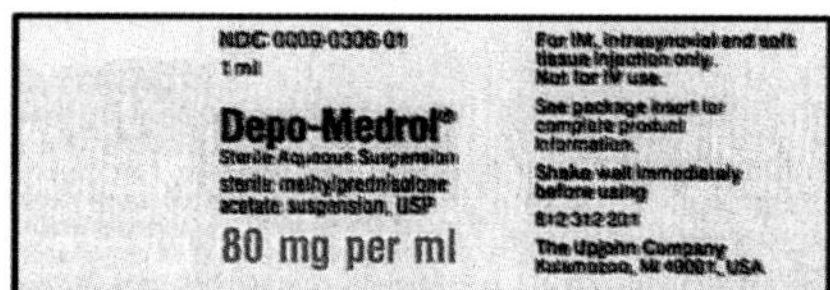

14. The licensed prescriber orders Tagamet 600 mg IV q 6 h. How many milliliters will the nurse administer? _______

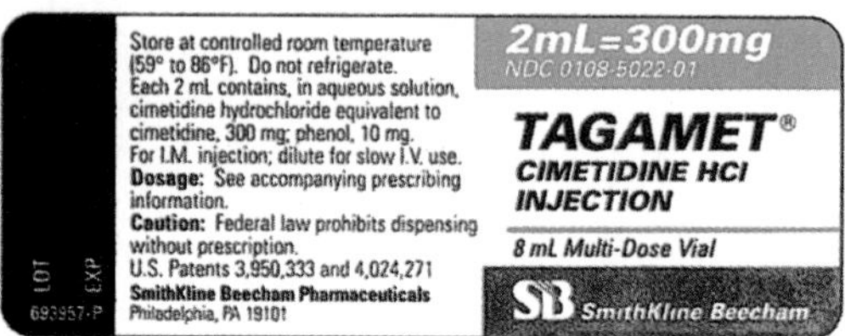

15. The licensed prescriber orders Ancef 300 mg IV q 8 h. You have Ancef 1 g/50 mL available. How many milliliters will you administer? _______

16. The licensed prescriber orders morphine 6 mg IM q 3 h prn. How many milliliters will the nurse administer? _______

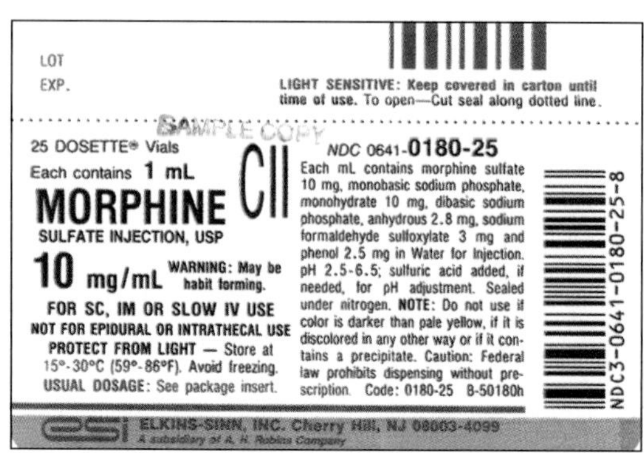

17. The licensed prescriber orders dexamethasone 6 mg IM STAT. You have dexamethasone 10 mg/mL. How many milliliters will you administer? _______

18. Your patient with congestive heart failure has furosemide 20 mg IV daily ordered. How many milliliters will you administer? _______

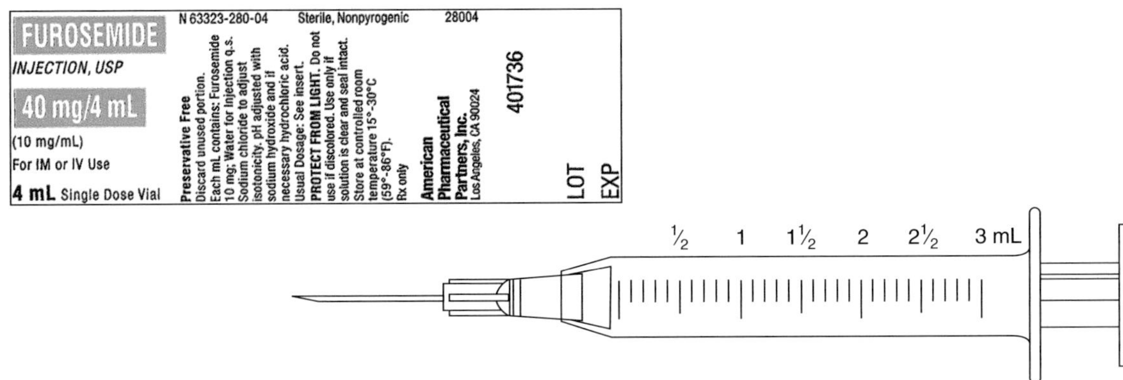

19. The licensed prescriber orders digoxin 0.3 mg IM now. How many milliliters will the nurse administer? _______

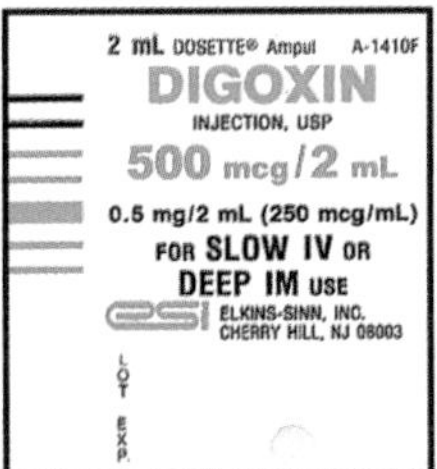

20. Mrs. Joyce has verapamil 5-mg IV bolus ordered to be given over 2 minutes now for dysrhythmia. Verapamil 2.5 mg/mL is supplied. How many milliliters will Mrs. Joyce receive? _______

ANSWERS ON PP. 342–344 AND 363–366.

NAME ______________________________

DATE ______________________________

ACCEPTABLE SCORE **19**

YOUR SCORE ______

CHAPTER 12
Parenteral Dosages

POSTTEST 2

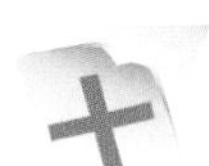

DIRECTIONS: The medication order is listed at the beginning of each problem. Calculate the parenteral doses. Show your work. Shade the syringe when provided to indicate the correct dose.

1. Your patient, who was involved in a motor vehicle accident, complains of pain and has Dilaudid 2 mg IM q 3 h prn ordered. How many milliliters will you administer? _______

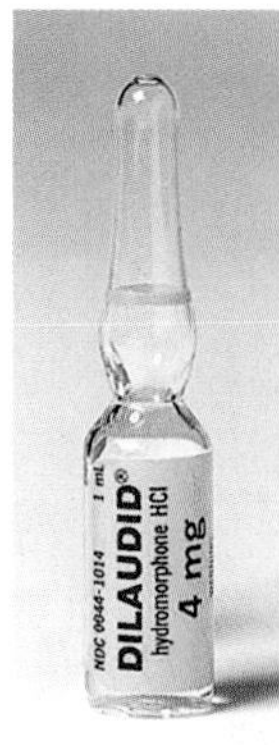

2. Your preoperative patient complains of anxiety and has Ativan 2 mg IM q 6 h ordered. Ativan is supplied 4 mg/mL. How many milliliters will you administer? _______

3. The licensed prescriber orders erythromycin 0.4 g IV today. The drug is supplied in vials containing 500 mg/10 mL. How many milliliters will the nurse prepare? _______

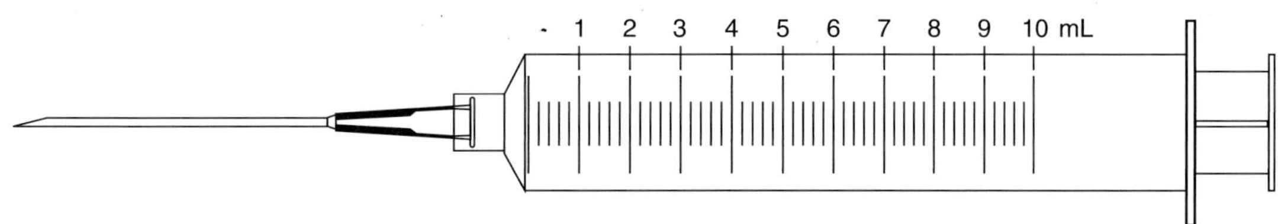

4. Mrs. Jesse has Cardizem 20 mg IV ordered STAT for hypertension. How many milliliters will the nurse administer? _______

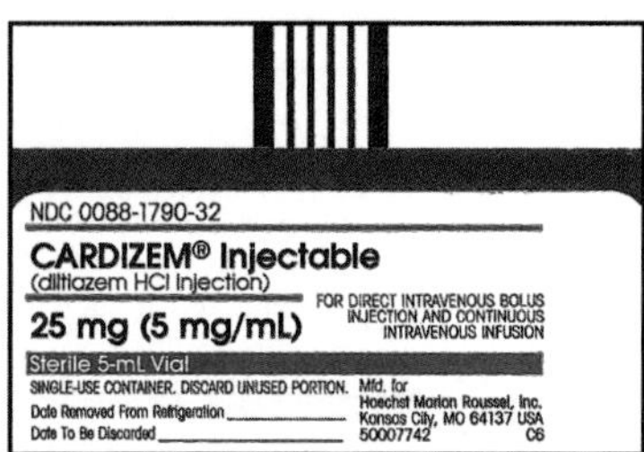

5. Your patient who has had a lumpectomy has codeine 60 mg IM q 3 h ordered. How many milliliters will you administer? _______

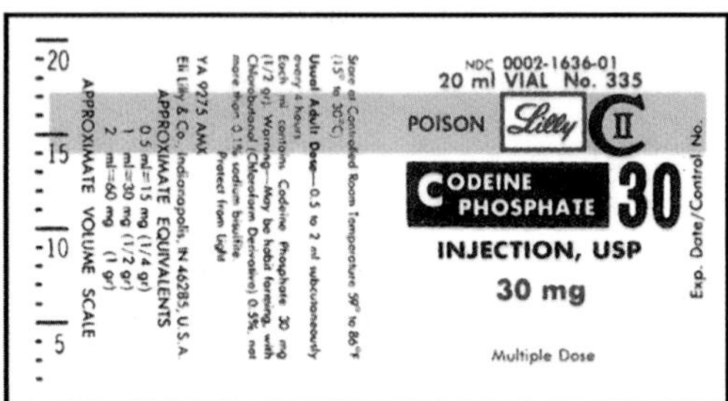

6. Mr. Ryan has Tigan 200 mg IM ordered three times a day for nausea and vomiting. How many milliliters will you administer? _______

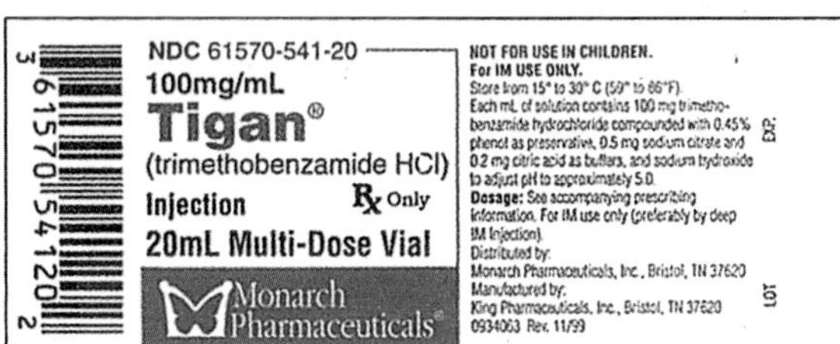

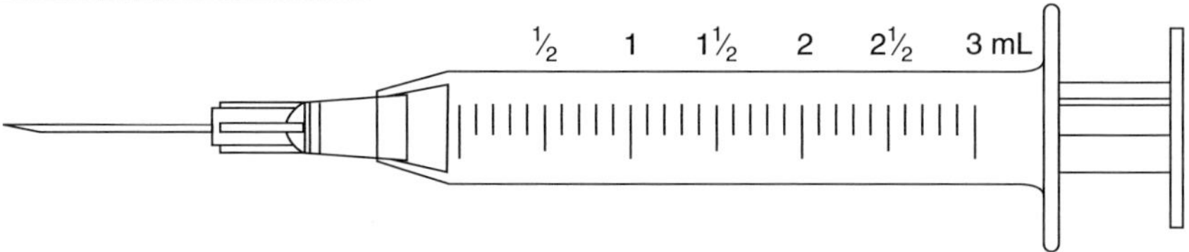

7. The licensed prescriber orders atropine 0.2 mg IM at 0600. How many milliliters will the nurse administer? _______

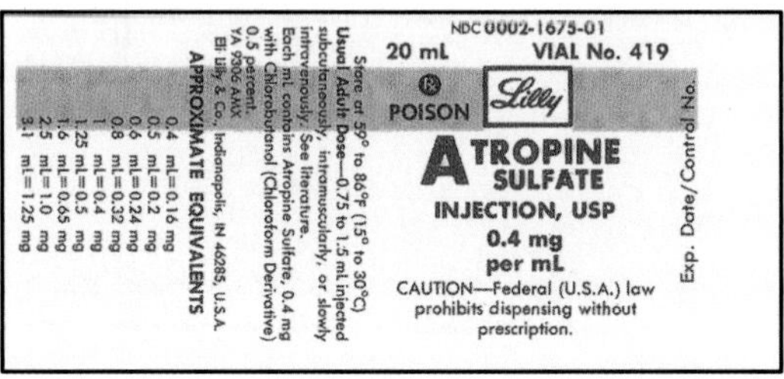

8. The licensed prescriber orders Benadryl 25 mg IV STAT for your patient with a mild medication reaction. How many milliliters will you prepare? _______

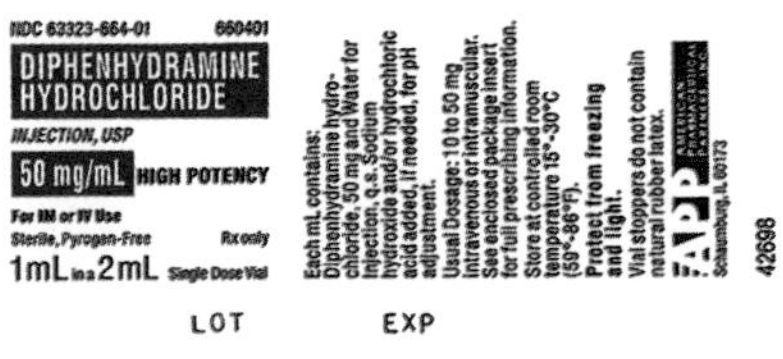

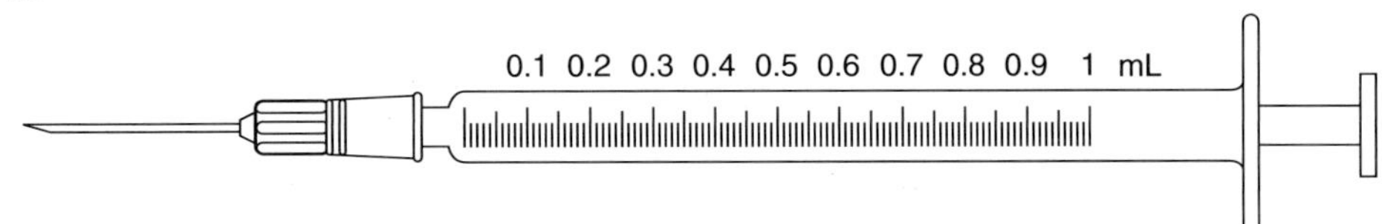

9. Ms. Straw has Anzemet 100 mg IV ordered to be given 30 minutes before her chemotherapy. Anzemet 20 mg/mL is available. How many milliliters will the nurse administer? _______

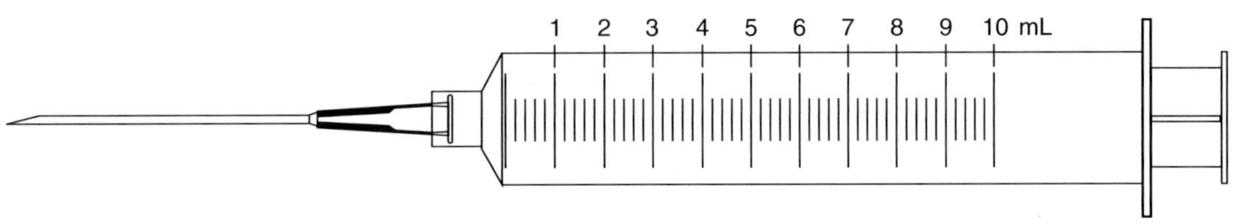

10. Mr. Trent has hydroxyzine 75 mg IM STAT ordered for severe motion sickness. You have hydroxyzine 50 mg/mL. How many milliliters will you administer? _______

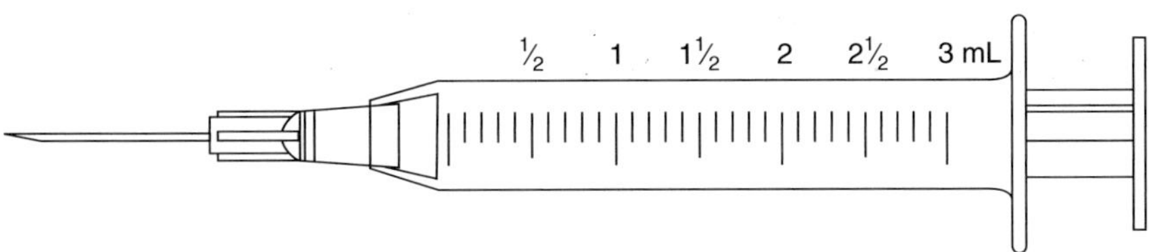

11. Your postsurgical patient has Sublimaze 70 mcg IM ordered q 2 h prn for pain. How many milliliters will you prepare? _______

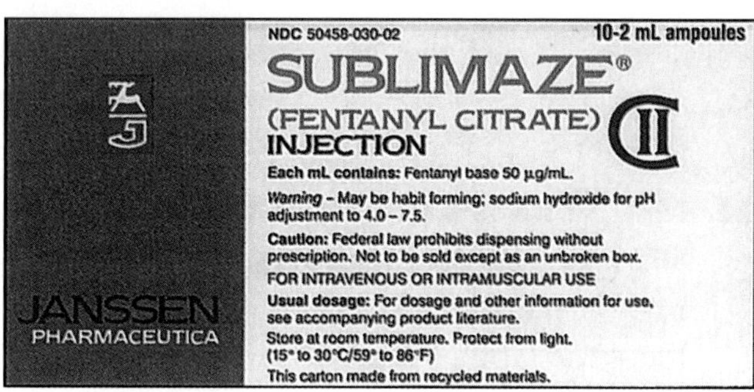

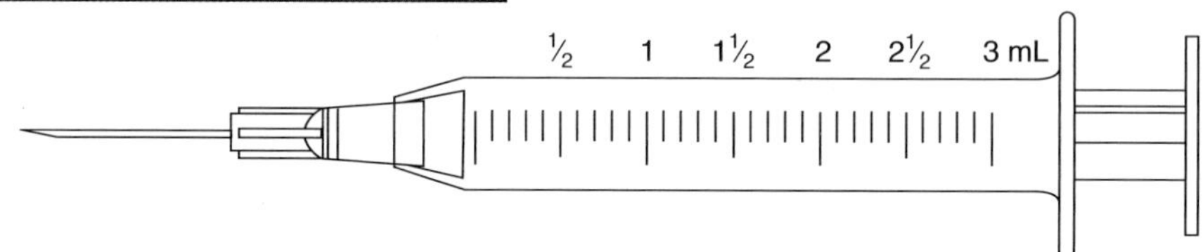

12. The licensed prescriber orders scopolamine 0.4 mg IM at 0700. Scopolamine 0.3 mg/mL is available. How many milliliters will the nurse administer? _______

13. The licensed prescriber orders piperacillin 2 g IV q 8 h for your patient with sepsis. Piperacillin 1 g/2.5 mL is available. How many milliliters will you prepare? _______

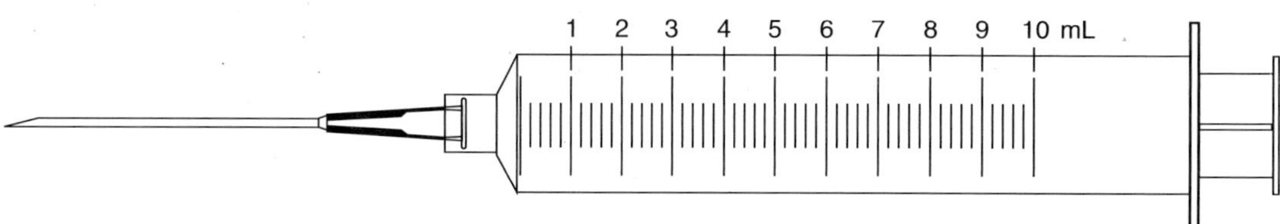

14. The licensed prescriber orders gentamicin 26 mg IV q 8 h. How many milliliters will the nurse prepare? _______

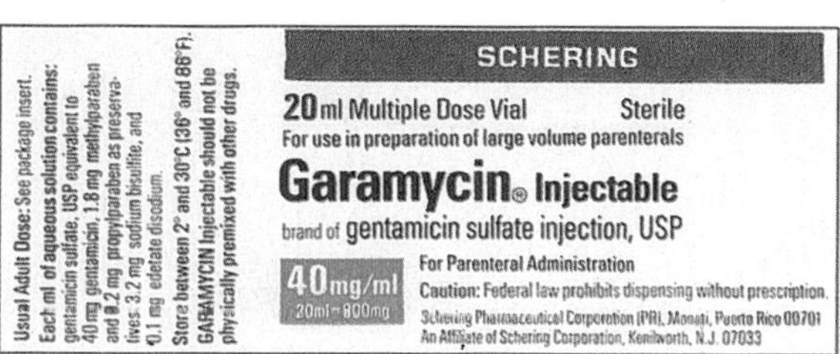

15. The licensed prescriber orders Lovenox 85 mg subcutaneous q 12 h. The drug is available as 40 mg/0.4 mL. How many milliliters will the nurse administer? _______

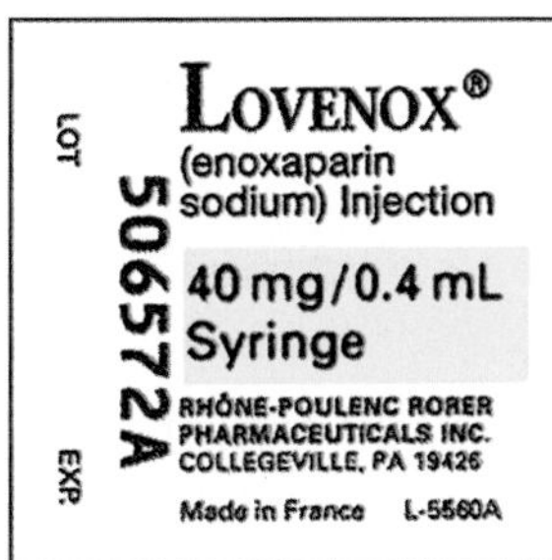

16. Your patient, who has undergone tricuspid valve repair, has Lanoxin 80 mcg IM twice a day ordered. How many milliliters will you administer? _______

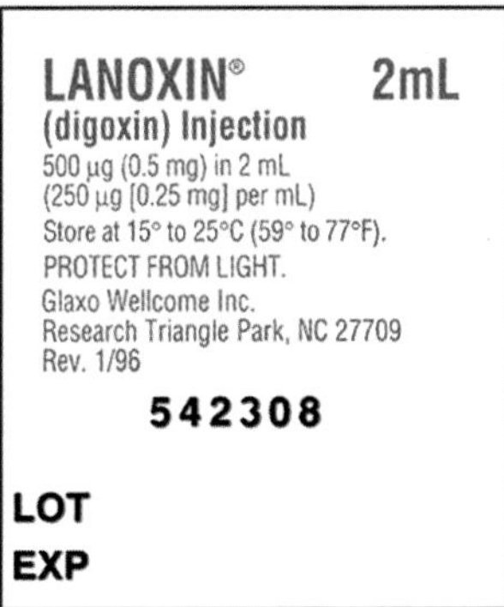

17. The licensed prescriber orders morphine 4 mg subcutaneous q 4 h prn. Morphine is supplied in a 1-mL ampule containing 8 mg. How many milliliters will the nurse administer? _______

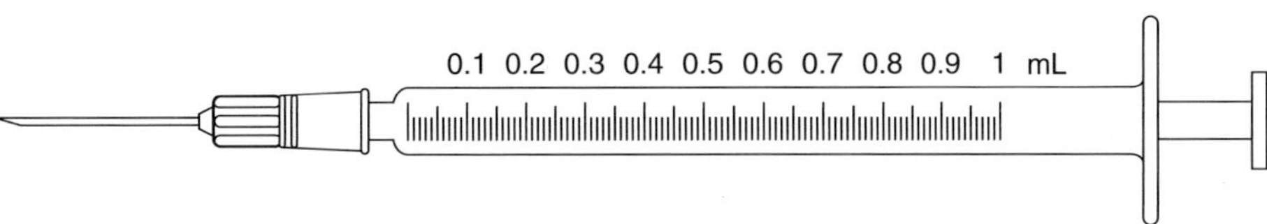

18. Your patient with a history of seizures has Dilantin 100 mg IV q 8 h ordered. Dilantin 50 mg/2 mL is available. How many milliliters will you prepare? _______

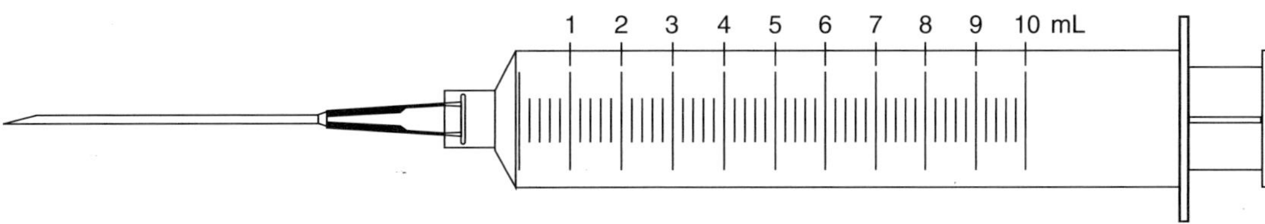

19. Mr. Richards has Floxin 300 mg IV q 12 h ordered to treat his prostatitis. Floxin 400 mg/100 mL is available. How many milliliters will the nurse administer? _______

20. The licensed prescriber orders D_5W 500 mL plus calcium chloride ($CaCl_2$) 10 mEq at 10 mL per hour IV. $CaCl_2$ is supplied in a 10-mL ampule containing 13.6 mEq. How many milliliters of $CaCl_2$ will be added to the 500 mL of D_5W? _______

ANSWERS ON PP. 344–346 AND 366–369.

evolve For additional practice problems, refer to the Parenteral Dosages section of *Elsevier's Interactive Drug Calculation Application*, version 1.

ANSWERS

CHAPTER 12 Dimensional Analysis—Worksheet, pp. 297–320

1. $x \text{ mL} = \frac{1 \text{ mL}}{400 \text{ mg}} \times \frac{500 \text{ mg}}{1} = 1.25 \text{ mL}$

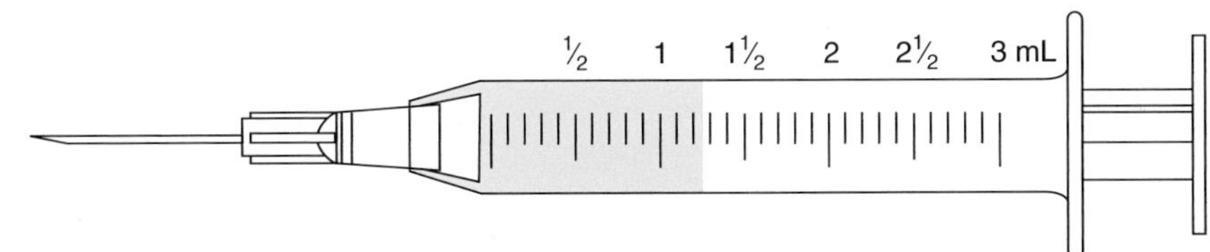

2. $x \text{ mL} = \frac{1 \text{ mL}}{0.25 \text{ mg}} \times \frac{1 \text{ mg}}{1000 \text{ mcg}} \times \frac{110 \text{ mcg}}{1} = 0.44 \text{ mL}$

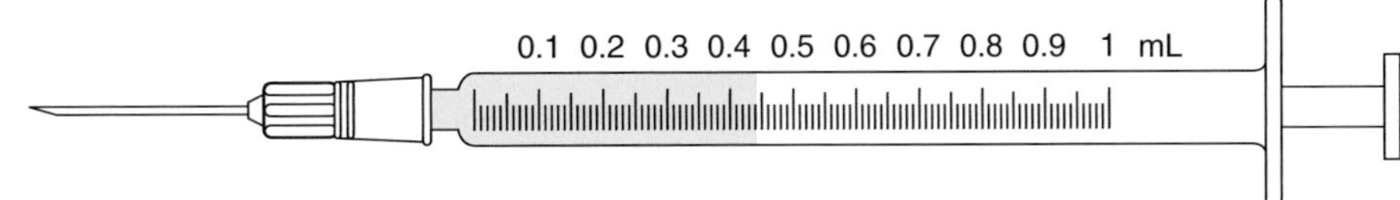

3. $x \text{ mL} = \frac{1 \text{ mL}}{0.4 \text{ mg}} \times \frac{0.3 \text{ mg}}{1} = 0.75 \text{ mL}$

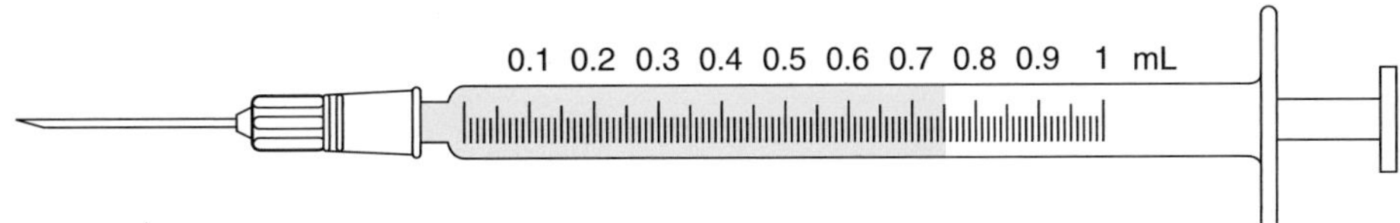

4. $x \text{ mL} = \frac{1 \text{ mL}}{5 \text{ mg}} \times \frac{10 \text{ mg}}{1} = 2 \text{ mL}$

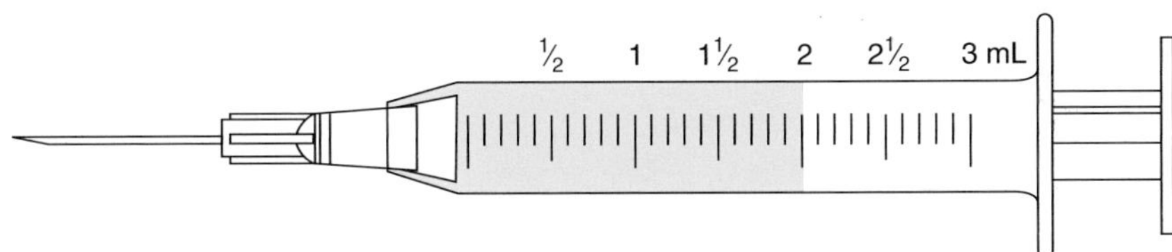

5. $x \text{ mL} = \frac{1 \text{ mL}}{25 \text{ mg}} \times \frac{50 \text{ mg}}{1} = 2 \text{ mL}$

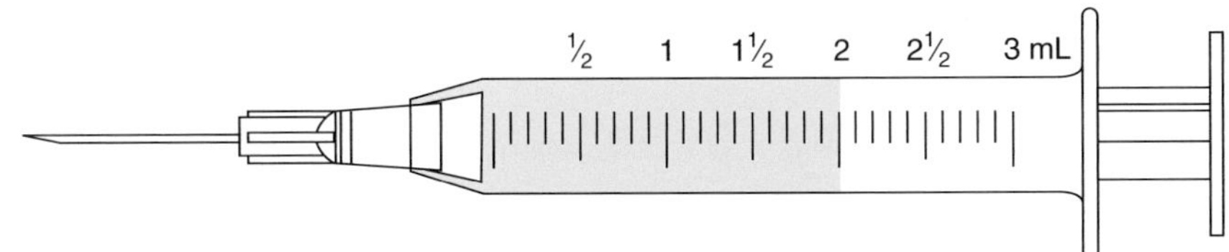

6. $x \text{ mL} = \frac{2.5 \text{ mL}}{1 \text{ g}} \times \frac{3 \text{ g}}{1} = 7.5 \text{ mL}$

7. $x \text{ mL} = \frac{1 \text{ mL}}{10 \text{ mg}} \times \frac{5 \text{ mg}}{1} = 0.5 \text{ mL}$

8. $x \text{ mL} = \frac{1 \text{ mL}}{5 \text{ mg}} \times \frac{4 \text{ mg}}{1} = 0.8 \text{ mL}$

9. $x \text{ mL} = \dfrac{1 \text{ mL}}{10 \text{ mg}} \times \dfrac{30 \text{ mg}}{1} = 3 \text{ mL}$

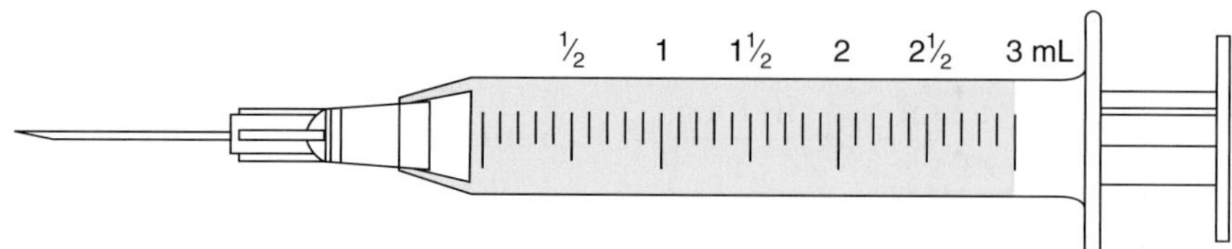

10. $x \text{ mL} = \dfrac{1 \text{ mL}}{30 \text{ mg}} \times \dfrac{15 \text{ mg}}{1} = 0.5 \text{ mL}$

11. $x \text{ mL} = \dfrac{50 \text{ mL}}{44.6 \text{ mg}} \times \dfrac{25.8 \text{ mg}}{1} = 28.9 \text{ mL}$

12. $x \text{ mL} = \dfrac{1 \text{ mL}}{25 \text{ mg}} \times \dfrac{100 \text{ mg}}{1} = 4 \text{ mL}$

13. $x \text{ mL} = \dfrac{20 \text{ mL}}{100 \text{ mg}} \times \dfrac{350 \text{ mg}}{1} = 70 \text{ mL}$

14. $x \text{ mL} = \dfrac{40 \text{ mL}}{400 \text{ mg}} \times \dfrac{300 \text{ mg}}{1} = 30 \text{ mL}$

15. $x \text{ mL} = \dfrac{2 \text{ mL}}{250 \text{ mg}} \times \dfrac{1000 \text{ mg}}{1 \text{ g}} \times \dfrac{0.05 \text{ g}}{1} = 0.4 \text{ mL}$

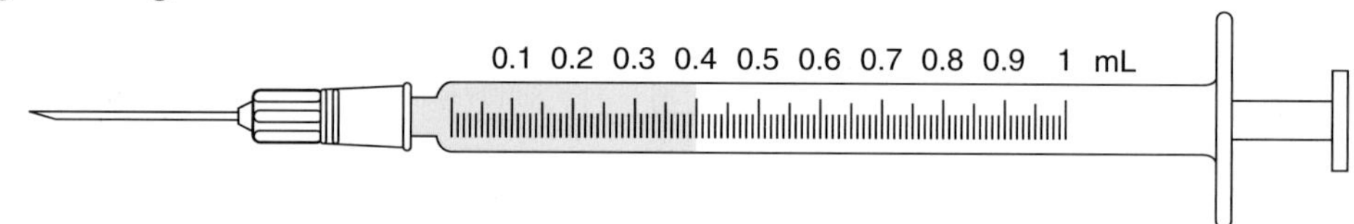

16. $x \text{ mL} = \dfrac{1 \text{ mL}}{0.4 \text{ mg}} \times \dfrac{0.6 \text{ mg}}{1} = 1.5 \text{ mL}$

17. $x \text{ mL} = \dfrac{2 \text{ mL}}{300 \text{ mg}} \times \dfrac{300 \text{ mg}}{1} = 2 \text{ mL}$

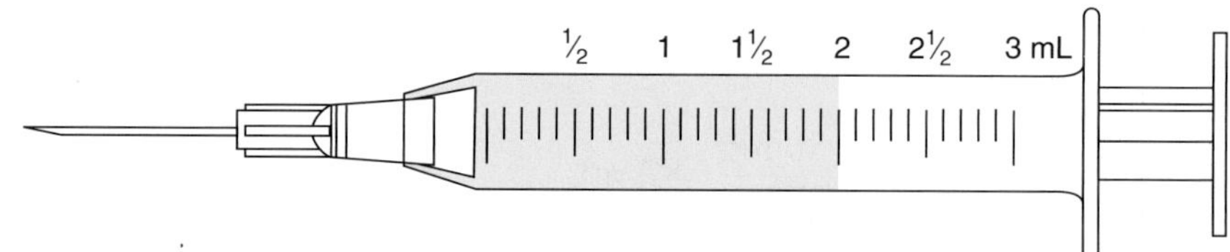

18. $x \text{ mL} = \dfrac{10 \text{ mL}}{10 \text{ mg}} \times \dfrac{6 \text{ mg}}{1} = 6 \text{ mL}$

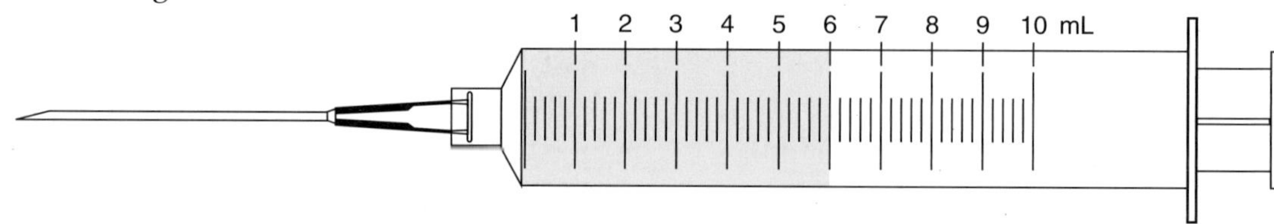

19. $x \text{ mL} = \dfrac{1 \text{ mL}}{50 \text{ mg}} \times \dfrac{25 \text{ mg}}{1} = 0.5 \text{ mL}$

20. $x \text{ mL} = \dfrac{1 \text{ mL}}{4 \text{ mg}} \times \dfrac{1 \text{ mg}}{1} = 0.25 \text{ mL}$

21. $x \text{ mL} = \dfrac{1 \text{ mL}}{20 \text{ mg}} \times \dfrac{10 \text{ mg}}{1} = 0.5 \text{ mL}$

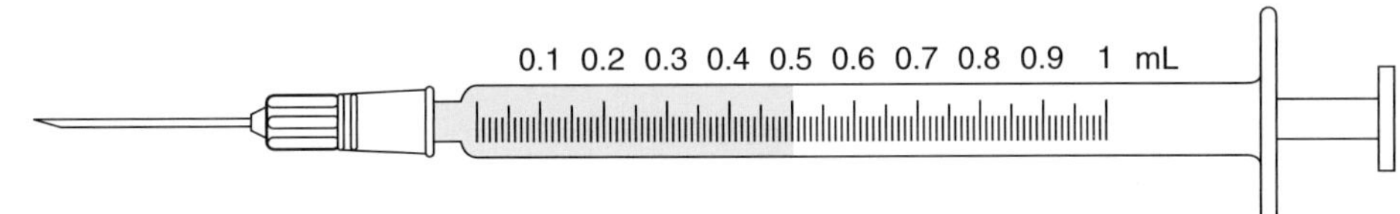

22. $x \text{ mL} = \dfrac{2 \text{ mL}}{500 \text{ mg}} \times \dfrac{400 \text{ mg}}{1} = 1.6 \text{ mL}$

23. $x \text{ mL} = \dfrac{1 \text{ mL}}{5 \text{ mg}} \times \dfrac{7.5 \text{ mg}}{1} = 1.5 \text{ mL}$

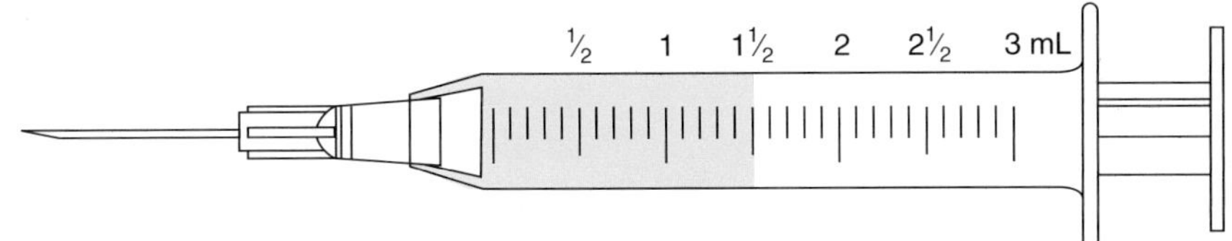

24. $x \text{ mL} = \dfrac{1 \text{ mL}}{30 \text{ mg}} \times \dfrac{15 \text{ mg}}{1} = 0.5 \text{ mL}$

25. $x \text{ mL} = \dfrac{1 \text{ mL}}{10 \text{ mg}} \times \dfrac{1000 \text{ mg}}{1 \text{ g}} \times \dfrac{0.01 \text{ g}}{1} = 1 \text{ mL}$

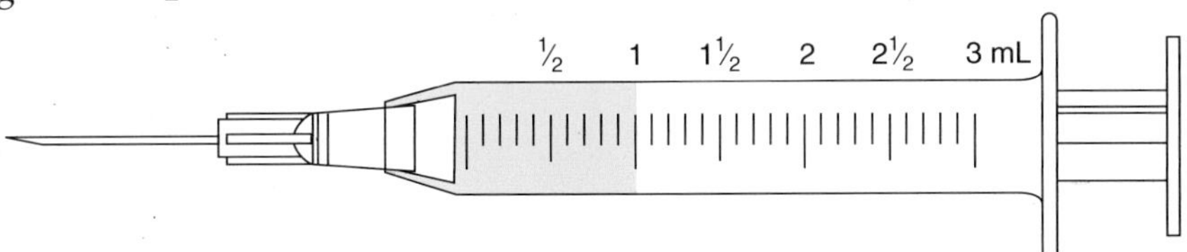

26. $x \text{ mL} = \dfrac{40 \text{ mL}}{400 \text{ mg}} \times \dfrac{1000 \text{ mg}}{1 \text{ g}} \times \dfrac{0.2 \text{ g}}{1} = 20 \text{ mL}$

27. $x \text{ mL} = \dfrac{1 \text{ mL}}{15 \text{ mg}} \times \dfrac{6 \text{ mg}}{1} = 0.4 \text{ mL}$

28. $x \text{ mL} = \dfrac{1 \text{ mL}}{50 \text{ mg}} \times \dfrac{100 \text{ mg}}{1} = 2 \text{ mL}$

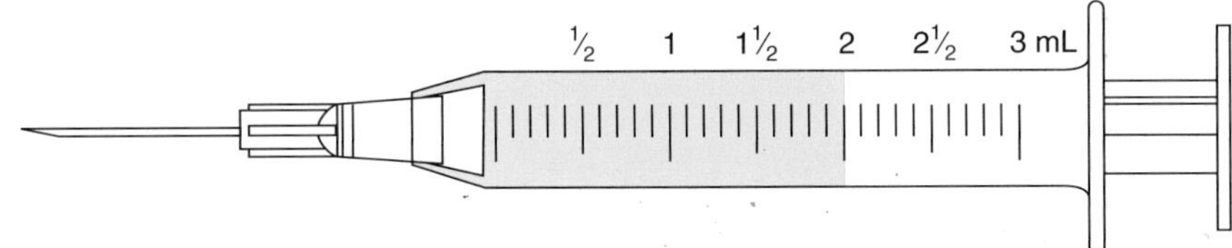

29. $x \text{ mL} = \dfrac{2 \text{ mL}}{0.5 \text{ mg}} \times \dfrac{1 \text{ mg}}{1000 \text{ mcg}} \times \dfrac{100 \text{ mcg}}{1} = 0.4 \text{ mL}$

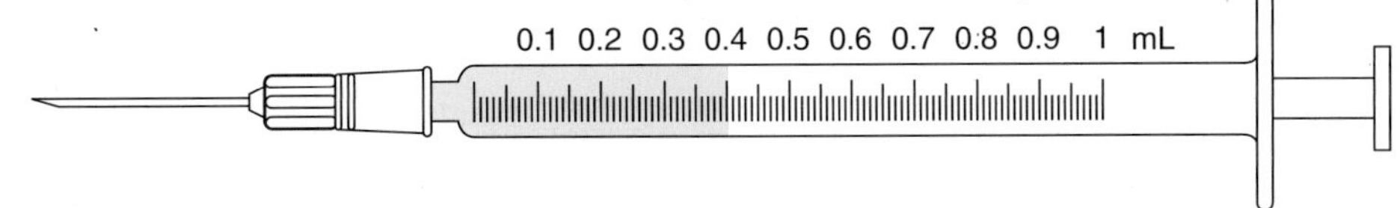

30. $x \text{ mL} = \dfrac{2 \text{ mL}}{500 \text{ mg}} \times \dfrac{700 \text{ mg}}{1} = 2.8 \text{ mL}$

31. $x \text{ mL} = \dfrac{1 \text{ mL}}{2 \text{ mg}} \times \dfrac{1.5 \text{ mg}}{1} = 0.75 \text{ mL}$

32. $x \text{ mL} = \dfrac{2 \text{ mL}}{250 \text{ mg}} \times \dfrac{100 \text{ mg}}{1} = 0.8 \text{ mL}$

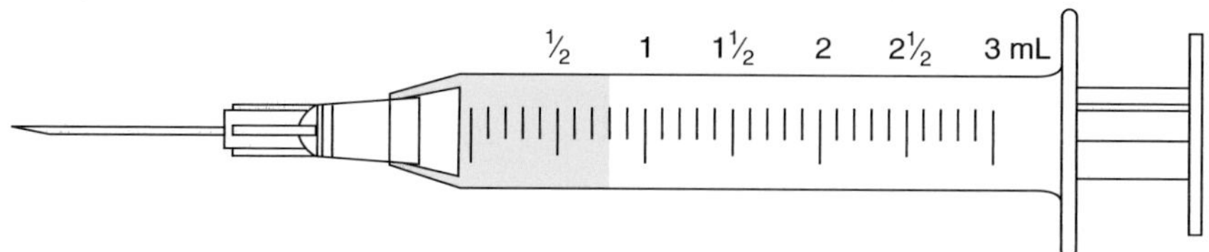

33. $x \text{ mL} = \dfrac{1 \text{ mL}}{2.5 \text{ mEq}} \times \dfrac{7.5 \text{ mEq}}{1} = 3 \text{ mL}$

34. $x \text{ mL} = \dfrac{1 \text{ mL}}{50 \text{ mg}} \times \dfrac{25 \text{ mg}}{1} = 0.5 \text{ mL}$

35. $x \text{ mL} = \dfrac{1 \text{ mL}}{0.4 \text{ mg}} \times \dfrac{0.6 \text{ mg}}{1} = 1.5 \text{ mL}$

36. $x \text{ mL} = \dfrac{1 \text{ mL}}{100 \text{ mg}} \times \dfrac{150 \text{ mg}}{1} = 1.5 \text{ mL}$

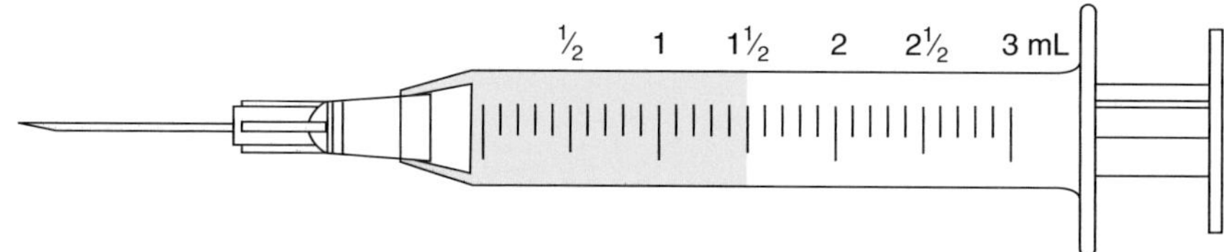

37. $x \text{ mL} = \dfrac{1 \text{ mL}}{0.25 \text{ mg}} \times \dfrac{0.5 \text{ mg}}{1} = 2 \text{ mL}$

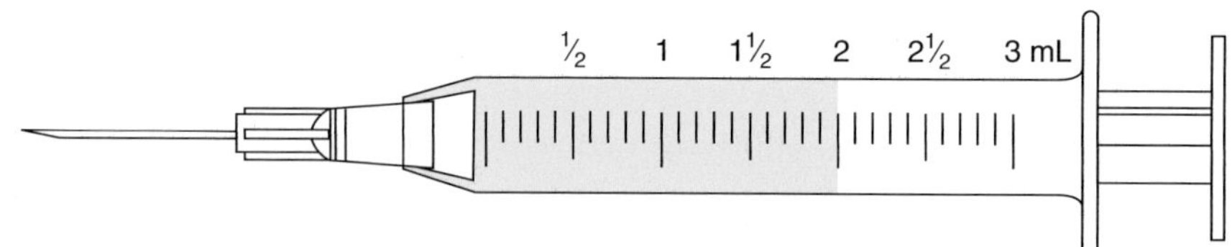

38. $x \text{ mL} = \dfrac{1 \text{ mL}}{25 \text{ mg}} \times \dfrac{75 \text{ mg}}{1} = 3 \text{ mL}$

39. $x \text{ mL} = \dfrac{1 \text{ mL}}{0.4 \text{ mg}} \times \dfrac{0.6 \text{ mg}}{1} = 1.5 \text{ mL}$

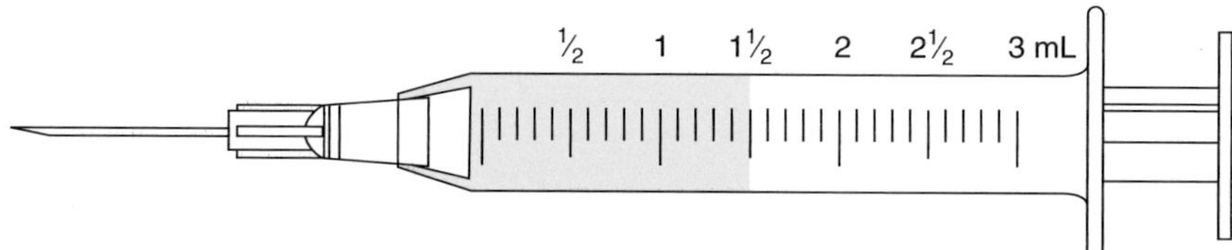

40. $x \text{ mL} = \dfrac{1 \text{ mL}}{5 \text{ mg}} \times \dfrac{10 \text{ mg}}{1} = 2 \text{ mL}$

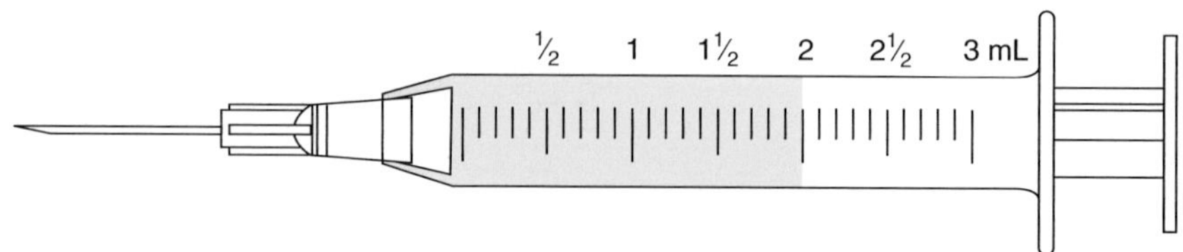

41. $x \text{ mL} = \dfrac{2 \text{ mL}}{100 \text{ mg}} \times \dfrac{25 \text{ mg}}{1} = 0.5 \text{ mL}$

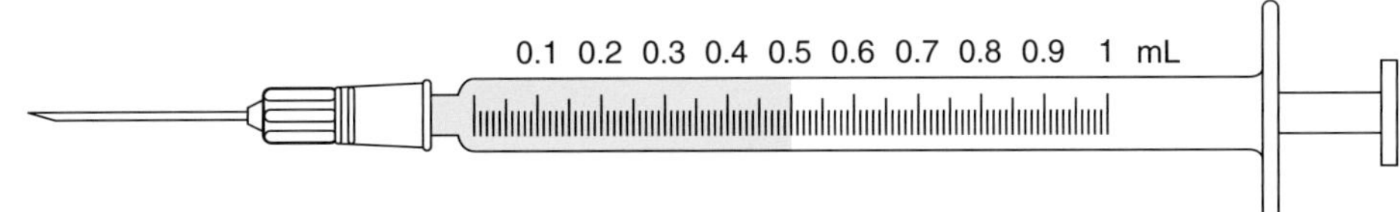

42. $x \text{ mL} = \dfrac{40 \text{ mL}}{400 \text{ mg}} \times \dfrac{200 \text{ mg}}{1} = 20 \text{ mL}$

43. $x \text{ mL} = \dfrac{1 \text{ mL}}{500 \text{ mg}} \times \dfrac{1000 \text{ mg}}{1 \text{ g}} \times \dfrac{0.25 \text{ g}}{1} = 0.5 \text{ mL}$

44. $x \text{ mL} = \dfrac{10 \text{ mL}}{13.6 \text{ mEq}} \times \dfrac{5 \text{ mEq}}{1} = 3.68 \text{ or } 3.7 \text{ mL}$

45. $x \text{ mL} = \dfrac{1 \text{ mL}}{130 \text{ mg}} \times \dfrac{70 \text{ mg}}{1} = 0.538 \text{ or } 0.54 \text{ mL}$

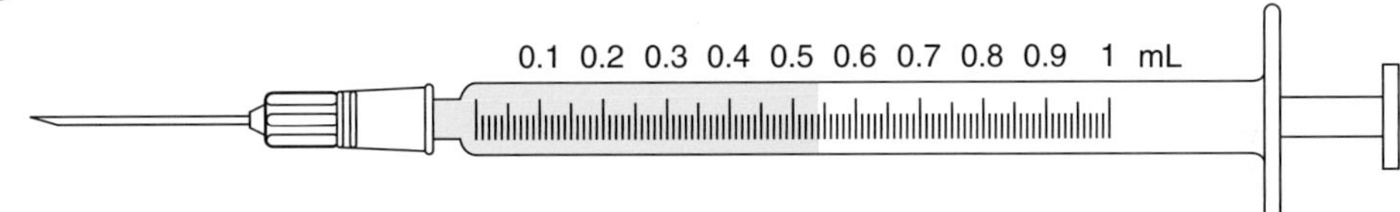

46. $x \text{ mL} = \dfrac{1 \text{ mL}}{10 \text{ mg}} \times \dfrac{200 \text{ mg}}{1} = 20 \text{ mL}$

47. $x \text{ mL} = \dfrac{1 \text{ mL}}{4 \text{ mg}} \times \dfrac{2 \text{ mg}}{1} = 0.5 \text{ mL}$

48. $x \text{ mL} = \dfrac{2 \text{ mL}}{0.5 \text{ mg}} \times \dfrac{0.2 \text{ mg}}{1} = 0.8 \text{ mL}$

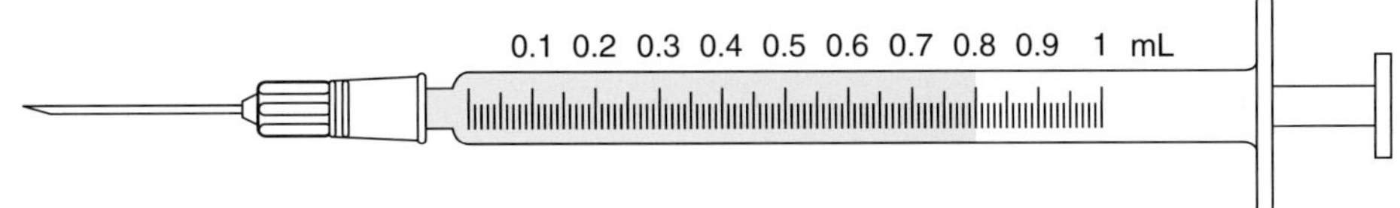

49. $x \text{ mL} = \dfrac{1 \text{ mL}}{15 \text{ mg}} \times \dfrac{10 \text{ mg}}{1} = 0.666 \text{ or } 0.67 \text{ mL}$

50. $x \text{ mL} = \dfrac{1 \text{ mL}}{50 \text{ mg}} \times \dfrac{25 \text{ mg}}{1} = 0.5 \text{ mL}$

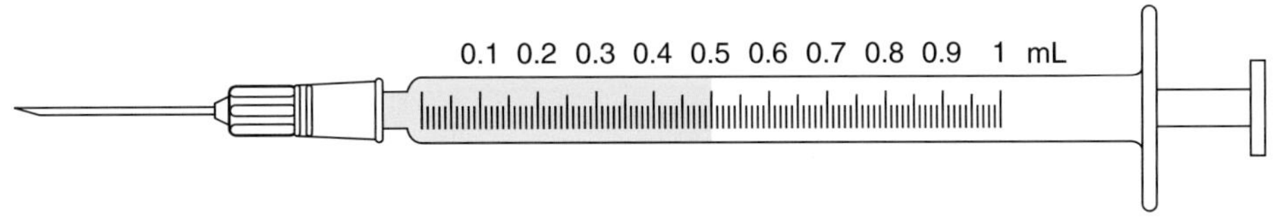

51. $x \text{ mL} = \dfrac{1.2 \text{ mL}}{500 \text{ mg}} \times \dfrac{600 \text{ mg}}{1} = 1.44 \text{ mL}$

52. $x \text{ mL} = \dfrac{1 \text{ mL}}{0.4 \text{ mg}} \times \dfrac{0.9 \text{ mg}}{1} = 2.25 \text{ mL}$

53. $x \text{ mL} = \dfrac{1 \text{ mL}}{30 \text{ mg}} \times \dfrac{30 \text{ mg}}{1} = 1 \text{ mL}$

54. $x \text{ mL} = \dfrac{1 \text{ mL}}{4 \text{ mg}} \times \dfrac{3 \text{ mg}}{1} = 0.75 \text{ mL}$

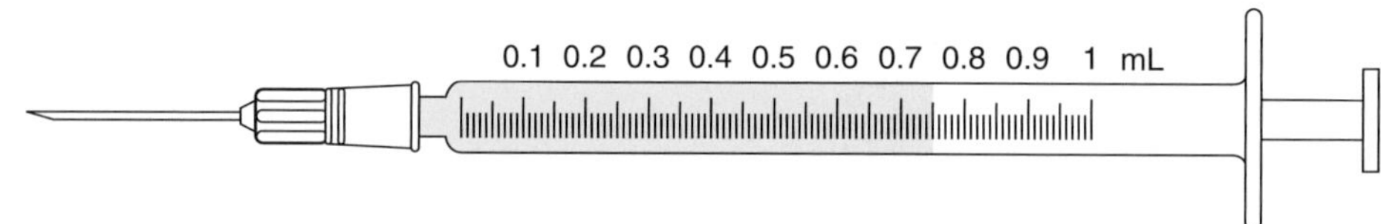

55. $x \text{ mL} = \dfrac{1 \text{ mL}}{0.89 \text{ mEq}} \times \dfrac{6 \text{ mEq}}{1} = 6.74 \text{ mL}$

56. $x \text{ mL} = \dfrac{1 \text{ mL}}{20 \text{ mg}} \times \dfrac{10 \text{ mg}}{1} = 0.5 \text{ mL}$

57. $x \text{ mL} = \dfrac{1 \text{ mL}}{25 \text{ mg}} \times \dfrac{5 \text{ mg}}{1} = 0.2 \text{ mL}$

58. $x \text{ mL} = \dfrac{1 \text{ mL}}{125 \text{ mg}} \times \dfrac{500 \text{ mg}}{1} = 4 \text{ mL}$

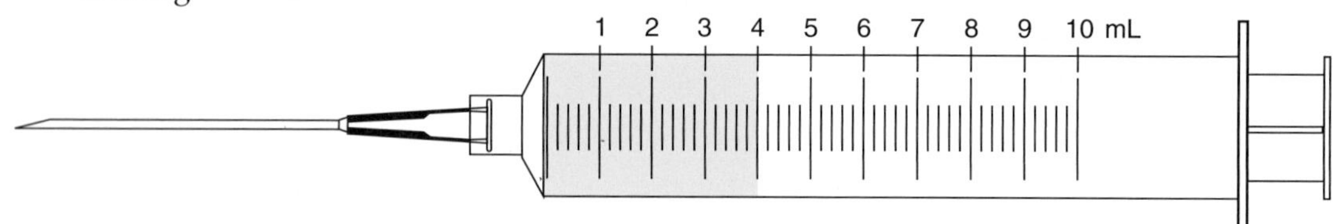

59. $x \text{ mL} = \dfrac{1 \text{ mL}}{0.25 \text{ mg}} \times \dfrac{0.2 \text{ mg}}{1} = 0.8 \text{ mL}$

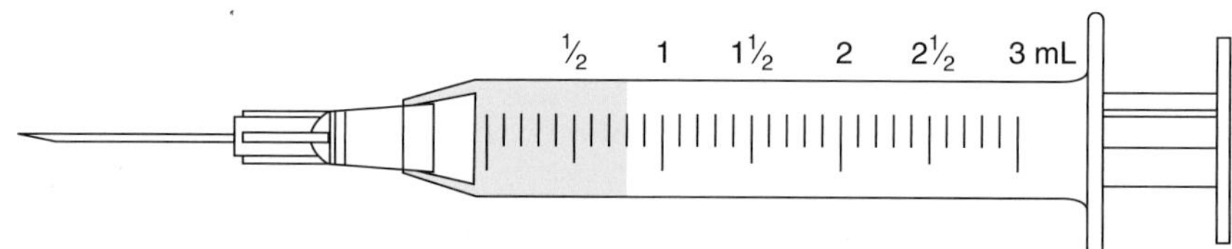

60. $x \text{ mL} = \dfrac{1 \text{ mL}}{2 \text{ mg}} \times \dfrac{0.5 \text{ mg}}{1} = 0.25 \text{ mL}$

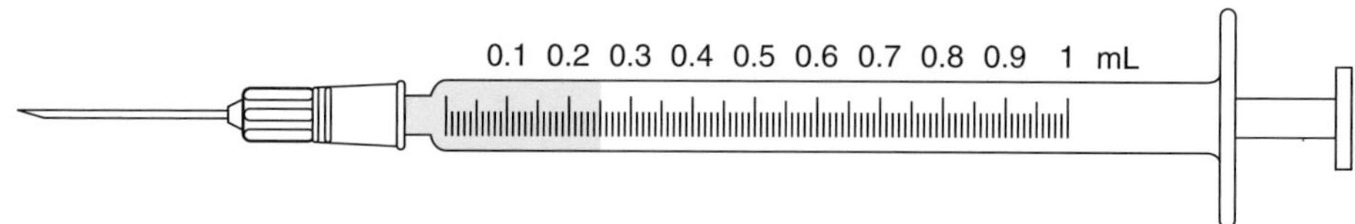

61. $x \text{ mL} = \dfrac{20 \text{ mL}}{500 \text{ mg}} \times \dfrac{1000 \text{ mg}}{1 \text{ g}} \times \dfrac{0.2 \text{ g}}{1} = 8 \text{ mL}$

62. $x \text{ mL} = \dfrac{1 \text{ mL}}{30 \text{ mg}} \times \dfrac{15 \text{ mg}}{1} = 0.5 \text{ mL}$

63. $x \text{ mL} = \dfrac{5 \text{ mL}}{250 \text{ mg}} \times \dfrac{100 \text{ mg}}{1} = 2 \text{ mL}$

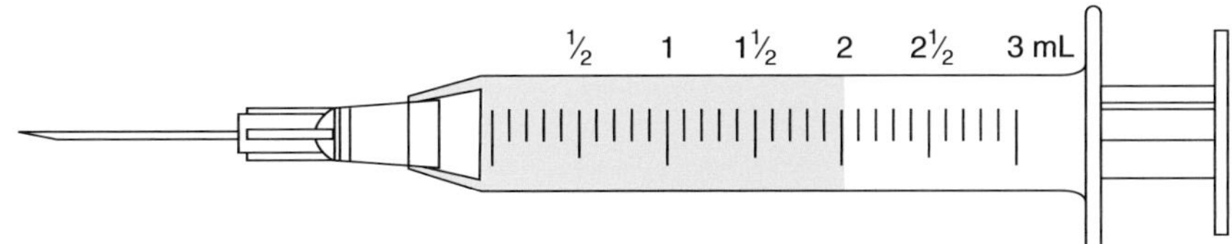

64. $x \text{ mL} = \dfrac{2 \text{ mL}}{0.5 \text{ mg}} \times \dfrac{0.25 \text{ mg}}{1} = 1 \text{ mL}$

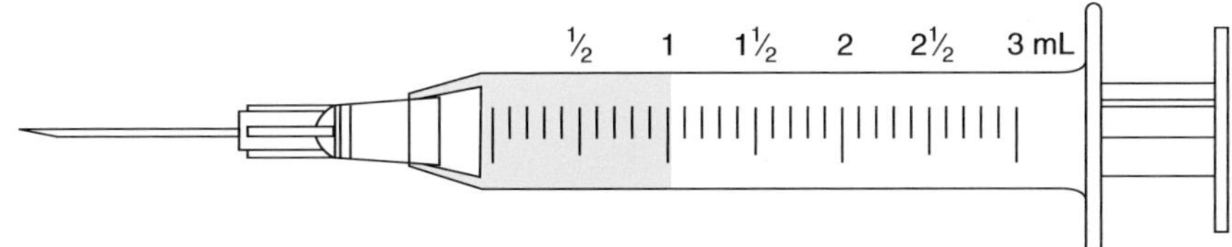

65. $x \text{ mL} = \dfrac{1 \text{ mL}}{1 \text{ mg}} \times \dfrac{1 \text{ mg}}{1000 \text{ mcg}} \times \dfrac{500 \text{ mcg}}{1} = 0.5 \text{ mL}$

66. $x \text{ mL} = \dfrac{10 \text{ mL}}{4.8 \text{ mEq}} \times \dfrac{5 \text{ mEq}}{1} = 10.416 \text{ or } 10.42 \text{ mL}$

67. $x \text{ mL} = \dfrac{1 \text{ mL}}{150 \text{ mg}} \times \dfrac{50 \text{ mg}}{1} = 0.333 \text{ mL}$

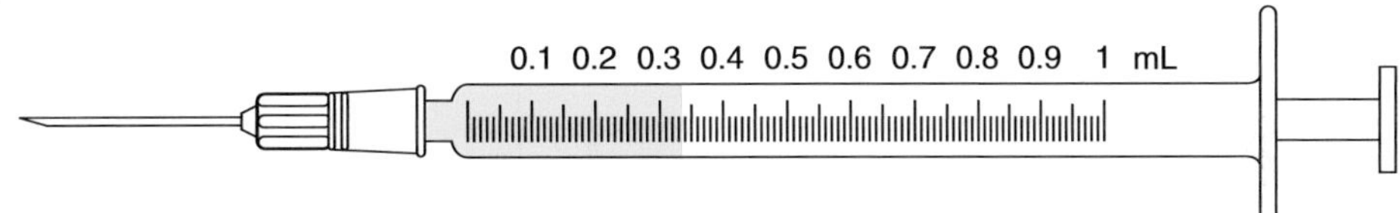

68. $x \text{ mL} = \dfrac{1 \text{ mL}}{0.4 \text{ mg}} \times \dfrac{0.2 \text{ mg}}{1} = 0.5 \text{ mL}$

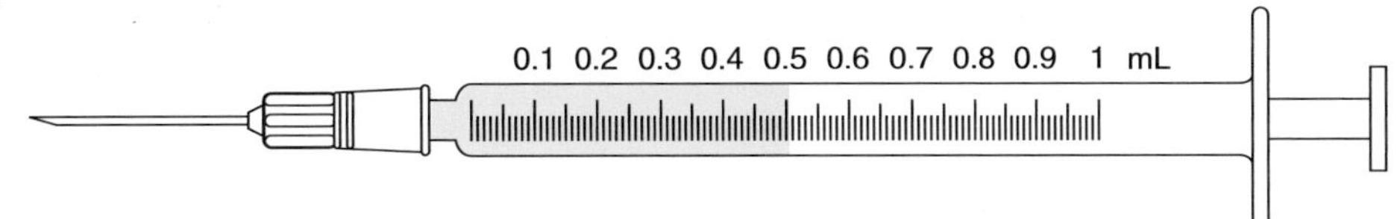

69. $x \text{ mL} = \dfrac{2 \text{ mL}}{80 \text{ mg}} \times \dfrac{55 \text{ mg}}{1} = 1.38 \text{ mL}$

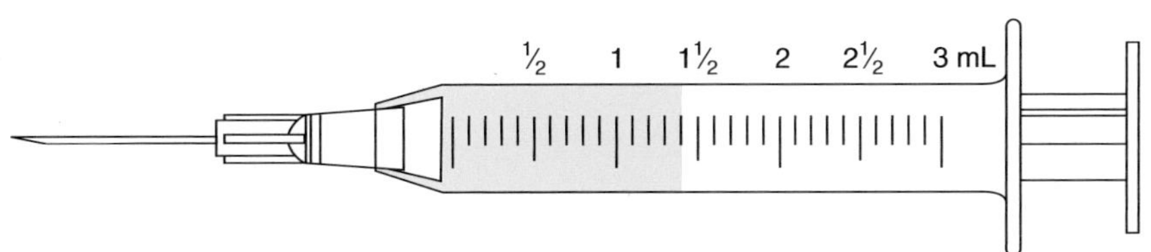

70. $x \text{ mL} = \dfrac{2 \text{ mL}}{500 \text{ mg}} \times \dfrac{600 \text{ mg}}{1} = 2.4 \text{ mL}$

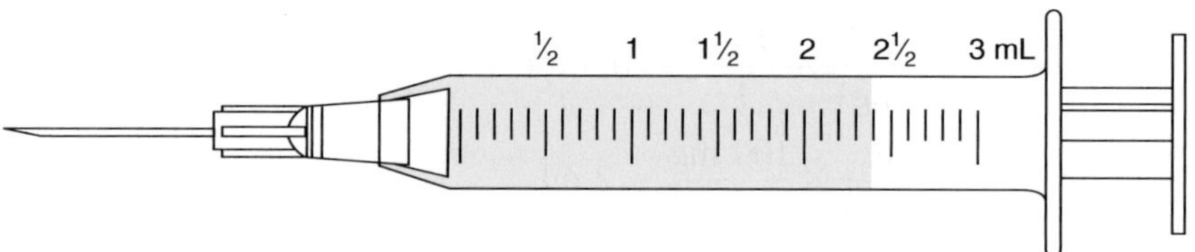

71. $x \text{ mL} = \dfrac{1 \text{ mL}}{15 \text{ mg}} \times \dfrac{6 \text{ mg}}{1} = 0.4 \text{ mL}$

72. $x \text{ mL} = \dfrac{1 \text{ mL}}{1000 \text{ mcg}} \times \dfrac{1000 \text{ mcg}}{1} = 1 \text{ mL}$

73. $x \text{ mL} = \dfrac{1 \text{ mL}}{325 \text{ mg}} \times \dfrac{800 \text{ mg}}{1} = 2.46 \text{ mL}$

74. $x \text{ mL} = \dfrac{1 \text{ mL}}{50 \text{ mg}} \times \dfrac{30 \text{ mg}}{1} = 0.6 \text{ mL}$

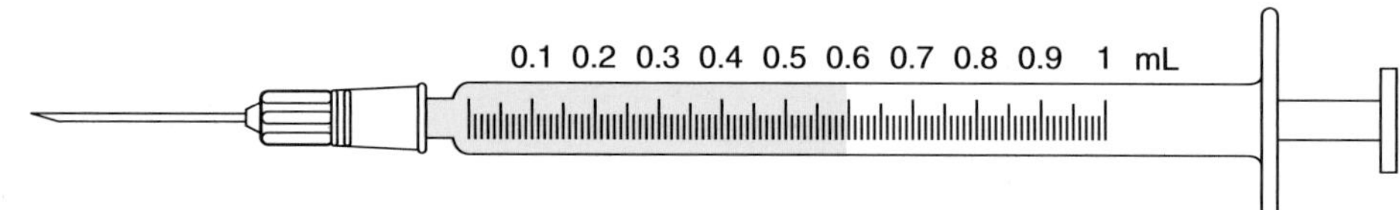

75. $x \text{ mL} = \dfrac{1 \text{ mL}}{0.2 \text{ mg}} \times \dfrac{0.28 \text{ mg}}{1} = 1.4 \text{ mL}$

76. $x \text{ mL} = \dfrac{1 \text{ mL}}{4 \text{ mg}} \times \dfrac{3 \text{ mg}}{1} = 0.75 \text{ mL}$

77. $x \text{ mL} = \dfrac{40 \text{ mL}}{100 \text{ mEq}} \times \dfrac{15 \text{ mEq}}{1} = 6 \text{ mL}$

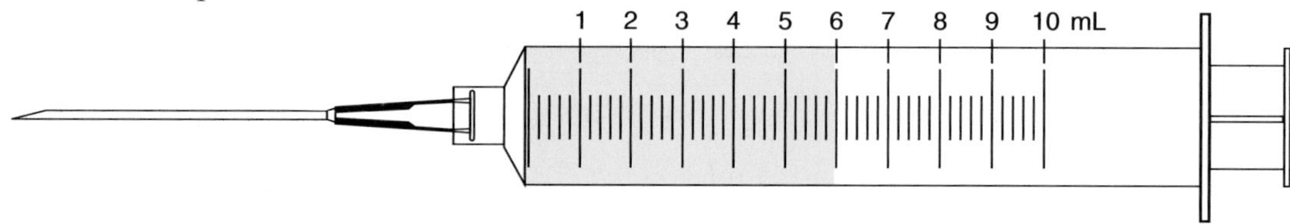

78. $x \text{ mL} = \dfrac{1 \text{ mL}}{225 \text{ mg}} \times \dfrac{250 \text{ mg}}{1} = 1.1 \text{ mL}$

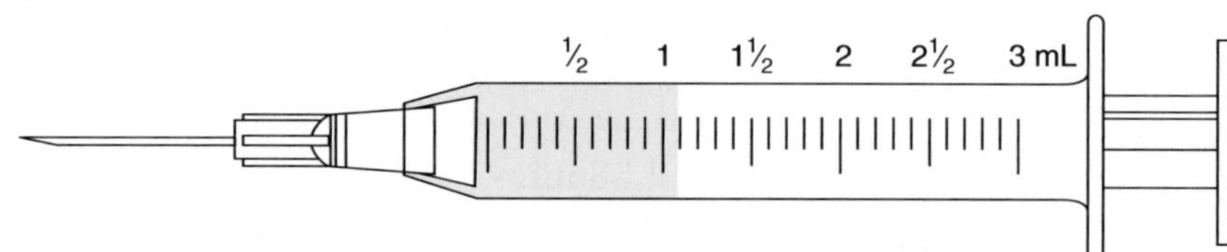

79. $x \text{ mL} = \dfrac{1 \text{ mL}}{150 \text{ mg}} \times \dfrac{300 \text{ mg}}{1} = 2 \text{ mL}$

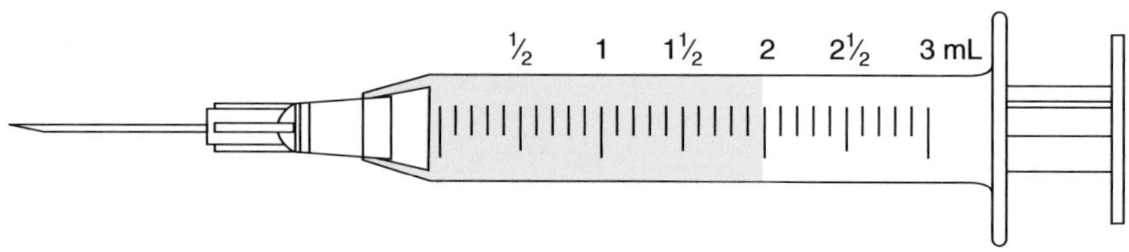

80. $x \text{ mL} = \frac{5 \text{ mL}}{100 \text{ mg}} \times \frac{75 \text{ mg}}{1} = 3.75 \text{ mL}$

81. $x \text{ mL} = \frac{2.6 \text{ mL}}{1 \text{ g}} \times \frac{0.8 \text{ g}}{1} = 2.08 \text{ mL}$

82. $x \text{ mL} = \frac{2 \text{ mL}}{125 \text{ mg}} \times \frac{100 \text{ mg}}{1} = 1.6 \text{ mL}$

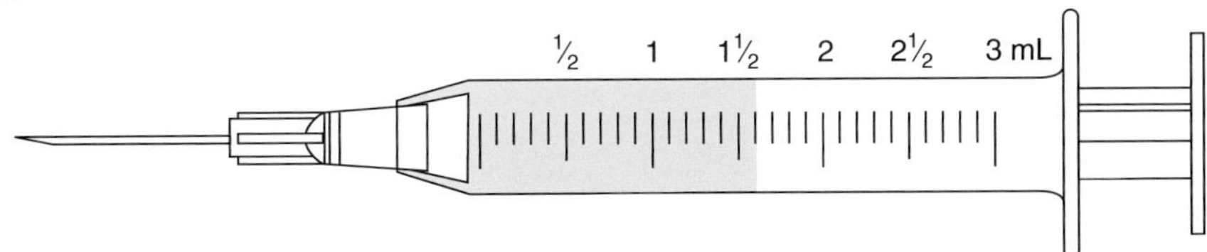

83. $x \text{ mL} = \frac{1 \text{ mL}}{75 \text{ mg}} \times \frac{300 \text{ mg}}{1} = 4 \text{ mL}$

84. $x \text{ mL} = \frac{1 \text{ mL}}{0.4 \text{ mg}} \times \frac{0.4 \text{ mg}}{1} = 1 \text{ mL}$

85. $x \text{ mL} = \frac{1 \text{ mL}}{50 \text{ mg}} \times \frac{10 \text{ mg}}{1} = 0.2 \text{ mL}$

86. $x \text{ mL} = \frac{1 \text{ mL}}{10 \text{ mg}} \times \frac{1 \text{ mg}}{1} = 0.1 \text{ mL}$

87. $x \text{ mL} = \frac{1 \text{ mL}}{50 \text{ mg}} \times \frac{50 \text{ mg}}{1} = 1 \text{ mL}$

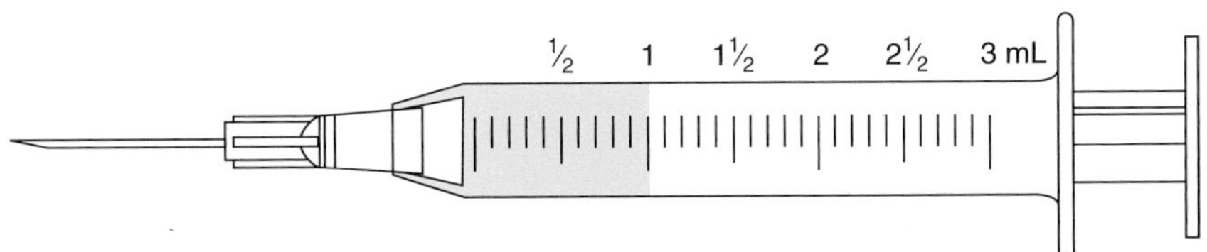

88. $x \text{ mL} = \frac{1 \text{ mL}}{50 \text{ mcg}} \times \frac{60 \text{ mcg}}{1} = 1.2 \text{ mL}$

89. $x \text{ mL} = \frac{1 \text{ mL}}{0.4 \text{ mg}} \times \frac{0.5 \text{ mg}}{1} = 1.25 \text{ mL}$

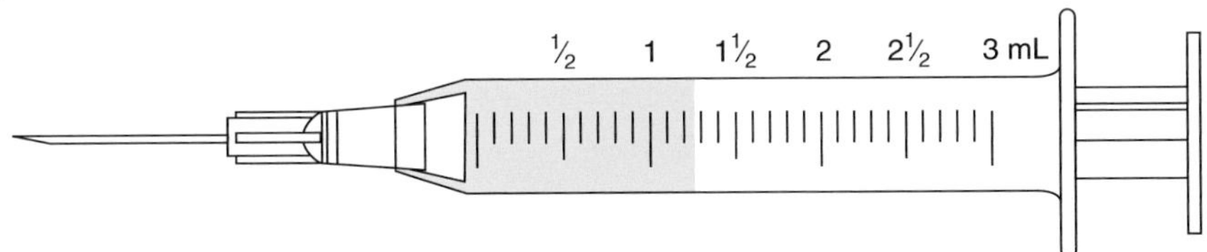

90. $x \text{ mL} = \frac{1 \text{ mL}}{25 \text{ mg}} \times \frac{15 \text{ mg}}{1} = 0.6 \text{ mL}$

91. $x \text{ mL} = \frac{1 \text{ mL}}{100 \text{ mg}} \times \frac{150 \text{ mg}}{1} = 1.5 \text{ mL}$

92. $x \text{ mL} = \frac{1 \text{ mL}}{0.2 \text{ mg}} \times \frac{1 \text{ mg}}{1000 \text{ mcg}} \times \frac{75 \text{ mcg}}{1} = 0.375 \text{ or } 0.38 \text{ mL}$

93. $x \text{ mL} = \frac{1 \text{ mL}}{5 \text{ mg}} \times \frac{2 \text{ mg}}{1} = 0.4 \text{ mL}$

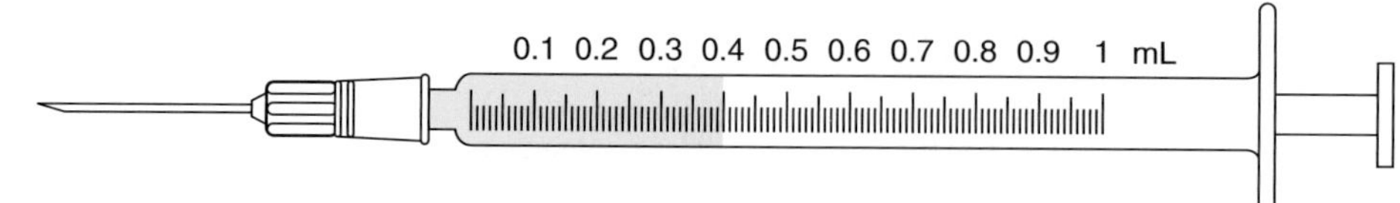

94. $x \text{ mL} = \frac{1 \text{ mL}}{100 \text{ mg}} \times \frac{500 \text{ mg}}{1} = 5 \text{ mL}$

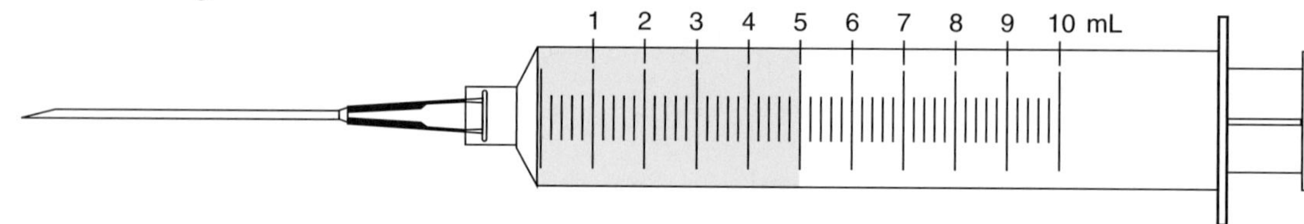

95. $x \text{ mL} = \frac{2.5 \text{ mL}}{1000 \text{ mg}} \times \frac{640 \text{ mg}}{1} = 1.6 \text{ mL}$

96. $x \text{ mL} = \frac{1 \text{ mL}}{250 \text{ mg}} \times \frac{500 \text{ mg}}{1} = 2 \text{ mL}$

97. $x \text{ mL} = \frac{1 \text{ mL}}{2 \text{ mg}} \times \frac{0.5 \text{ mg}}{1} = 0.25 \text{ mL}$

98. $x \text{ mL} = \frac{0.5 \text{ mL}}{25 \text{ mg}} \times \frac{100 \text{ mg}}{1} = 2 \text{ mL}$

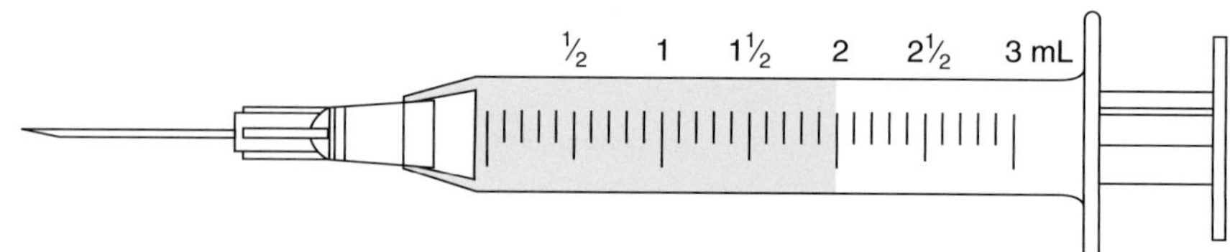

99. $x \text{ mL} = \frac{1 \text{ mL}}{50 \text{ mg}} \times \frac{10 \text{ mg}}{1} = 0.2 \text{ mL}$

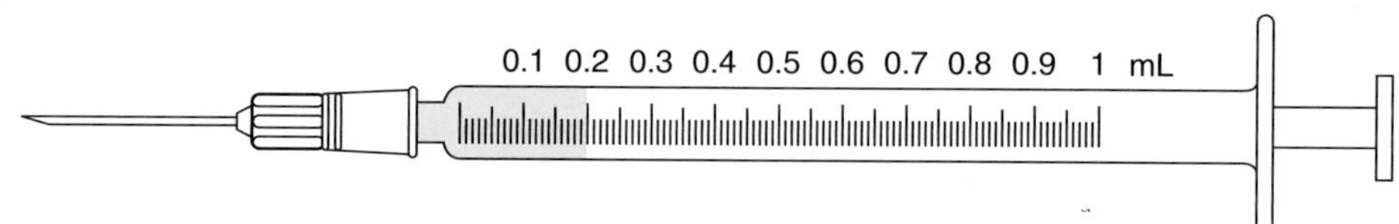

100. $x \text{ mL} = \frac{1 \text{ mL}}{1 \text{ mg}} \times \frac{3.5 \text{ mg}}{1} = 3.5 \text{ mL}$

CHAPTER 12 Dimensional Analysis—Posttest 1, pp. 321–325

1. $x \text{ mL} = \frac{1 \text{ mL}}{50 \text{ mg}} \times \frac{25 \text{ mg}}{1} = 0.5 \text{ mL}$

2. $x \text{ mL} = \frac{1 \text{ mL}}{50 \text{ mg}} \times \frac{25 \text{ mg}}{1} = 0.5 \text{ mL}$

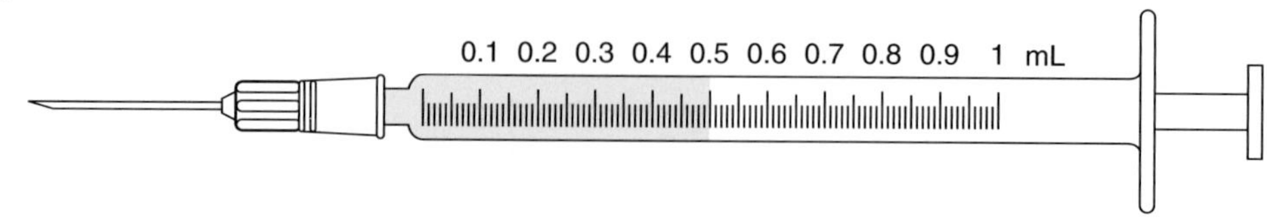

3. $x \text{ mL} = \frac{1 \text{ mL}}{15 \text{ mg}} \times \frac{30 \text{ mg}}{1} = 2 \text{ mL}$

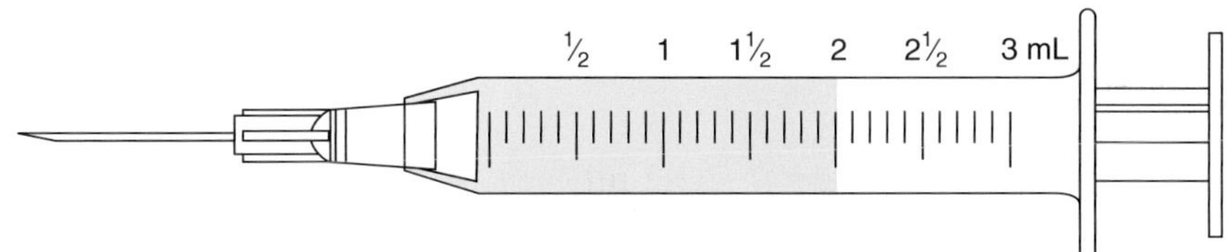

4. $x \text{ mL} = \frac{10 \text{ mL}}{1 \text{ g}} \times \frac{1 \text{ g}}{1000 \text{ mg}} \times \frac{500 \text{ mg}}{1} = 5 \text{ mL}$

5. $x \text{ mL} = \frac{2 \text{ mL}}{100 \text{ mg}} \times \frac{50 \text{ mg}}{1} = 1 \text{ mL}$

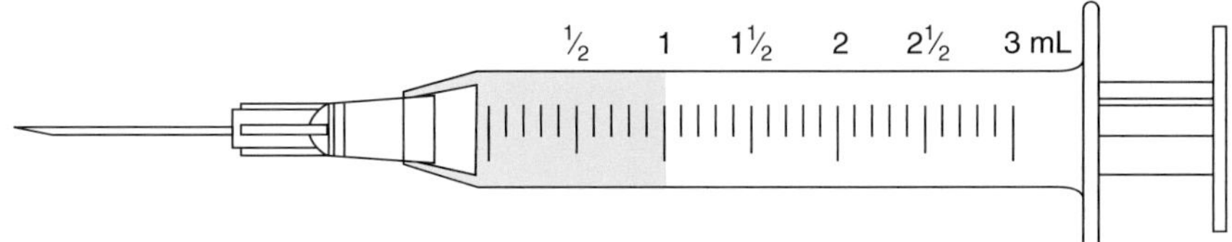

6. $x \text{ mL} = \frac{1 \text{ mL}}{2 \text{ mg}} \times \frac{0.5 \text{ mg}}{1} = 0.25 \text{ mL}$

7. $x \text{ mL} = \frac{1 \text{ mL}}{30 \text{ mg}} \times \frac{15 \text{ mg}}{1} = 0.5 \text{ mL}$

8. $x \text{ mL} = \frac{1 \text{ mL}}{0.4 \text{ mg}} \times \frac{0.2 \text{ mg}}{1} = 0.5 \text{ mL}$

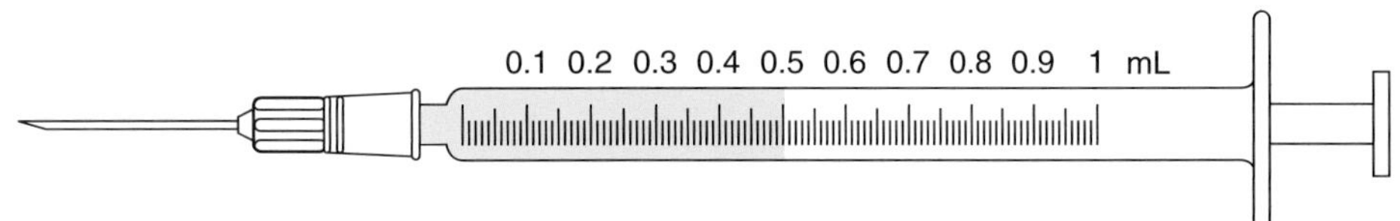

9. $x \text{ mL} = \frac{1 \text{ mL}}{25 \text{ mg}} \times \frac{100 \text{ mg}}{1} = 4 \text{ mL}$

10. $x \text{ mL} = \frac{1 \text{ mL}}{5 \text{ mg}} \times \frac{2 \text{ mg}}{1} = 0.4 \text{ mL}$

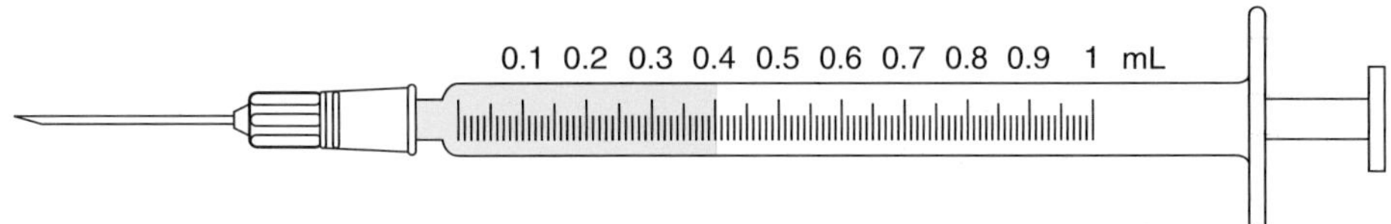

11. $x \text{ mL} = \frac{1 \text{ mL}}{0.5 \text{ mg}} \times \frac{0.7 \text{ mg}}{1} = 1.4 \text{ mL}$

12. $x \text{ mL} = \frac{1 \text{ mL}}{50 \text{ mg}} \times \frac{25 \text{ mg}}{1} = 0.5 \text{ mL}$

13. $x \text{ mL} = \frac{1 \text{ mL}}{80 \text{ mg}} \times \frac{50 \text{ mg}}{1} = 0.625 \text{ or } 0.63 \text{ mL}$

14. $x \text{ mL} = \frac{2 \text{ mL}}{300 \text{ mg}} \times \frac{600 \text{ mg}}{1} = 4 \text{ mL}$

15. $x \text{ mL} = \frac{50 \text{ mL}}{1 \text{ g}} \times \frac{1 \text{ g}}{1000 \text{ mg}} \times \frac{300 \text{ mg}}{1} = 15 \text{ mL}$

16. $x \text{ mL} = \dfrac{1 \text{ mL}}{10 \text{ mg}} \times \dfrac{6 \text{ mg}}{1} = 0.6 \text{ mL}$

17. $x \text{ mL} = \dfrac{1 \text{ mL}}{10 \text{ mg}} \times \dfrac{6 \text{ mg}}{1} = 0.6 \text{ mL}$

18. $x \text{ mL} = \dfrac{1 \text{ mL}}{10 \text{ mg}} \times \dfrac{20 \text{ mg}}{1} = 2 \text{ mL}$

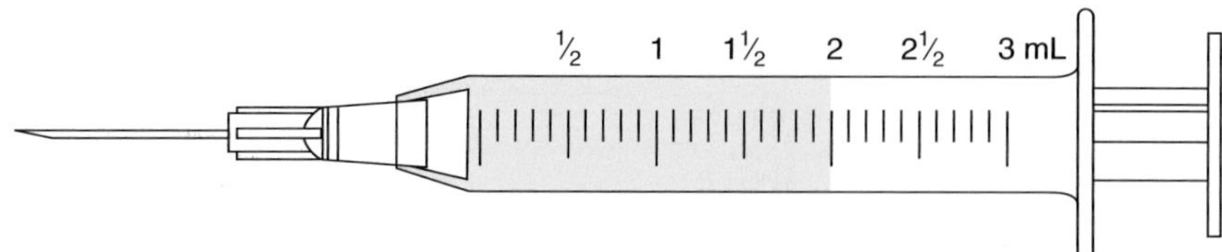

19. $x \text{ mL} = \dfrac{2 \text{ mL}}{0.5 \text{ mg}} \times \dfrac{0.3 \text{ mg}}{1} = 1.2 \text{ mL}$

20. $x \text{ mL} = \dfrac{1 \text{ mL}}{2.5 \text{ mg}} \times \dfrac{5 \text{ mg}}{1} = 2 \text{ mL}$

CHAPTER 12 Dimensional Analysis—Posttest 2, pp. 327–332

1. $x \text{ mL} = \dfrac{1 \text{ mL}}{4 \text{ mg}} \times \dfrac{2 \text{ mg}}{1} = 0.5 \text{ mL}$

2. $x \text{ mL} = \dfrac{1 \text{ mL}}{4 \text{ mg}} \times \dfrac{2 \text{ mg}}{1} = 0.5 \text{ mL}$

3. $x \text{ mL} = \dfrac{10 \text{ mL}}{500 \text{ mg}} \times \dfrac{1000 \text{ mg}}{1 \text{ g}} \times \dfrac{0.4 \text{ g}}{1} = 8 \text{ mL}$

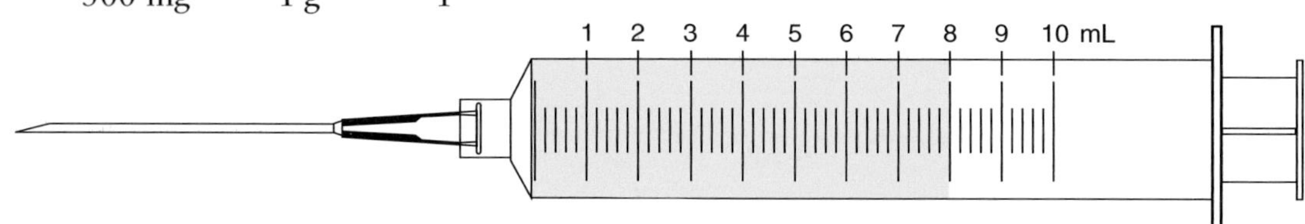

4. $x \text{ mL} = \dfrac{1 \text{ mL}}{5 \text{ mg}} \times \dfrac{20 \text{ mg}}{1} = 4 \text{ mL}$

5. $x \text{ mL} = \dfrac{1 \text{ mL}}{30 \text{ mg}} \times \dfrac{60 \text{ mg}}{1} = 2 \text{ mL}$

6. $x \text{ mL} = \dfrac{1 \text{ mL}}{100 \text{ mg}} \times \dfrac{200 \text{ mg}}{1} = 2 \text{ mL}$

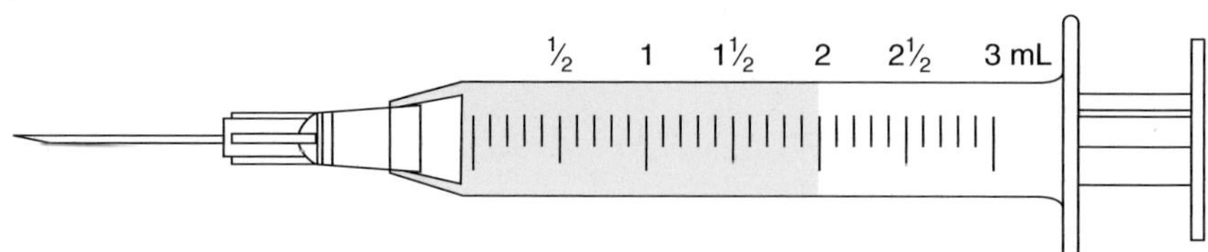

7. $x \text{ mL} = \dfrac{1 \text{ mL}}{0.4 \text{ mg}} \times \dfrac{0.2 \text{ mg}}{1} = 0.5 \text{ mL}$

8. $x \text{ mL} = \dfrac{1 \text{ mL}}{50 \text{ mg}} \times \dfrac{25 \text{ mg}}{1} = 0.5 \text{ mL}$

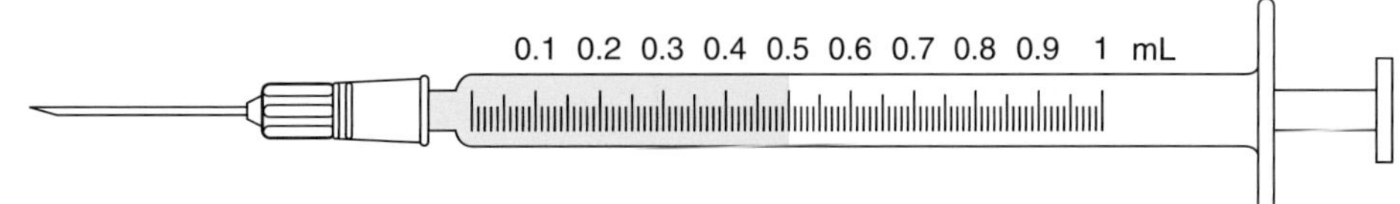

9. $x \text{ mL} = \dfrac{1 \text{ mL}}{20 \text{ mg}} \times \dfrac{100 \text{ mg}}{1} = 5 \text{ mL}$

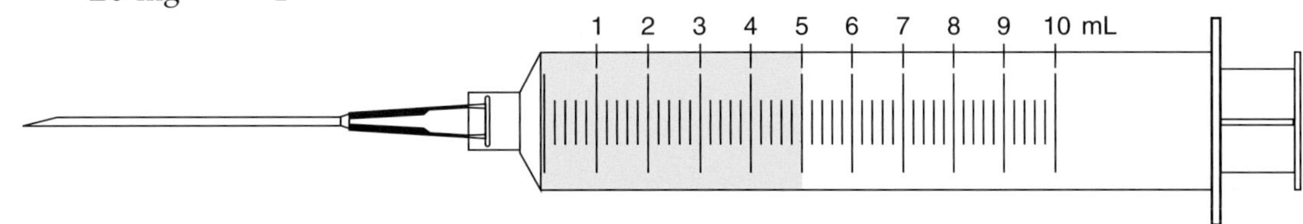

10. $x \text{ mL} = \dfrac{1 \text{ mL}}{50 \text{ mg}} \times \dfrac{75 \text{ mg}}{1} = 1.5 \text{ mL}$

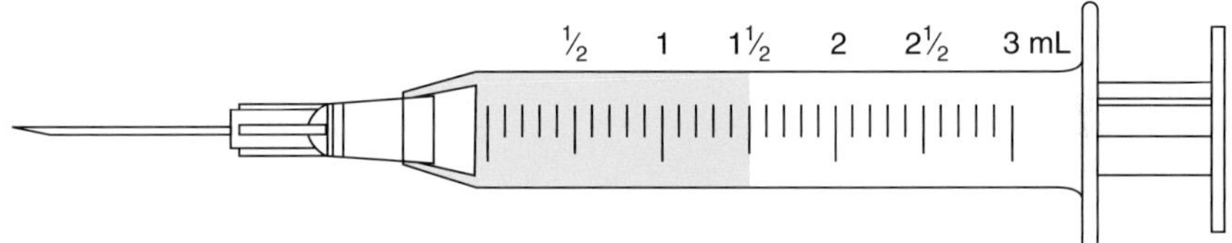

11. $x \text{ mL} = \dfrac{1 \text{ mL}}{50 \text{ mcg}} \times \dfrac{70 \text{ mcg}}{1} = 1.4 \text{ mL}$

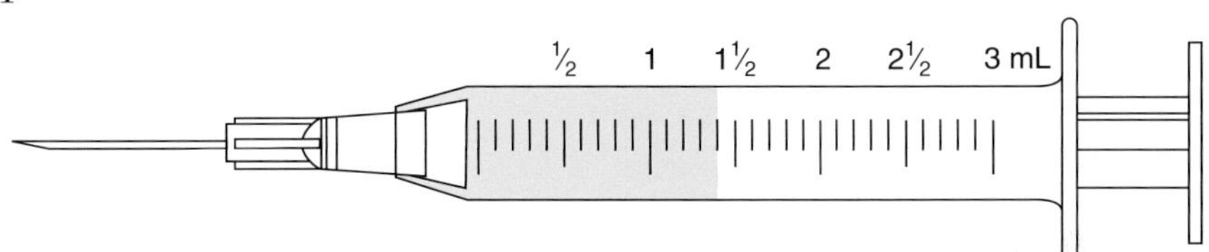

12. $x \text{ mL} = \dfrac{1 \text{ mL}}{0.3 \text{ mg}} \times \dfrac{0.4 \text{ mg}}{1} = 1.33 \text{ mL}$

13. $x \text{ mL} = \dfrac{2.5 \text{ mL}}{1 \text{ g}} \times \dfrac{2 \text{ g}}{1} = 5 \text{ mL}$

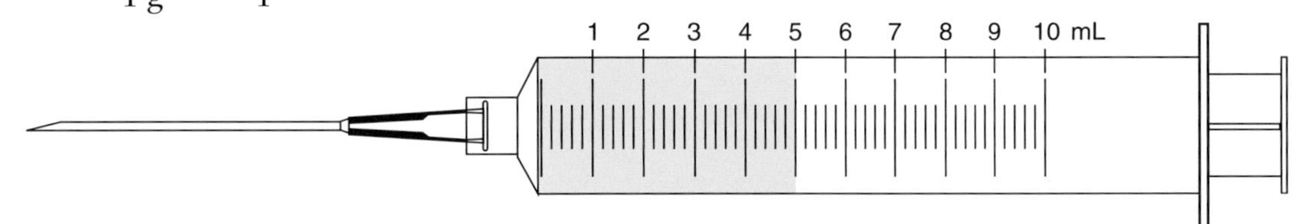

14. $x \text{ mL} = \dfrac{1 \text{ mL}}{40 \text{ mg}} \times \dfrac{26 \text{ mg}}{1} = 0.65 \text{ mL}$

ANSWERS

15. $x \text{ mL} = \dfrac{0.4 \text{ mL}}{40 \text{ mg}} \times \dfrac{85 \text{ mg}}{1} = 0.85 \text{ mL}$

16. $x \text{ mL} = \dfrac{1 \text{ mL}}{0.25 \text{ mg}} \times \dfrac{1 \text{ mg}}{1000 \text{ mcg}} \times \dfrac{80 \text{ mcg}}{1} = 0.32 \text{ mL}$

17. $x \text{ mL} = \dfrac{1 \text{ mL}}{8 \text{ mg}} \times \dfrac{4 \text{ mg}}{1} = 0.5 \text{ mL}$

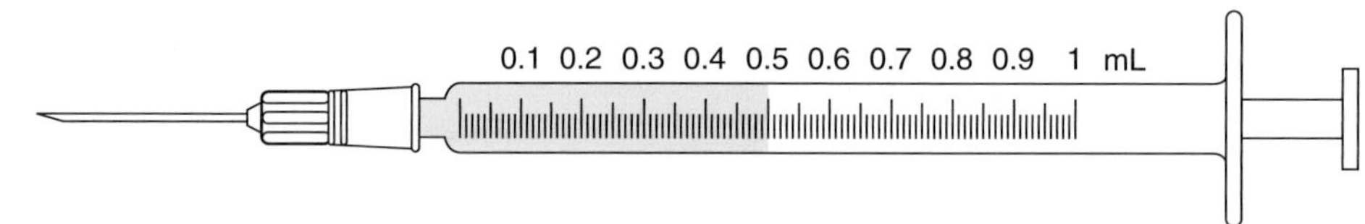

18. $x \text{ mL} = \dfrac{2 \text{ mL}}{50 \text{ mg}} \times \dfrac{100 \text{ mg}}{1} = 4 \text{ mL}$

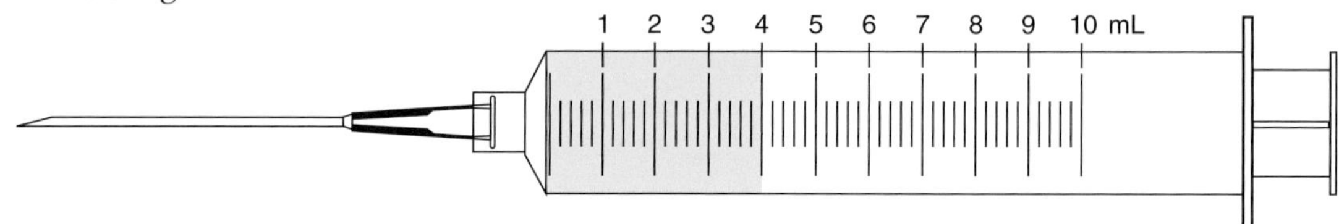

19. $x \text{ mL} = \dfrac{100 \text{ mL}}{400 \text{ mg}} \times \dfrac{300 \text{ mg}}{1} = 75 \text{ mL}$

20. $x \text{ mL} = \dfrac{10 \text{ mL}}{13.6 \text{ mEq}} \times \dfrac{10 \text{ mEq}}{1} = 7.35 \text{ mL}$

CHAPTER 12 Proportion/Formula Method—Worksheet, pp. 297–320

Proportion	**Formula**
1. 400 mg : 1 mL :: 500 mg : x mL $400x = 500$ $x = \dfrac{500}{400}$ $x = 1.25$ mL or 1.3 mL	$\dfrac{500 \text{ mg}}{400 \text{ mg}} \times 1 \text{ mL} = 1.25 \text{ mL or } 1.3 \text{ mL}$

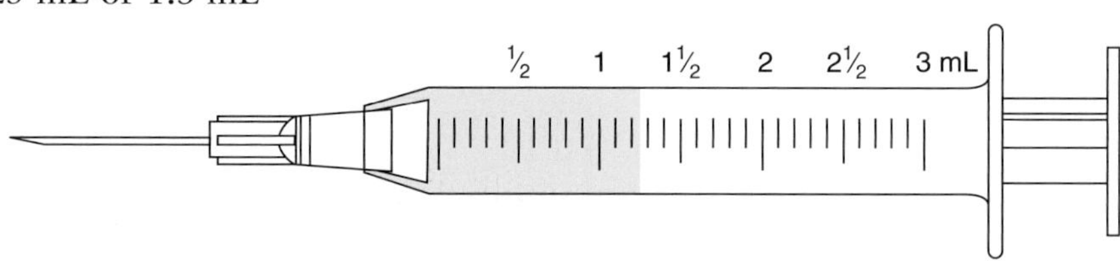

ANSWERS

Proportion	**Formula**
2. 500 mcg : 2 mL :: 110 mcg : x mL $500x = 220$ $x = \frac{220}{500}$ $x = 0.44$ mL	$\frac{110\text{ mcg}}{500\text{ mcg}} \times 2\text{ mL} = \frac{220}{500} = 0.44\text{ mL}$

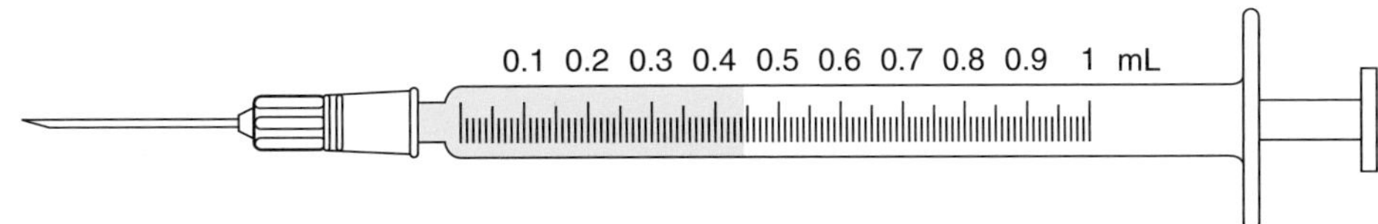

3. 0.4 mg : 1 mL :: 0.3 mg : x mL $0.4x = 0.3$ $x = \frac{0.3}{0.4}$ $x = 0.75$ mL	$\frac{0.3\text{ mg}}{0.4\text{ mg}} \times 1\text{ mL} = 0.75\text{ mL}$

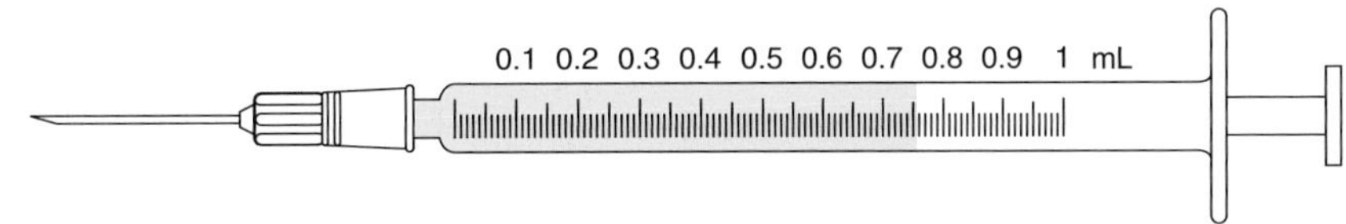

4. 5 mg : 1 mL :: 10 mg : x mL $5x = 10$ $x = \frac{10}{5}$ $x = 2$ mL	$\frac{10\text{ mg}}{5\text{ mg}} \times 1\text{ mL} = 2\text{ mL}$

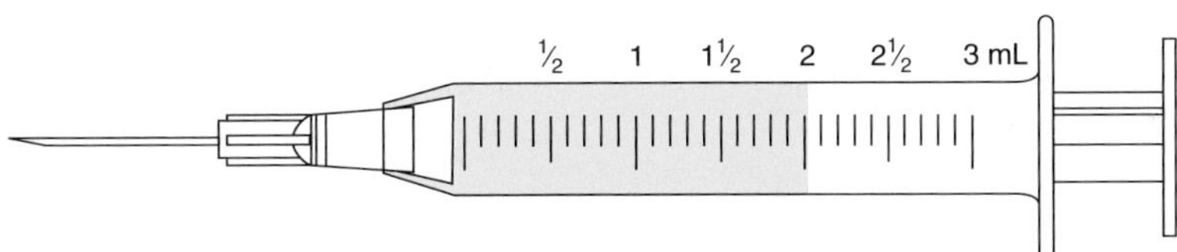

5. 25 mg : 1 mL :: 50 mg : x mL $25x = 50$ $x = \frac{50}{25}$ $x = 2$ mL	$\frac{50\text{ mg}}{25\text{ mg}} \times 1\text{ mL} = \frac{50}{25} = 2\text{ mL}$

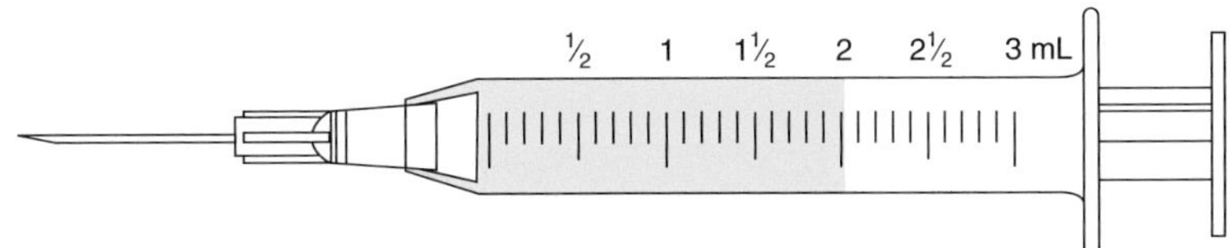

6. 1 g : 2.5 mL :: 3 g : x mL $x = 2.5 \times 3$ $x = 7.5$ mL	$\frac{3\text{ g}}{1\text{ g}} \times 2.5\text{ mL} = 7.5\text{ mL}$
7. 10 mg : 1 mL :: 5 mg : x mL $10x = 5$ $x = \frac{5}{10}$ $x = 0.5$ mL	$\frac{5\text{ mg}}{10\text{ mg}} \times 1\text{ mL} = 0.5\text{ mL}$

Proportion	Formula
8. 5 mg : 1 mL :: 4 mg : x mL $5x = 4$ $x = \frac{4}{5}$ $x = 0.8$ mL	$\frac{4 \text{ mg}}{5 \text{ mg}} \times 1 \text{ mL} = \frac{4}{5} = 0.8 \text{ mL}$
9. 40 mg : 4 mL :: 30 mg : x mL $40x = 120$ $x = \frac{120}{40}$ $x = 3$ mL	$\frac{30 \text{ mg}}{\cancel{40}_{10} \text{ mg}} \times \frac{\cancel{4}^{1} \text{ mL}}{1} = \frac{30}{10} = 3 \text{ mL}$

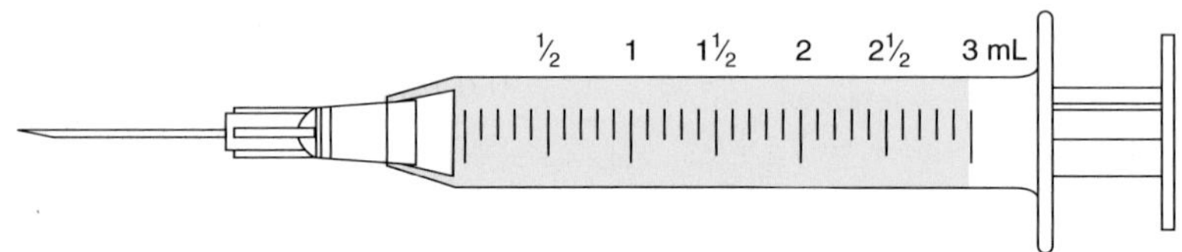

Proportion	Formula
10. 30 mg : 1 mL :: 15 mg : x mL $30x = 15$ $x = \frac{15}{30}$ $x = 0.5$ mL	$\frac{\cancel{15}^{1} \text{ mg}}{\cancel{30}_{2} \text{ mg}} \times 1 \text{ mL} = \frac{1}{2} \text{ or } 0.5 \text{ mL}$
11. 44.6 mEq : 50 mL :: 25.8 mEq : x mL $44.6x = 1290$ $x = \frac{1290}{44.6}$ $x = 28.9$ mL or 29 mL	$\frac{25.8 \text{ mEq}}{44.6 \text{ mEq}} \times 50 \text{ mL} =$ $0.58 \times 50 = 28.9 \text{ mL or } 29 \text{ mL}$
12. 25 mg : 1 mL :: 100 mg : x mL $25x = 100$ $x = \frac{100}{25}$ $x = 4$ mL	$\frac{100 \text{ mg}}{25 \text{ mg}} \times 1 \text{ mL} = 4 \text{ mL}$
13. 100 mg : 20 mL :: 350 mg : x mL $100x = 7000$ $x = \frac{7000}{100}$ $x = 70$ mL	$\frac{\cancel{350}^{70} \text{ mg}}{\cancel{100}_{\cancel{5}\ 1} \text{ mg}} \times \frac{\cancel{20}^{1} \text{ mL}}{1} =$ $\frac{70}{1} = 70 \text{ mL}$
14. 400 mg : 40 mL :: 300 mg : x mL $400x = 12{,}000$ $x = \frac{12{,}000}{400}$ $x = 30$ mL	$\frac{300 \text{ mg}}{400 \text{ mg}} \times 40 \text{ mL} =$ $\frac{300}{\cancel{400}_{10}} \times \frac{\cancel{40}^{1}}{1} =$ $\frac{300}{10} = 30 \text{ mL}$

ANSWERS

Proportion	**Formula**

15. 250 mg : 2 mL :: 50 mg : x mL

$$250x = 100$$
$$x = \frac{100}{250}$$
$$x = 0.4 \text{ mL}$$

$$\frac{50 \text{ mg}}{\cancel{250}_{125} \text{ mg}} \times \frac{\cancel{2}^{1} \text{ mL}}{1} = \frac{50}{125} = 0.4 \text{ mL}$$

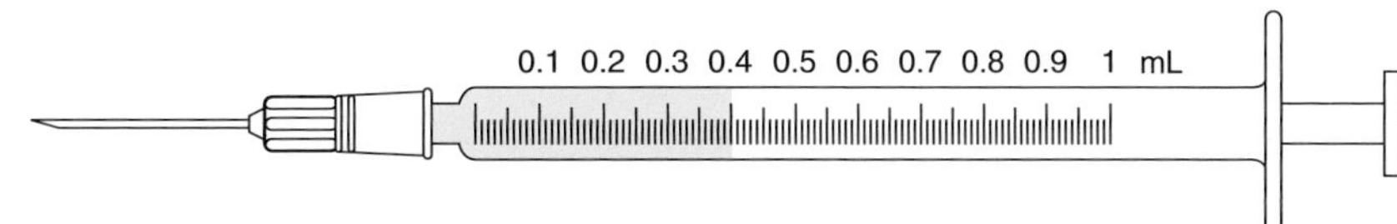

16. 0.4 mg : 1 mL :: 0.6 mg : x mL

$$0.4x = 0.6$$
$$x = \frac{0.6}{0.4}$$
$$x = 1.5 \text{ mL}$$

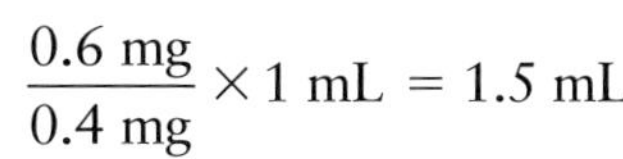

$$\frac{0.6 \text{ mg}}{0.4 \text{ mg}} \times 1 \text{ mL} = 1.5 \text{ mL}$$

17. 300 mg : 2 mL :: 300 mg : x mL

$$300x = 600$$
$$x = \frac{600}{300}$$
$$x = 2 \text{ mL}$$

$$\frac{300 \text{ mg}}{300 \text{ mg}} \times 2 \text{ mL} = 2 \text{ mL}$$

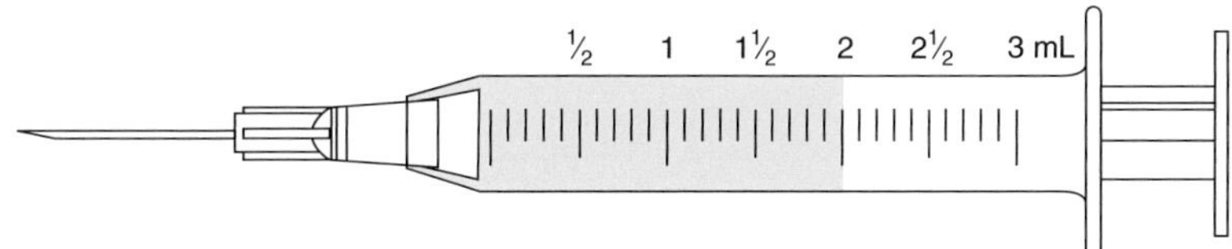

18. 10 mg : 10 mL :: 6 mg : x mL

$$10x = 60$$
$$x = \frac{60}{10}$$
$$x = 6 \text{ mL}$$

$$\frac{6 \text{ mg}}{10 \text{ mg}} \times 10 \text{ mL} =$$
$$\frac{6}{\cancel{10}_{1}} \times \frac{\cancel{10}^{1}}{1} = 6 \text{ mL}$$

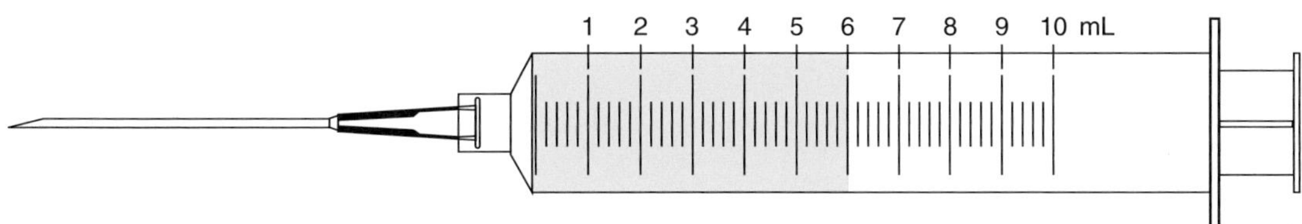

19. 50 mg : 1 mL :: 25 mg : x mL

$$50x = 25$$
$$x = \frac{25}{50}$$
$$x = 0.5 \text{ mL}$$

$$\frac{25 \text{ mg}}{50 \text{ mg}} \times 1 \text{ mL} = 0.5 \text{ mL}$$

20. 4 mg : 1 mL :: 1 mg : x mL

$$4x = 1$$
$$x = \frac{1}{4}$$
$$x = 0.25 \text{ mL}$$

$$\frac{1 \text{ mg}}{4 \text{ mg}} \times 1 \text{ mL} = 0.25 \text{ mL}$$

Proportion	Formula
21. $20 \text{ mg} : 1 \text{ mL} :: 10 \text{ mg} : x \text{ mL}$ $20x = 10$ $x = \frac{10}{20}$ $x = 0.5 \text{ mL}$	$\frac{10 \text{ mg}}{20 \text{ mg}} \times 1 \text{ mL} = 0.5 \text{ mL}$

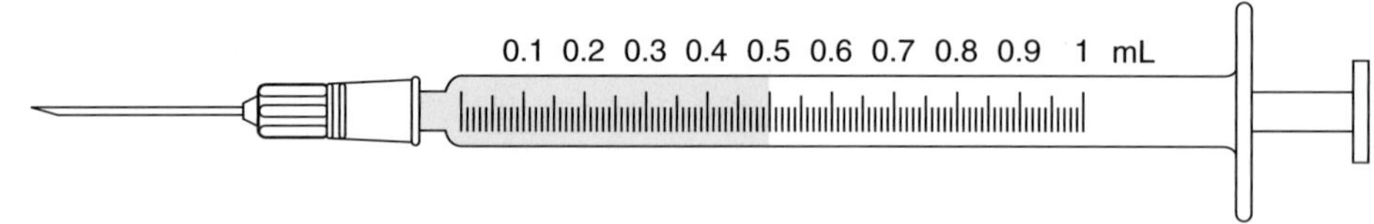

Proportion	Formula
22. $500 \text{ mg} : 2 \text{ mL} :: 400 \text{ mg} : x \text{ mL}$ $500x = 800$ $x = \frac{800}{500}$ $x = 1.6 \text{ mL}$	$\frac{400 \text{ mg}}{500 \text{ mg}} \times 2 \text{ mL} =$ $\frac{800}{500} = 1.6 \text{ mL}$
23. $5 \text{ mg} : 1 \text{ mL} :: 7.5 \text{ mg} : x \text{ mL}$ $5x = 7.5$ $x = \frac{7.5}{5}$ $x = 1.5 \text{ mL}$	$\frac{7.5 \text{ mg}}{5 \text{ mg}} \times 1 \text{ mL} = 1.5 \text{ mL}$
24. $30 \text{ mg} : 1 \text{ mL} :: 15 \text{ mg} : x \text{ mL}$ $30x = 15$ $x = \frac{15}{30}$ $x = \frac{1}{2}$ $x = 0.5 \text{ mL}$	$\frac{15 \text{ mg}}{30 \text{ mg}} \times 1 \text{ mL} = 0.5 \text{ mL}$
25. $10 \text{ mg} : 1 \text{ mL} :: 10 \text{ mg} : x \text{ mL}$ $10x = 10$ $x = \frac{10}{10}$ $x = 1 \text{ mL}$	$\frac{10 \text{ mg}}{10 \text{ mg}} \times 1 \text{ mL} = 1 \text{ mL}$

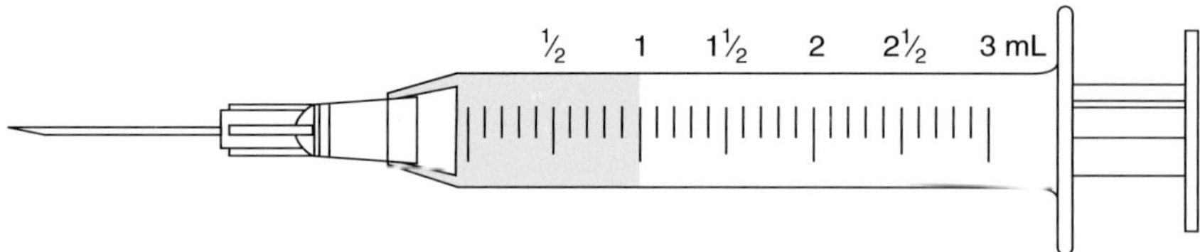

Proportion	Formula
26. $400 \text{ mg} : 40 \text{ mL} :: 200 \text{ mg} : x \text{ mL}$ $400x = 8000$ $x = \frac{8000}{400}$ $x = 20 \text{ mL}$	$\frac{200 \text{ mg}}{400 \text{ mg}} \times \frac{40 \text{ mL}}{1} = 20 \text{ mL}$

Proportion | **Formula**

27. 15 mg : 1 mL :: 6 mg : x mL

$$15x = 6$$
$$x = \frac{6}{15}$$
$$x = 0.4\text{ mL}$$

$$\frac{6\text{ mg}}{15\text{ mg}} \times 1\text{ mL} = 0.4\text{ mL}$$

28. 50 mg : 1 mL :: 100 mg : x mL

$$50x = 100$$
$$x = \frac{100}{50}$$
$$x = 2\text{ mL}$$

$$\frac{100\text{ mg}}{50\text{ mg}} \times 1\text{ mL} = 2\text{ mL}$$

29. 500 mcg : 2 mL :: 100 mcg : x mL

$$500x = 200$$
$$x = \frac{200}{500}$$
$$x = 0.4\text{ mL}$$

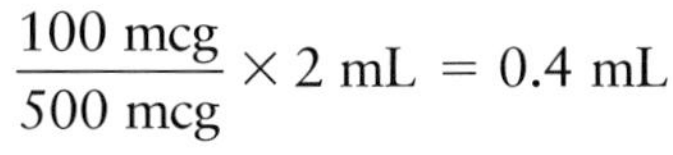

$$\frac{100\text{ mcg}}{500\text{ mcg}} \times 2\text{ mL} = 0.4\text{ mL}$$

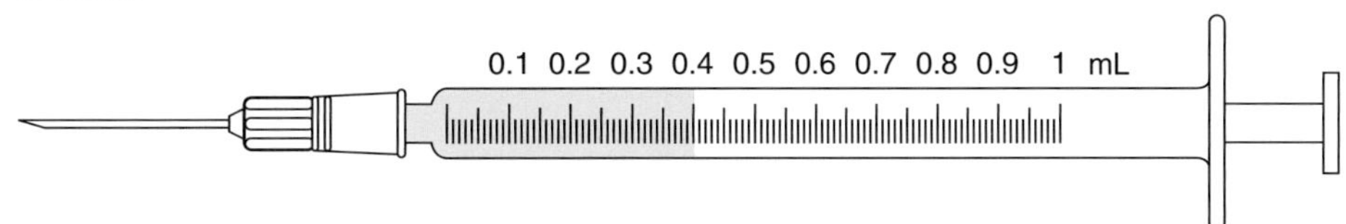

30. 500 mg : 2 mL :: 700 mg : x mL

$$500x = 1400$$
$$x = \frac{1400}{500}$$
$$x = 2.8\text{ mL}$$

$$\frac{700\text{ mg}}{500\text{ mg}} \times 2\text{ mL} = \frac{1400}{500} = 2.8\text{ mL}$$

31. 2 mg : 1 mL :: 1.5 mg : x mL

$$2x = 1.5$$
$$x = \frac{1.5}{2}$$
$$x = 0.75\text{ mL}$$

$$\frac{1.5\text{ mg}}{2\text{ mg}} \times 1\text{ mL} = 0.75\text{ mL}$$

32. 250 mg : 2 mL :: 100 mg : x mL

$$250x = 200$$
$$x = \frac{200}{250}$$
$$x = 0.8\text{ mL}$$

$$\frac{100\text{ mg}}{\underset{125}{\cancel{250}}\text{ mg}} \times \frac{\overset{1}{\cancel{2}}\text{ mL}}{1} = 0.8\text{ mL}$$

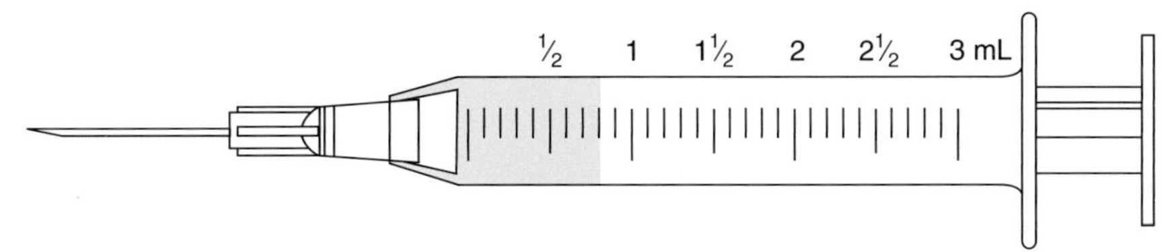

ANSWERS

Proportion	Formula
33. $2.5 \text{ mEq} : 1 \text{ mL} :: 7.5 \text{ mEq} : x \text{ mL}$ $2.5x = 7.5$ $x = \frac{7.5}{2.5}$ $x = 3 \text{ mL}$	$\frac{7.5 \text{ mEq}}{2.5 \text{ mEq}} \times 1 \text{ mL} = 3 \text{ mL}$
34. $50 \text{ mg} : 1 \text{ mL} :: 25 \text{ mg} : x \text{ mL}$ $50x = 25$ $x = \frac{25}{50}$ $x = 0.5 \text{ mL}$	$\frac{25 \text{ mg}}{50 \text{ mg}} \times 1 \text{ mL} = 0.5 \text{ mL}$
35. $0.4 \text{ mg} : 1 \text{ mL} :: 0.6 \text{ mg} : x \text{ mL}$ $0.4x = 0.6$ $x = \frac{0.6}{0.4}$ $x = 1.5 \text{ mL}$	$\frac{0.6 \text{ mg}}{0.4 \text{ mg}} \times 1 \text{ mL} = 1.5 \text{ mL}$
36. $100 \text{ mg} : 1 \text{ mL} :: 150 \text{ mg} : x \text{ mL}$ $100x = 150$ $x = \frac{150}{100}$ $x = 1.5 \text{ mL}$	$\frac{150 \text{ mg}}{100 \text{ mg}} \times 1 \text{ mL} = 1.5 \text{ mL}$

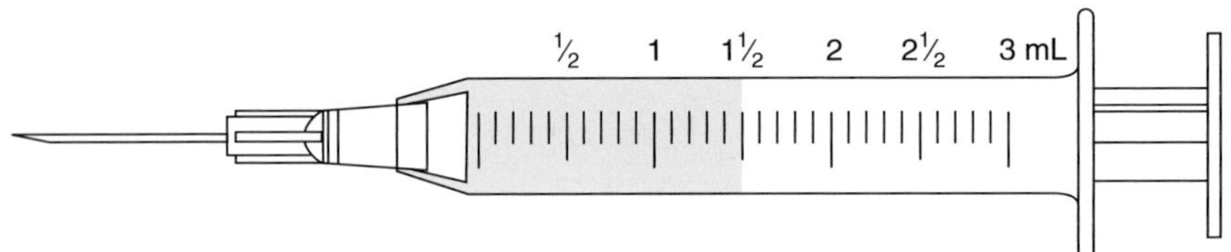

Proportion	Formula
37. $0.25 \text{ mg} : 1 \text{ mL} :: 0.5 \text{ mg} : x \text{ mL}$ $0.25x = 0.5$ $x = \frac{0.5}{0.25}$ $x = 2 \text{ mL}$	$\frac{0.5 \text{ mg}}{0.25 \text{ mg}} \times 1 \text{ mL} = 2 \text{ mL}$

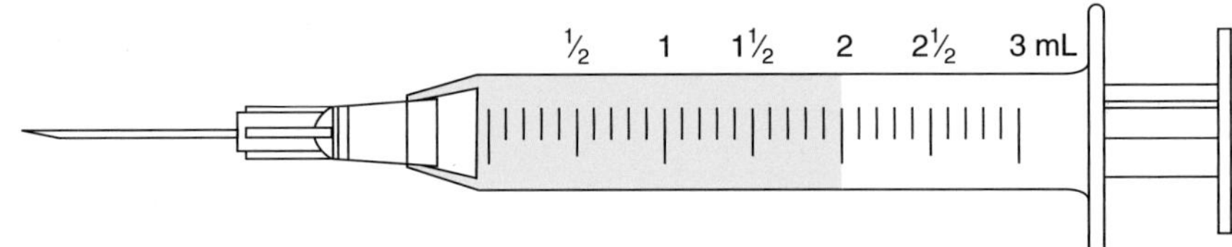

Proportion	Formula
38. $25 \text{ mg} : 1 \text{ mL} :: 75 \text{ mg} : x \text{ mL}$ $25x = 75$ $x = \frac{75}{25}$ $x = 3 \text{ mL}$	$\frac{75 \text{ mg}}{25 \text{ mg}} \times 1 \text{ mL} = 3 \text{ mL}$

Proportion / **Formula**

39. 0.4 mg : 1 mL :: 0.6 mg : x mL

$$0.4x = 0.6$$
$$x = \frac{0.6}{0.4}$$
$$x = 1.5 \text{ mL}$$

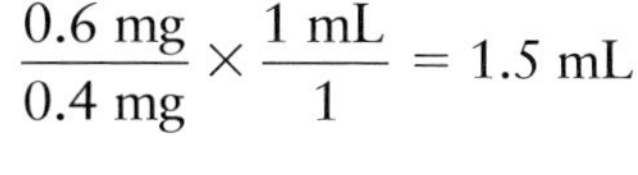

$$\frac{0.6 \text{ mg}}{0.4 \text{ mg}} \times \frac{1 \text{ mL}}{1} = 1.5 \text{ mL}$$

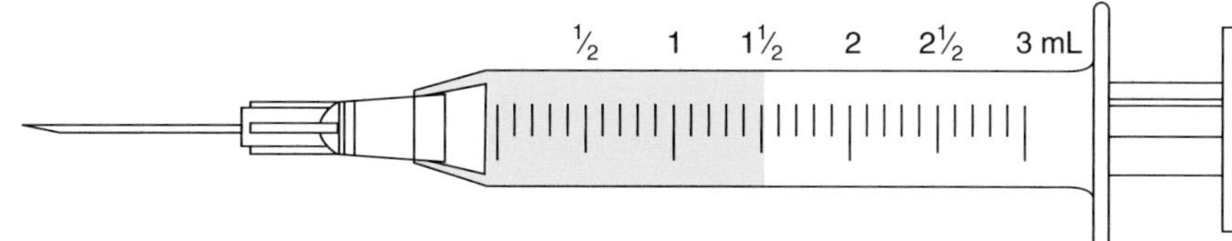

40. 5 mg : 1 mL :: 10 mg : x mL

$$5x = 10$$
$$x = \frac{10}{5}$$
$$x = 2 \text{ mL}$$

$$\frac{10 \text{ mg}}{5 \text{ mg}} \times 1 \text{ mL} = 2 \text{ mL}$$

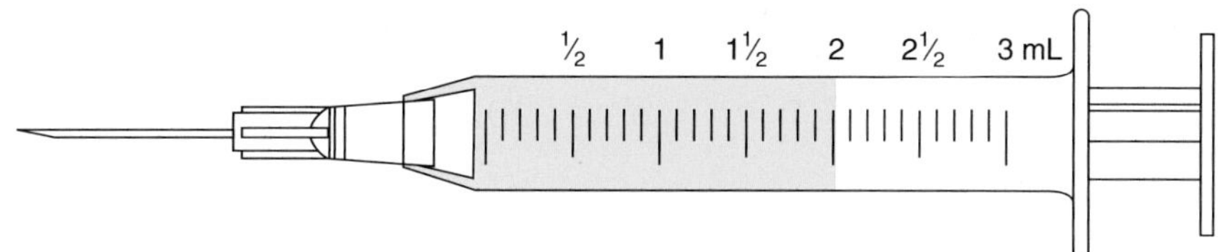

41. 100 mg : 2 mL :: 25 mg : x mL

$$100x = 50$$
$$x = \frac{50}{100}$$
$$x = 0.5 \text{ mL}$$

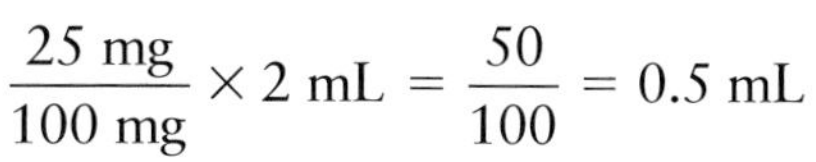

$$\frac{25 \text{ mg}}{100 \text{ mg}} \times 2 \text{ mL} = \frac{50}{100} = 0.5 \text{ mL}$$

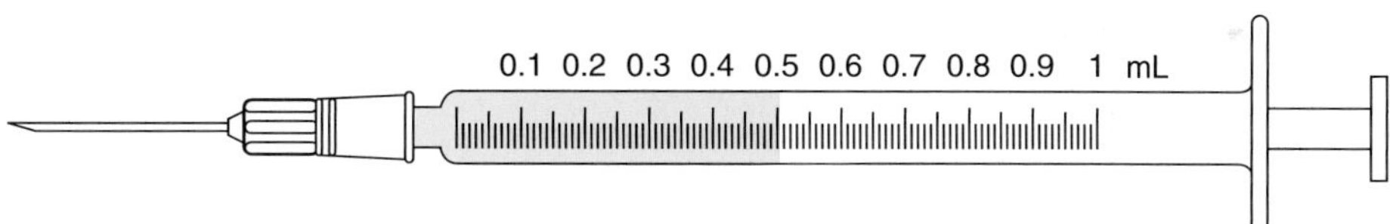

42. 400 mg : 40 mL :: 200 mg : x mL

$$400x = 8000$$
$$x = \frac{8000}{400}$$
$$x = 20 \text{ mL}$$

$$\frac{200 \text{ mg}}{400 \text{ mg}} \times 40 \text{ mL} =$$
$$\frac{200}{\cancel{400}_{10}} \times \frac{\cancel{40}^{1}}{1} = \frac{200}{10}$$
$$\frac{200}{10} = 20 \text{ mL}$$

43. 500 mg : 1 mL :: 250 mg : x mL

$$500x = 250$$
$$x = \frac{250}{500}$$
$$x = 0.5 \text{ mL}$$

$$\frac{250 \text{ mg}}{500 \text{ mg}} \times 1 \text{ mL} = 0.5 \text{ mL}$$

Proportion	Formula
44. 13.6 mEq : 10 mL :: 5 mEq : x mL $13.6x = 50$ $x = \frac{50}{13.6}$ $x = 3.68$ mL or 3.7 mL	$\frac{5 \text{ mEq}}{13.6 \text{ mEq}} \times 10 \text{ mL} = \frac{50}{13.6}$ $= 3.68$ mL or 3.7 mL
45. 130 mg : 1 mL :: 70 mg : x mL $130x = 70$ $x = \frac{70}{130}$ $x = 0.538$ or 0.54 mL	$\frac{70 \text{ mg}}{130 \text{ mg}} \times 1 \text{ mL} = 0.538$ or 0.54 mL

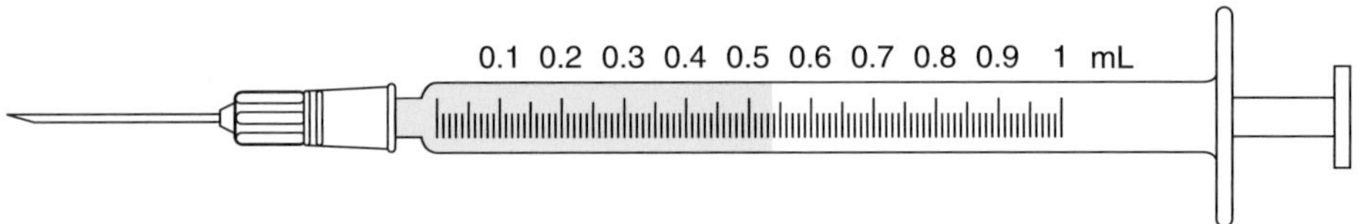

Proportion	Formula
46. 10 mg : 1 mL :: 200 mg : x mL $10x = 200$ $x = \frac{200}{10}$ $x = 20$ mL	$\frac{200 \text{ mg}}{10 \text{ mg}} \times 1 \text{ mL} = 20$ mL
47. 4 mg : 1 mL :: 2 mg : x mL $4x = 2$ $x = \frac{2}{4} = 0.5$ mL	$\frac{2 \text{ mg}}{4 \text{ mg}} \times 1 \text{ mL} = \frac{2}{4} = 0.5$ mL
48. 0.5 mg : 2 mL :: 0.2 mg : x mL $0.5x = 0.4$ $x = \frac{0.4}{0.5}$ $x = 0.8$ mL	$\frac{0.2 \text{ mg}}{0.5 \text{ mg}} \times 2 \text{ mL} = \frac{0.4}{0.5} = 0.8$ mL

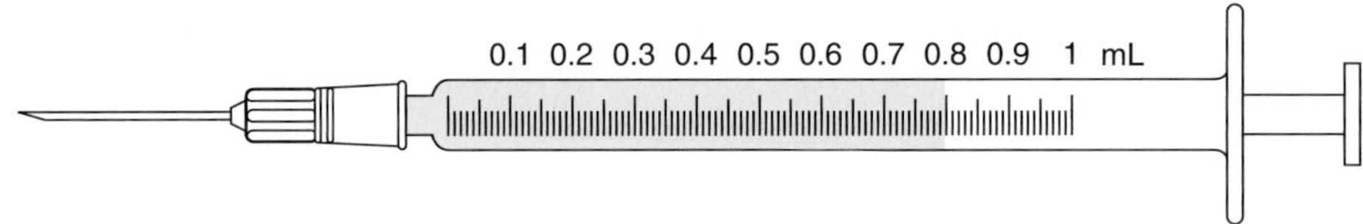

Proportion	Formula
49. 15 mg : 1 mL :: 10 mg : x mL $15x = 10$ $x = \frac{10}{15}$ $x = 0.67$ mL	$\frac{10 \text{ mg}}{15 \text{ mg}} \times 1 \text{ mL} = 0.67$ mL

Proportion	Formula
50. $50 \text{ mg} : 1 \text{ mL} :: 25 \text{ mg} : x \text{ mL}$ $50x = 25$ $x = \frac{25}{50}$ $x = 0.5 \text{ mL}$	$\frac{25 \text{ mg}}{50 \text{ mg}} \times 1 \text{ mL} = 0.5 \text{ mL}$

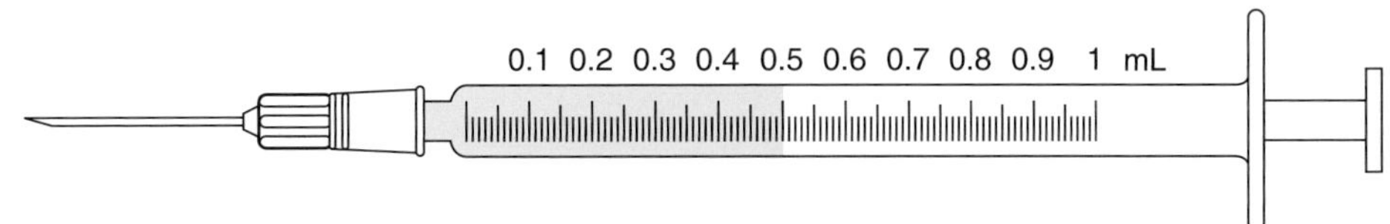

Proportion	Formula
51. $500 \text{ mg} : 1.2 \text{ mL} :: 600 \text{ mg} : x \text{ mL}$ $500x = 720$ $x = \frac{720}{500}$ $x = 1.44 \text{ mL or } 1.4 \text{ mL}$	$\frac{600 \text{ mg}}{500 \text{ mg}} \times 1.2 \text{ mL} = 1.44 \text{ mL or } 1.4 \text{ mL}$
52. $0.4 \text{ mg} : 1 \text{ mL} :: 0.9 \text{ mg} : x \text{ mL}$ $0.4x = 0.9$ $x = \frac{0.9}{0.4}$ $x = 2.25 \text{ mL or } 2.3 \text{ mL}$	$\frac{0.9 \text{ mg}}{0.4 \text{ mg}} \times 1 \text{ mL} = 2.25 \text{ mL or } 2.3 \text{ mL}$
53. $30 \text{ mg} : 1 \text{ mL} :: 30 \text{ mg} : x \text{ mL}$ $30x = 30$ $x = \frac{30}{30}$ $x = 1 \text{ mL}$	$\frac{30 \text{ mg}}{30 \text{ mg}} \times 1 \text{ mL} = 1 \text{ mL}$
54. $4 \text{ mg} : 1 \text{ mL} :: 3 \text{ mg} : x \text{ mL}$ $4x = 3$ $x = \frac{3}{4}$ $x = 0.75 \text{ mL}$	$\frac{3 \text{ mg}}{4 \text{ mg}} \times 1 \text{ mL} = 0.75 \text{ mL}$

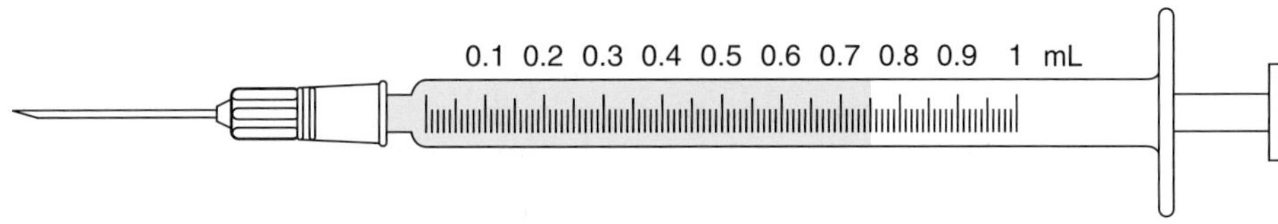

Proportion	Formula
55. $0.89 \text{ mEq} : 1 \text{ mL} :: 6 \text{ mEq} : x \text{ mL}$ $0.89x = 6$ $x = \frac{6}{0.89}$ $x = 6.74 \text{ mL or } 6.7 \text{ mL}$	$\frac{6 \text{ mEq}}{0.89 \text{ mEq}} \times 1 \text{ mL} = 6.74 \text{ mL or } 6.7 \text{ mL}$

ANSWERS

Proportion	Formula
56. $20 \text{ mg} : 1 \text{ mL} :: 10 \text{ mg} : x \text{ mL}$ $20x = 10$ $x = \frac{10}{20}$ $x = 0.5 \text{ mL}$	$\frac{10 \text{ mg}}{20 \text{ mg}} \times 1 \text{ mL} = 0.5 \text{ mL}$
57. $25 \text{ mg} : 1 \text{ mL} :: 5 \text{ mg} : x \text{ mL}$ $25x = 5$ $x = \frac{5}{25}$ $x = 0.2 \text{ mL}$	$\frac{5 \text{ mg}}{25 \text{ mg}} \times 1 \text{ mL} = 0.2 \text{ mL}$
58. $125 \text{ mg} : 1 \text{ mL} :: 500 \text{ mg} : x \text{ mL}$ $125x = 500$ $x = \frac{500}{125}$ $x = 4 \text{ mL}$	$\frac{500 \text{ mg}}{125 \text{ mg}} \times 1 \text{ mL} = 4 \text{ mL}$

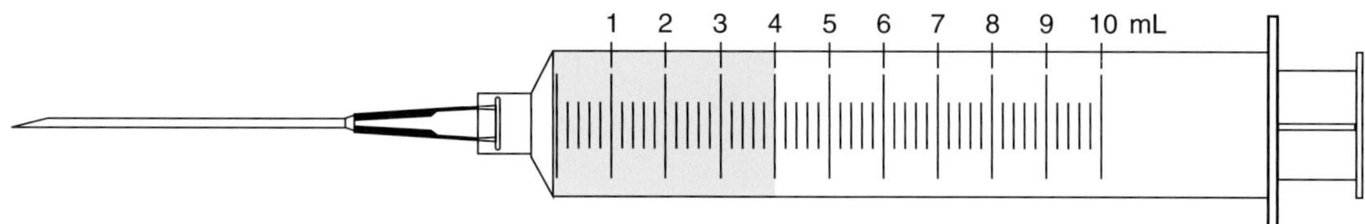

59. $0.25 \text{ mg} : 1 \text{ mL} :: 0.2 \text{ mg} : x \text{ mL}$
$0.25x = 0.2$
$x = \frac{0.2}{0.25}$
$x = 0.8 \text{ mL}$

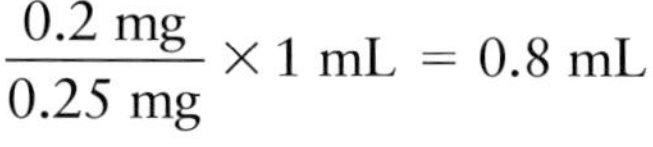
$\frac{0.2 \text{ mg}}{0.25 \text{ mg}} \times 1 \text{ mL} = 0.8 \text{ mL}$

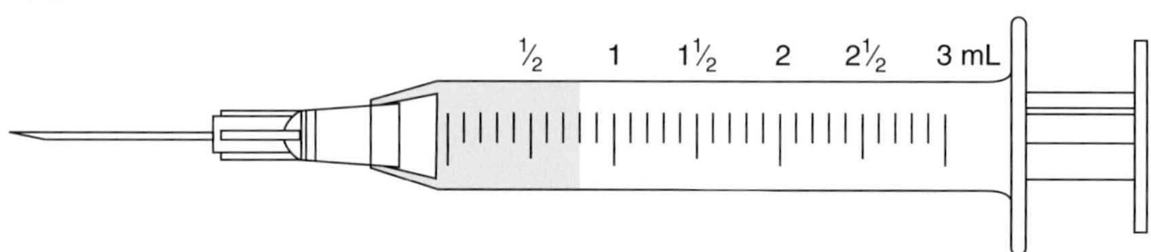

60. $2 \text{ mg} : 1 \text{ mL} :: 0.5 \text{ mg} : x \text{ mL}$
$2x = 0.5$
$x = \frac{0.5}{2}$
$x = 0.25 \text{ mL}$

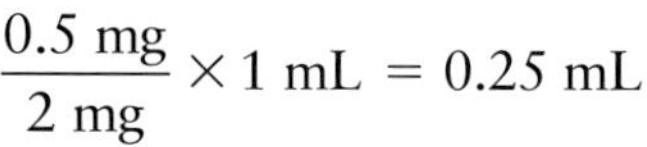
$\frac{0.5 \text{ mg}}{2 \text{ mg}} \times 1 \text{ mL} = 0.25 \text{ mL}$

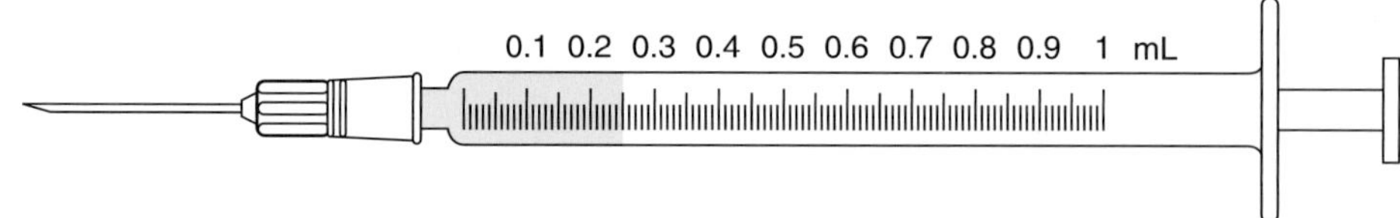

Proportion	Formula
61. $0.5 \text{ g} : 20 \text{ mL} :: 0.2 \text{ g} : x \text{ mL}$ $0.5x = 4$ $x = \frac{4}{0.5}$ $x = 8 \text{ mL}$	$\frac{0.2 \text{ g}}{0.5 \text{ g}} \times 20 \text{ mL} = \frac{4}{0.5} = 8 \text{ mL}$

ANSWERS

Proportion / **Formula**

62. $30 \text{ mg} : 1 \text{ mL} :: 15 \text{ mg} : x \text{ mL}$

$$30x = 15$$
$$x = \frac{15}{30}$$
$$x = 0.5 \text{ mL}$$

$$\frac{15 \text{ mg}}{30 \text{ mg}} \times 1 \text{ mL} = 0.5 \text{ mL}$$

63. $250 \text{ mg} : 5 \text{ mL} :: 100 \text{ mg} : x \text{ mL}$

$$250x = 500$$
$$x = \frac{500}{250}$$
$$x = 2 \text{ mL}$$

$$\frac{100 \text{ mg}}{250 \text{ mg}} \times 5 \text{ mL} = 2 \text{ mL}$$

½ 1 1½ 2 2½ 3 mL

64. $0.5 \text{ mg} : 2 \text{ mL} :: 0.25 : x \text{ mL}$

$$0.5x = 0.5$$
$$x = \frac{0.5}{0.5}$$
$$x = 1 \text{ mL}$$

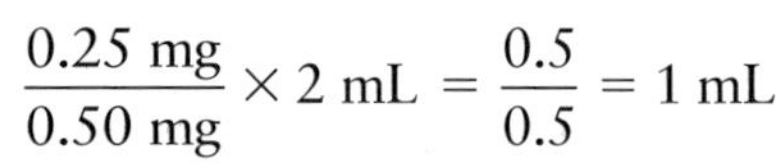

$$\frac{0.25 \text{ mg}}{0.50 \text{ mg}} \times 2 \text{ mL} = \frac{0.5}{0.5} = 1 \text{ mL}$$

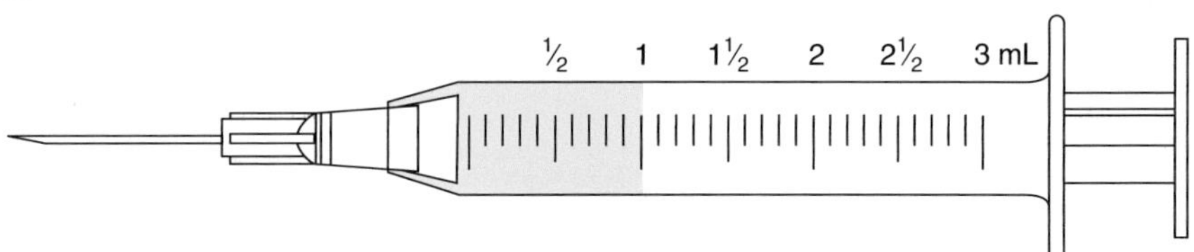

65. $1000 \text{ mcg} : 1 \text{ mL} :: 500 \text{ mcg} : x \text{ mL}$

$$1000x = 500$$
$$x = \frac{500}{1000}$$
$$x = 0.5 \text{ mL}$$

$$\frac{500 \text{ mcg}}{1000 \text{ mcg}} \times 1 \text{ mL} = 0.5 \text{ mL}$$

66. $4.8 \text{ mEq} : 10 \text{ mL} :: 5 \text{ mEq} : x \text{ mL}$

$$4.8x = 50$$
$$x = \frac{50}{4.8}$$
$$x = 10.42 \text{ mL or } 10.4 \text{ mL}$$

$$\frac{5 \text{ mEq}}{4.8 \text{ mEq}} \times 10 \text{ mL} = \frac{50}{4.8}$$
$$= 10.42 \text{ mL or } 10.4 \text{ mL}$$

67. $150 \text{ mg} : 1 \text{ mL} :: 50 \text{ mg} : x \text{ mL}$

$$150x = 50$$
$$x = \frac{50}{150}$$
$$x = 0.33 \text{ mL}$$

$$\frac{50 \text{ mg}}{150 \text{ mg}} \times 1 \text{ mL} = 0.33 \text{ mL}$$

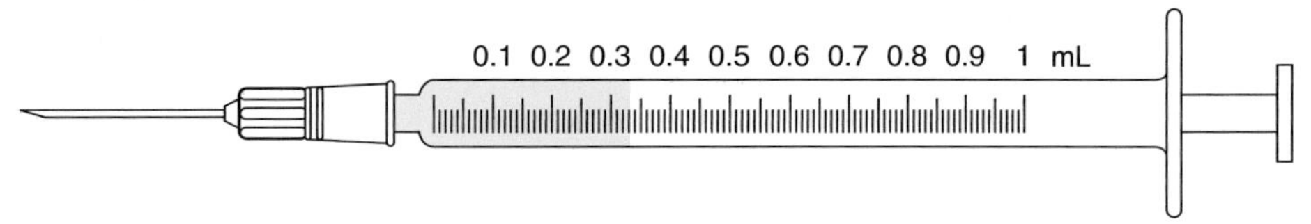

ANSWERS

Proportion	Formula

68. 0.4 mg : 1 mL :: 0.2 mg : x mL

$$0.4x = 0.2$$
$$x = \frac{0.2}{0.4}$$
$$x = 0.5 \text{ mL}$$

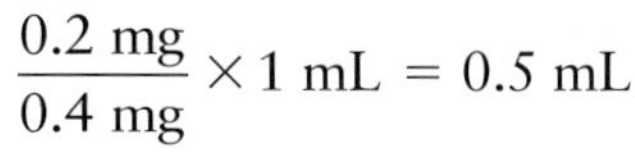

$$\frac{0.2 \text{ mg}}{0.4 \text{ mg}} \times 1 \text{ mL} = 0.5 \text{ mL}$$

69. 80 mg : 2 mL :: 55 mg : x mL

$$80x = 110$$
$$x = \frac{110}{80}$$
$$x = 1.38 \text{ mL or } 1.4 \text{ mL}$$

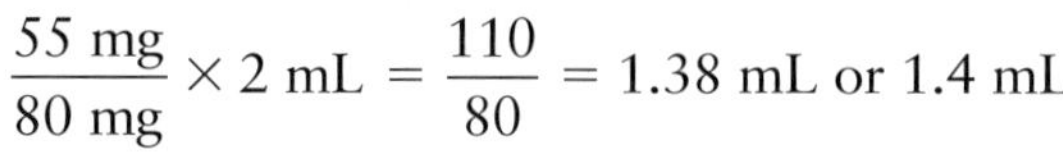

$$\frac{55 \text{ mg}}{80 \text{ mg}} \times 2 \text{ mL} = \frac{110}{80} = 1.38 \text{ mL or } 1.4 \text{ mL}$$

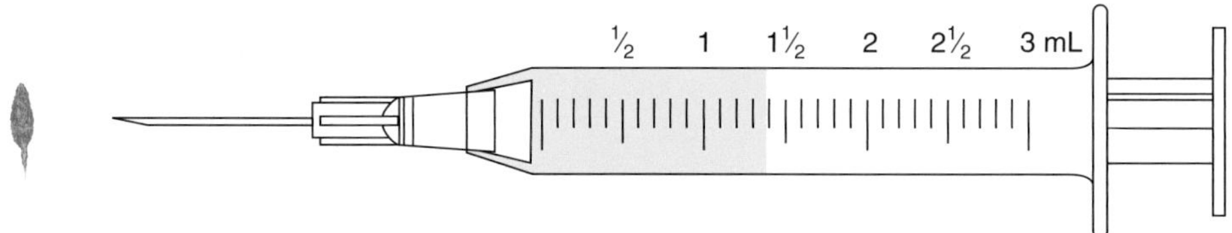

70. 500 mg : 2 mL :: 600 mg : x mL

$$500x = 1200$$
$$x = \frac{1200}{500}$$
$$x = 2.4 \text{ mL}$$

$$\frac{600 \text{ mg}}{500 \text{ mg}} \times 2 \text{ mL} =$$
$$\frac{600}{\cancel{500}_{250}} \times \frac{\cancel{2}^{1}}{1} = \frac{600}{250}$$
$$x = 2.4 \text{ mL}$$

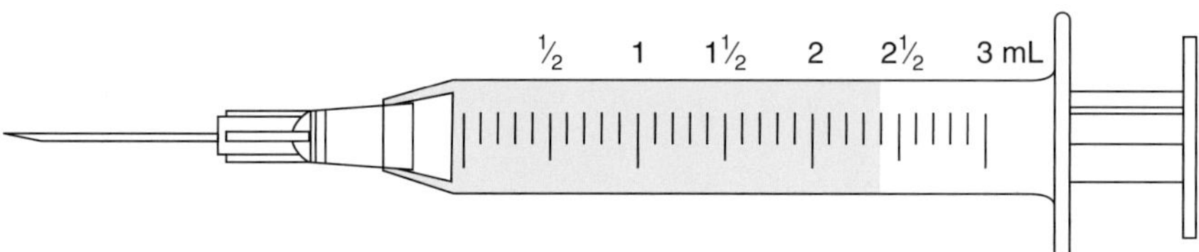

71. 15 mg : 1 mL :: 6 mg : x mL

$$15x = 6$$
$$x = \frac{6}{15}$$
$$x = 0.4 \text{ mL}$$

$$\frac{6 \text{ mg}}{15 \text{ mg}} \times 1 \text{ mL} = 0.4 \text{ mL}$$

72. 1000 mcg : 1 mL :: 1000 mcg : x mL

$$1000x = 1000$$
$$x = \frac{1000}{1000}$$
$$x = 1 \text{ mL}$$

$$\frac{1000 \text{ mcg}}{1000 \text{ mcg}} \times 1 \text{ mL} = 1 \text{ mL}$$

73. 325 mg : 1 mL :: 800 mg : x mL

$$325x = 800$$
$$x = \frac{800}{325}$$
$$x = 2.46 \text{ mL or } 2.5 \text{ mL}$$

$$\frac{800 \text{ mg}}{325 \text{ mg}} \times 1 \text{ mL} = 2.46 \text{ mL or } 2.5 \text{ mL}$$

Proportion | **Formula**

74. 50 mg : 1 mL :: 30 mg : x mL

$$50x = 30$$
$$x = \frac{30}{50}$$
$$x = 0.6 \text{ mL}$$

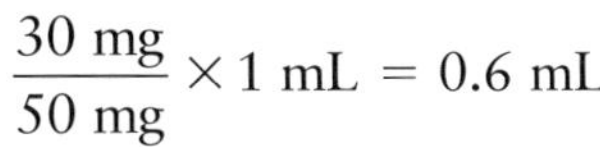

$$\frac{30 \text{ mg}}{50 \text{ mg}} \times 1 \text{ mL} = 0.6 \text{ mL}$$

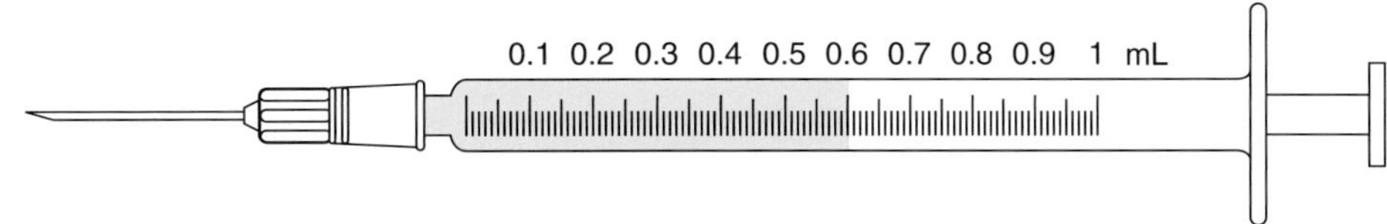

75. 0.2 mg : 1 mL :: 0.28 mg : x mL

$$0.2x = 0.28$$
$$x = \frac{0.28}{0.2}$$
$$x = 1.4 \text{ mL}$$

$$\frac{0.28 \text{ mg}}{0.2 \text{ mg}} \times 1 \text{ mL} = 1.4 \text{ mL}$$

76. 4 mg : 1 mL :: 3 mg : x mL

$$4x = 3$$
$$x = \frac{3}{4}$$
$$x = 0.75 \text{ mL}$$

$$\frac{3 \text{ mg}}{4 \text{ mg}} \times 1 \text{ mL} = 0.75 \text{ mL}$$

77. 100 mEq : 40 mL :: 15 mEq : x mL

$$100x = 600$$
$$x = \frac{600}{100}$$
$$x = 6 \text{ mL}$$

$$\frac{15 \text{ mEq}}{100 \text{ mEq}} \times 40 \text{ mL} = \frac{600}{100} = 6 \text{ mL}$$

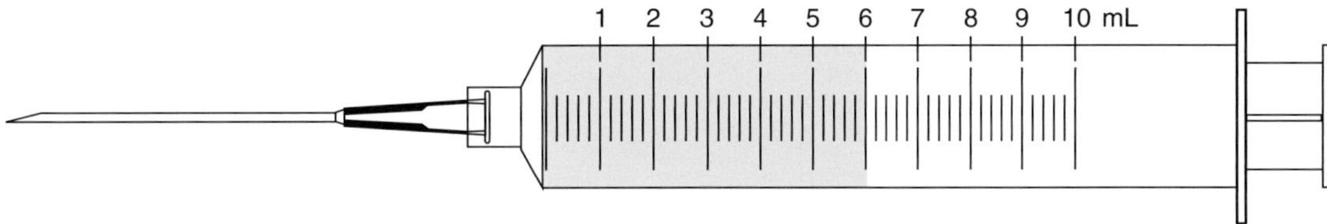

78. 225 mg : 1 mL :: 250 mg : x mL

$$225x = 250$$
$$x = \frac{250}{225}$$
$$x = 1.1 \text{ mL}$$

$$\frac{250 \text{ mg}}{225 \text{ mg}} \times 1 \text{ mL} = 1.1 \text{ mL}$$

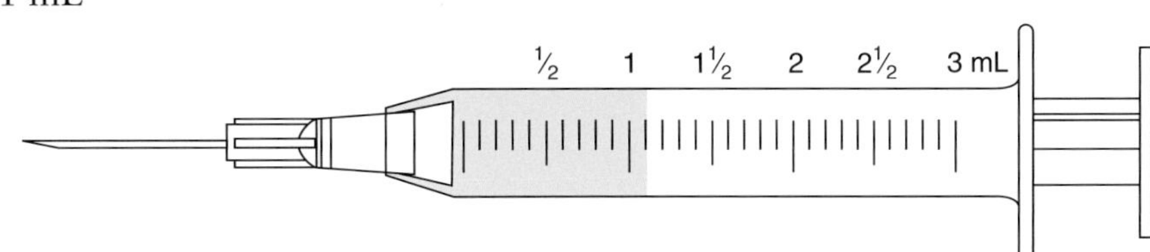

Proportion	Formula
79. $150 \text{ mg} : 1 \text{ mL} :: 300 \text{ mg} : x \text{ mL}$ $150x = 300$ $x = \frac{300}{150}$ $x = 2 \text{ mL}$	$\frac{300 \text{ mg}}{150 \text{ mg}} \times 1 \text{ mL} = 2 \text{ mL}$

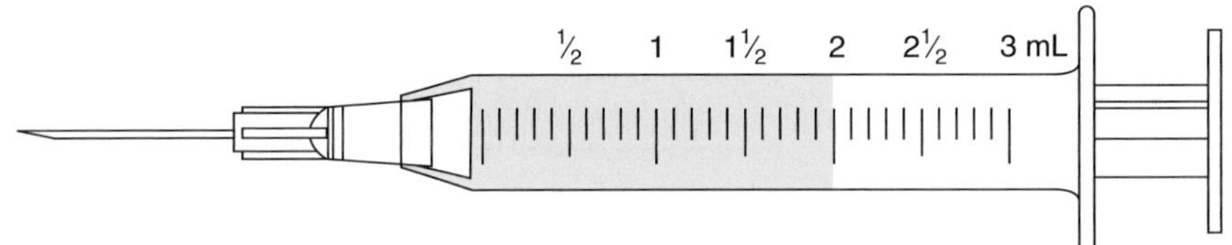

Proportion	Formula
80. $100 \text{ mg} : 5 \text{ mL} :: 75 \text{ mg} : x \text{ mL}$ $100x = 375$ $x = \frac{375}{100}$ $x = 3.75 \text{ mL or } 3.8 \text{ mL}$	$\frac{75 \text{ mg}}{100 \text{ mg}} \times 5 \text{ mL} = \frac{375}{100} = 3.75 \text{ mL or } 3.8 \text{ mL}$
81. $1 \text{ g} : 2.6 \text{ mL} :: 0.8 \text{ g} : x \text{ mL}$ $x = 2.08 \text{ mL or } 2.1 \text{ mL}$	$\frac{0.8 \text{ g}}{1 \text{ g}} \times 2.6 \text{ mL} = 2.08 \text{ mL or } 2.1 \text{ mL}$
82. $125 \text{ mg} : 2 \text{ mL} :: 100 \text{ mg} : x \text{ mL}$ $125x = 200$ $x = \frac{200}{125}$ $x = 1.6 \text{ mL}$	$\frac{\overset{4}{\cancel{100}} \text{ mg}}{\underset{5}{\cancel{125}} \text{ mg}} \times 2 \text{ mL} = \frac{8}{5} = 1.6 \text{ mL}$

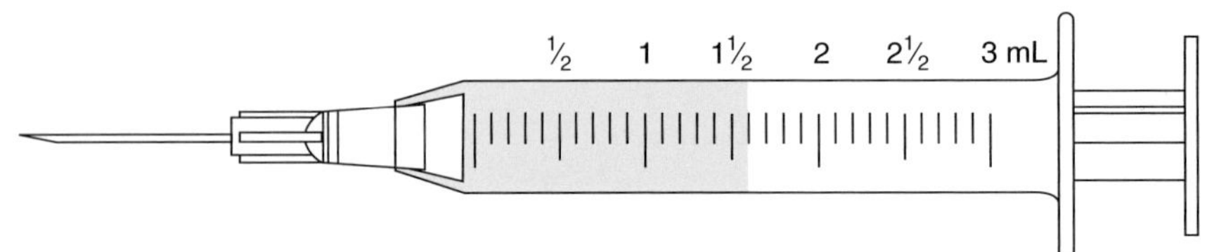

Proportion	Formula
83. $75 \text{ mg} : 1 \text{ mL} :: 300 \text{ mg} : x \text{ mL}$ $75x = 300$ $x = \frac{300}{75}$ $x = 4 \text{ mL}$	$\frac{300 \text{ mg}}{75 \text{ mg}} \times 1 \text{ mL} = 4 \text{ mL}$
84. $0.4 \text{ mg} : 1 \text{ mL} :: 0.4 \text{ mg} : x \text{ mL}$ $0.4x = 0.4$ $x = \frac{0.4}{0.4}$ $x = 1 \text{ mL}$	$\frac{0.4 \text{ mg}}{0.4 \text{ mg}} \times 1 \text{ mL} = 1 \text{ mL}$
85. $50 \text{ mg} : 1 \text{ mL} :: 10 \text{ mg} : x \text{ mL}$ $50x = 10$ $x = \frac{10}{50}$ $x = 0.2 \text{ mL}$	$\frac{10 \text{ mg}}{50 \text{ mg}} \times 1 \text{ mL} = 0.2 \text{ mL}$

Proportion	Formula
86. 10 mg : 1 mL :: 1 mg : x mL $10x = 1$ $x = \frac{1}{10}$ or 0.1 mL	$\frac{1 \text{ mg}}{10 \text{ mg}} \times 1 \text{ mL} = 0.1 \text{ mL}$
87. 50 mg : 1 mL :: 50 mg : x mL $50x = 50$ $x = \frac{50}{50}$ $x = 1$ mL	$\frac{50 \text{ mg}}{50 \text{ mg}} \times 1 \text{ mL} = 1 \text{ mL}$

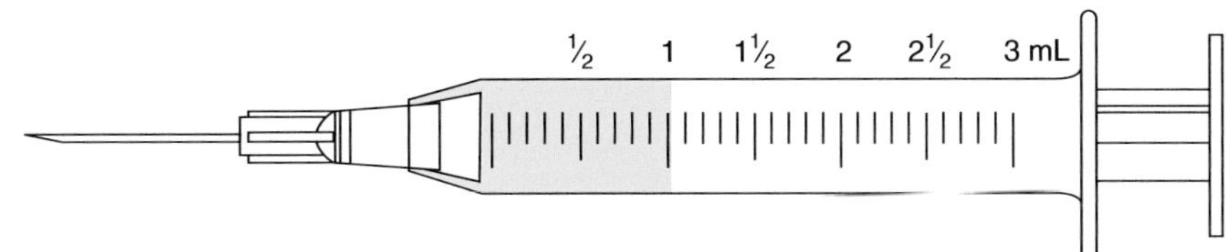

Proportion	Formula
88. 50 mcg : 1 mL :: 60 mcg : x mL $50x = 60$ $x = \frac{60}{50}$ $x = 1.2$ mL	$\frac{60 \text{ mcg}}{50 \text{ mcg}} \times 1 \text{ mL} = 1.2 \text{ mL}$
89. 0.4 mg : 1 mL :: 0.5 mg : x mL $0.4x = 0.5$ $x = \frac{0.5}{0.4}$ $x = 1.25$ mL or 1.3 mL	$\frac{0.5 \text{ mg}}{0.4 \text{ mg}} \times 1 \text{ mL} = 1.25 \text{ mL or } 1.3 \text{ mL}$

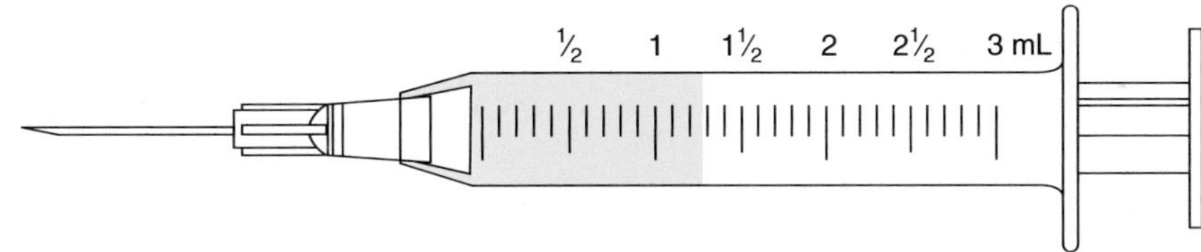

Proportion	Formula
90. 25 mg : 1 mL :: 15 mg : x mL $25x = 15$ $x = \frac{15}{25}$ $x = 0.6$ mL	$\frac{15 \text{ mg}}{25 \text{ mg}} \times 1 \text{ mL} = 0.6 \text{ mL}$
91. 100 mg : 1 mL :: 150 mg : x mL $100x = 150$ $x = \frac{150}{100}$ $x = 1.5$ mL	$\frac{150 \text{ mg}}{100 \text{ mg}} \times 1 \text{ mL} = \frac{150}{100} = 1.5 \text{ mL}$
92. 200 mcg : 1 mL :: 75 mcg : x mL $200x = 75$ $x = \frac{75}{200}$ $x = 0.375$ or 0.38 mL	$\frac{75 \text{ mcg}}{200 \text{ mcg}} \times 1 \text{ mL} = 0.375 \text{ or } 0.38 \text{ mL}$

Proportion	Formula
93. 5 mg : 1 mL :: 2 mg : x mL $5x = 2$ $x = \frac{2}{5}$ $x = 0.4$ mL	$\frac{2\text{ mg}}{5\text{ mg}} \times 1\text{ mL} = 0.4\text{ mL}$

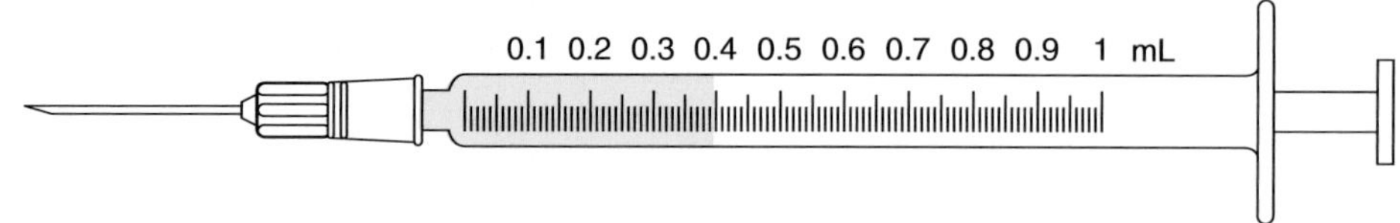

Proportion	Formula
94. 100 mg : 1 mL :: 500 mg : x mL $100x = 500$ $x = \frac{500}{100}$ $x = 5$ mL	$\frac{500\text{ mg}}{100\text{ mg}} \times 1\text{ mL} = 5\text{ mL}$

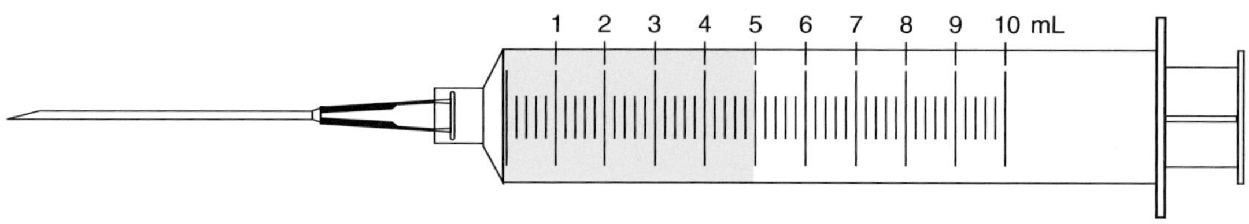

Proportion	Formula
95. 400 mg : 1 mL :: 640 mg : x mL $400x = 640$ $x = \frac{640}{400}$ $x = 1.6$ mL	$\frac{640\text{ mg}}{400\text{ mg}} \times 1\text{ mL} = 1.6\text{ mL}$
96. 250 mg : 1 mL :: 500 mg : x mL $250x = 500$ $x = \frac{500}{250}$ $x = 2$ mL	$\frac{500\text{ mg}}{250\text{ mg}} \times 1\text{ mL} = 2\text{ mL}$
97. 2 mg : 1 mL :: 0.5 mg : x mL $2x = 0.5$ $x = \frac{0.5}{2}$ $x = 0.25$ mL	$\frac{0.5\text{ mg}}{2\text{ mg}} \times 1\text{ mL} = 0.25\text{ mL}$
98. 25 mg : 0.5 mL :: 100 mg : x mL $25x = 50$ $x = \frac{50}{25}$ $x = 2$ mL	$\frac{100\text{ mg}}{25\text{ mg}} \times 0.5\text{ mL} = \frac{50}{25} = 2\text{ mL}$

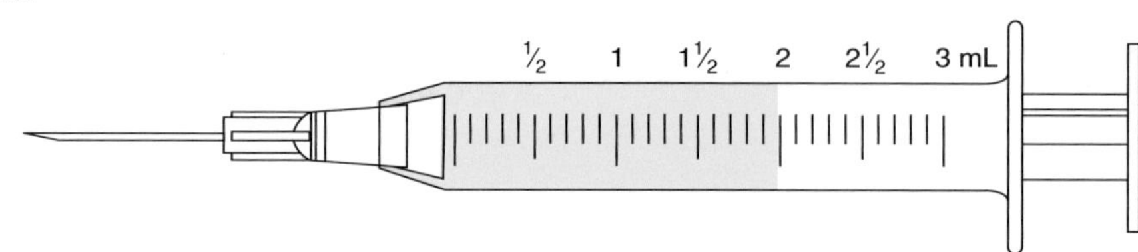

Proportion	**Formula**

99. 50 mg : 1 mL :: 10 mg : x mL
$50x = 10$
$x = \frac{10}{50}$
$x = 0.2$ mL

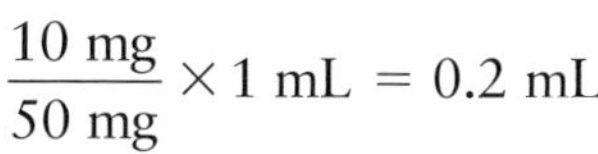

$\frac{10 \text{ mg}}{50 \text{ mg}} \times 1 \text{ mL} = 0.2 \text{ mL}$

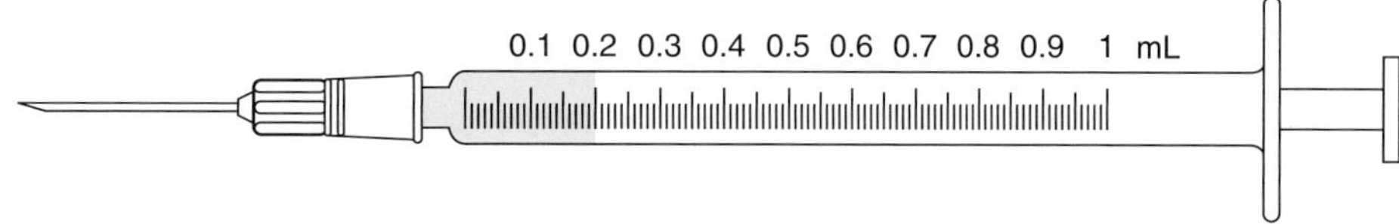

100. 1 mg : 1 mL :: 3.5 mg : x mL
$1x = 3.5$
$x = \frac{3.5}{1}$
$x = 3.5$ mL

$\frac{3.5 \text{ mg}}{1 \text{ mg}} \times 1 \text{ mL} = 3.5 \text{ mL}$

CHAPTER 12 Proportion/Formula Method—Posttest 1, pp. 321–325

Proportion	**Formula**

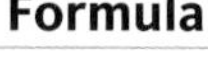

1. 50 mg : 1 mL :: 25 mg : x mL
$50x = 25$
$x = \frac{25}{50}$
$x = 0.5$ mL

$\frac{25 \text{ mg}}{50 \text{ mg}} \times 1 \text{ mL} = 0.5 \text{ mL}$

2. 50 mg : 1 mL :: 25 mg : x mL
$50x = 25$
$x = \frac{25}{50}$
$x = 0.5$ mL

$\frac{25 \text{ mg}}{50 \text{ mg}} \times 1 \text{ mL} = 0.5 \text{ mL}$

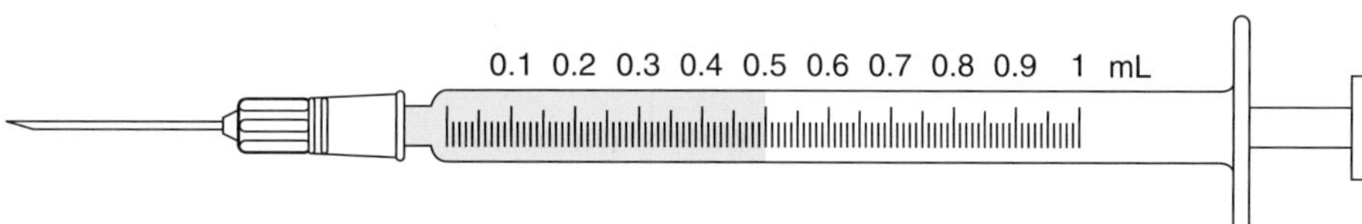

3. 15 mg : 1 mL :: 30 mg : x mL
$15x = 30$
$x = \frac{30}{15}$
$x = 2$ mL

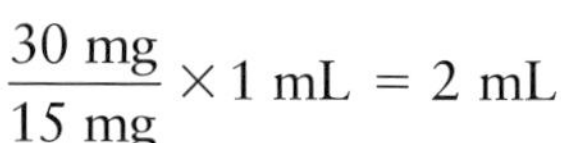

$\frac{30 \text{ mg}}{15 \text{ mg}} \times 1 \text{ mL} = 2 \text{ mL}$

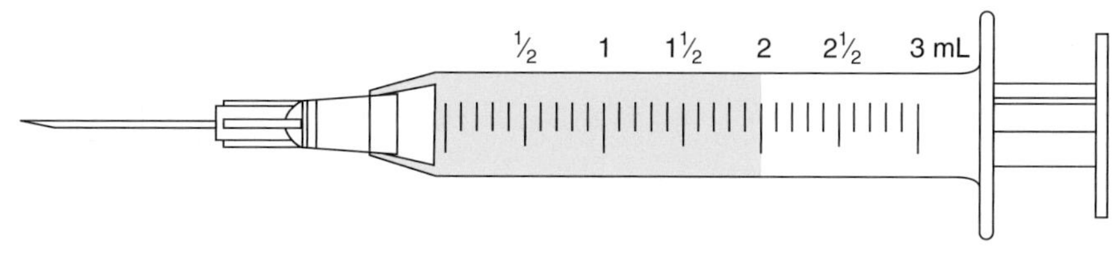

Proportion	**Formula**
4. $1000 \text{ mg} : 10 \text{ mL} :: 500 \text{ mg} : x \text{ mL}$ $1000x = 5000$ $x = \dfrac{5000}{1000}$ $x = 5 \text{ mL}$	$\dfrac{\overset{1}{\cancel{500}} \text{ mg}}{\underset{2}{\cancel{1000}} \text{ mg}} \times 10 \text{ mL} = \dfrac{10}{2} = 5 \text{ mL}$
5. $100 \text{ mg} : 2 \text{ mL} :: 50 \text{ mg} : x \text{ mL}$ $100x = 100$ $x = \dfrac{100}{100}$ $x = 1 \text{ mL}$	$\dfrac{50 \text{ mg}}{100 \text{ mg}} \times 2 \text{ mL} = \dfrac{100}{100} = 1 \text{ mL}$

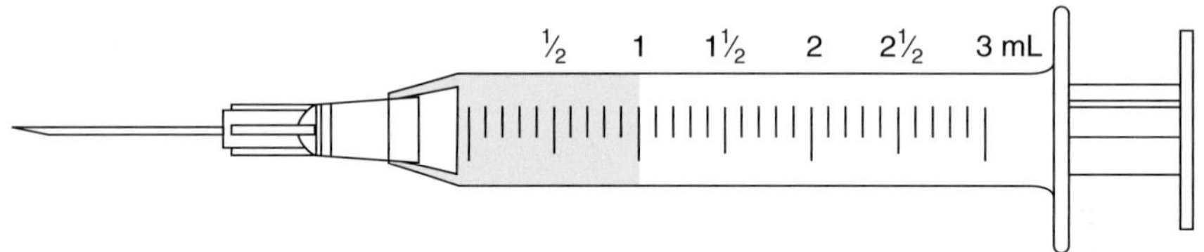

Proportion	**Formula**
6. $2 \text{ mg} : 1 \text{ mL} :: 0.5 \text{ mg} : x \text{ mL}$ $2x = 0.5$ $x = \dfrac{0.5}{2}$ $x = 0.25 \text{ mL}$	$\dfrac{0.5 \text{ mg}}{2 \text{ mg}} \times 1 \text{ mL} = 0.25 \text{ mL}$
7. $30 \text{ mg} : 1 \text{ mL} :: 15 \text{ mg} : x \text{ mL}$ $30x = 15$ $x = \dfrac{15}{30}$ $x = 0.5 \text{ mL}$	$\dfrac{15 \text{ mg}}{30 \text{ mg}} \times 1 \text{ mL} = 0.5 \text{ mL}$
8. $0.4 \text{ mg} : 1 \text{ mL} :: 0.2 \text{ mg} : x \text{ mL}$ $0.4x = 0.2$ $x = \dfrac{0.2}{0.4}$ $x = 0.5 \text{ mL}$	$\dfrac{0.2 \text{ mg}}{0.4 \text{ mg}} \times 1 \text{ mL} = 0.5 \text{ mL}$

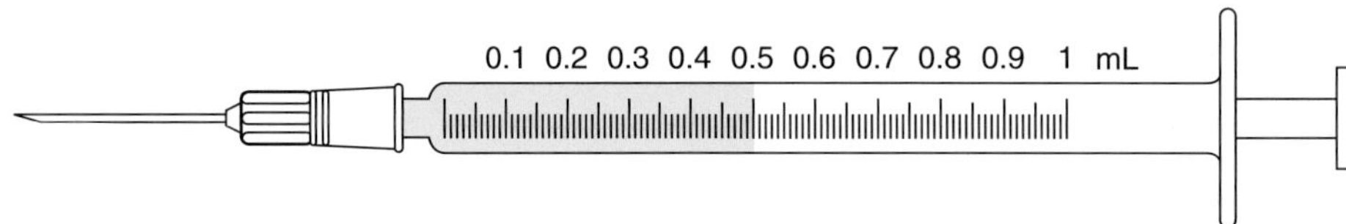

Proportion	**Formula**
9. $25 \text{ mg} : 1 \text{ mL} :: 100 \text{ mg} : x \text{ mL}$ $25x = 100$ $x = \dfrac{100}{25}$ $x = 4 \text{ mL}$	$\dfrac{100 \text{ mg}}{25 \text{ mg}} \times 1 \text{ mL} = 4 \text{ mL}$

Proportion	**Formula**

10. $5 \text{ mg} : 1 \text{ mL} :: 2 \text{ mg} : x \text{ mL}$

$$5x = 2$$
$$x = \frac{2}{5}$$
$$x = 0.4 \text{ mL}$$

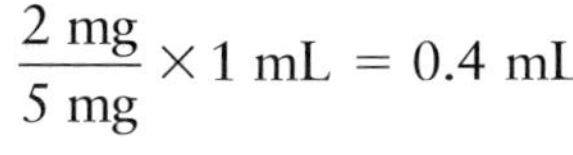

$$\frac{2 \text{ mg}}{5 \text{ mg}} \times 1 \text{ mL} = 0.4 \text{ mL}$$

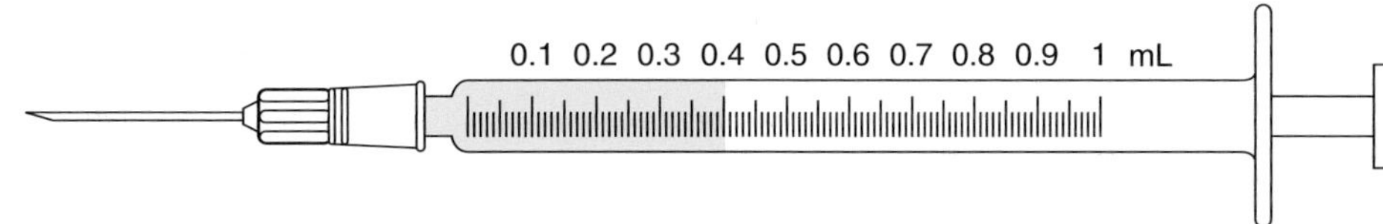

11. $0.5 \text{ mg} : 1 \text{ mL} :: 0.7 \text{ mg} : x \text{ mL}$

$$0.5x = 0.7$$
$$x = \frac{0.7}{0.5}$$
$$x = 1.4 \text{ mL}$$

$$\frac{0.7 \text{ mg}}{0.5 \text{ mg}} \times 1 \text{ mL} = 1.4 \text{ mL}$$

12. $50 \text{ mg} : 1 \text{ mL} :: 25 \text{ mg} : x \text{ mL}$

$$50x = 25$$
$$x = \frac{25}{50}$$
$$x = 0.5 \text{ mL}$$

$$\frac{25 \text{ mg}}{50 \text{ mg}} \times 1 \text{ mL} = 0.5 \text{ mL}$$

13. $80 \text{ mg} : 1 \text{ mL} : 50 \text{ mg} : x \text{ mL}$

$$80x = 50$$
$$x = \frac{50}{80}$$
$$x = 0.625 \text{ mL or } 0.63 \text{ mL}$$

$$\frac{50 \text{ mg}}{80 \text{ mg}} \times 1 \text{ mL} = 0.625 \text{ mL or } 0.63 \text{ mL}$$

14. $300 \text{ mg} : 2 \text{ mL} :: 600 \text{ mg} : x \text{ mL}$

$$300x = 1200$$
$$x = \frac{1200}{300}$$
$$x = 4 \text{ mL}$$

$$\frac{600 \text{ mg}}{300 \text{ mg}} \times 2 \text{ mL} = \frac{1200}{300} = 4 \text{ mL}$$

15. $1000 \text{ mg} : 50 \text{ mL} :: 300 \text{ mg} : x \text{ mL}$

$$1000x = 15{,}000$$
$$x = \frac{15{,}000}{1000}$$
$$x = 15 \text{ mL}$$

$$\frac{300 \text{ mg}}{\overset{}{\cancel{1000}}_{20} \text{ mg}} \times \frac{\overset{1}{\cancel{50}} \text{ mL}}{1} = \frac{300}{20} = 15 \text{ mL}$$

16. $10 \text{ mg} : 1 \text{ mL} :: 6 \text{ mg} : x \text{ mL}$

$$10x = 6$$
$$x = \frac{6}{10}$$
$$x = 0.6 \text{ mL}$$

$$\frac{6 \text{ mg}}{10 \text{ mg}} \times 1 \text{ mL} = 0.6 \text{ mL}$$

17. $10 \text{ mg} : 1 \text{ mL} :: 6 \text{ mg} : x \text{ mL}$

$$10x = 6$$
$$x = \frac{6}{10}$$
$$x = 0.6 \text{ mL}$$

$$\frac{6 \text{ mg}}{10 \text{ mg}} \times 1 \text{ mL} = 0.6 \text{ mL}$$

Proportion	Formula
18. 40 mg : 4 mL :: 20 mg : x mL $40x = 80$ $x = \frac{80}{40}$ $x = 2$ mL	$\frac{20 \text{ mg}}{40 \text{ mg}} \times 4 \text{ mL} =$ $\frac{20}{\cancel{40}_{4}} \times \frac{\cancel{4}^{1}}{1} = \frac{20}{10}$ $\frac{20}{10} = 2$ mL

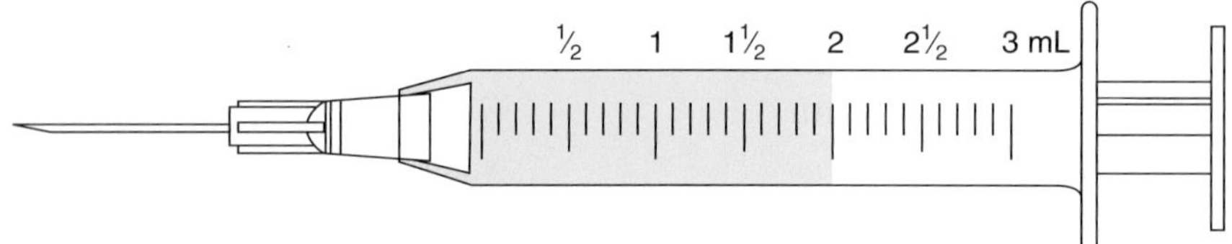

Proportion	Formula
19. 0.5 mg : 2 mL :: 0.3 mg : x mL $0.5x = 0.6$ $x = \frac{0.6}{0.5}$ $x = 1.2$ mL	$\frac{0.3 \text{ mg}}{0.5 \text{ mg}} \times 2 \text{ mL} = \frac{0.6}{0.5} = 1.2$ mL
20. 2.5 mg : 1 mL :: 5 mg : x mL $2.5x = 5$ $x = \frac{5}{2.5}$ $x = 2$ mL	$\frac{5 \text{ mg}}{2.5 \text{ mg}} \times 1 \text{ mL} = 2$ mL

CHAPTER 12 Proportion/Formula Method—Posttest 2, pp. 327–332

Proportion	Formula
1. 4 mg : 1 mL :: 2 mg : x mL $4x = 2$ $x = \frac{2}{4}$ $x = 0.5$ mL	$\frac{2 \text{ mg}}{4 \text{ mg}} \times 1 \text{ mL} = 0.5$ mL
2. 4 mg : 1 mL :: 2 mg : x mL $4x = 2$ $x = \frac{2}{4}$ $x = 0.5$ mL	$\frac{2 \text{ mg}}{4 \text{ mg}} \times 1 \text{ mL} = 0.5$ mL
3. 500 mg : 10 mL :: 400 mg : x mL $500x = 4000$ $x = \frac{4000}{500}$ $x = 8$ mL	$\frac{\cancel{400}^{4} \text{ mg}}{\cancel{500}_{5} \text{ mg}} \times 10 \text{ mL} = \frac{40}{5} = 8$ mL

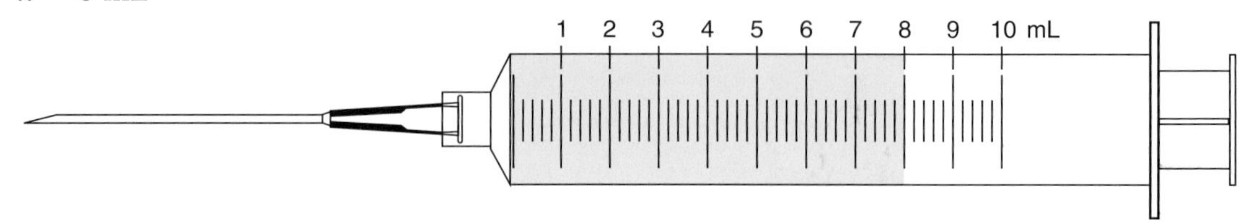

ANSWERS

Proportion	Formula
4. $5 \text{ mg} : 1 \text{ mL} :: 20 \text{ mg} : x \text{ mL}$ $5x = 20$ $x = \frac{20}{5}$ $x = 4 \text{ mL}$	$\frac{20 \text{ mg}}{5 \text{ mg}} \times 1 \text{ mL} = 4 \text{ mL}$
5. $30 \text{ mg} : 1 \text{ mL} :: 60 \text{ mg} : x \text{ mL}$ $30x = 60$ $x = \frac{60}{30}$ $x = 2 \text{ mL}$	$\frac{60 \text{ mg}}{30 \text{ mg}} \times 1 \text{ mL} = 2 \text{ mL}$
6. $100 \text{ mg} : 1 \text{ mL} :: 200 \text{ mg} : x \text{ mL}$ $100x = 200$ $x = \frac{200}{100}$ $x = 2 \text{ mL}$	$\frac{200 \text{ mg}}{100 \text{ mg}} \times 1 \text{ mL} = 2 \text{ mL}$

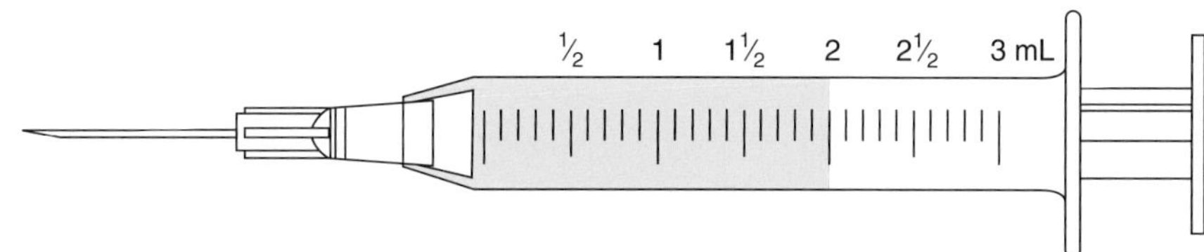

Proportion	Formula
7. $0.4 \text{ mg} : 1 \text{ mL} :: 0.2 \text{ mg} : x \text{ mL}$ $0.4x = 0.2$ $x = \frac{0.2}{0.4}$ $x = 0.5 \text{ mL}$	$\frac{0.2 \text{ mg}}{0.4 \text{ mg}} \times 1 \text{ mL} = 0.5 \text{ mL}$
8. $50 \text{ mg} : 1 \text{ mL} :: 25 \text{ mg} : x \text{ mL}$ $50x = 25$ $x = \frac{25}{50}$ $x = 0.5 \text{ mL}$	$\frac{25 \text{ mg}}{50 \text{ mg}} \times 1 \text{ mL} = 0.5 \text{ mL}$

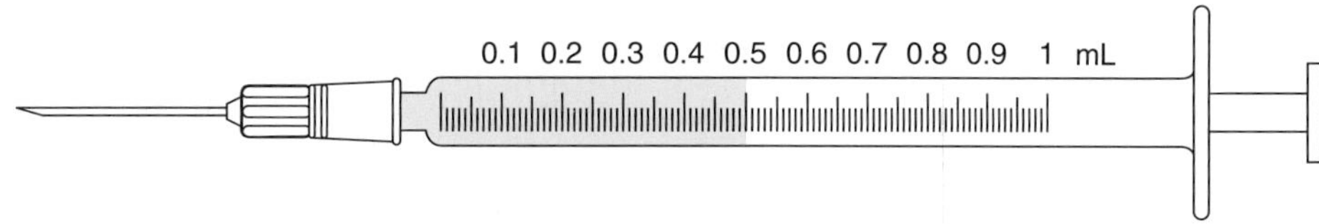

Proportion	Formula
9. $20 \text{ mg} : 1 \text{ mL} :: 100 \text{ mg} : x \text{ mL}$ $20x = 100$ $x = \frac{100}{20}$ $x = 5 \text{ mL}$	$\frac{100 \text{ mg}}{20 \text{ mg}} \times 1 \text{ mL} = 5 \text{ mL}$

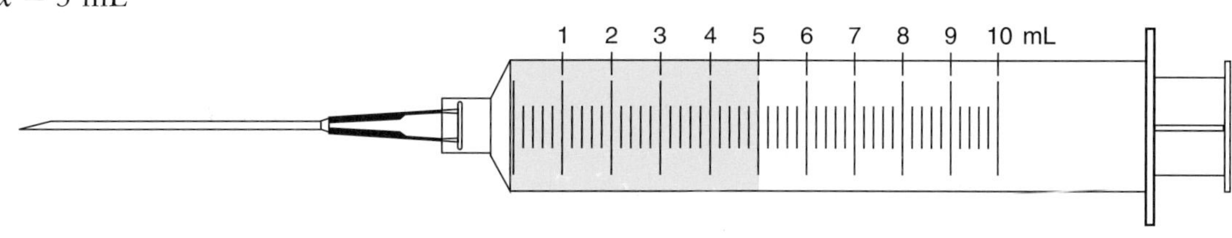

Proportion	Formula
10. 50 mg : 1 mL :: 75 mg : x mL $50x = 75$ $x = \frac{75}{50}$ $x = 1.5$ mL	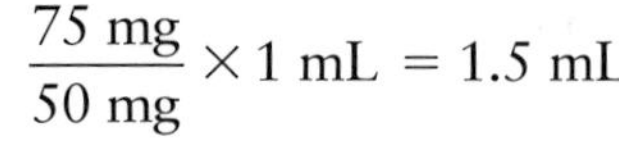 $\frac{75\text{ mg}}{50\text{ mg}} \times 1\text{ mL} = 1.5\text{ mL}$

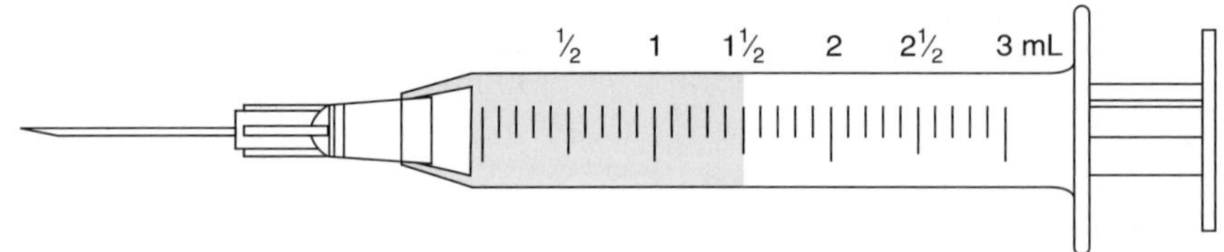

11. 50 mcg : 1 mL :: 70 mcg : x mL $50x = 70$ $x = \frac{70}{50}$ $x = 1.4$ mL	$\frac{70\text{ mcg}}{50\text{ mcg}} \times 1\text{ mL} = 1.4\text{ mL}$

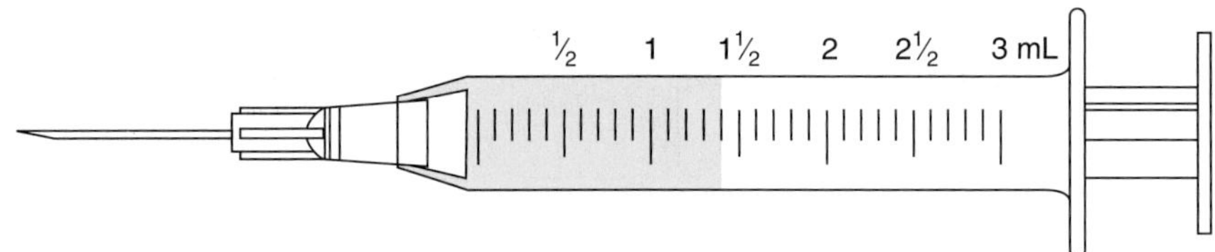

12. 0.3 mg : 1 mL :: 0.4 mg : x mL $0.3x = 0.4$ $x = \frac{0.4}{0.3}$ $x = 1.33$ mL or 1.3 mL	$\frac{0.4\text{ mg}}{0.3\text{ mg}} \times 1\text{ mL} = 1.33\text{ mL or } 1.3\text{ mL}$
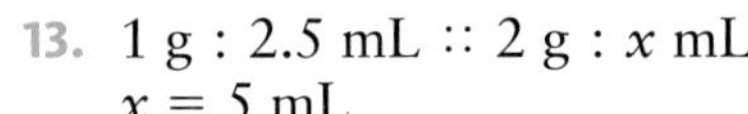 13. 1 g : 2.5 mL :: 2 g : x mL $x = 5$ mL	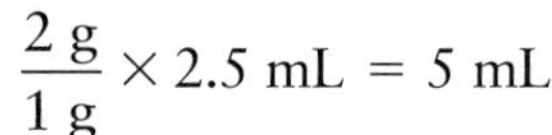 $\frac{2\text{ g}}{1\text{ g}} \times 2.5\text{ mL} = 5\text{ mL}$

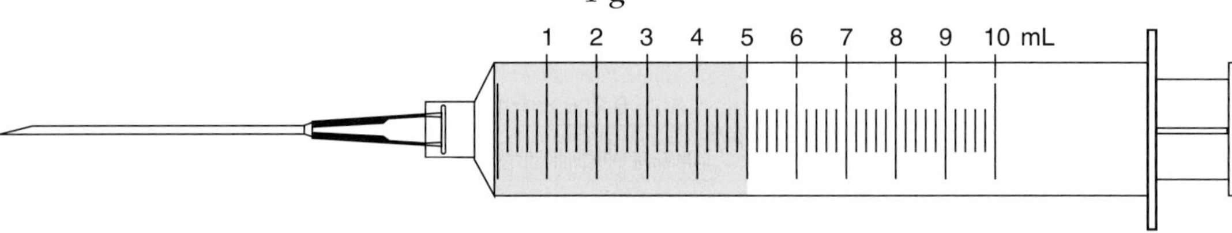

14. 40 mg : 1 mL :: 26 mg : x mL $40x = 26$ $x = \frac{26}{40}$ $x = 0.65$ mL	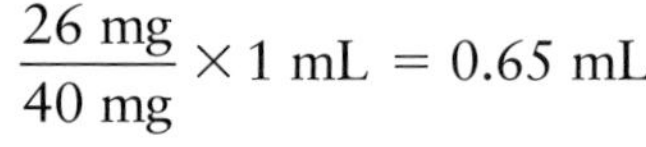 $\frac{26\text{ mg}}{40\text{ mg}} \times 1\text{ mL} = 0.65\text{ mL}$

ANSWERS

Proportion	Formula
15. 40 mg : 0.4 mL :: 85 mg : x mL $40x = 34$ $x = \frac{34}{40}$ $x = 0.85$ mL	$\frac{85 \text{ mg}}{100 \text{ mg}} \times 1 \text{ mL} = 0.85 \text{ mL}$
16. 500 mcg : 2 mL :: 80 mcg : x mL $500x = 160$ $x = \frac{160}{500}$ $x = 0.32$ mL	$\frac{80 \text{ mcg}}{500 \text{ mcg}} \times 2 \text{ mL} = \frac{160}{500} = 0.32 \text{ mL}$
17. 8 mg : 1 mL :: 4 mg : x mL $8x = 4$ $x = \frac{4}{8}$ $x = 0.5$ mL	$\frac{4 \text{ mg}}{8 \text{ mg}} \times 1 \text{ mL} = 0.5 \text{ mL}$

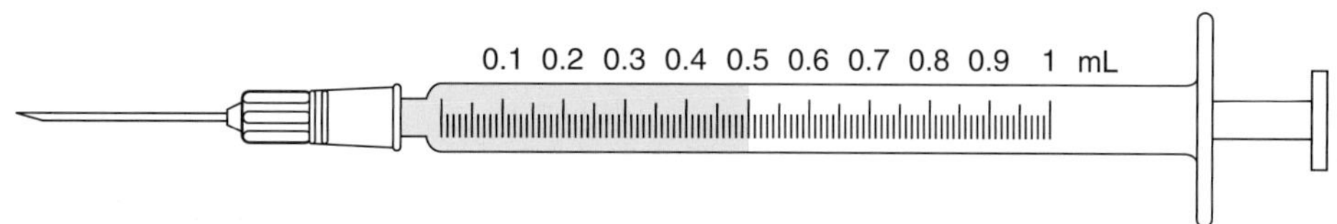

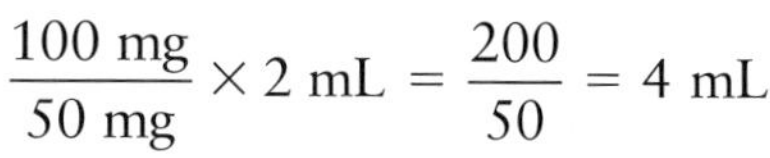

Proportion	Formula
18. 50 mg : 2 mL :: 100 mg : x mL $50x = 200$ $x = \frac{200}{50}$ $x = 4$ mL	$\frac{100 \text{ mg}}{50 \text{ mg}} \times 2 \text{ mL} = \frac{200}{50} = 4 \text{ mL}$

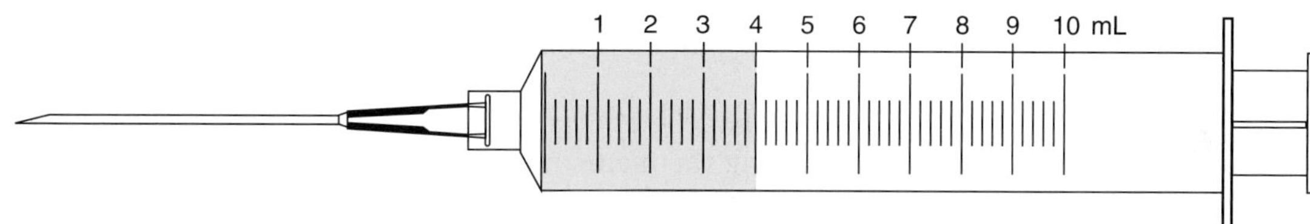

Proportion	Formula
19. 400 mg : 100 mL :: 300 mg : x mL $400x = 30{,}000$ $x = \frac{30{,}000}{400}$ $x = 75$ mL	$\frac{300 \text{ mg}}{400 \text{ mg}} \times 100 \text{ mL} =$ $\frac{300}{\underset{4}{\cancel{400}}} \times \frac{\overset{1}{\cancel{100}}}{1} = \frac{300}{4}$ $\frac{300}{40} = 75 \text{ mL}$
20. 13.6 mEq : 10 mL :: 10 mEq : x mL $13.6x = 100$ $x = \frac{100}{13.6}$ $x = 7.35$ mL or 7.4 mL	$\frac{10 \text{ mEq}}{13.6 \text{ mEq}} \times 10 \text{ mL} = \frac{100}{13.6}$ $= 7.35$ mL or 7.4 mL

ANSWERS

CHAPTER 13

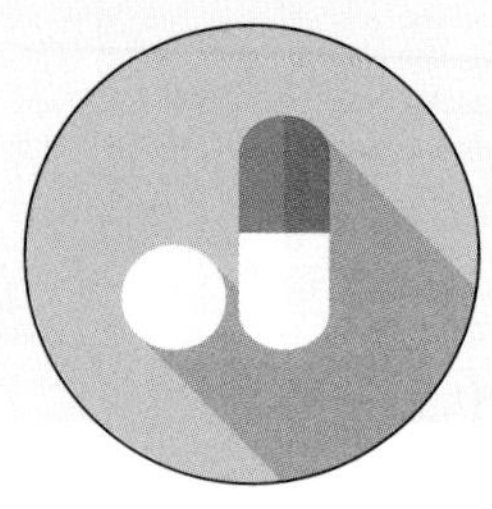

Dosages Measured in Units

LEARNING OBJECTIVES

Upon completion of the materials provided in this chapter, you will be able to perform computations accurately by mastering the following mathematical concepts:

1. Solving problems involving drugs measured in unit dosages
2. Drawing a line through an insulin syringe to indicate the number of units desired

A unit is the amount of a drug needed to produce a given result. Various drugs are measured in units; the examples used in this chapter are among the more common drugs prescribed.

Drugs used in this chapter include:

Epogen—A drug that increases the production of red blood cells
Fragmin—An anticoagulant that prevents the clotting of blood
Heparin—An anticoagulant that inhibits clotting of the blood
Insulin—A hormone secreted by the pancreas that lowers blood glucose

Epogen is a drug that helps to combat the effects of anemia caused by chemotherapy or chronic renal failure. After administering the medicine, the nurse should monitor the patient's blood pressure and laboratory results on a routine basis.

Fragmin is used in the prevention of deep vein thrombosis after abdominal surgery, hip replacements, and unstable angina/non–Q wave myocardial infarction. It may also be used with patients who have restricted mobility during an acute illness. Fragmin may only be given by subcutaneous injections—never intramuscularly or intravenously. The patient's blood studies must be monitored on a routine basis during treatment with Fragmin.

Because heparin prolongs the time blood takes to clot, the dosage must be accurate. A larger dose may cause hemorrhage, and an insufficient dose may not have the desired result. After administering the drug, the nurse should observe the patient for signs of hemorrhage.

INSULIN

Insulin is used in the treatment of diabetes mellitus. Accuracy is important in the preparation of insulin. A higher dosage than needed may cause insulin shock. An insufficient amount of insulin may result in diabetic coma. Both conditions are extremely serious, and the nurse must be able to recognize the symptoms of each condition so that immediate treatment can be initiated to stabilize the patient. In many institutions, both insulin and heparin dosages are checked for accuracy by another nurse before the drug is administered to the patient. Figure 13-1 shows examples of different types of insulin.

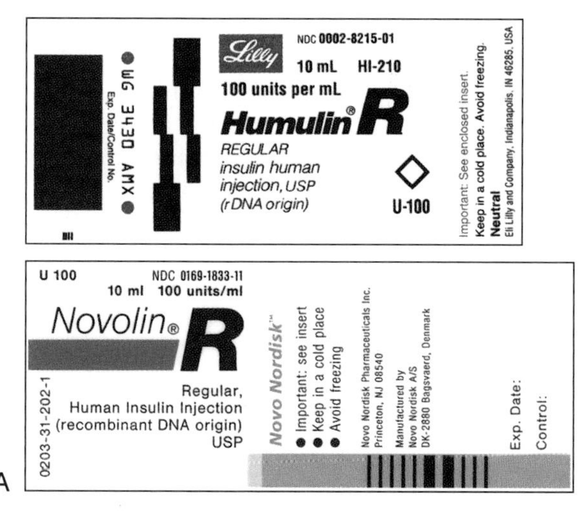

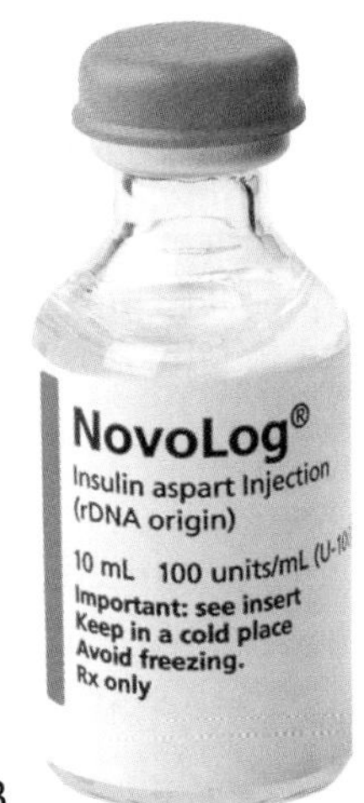

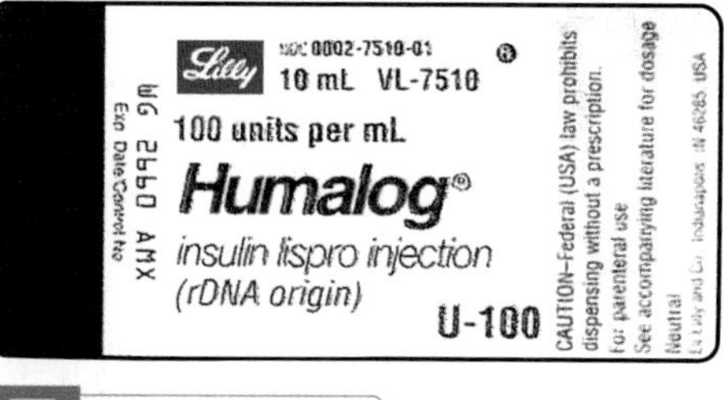

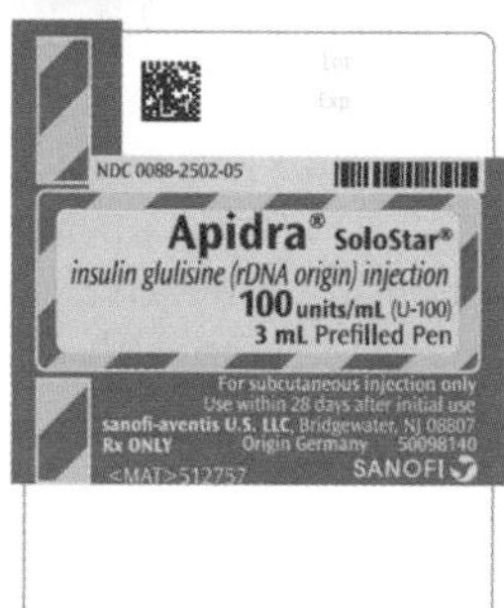

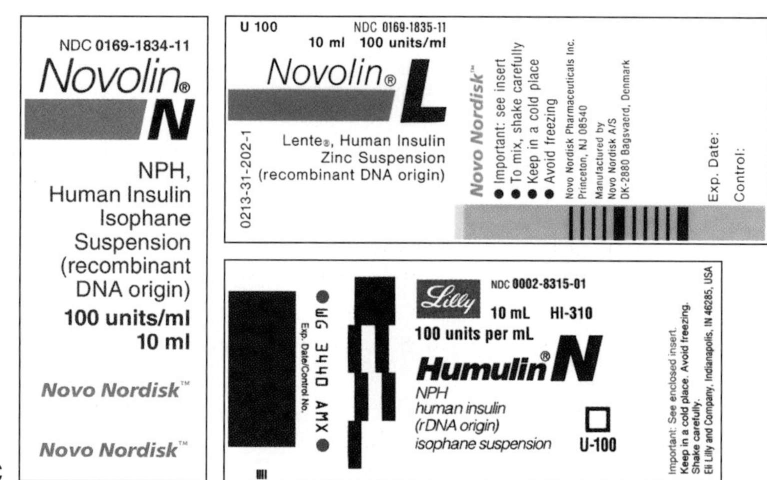

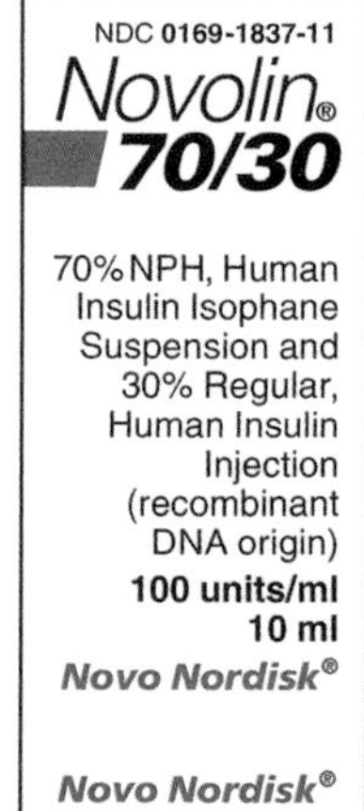

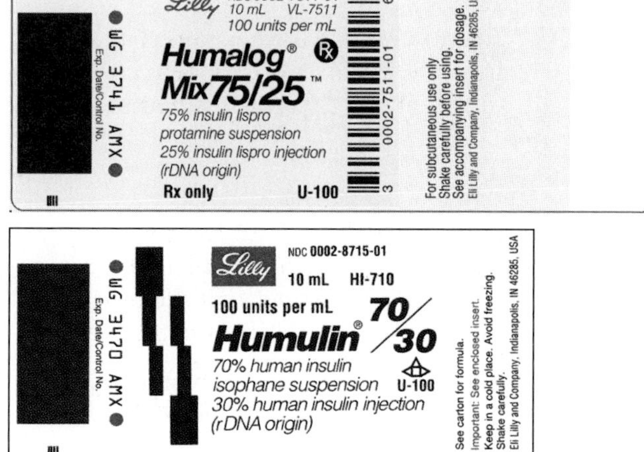

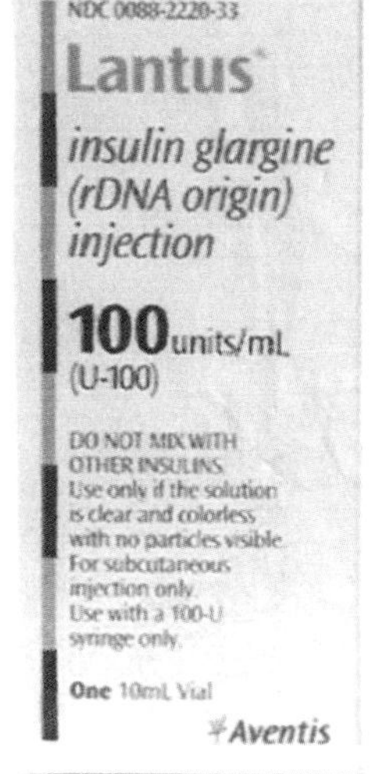

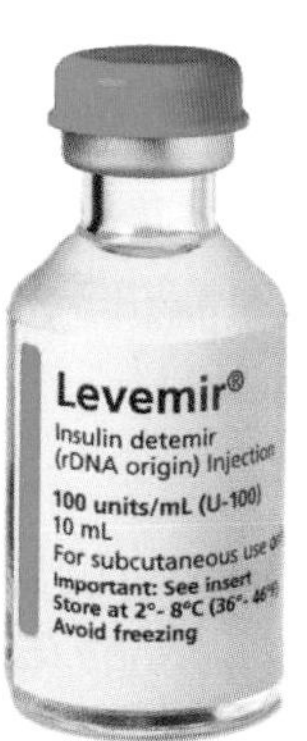

FIGURE 13-1 Examples of different types of insulins. **A,** Short-acting. **B,** Rapid-acting. **C,** Intermediate-acting. **D,** Intermediate- and rapid-acting mixture. **E,** Long-acting. (**B** and **E,** from Novo Nordisk Inc., Princeton, NJ.)

Insulin Syringes

Insulin syringes were developed specifically for the administration of insulin. They are calibrated in units and are available in 30 units, 50 units, and 100 units (Figure 13-2). A U-100 insulin syringe and U-100 insulin are necessary to ensure an accurate insulin dosage. U-100 insulin means that 100 units of insulin are contained in 1 mL of liquid. U-100 insulin is a universal insulin preparation that all persons requiring insulin can use. Another type of U-100 syringe is the U-100 Lo-Dose syringe, which measures 50 units; however, for accuracy, no more than 40 units should be measured in the U-100 Lo-Dose syringe. Because the doses are minute, the U-100 syringe provides the most accurate measurement of insulin dosages. The 30-unit U-100 syringe is used for insulin doses that equal less than 30 units.

IMPORTANT NOTE: Only insulin is measured and given in the syringes that are marked in units. Only regular insulin can be given intravenously. Heparin and other medication measured in units can be measured and given only in syringes marked in milliliters.

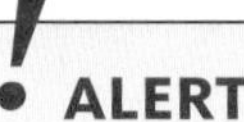

ALERT

Only insulin is measured and given in insulin syringes.

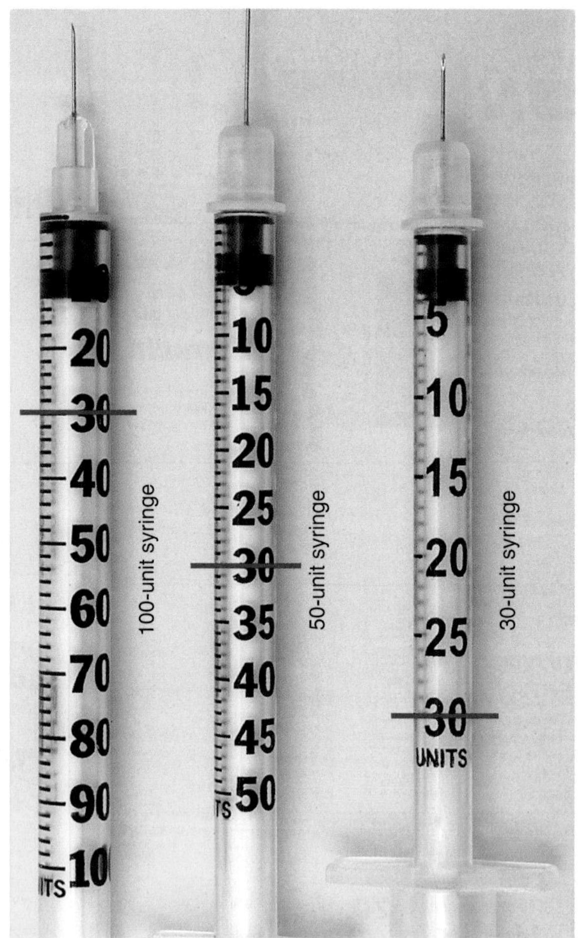

FIGURE 13-2 *Left to right:* 30 units measured on a 100-unit syringe (each calibration is 2 units), a 50-unit syringe (each calibration is 1 unit), and 30-unit syringe (each calibration is 1 unit). (From Macklin D, Chernecky C, Infortuna H: *Math for clinical practice,* ed 2, St Louis, 2011, Mosby.)

Insulin Pens

Insulin is also available in prefilled insulin pens. The insulin pens require a special needle to be attached. Each insulin pen contains a dial for choosing the desired number of units to be administered. For example, if 6 units of NovoLog insulin are desired, the dial on the NovoLog insulin pen would be turned to the Number 6. See Figure 13-3 for examples of insulin pens.

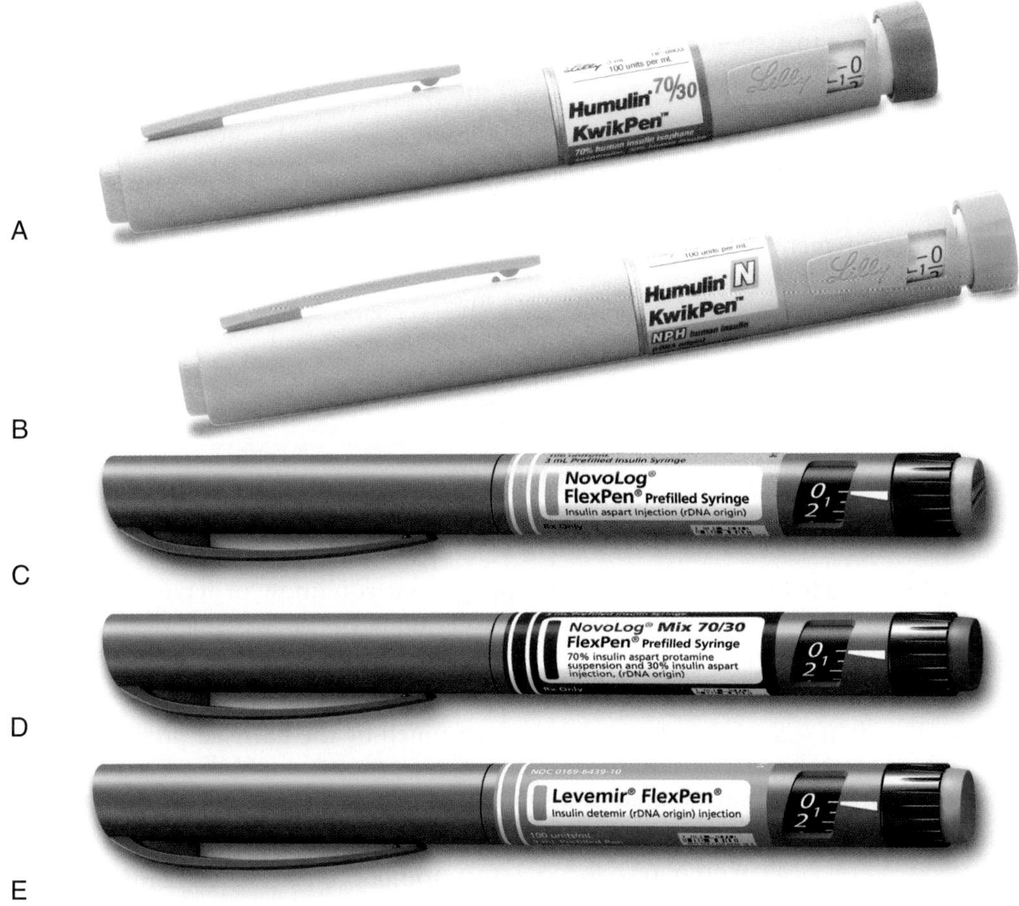

FIGURE 13-3 Prefilled insulin pens. **A,** Humulin 70/30 KwikPen™ short- and intermediate acting. **B,** Humulin KwikPen™ intermediate-acting. **C,** NovoLog® rapid-acting. **D,** NovoLog® 70/30 short- and intermediate-acting. **E,** Levemir® long-acting. (**A** and **B**, Copyright Eli Lilly and Company. All rights reserved. Used with permission. **C-E**, From Novo Nordisk Inc., Princeton, NJ.)

Dosages Measured in Units Involving Oral Medications

EXAMPLE: The licensed prescriber orders mycostatin 400,000 units po four times a day. The drug is supplied as 100,000 units/mL after reconstitution. How many milliliters will the nurse administer?

Using the Dimensional Analysis Method

Step 1. On the left side of the equation, place what you are solving for:

$$x \text{ mL} =$$

Step 2. On the right side of the equation, place the available information related to the measurement or abbreviation that was placed on the left side. In this example, the measurement we are solving for is *mL*. This information is placed in the equation as part of a fraction; match the appropriate abbreviation. Remember that the abbreviation that matches the x quantity must be placed in the numerator.

$$x\ \textbf{mL} = \frac{\textbf{1 mL}}{\text{100,000 units}}$$

Step 3. Next, find the information that matches the measurement used in the denominator of the fraction you created. In this example, *units* is in the denominator, so 400,000 units is used.

$$x\ \text{mL} = \frac{1\ \text{mL}}{100{,}000\ \text{units}} \times \frac{400{,}000\ \text{units}}{1}$$

Step 4. Then cancel out the abbreviations on the right side of the equation. If you have set up the problem correctly, the remaining measurement should match the measurement on the left side of the equation. Now solve for x.

$$x\ \text{mL} = \frac{1\ \text{mL}}{100{,}000\ \cancel{\text{units}}} \times \frac{400{,}000\ \cancel{\text{units}}}{1}$$

$$x\ \text{mL} = \frac{400{,}000}{100{,}000}$$

$$x = 4\ \text{mL}$$

Using the Proportion Method

Step 1. On the left side of the proportion, place what you know or have available. In this example, each milliliter contains 100,000 units. So the left side of the proportion would be

$$100{,}000\ \text{units} : 1\ \text{mL} ::$$

Step 2. The right side of the proportion is determined by the licensed prescriber's order and the abbreviations on the left side of the proportion. Only *two* different abbreviations may be used in a single proportion. The abbreviations must be in the same position on the right side as on the left side.

$$100{,}000\ \text{units} : 1\ \text{mL} :: 400{,}000\ \text{units} : \underline{\hspace{2em}}\ \text{mL}$$

We need to find the number of milliliters to be administered, so we use the symbol x to represent the unknown.

$$100{,}000\ \text{units} : 1\ \text{mL} :: 400{,}000\ \text{units} : x\ \text{mL}$$

Step 3. Rewrite the proportion without the abbreviations.

$$100{,}000 : 1 :: 400{,}000 : x$$

Step 4. Solve for x.

$$100{,}000 : 1 :: 400{,}000 : x$$

$$100{,}000x = 400{,}000$$

$$x = \frac{400{,}000}{100{,}000}$$

$$x = 4$$

Step 5. Label your answer as determined by the abbreviation placed next to x in the original proportion.

$$x = 4\ \text{mL}$$

The nurse would measure 4 mL to administer 400,000 units of mycostatin.

Dosages Measured in Units Involving Parenteral Medications

EXAMPLE: The licensed prescriber orders heparin 4000 units subcutaneous q 8 h. How many milliliters will the nurse administer?

Using the Dimensional Analysis Method

Step 1. On the left side of the equation, place what you are solving for:

$$x \text{ mL} =$$

Step 2. On the right side of the equation, place the available information related to the measurement or abbreviation that was placed on the left side. In this example, the measurement we are solving for is *mL*. This information is placed in the equation as part of a fraction; match the appropriate abbreviation. Remember that the abbreviation that matches the *x* quantity must be placed in the numerator.

$$x\ \mathbf{mL} = \frac{\mathbf{1\ mL}}{5000 \text{ units}}$$

Step 3. Next, find the information that matches the measurement used in the denominator of the fraction you created. In this example, *units* is in the denominator, so 4000 units is used.

$$x \text{ mL} = \frac{1 \text{ mL}}{5000 \text{ units}} \times \frac{4000 \text{ units}}{1}$$

Step 4. Then cancel out the abbreviations on the right side of the equation. If you have set up the problem correctly, the remaining measurement should match the measurement on the left side of the equation. Now solve for *x*.

$$x \text{ mL} = \frac{1 \text{ mL}}{5000 \cancel{\text{units}}} \times \frac{4000 \cancel{\text{units}}}{1}$$

$$x \text{ mL} = \frac{4000}{5000}$$

$$x = 0.8 \text{ mL}$$

Using the Proportion Method

Step 1. 5000 units : 1 mL ::

Step 2. 5000 units : 1 mL :: _______ units : _______ mL

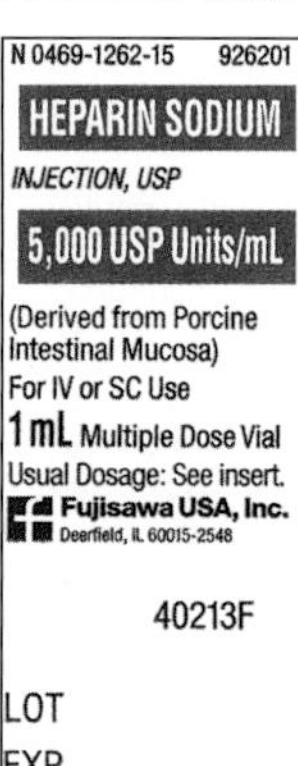

5000 units : 1 mL :: 4000 units : *x* mL

Step 3. $5000 : 1 :: 4000 : x$

Step 4. $5000x = 4000$

$$x = \frac{4000}{5000}$$

$$x = 0.8$$

Step 5. $x = 0.8$ mL

Therefore 0.8 mL of heparin would be the amount of each individual dose of heparin given q 8 h.

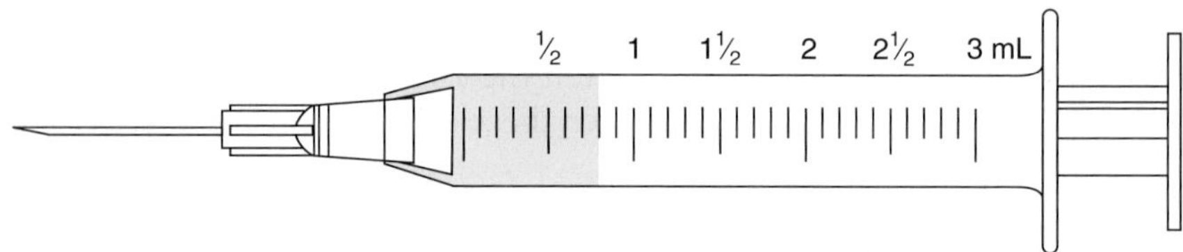

Insulin Given with a Lo-Dose Insulin Syringe

EXAMPLE: The licensed prescriber orders Lantus U-100 insulin 36 units subcutaneous injection in AM. A U-100 Lo-Dose syringe is available. Shade the syringe to indicate the correct dose.

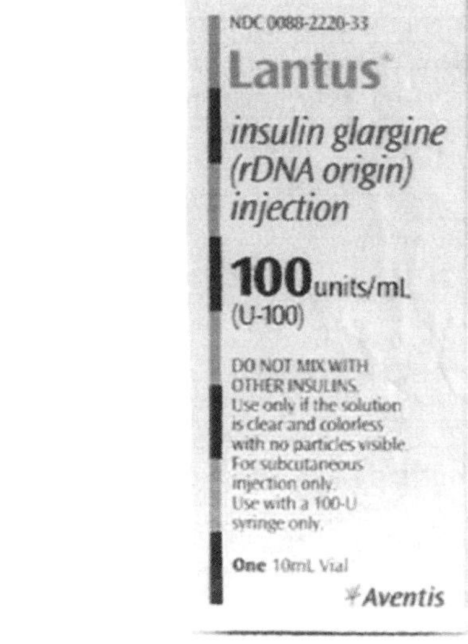

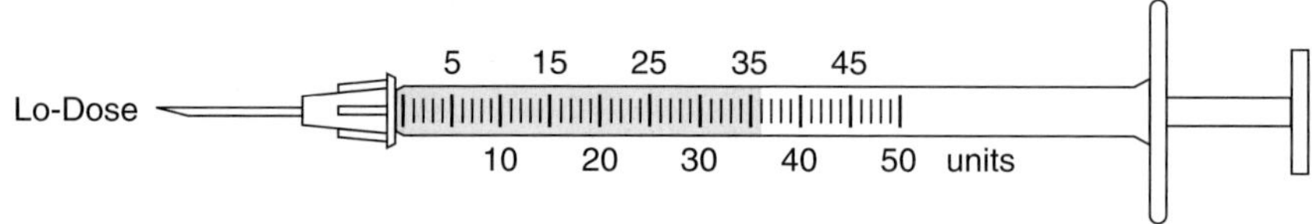

With a Lo-Dose insulin syringe, 36 units of U-100 insulin would be measured as indicated.

Mixed Insulin Administration

The licensed prescriber may prescribe two types of insulin to be administered at the same time. As long as they are compatible, these insulins will be drawn up in the same syringe to avoid injecting the patient twice. The practice of mixing insulins is diminishing as the use of Lantus insulin increases.

Several guidelines apply to this type of administration:

1. Air equal to the amount of insulin being withdrawn should be injected into each vial. Do *not* touch the solution with the tip of the needle.
2. Using the same syringe, draw up the desired amount of insulin from the **regular** insulin bottle first.
3. Remove the syringe from the regular insulin bottle. Check the syringe for any air bubbles and remove them.
4. Using the same syringe, draw up the amount of cloudy insulin to the desired dose.
5. Hospitals usually require that you check your insulin dosages with another nurse before administration. Consult your hospital policy and procedures.

EXAMPLE 1: The licensed prescriber orders Humulin Regular U-100 10 units plus Humulin NPH U-100 20 units subcutaneous now. The syringe is shaded in yellow to indicate the amount of Humulin regular insulin to be given, and in a different color to indicate the total dose.

The total amount of insulin is 30 units (10 units + 20 units = 30 units).

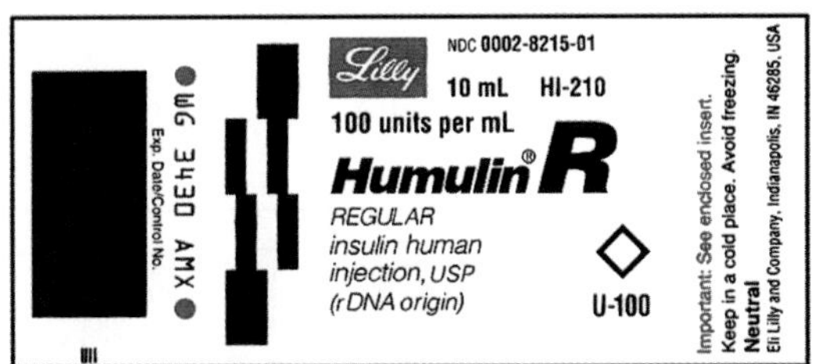

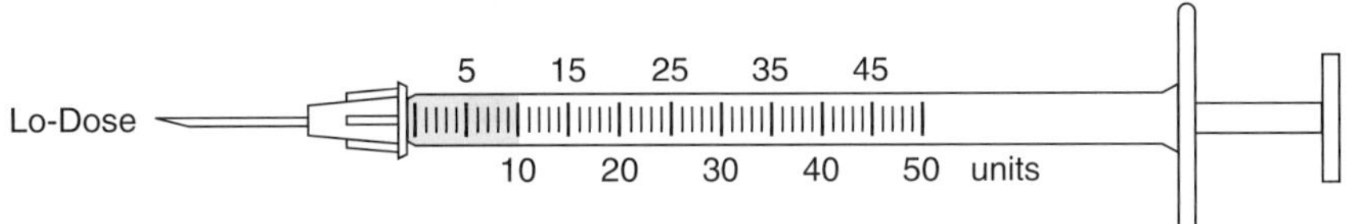

10 units of regular insulin is drawn up first; then 20 units of NPH insulin is drawn up.

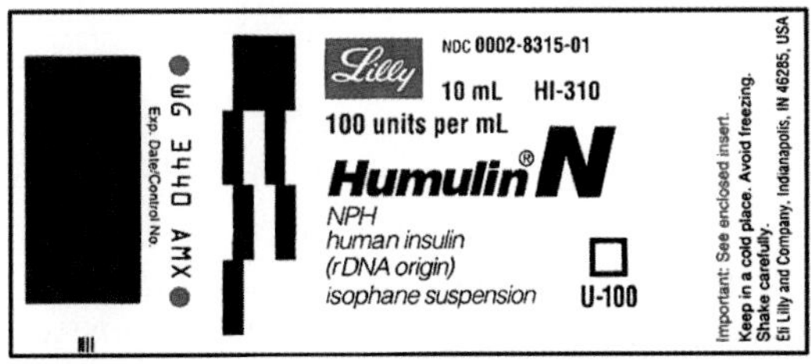

10 units of regular insulin + 20 units of NPH insulin = 30 units of insulin.

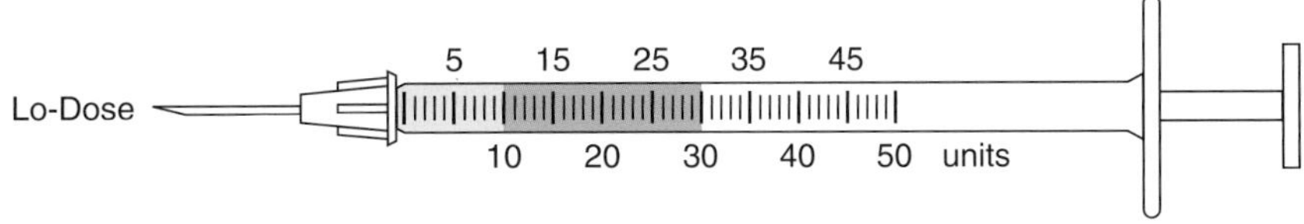

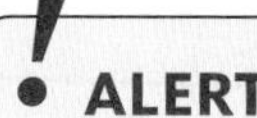

ALERT

Some insulins such as Lantus should never be mixed. Be sure to always check whether an insulin can be mixed with another insulin.

EXAMPLE 2: The licensed prescriber orders Humulin Lente U-100 46 units subcutaneous daily, plus regular Humulin U-100 20 units. A U-100 insulin syringe is available. The syringe is shaded in yellow to indicate the amount of Humulin regular insulin to be given, and in a different color to indicate the total dose.

The total amount of insulin is 66 units (46 units + 20 units = 66 units).

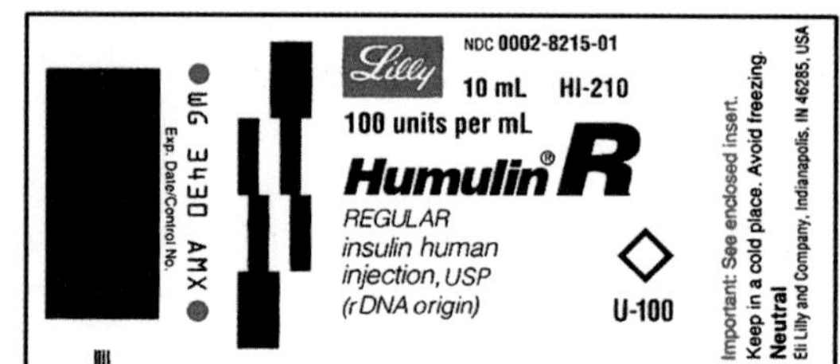

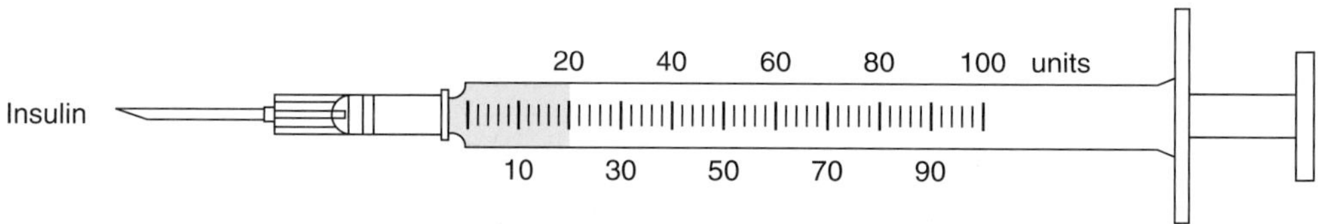

20 units of regular insulin is drawn up first; then 46 units of Lente insulin is drawn up.

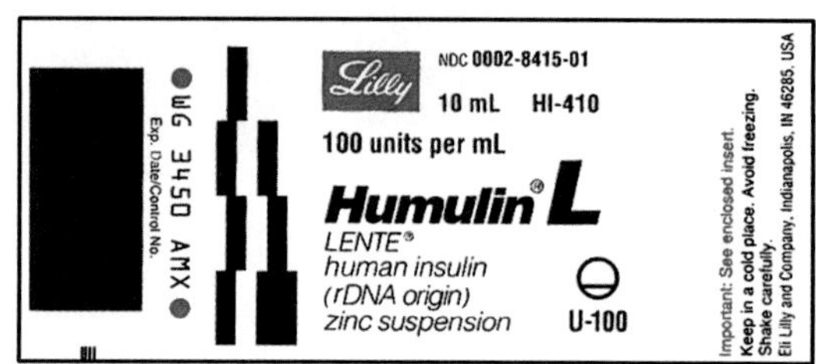

20 units of regular insulin + 46 units of Lente insulin = 66 units of insulin.

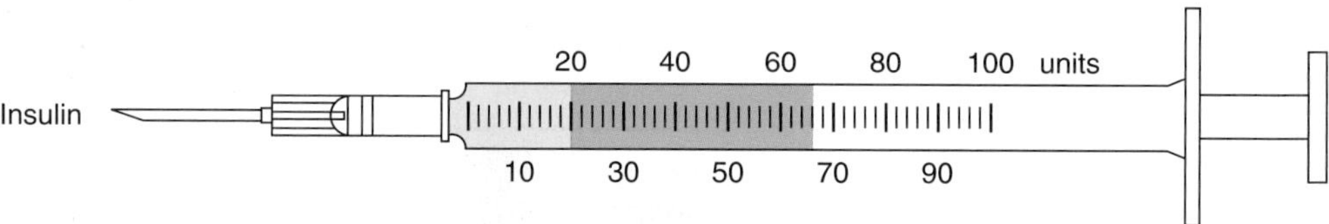

Complete the following work sheet, which provides for extensive practice in the calculation of dosages measured in units. Check your answers. If you have difficulties, go back and review the necessary material. When you feel ready to evaluate your learning, take the first posttest. Check your answers. An acceptable score as indicated on the posttest signifies that you have successfully completed this chapter. An unacceptable score signifies a need for further study before taking the second posttest.

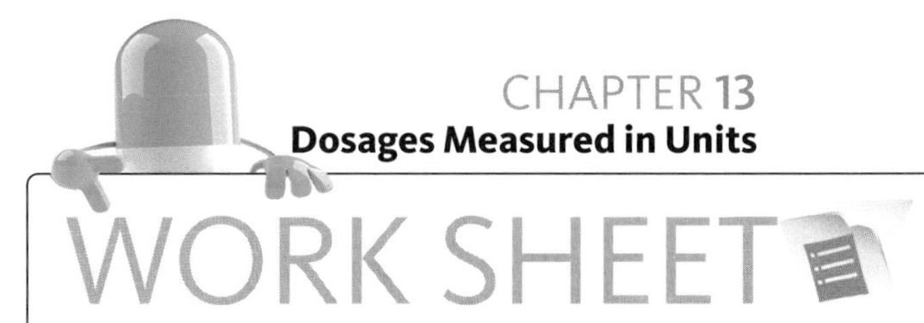

WORK SHEET

DIRECTIONS: The medication order is listed at the beginning of each problem. Calculate the doses. Show your work. Mark the syringe when provided to indicate the correct dose.

1. Mr. Curtis has Epogen 12,000 units subcutaneous injection three times a week to treat anemia related to chemotherapy. How many milliliters will you administer? ______

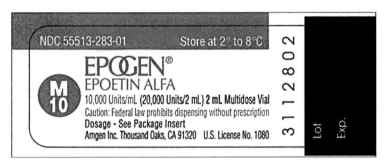

2. The licensed prescriber orders Humalog U-100 insulin 10 units subcutaneous daily at 0800. Draw a vertical line through the syringe to indicate the amount of NPH insulin to be given.

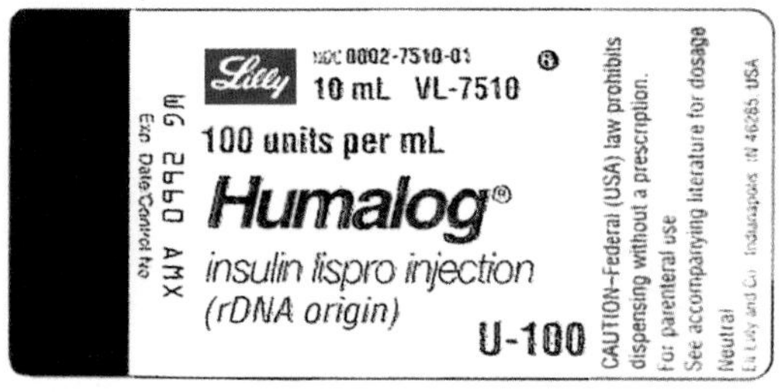

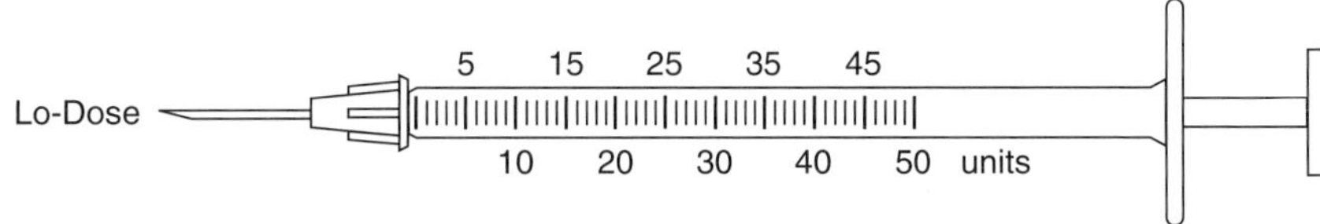

3. Following a right total hip replacement, Mr. Stephens has Fragmin 5000 international units by subcutaneous injection daily ordered. How many milliliters will the nurse administer? ______

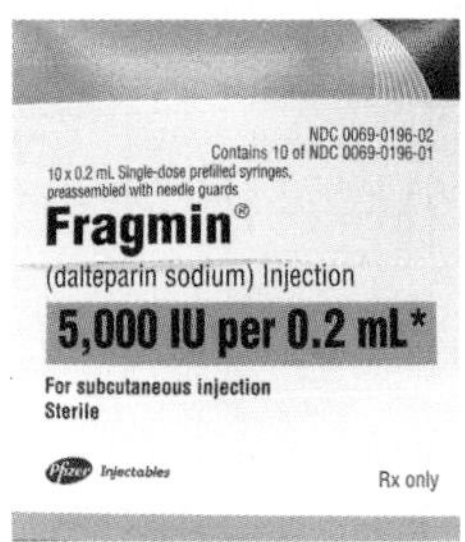

4. The licensed prescriber orders regular Humulin insulin 2 units subcutaneous daily at 1900. Draw a vertical line through the syringe to indicate the dose.

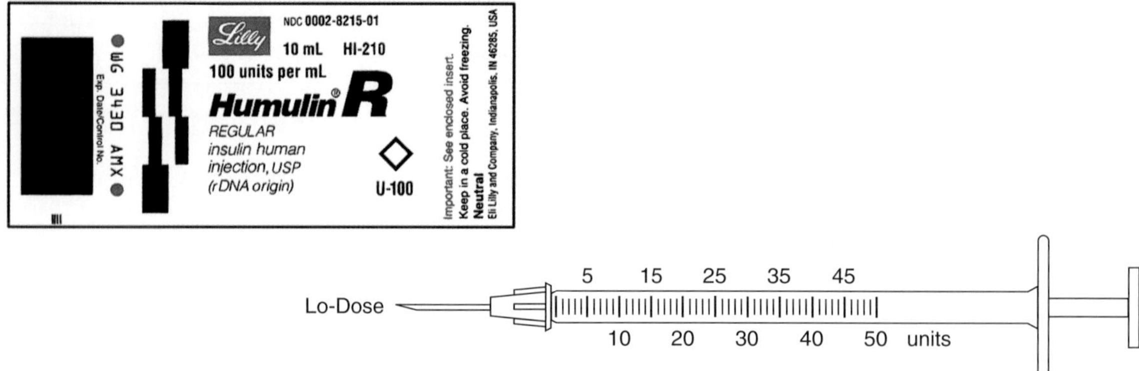

5. Your postoperative patient receives heparin 3000 units subcutaneous q 8 h to prevent deep vein thrombosis. How many milliliters will you administer? ______

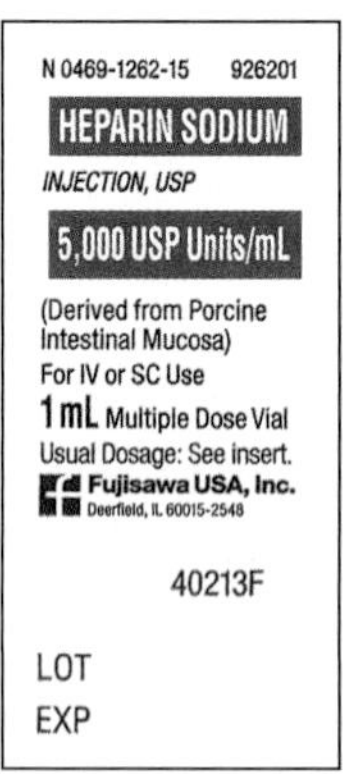

6. The licensed prescriber orders Lente insulin 14 units, regular insulin 6 units subcutaneous every morning. Lente insulin U-100, regular insulin U-100, and a U-100 Lo-Dose syringe are supplied. Draw a vertical line through the syringe to indicate the amount of regular insulin to be given and a second line to indicate the total dose.

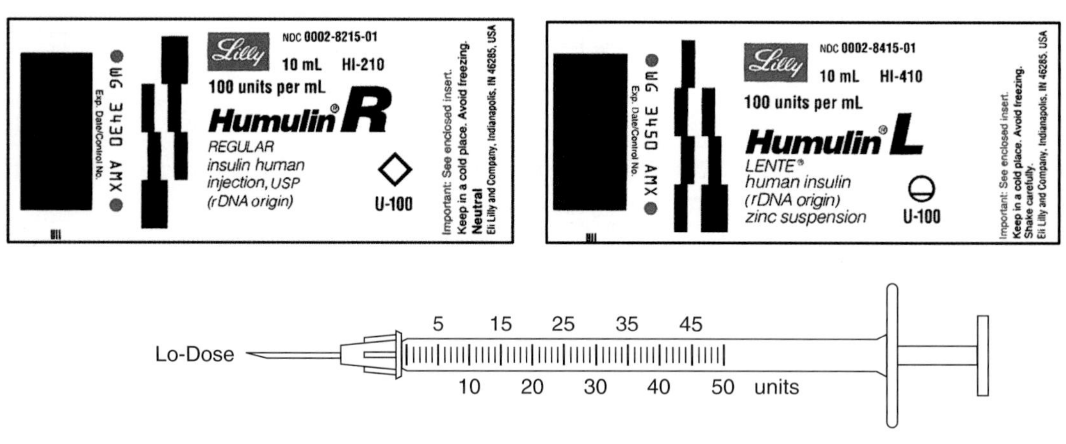

7. Mrs. Alvarez has Epogen 4500 units subcutaneous injection three times a week ordered for anemia caused by chronic renal failure. How many milliliters will you administer? (Round your final answer to the nearest hundredth.) ______

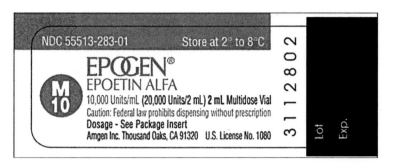

8. The licensed prescriber orders Humulin regular insulin 18 units subcutaneous at 0700 daily. Draw a vertical line through the syringe to indicate the dose.

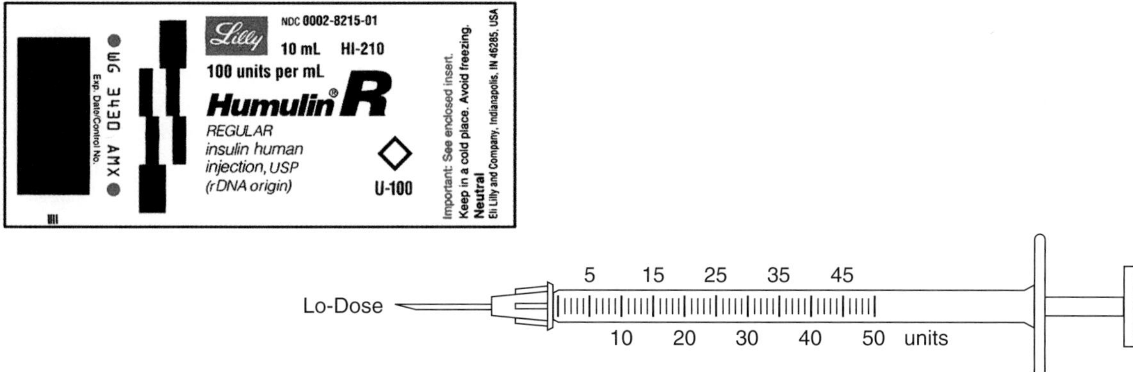

9. The licensed prescriber orders Humulin 70/30 insulin 32 units subcutaneous tomorrow at 0745. Draw a vertical line through the syringe to indicate the dose.

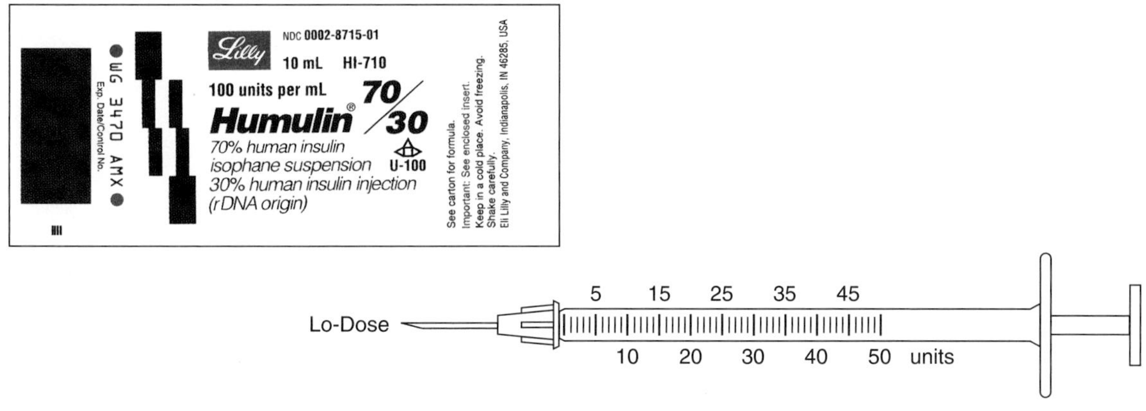

10. Your patient with a stapedectomy receives penicillin V 300,000 units po four times a day. The drug is supplied in oral solution 200,000 units/5 mL. How many milliliters will you administer? ______

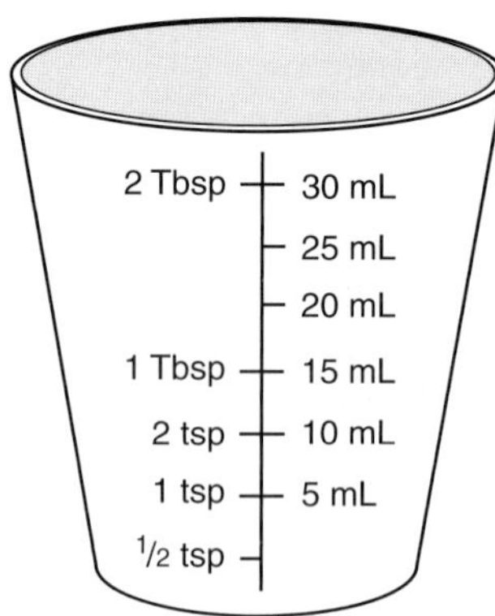

11. Your patient with insulin-dependent diabetes receives Humulin U Insulin 24 units subcutaneously every morning. Draw a vertical line through the syringe to indicate the dose.

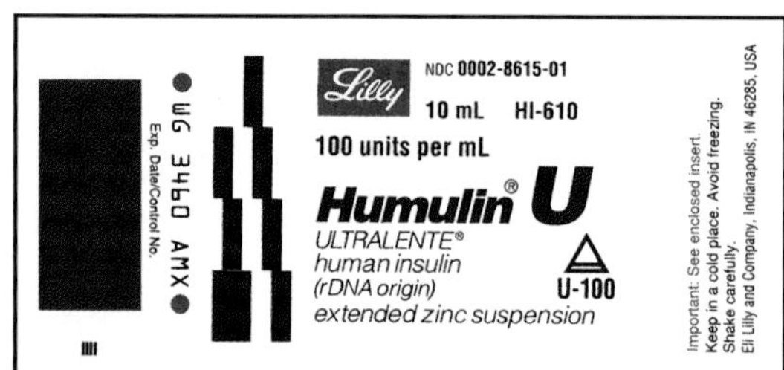

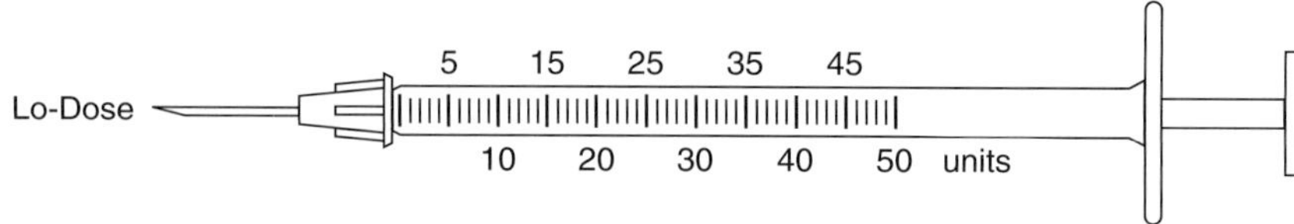

12. Your postoperative patient receives heparin 4000 units subcutaneous injection now. Draw a vertical line through the syringe to indicate the dose.

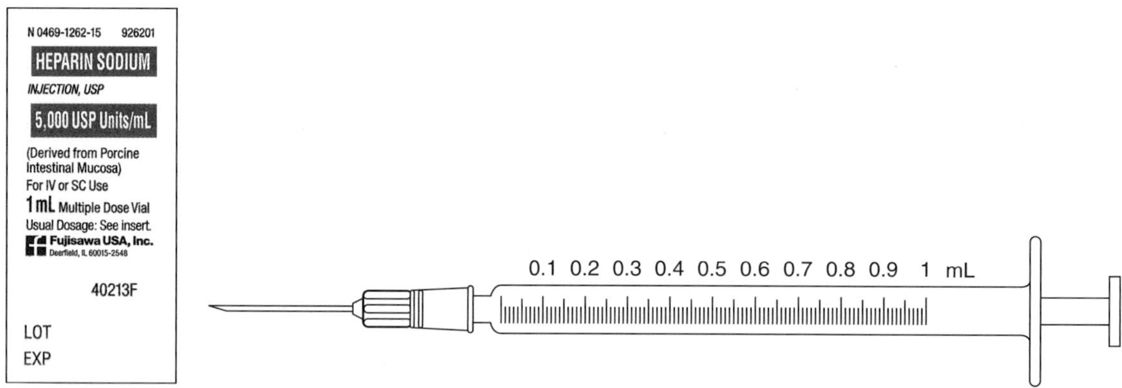

13. Your patient with a gastric pull-up receives penicillin G 200,000 units IM q 6 h. You have penicillin G 250,000 units/mL available. How many milliliters will you administer? ______ Draw a vertical line through the syringe to indicate the dose.

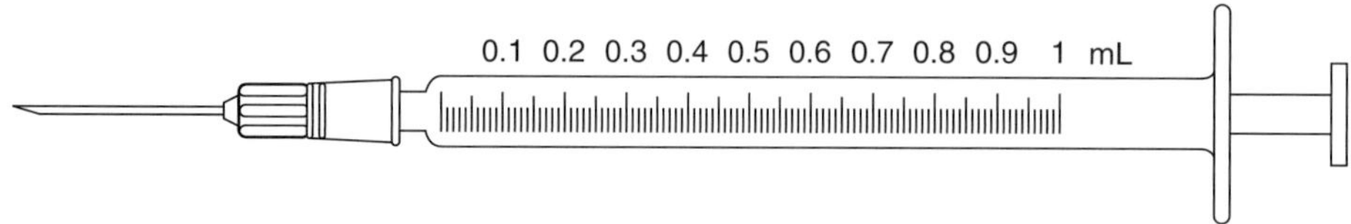

14. Mrs. Schroeder has orders for Fragmin 5500 international units by subcutaneous injection twice a day for system anticoagulation. You have Fragmin 10,000 international units/mL. How many milliliters will you administer? (Round your final answer to the nearest hundredth.) ______

15. The licensed prescriber orders Humulin regular insulin 40 units and Humulin NPH 35 units every morning before breakfast. Draw a vertical line through the syringe to indicate the dosage for regular Humulin first; then draw a second line to indicate the total dose with the Humulin NPH.

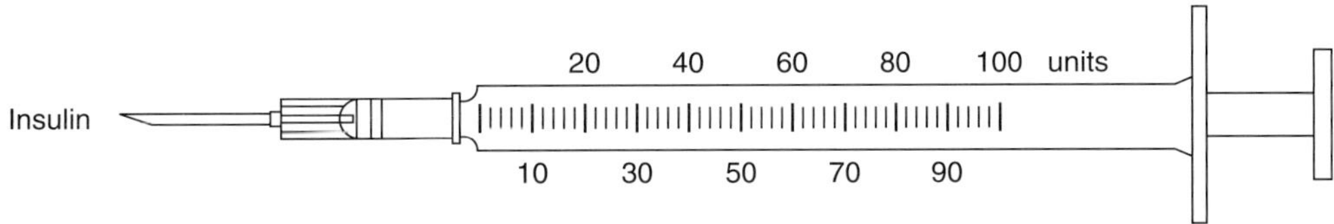

16. The licensed prescriber orders heparin 2500 units subcutaneous q 12 h for your patient with a jejunostomy. How many milliliters will you administer? ______ Draw a vertical line through the syringe to indicate the dose.

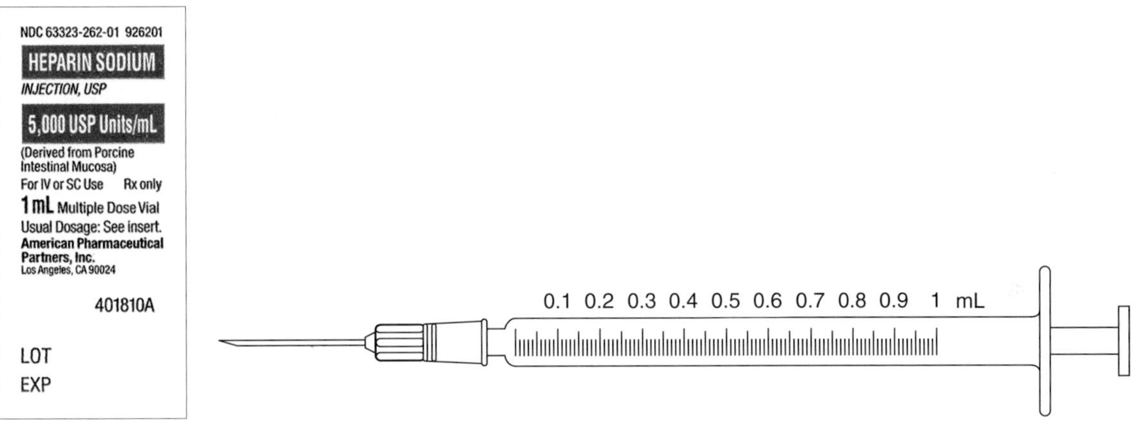

17. The licensed prescriber orders 24 units Humulin U subcutaneous injection now. Draw a vertical line through the syringe to indicate the dose.

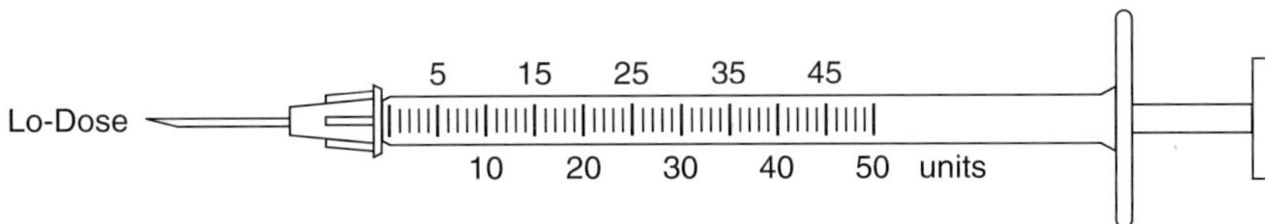

18. The licensed prescriber orders Humulin 50/50 70 units subcutaneous injection. Draw a vertical line through the syringe to indicate the dose.

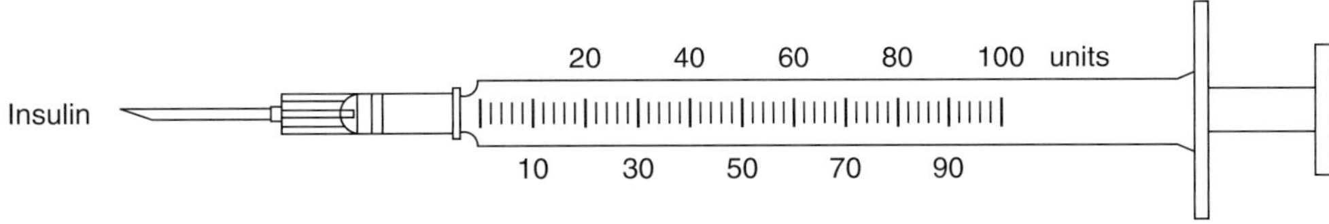

19. The licensed prescriber orders 60 units Lantus U-100 subcutaneous injection daily at bedtime. Draw a vertical line through the syringe to indicate the dose.

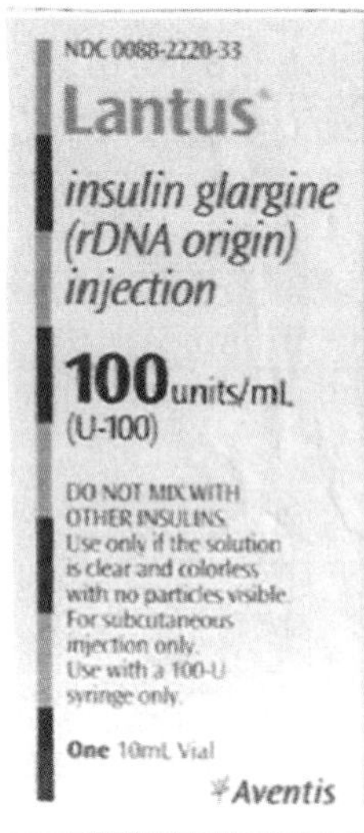

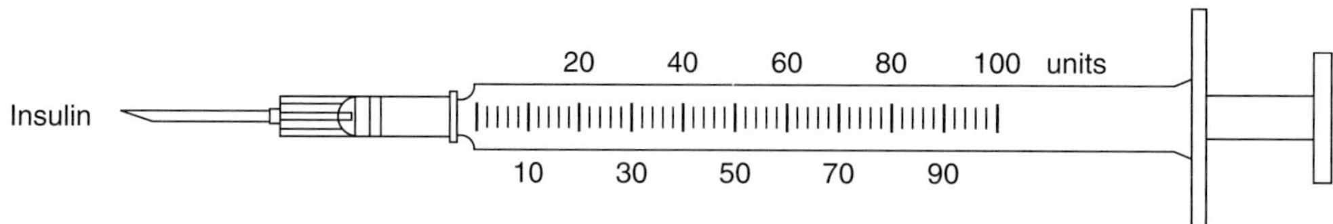

20. The licensed prescriber orders 14 units NovoLog U-100 subcutaneous injection daily at bedtime. Draw a vertical line through the syringe to indicate the dose.

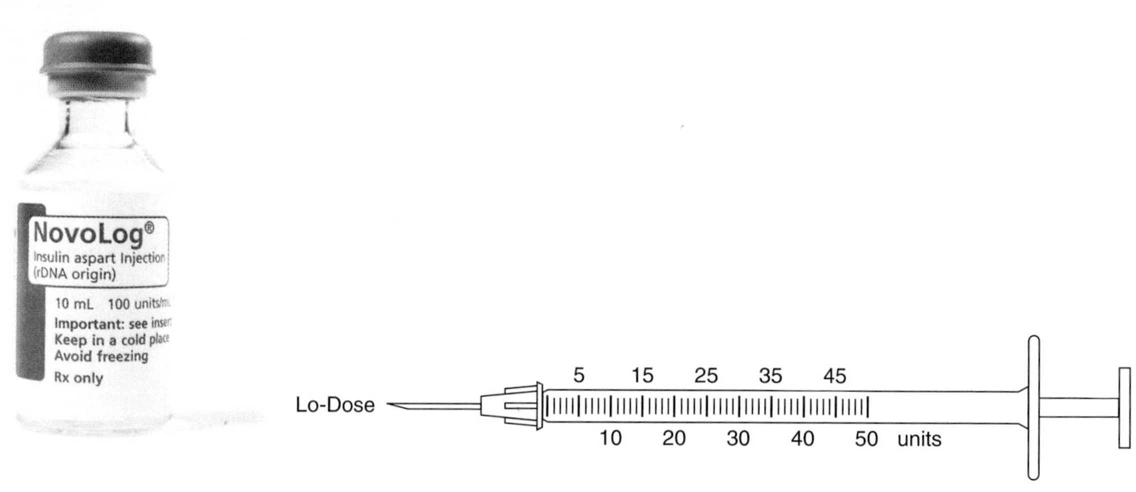

Used with permission from Novo Nordisk Inc.

ANSWERS ON PP. 396–398 AND 401–403.

NAME ______________________

DATE ______________________

ACCEPTABLE SCORE 14

YOUR SCORE ______

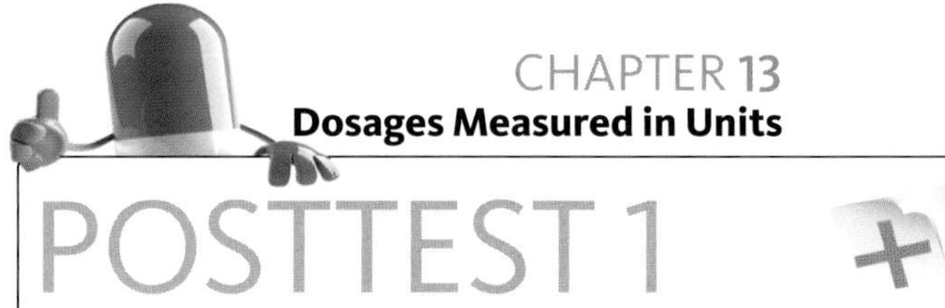

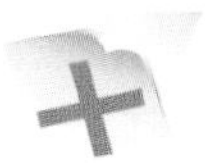

DIRECTIONS: The medication order is listed at the beginning of each problem. Calculate the doses. Show your work. Mark the syringe when provided to indicate the correct dose.

1. The licensed prescriber orders penicillin V 500,000 units po four times a day for your patient with a hysterectomy. Penicillin V pediatric suspension 400,000 units/5 mL is supplied. How many milliliters will you administer? ______ Draw a vertical line through the syringe to indicate the dose.

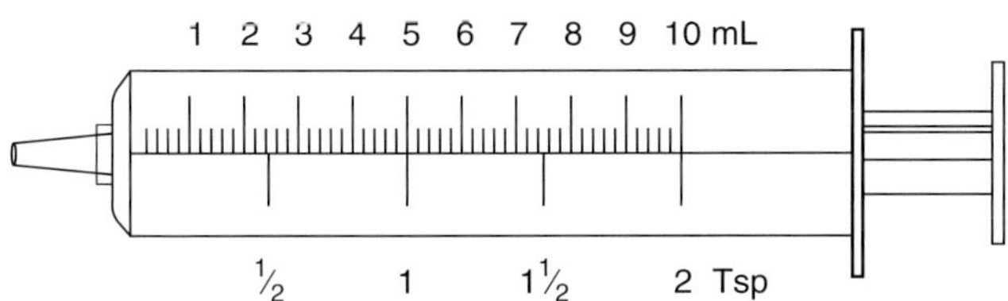

2. The licensed prescriber orders Lantus insulin 40 units subcutaneous daily. Draw a vertical line through the syringe to indicate the dose.

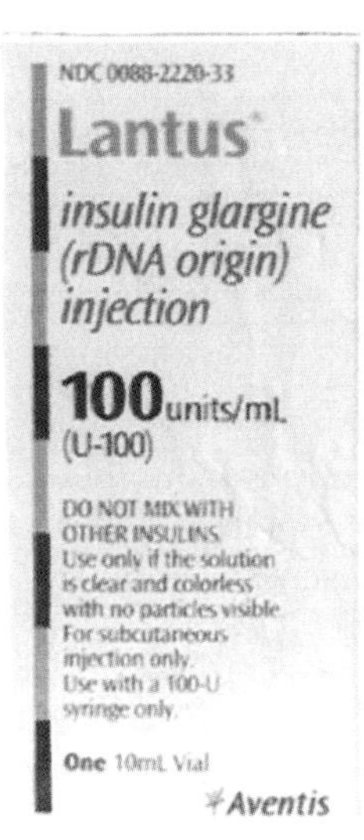

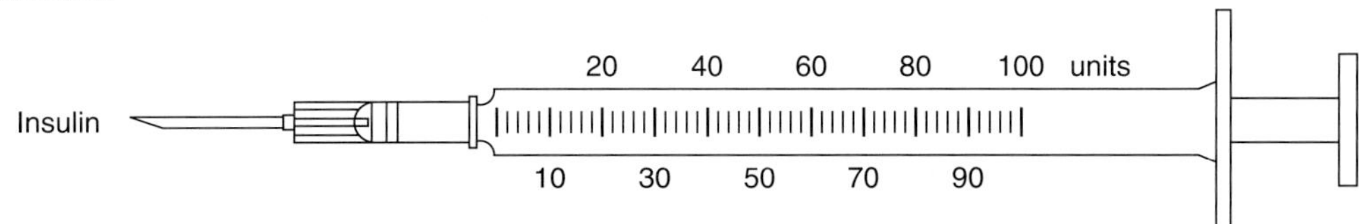

3. In preparation for his upcoming hip replacement surgery, Mr. Stone has Epogen 36,000 units subcutaneous injection once 3 weeks before his surgery. Epogen 40,000 units/mL is available. How many milliliters will the nurse administer? ______

4. The licensed prescriber orders Humulin 50/50 insulin 6 units subcutaneous now. Draw a vertical line through the syringe to indicate the dose.

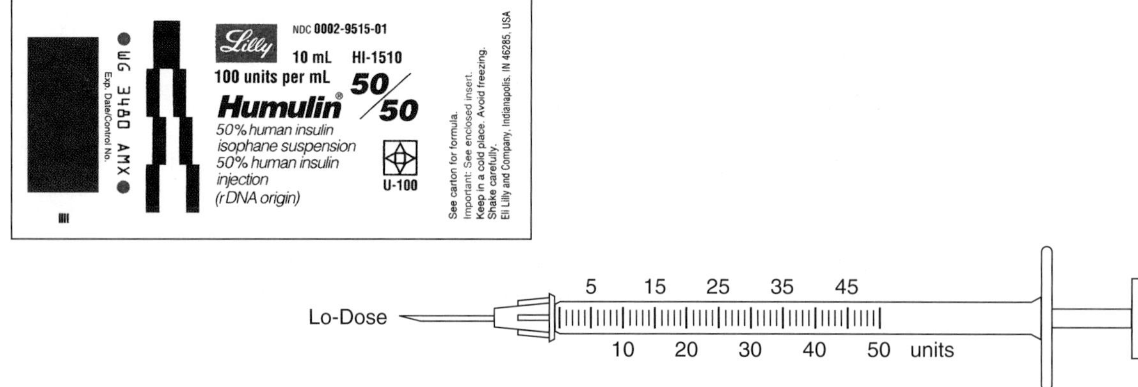

5. Your patient with insulin-dependent diabetes has orders for Humalog insulin 12 units subcutaneous four times a day. You have Humalog insulin U-100 and a U-100 syringe. Draw a vertical line through the syringe to indicate the dose.

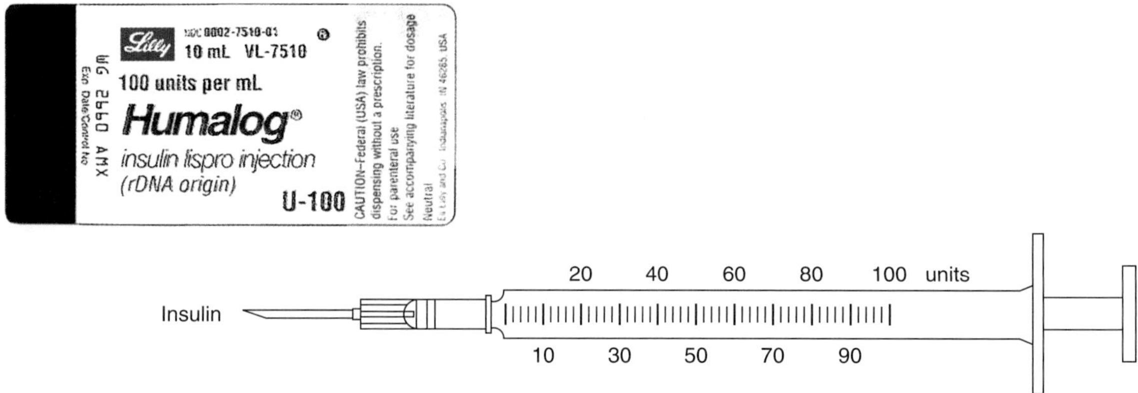

6. The licensed prescriber orders Lente insulin 38 units, regular insulin 18 units subcutaneous daily. Lente U-100, regular insulin U-100, and a U-100 syringe are supplied. Draw a vertical line through the syringe to indicate the amount of regular insulin to be given and a second line to indicate the total dose.

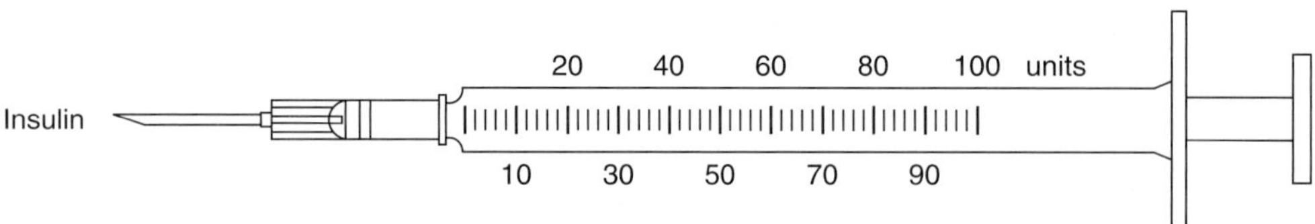

7. The licensed prescriber orders penicillin V 300,000 units po four times a day for your patient with chronic otitis. The drug is supplied in oral solution 200,000 units/5 mL. How many milliliters will you administer? ______

8. Your patient with a sacral decubitus receives penicillin V 200,000 units po four times a day. You have penicillin V oral solution 400,000 units/5 mL. How many milliliters will you administer? ______

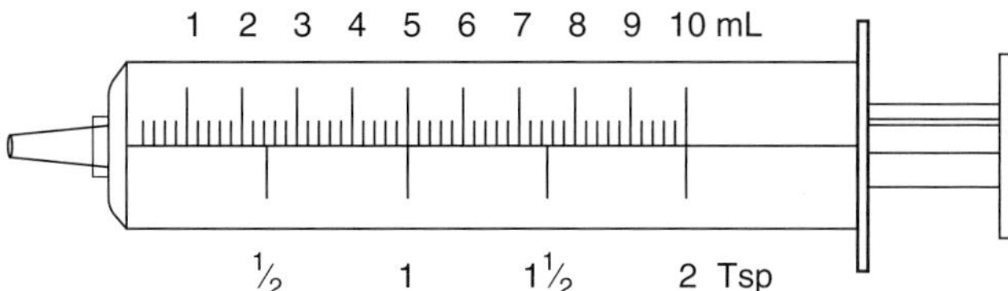

9. Your postoperative patient receives heparin 5000 units subcutaneous q 12 h. Heparin 2500 units/mL is available. How many milliliters will you administer? ______

10. Mrs. Tanaka has been admitted with unstable angina. The licensed prescriber orders Fragmin 8700 international units subcutaneous injection q 12 h. How many milliliters will be administered? (Round your final answer to the nearest hundredth.) ______

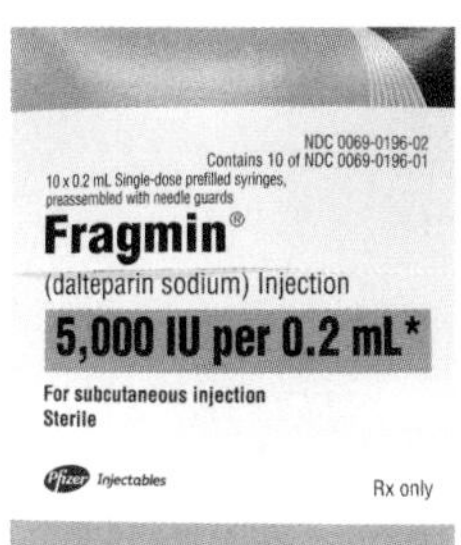

11. Mrs. Daisy receives nystatin oral suspension 600,000 units po four times a day. How many milliliters will the nurse administer? ______

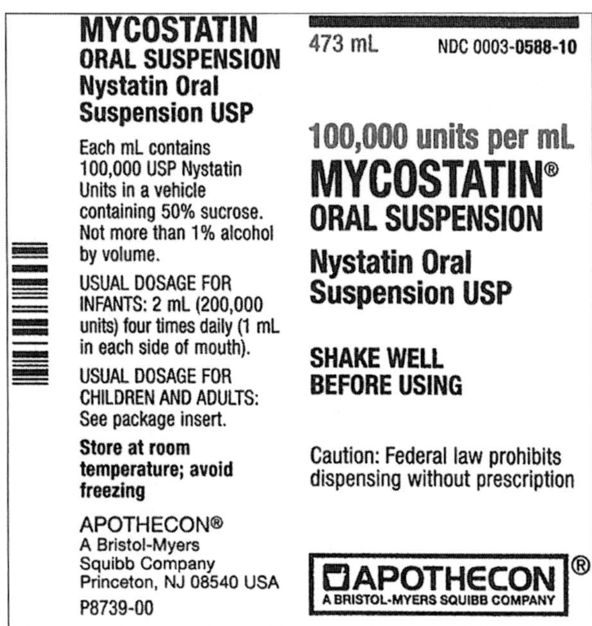

12. Ms. Sanders has Epogen 2200 units subcutaneous injection three times a week ordered for anemia caused by chronic renal failure. Epogen 3000 units/mL is available. How many milliliters will the patient receive for each dose? ______

13. The licensed prescriber orders 40 units Lantus U 100 subcutaneous injection daily at bedtime. Draw a vertical line through the syringe to indicate the dose.

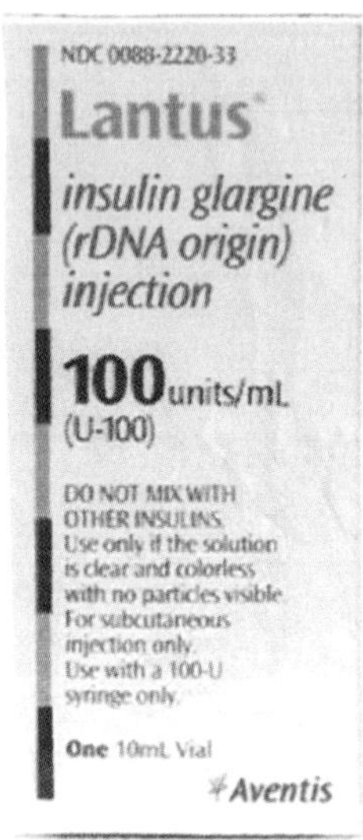

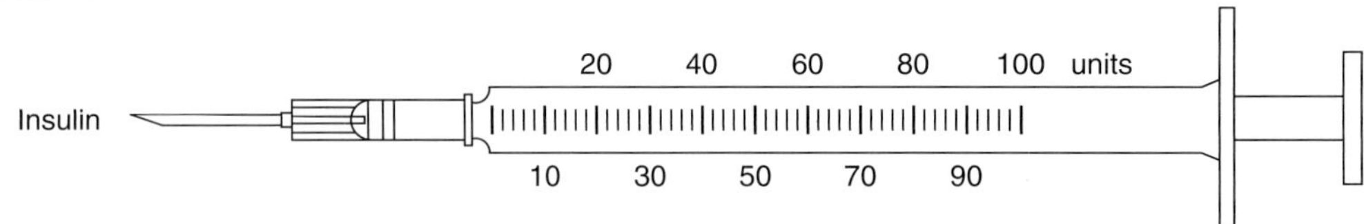

14. The licensed prescriber orders 8 units NovoLog U-100 subcutaneous injection daily at bedtime. Draw a vertical line through the syringe to indicate the dose.

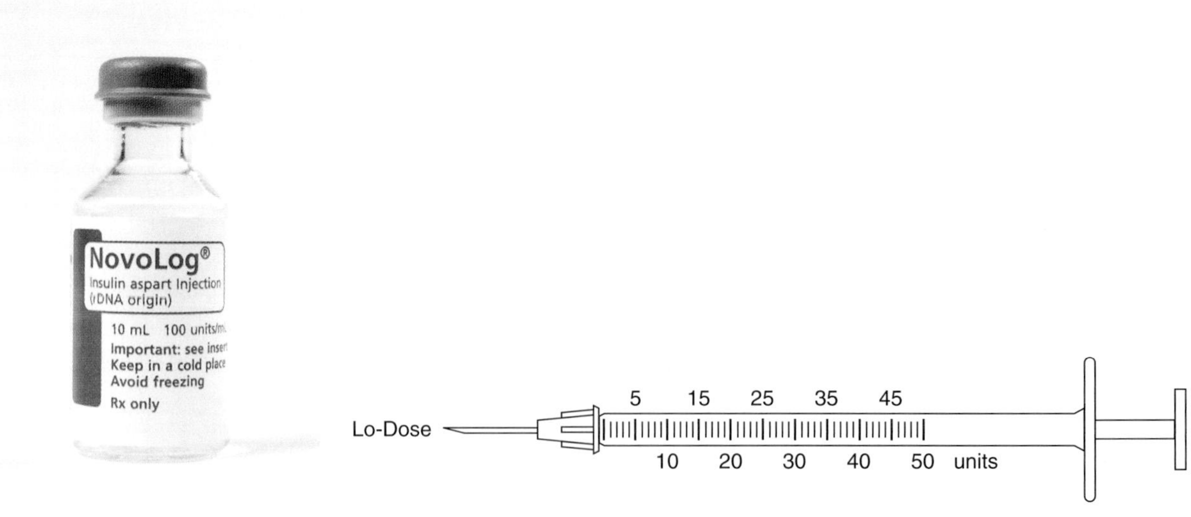

Used with permission from Novo Nordisk Inc.

15. The licensed prescriber orders NPH insulin 12 units and regular insulin 8 units subcutaneous daily before breakfast and dinner. Draw a vertical line through the syringe to indicate the amount of regular insulin to be given and a second line to indicate the total dose.

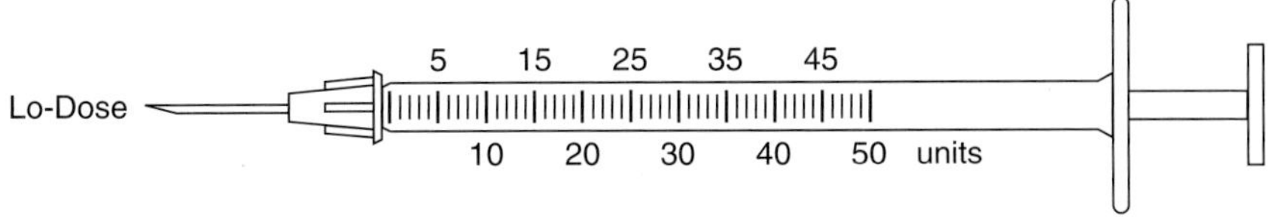

ANSWERS ON PP. 398–399 AND 404–405.

NAME ______________________

DATE ______________________

ACCEPTABLE SCORE 14

YOUR SCORE ______

CHAPTER 13
Dosages Measured in Units

POSTTEST 2

DIRECTIONS: The medication order is listed at the beginning of each problem. Calculate the doses. Show your work. Mark the syringe when provided to indicate the correct dose.

1. The licensed prescriber orders regular insulin 10 units subcutaneous. Regular insulin U-100 and a U-100 Lo-Dose syringe are supplied. Draw a vertical line through the syringe to indicate the dose.

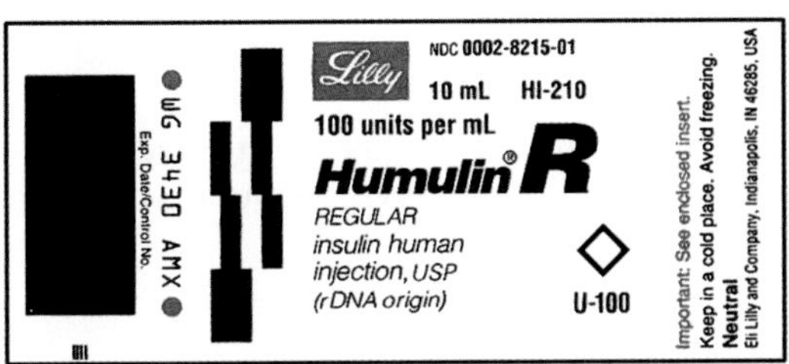

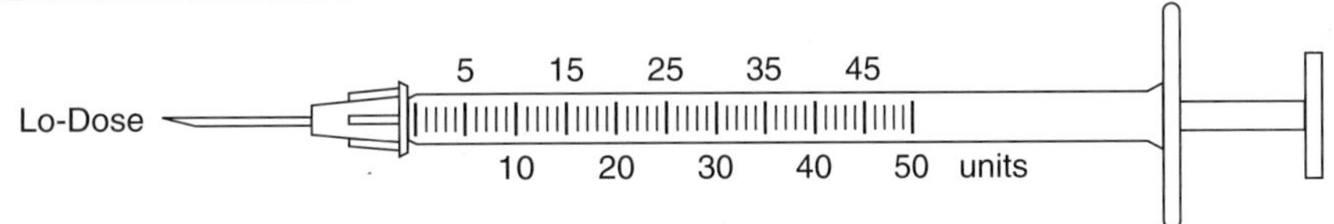

2. Mr. Blackwell has 14,000 units Epogen subcutaneous injection ordered three times a week for anemia related to his chemotherapy. How many milliliters will he receive each time? ______

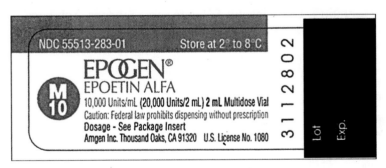

3. Your patient with a septoplasty receives V-Cillin K 500,000 units po q 6 h. You have 200,000 units/5 mL available. How many milliliters will you administer? ______

4. The licensed prescriber orders Novolin L insulin 28 units subcutaneous at 0745. Draw a vertical line through the syringe to indicate the dose of NPH insulin to be given.

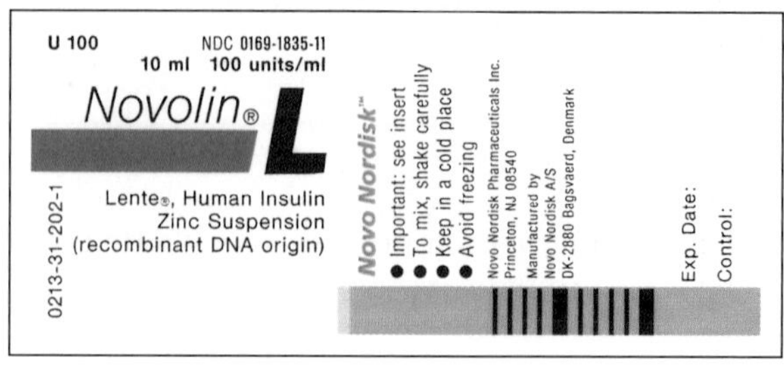

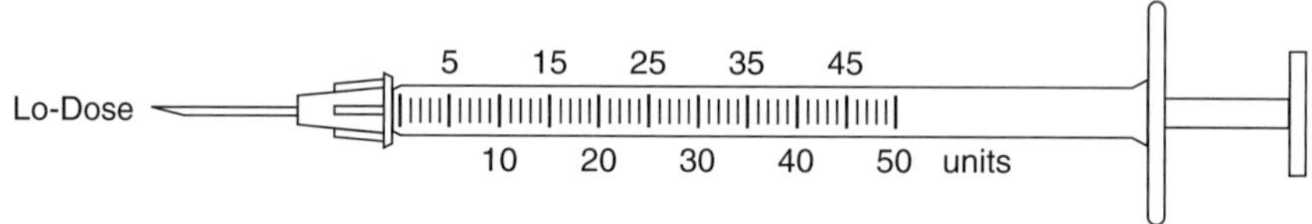

5. Mr. Noah has orders for Fragmin 2500 international units subcutaneous 2 hours before surgery for a total hip replacement. How many milliliters will he receive? (Round your final answer to the nearest hundredth.) ______

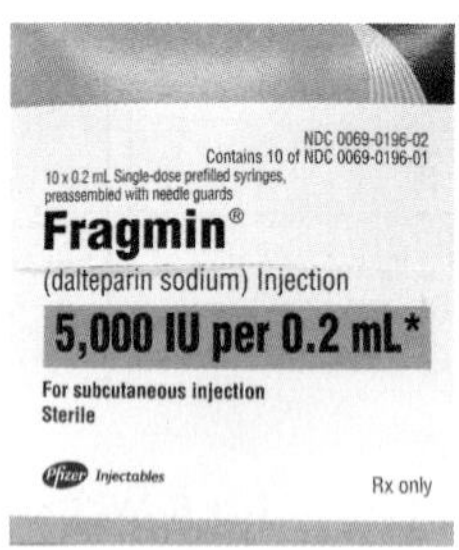

6. The licensed prescriber orders Humulin L Lente insulin 54 units subcutaneous. You have Lente insulin U-100 and a U-100 syringe. Draw a vertical line through the syringe to indicate the amount of Lente insulin to be given.

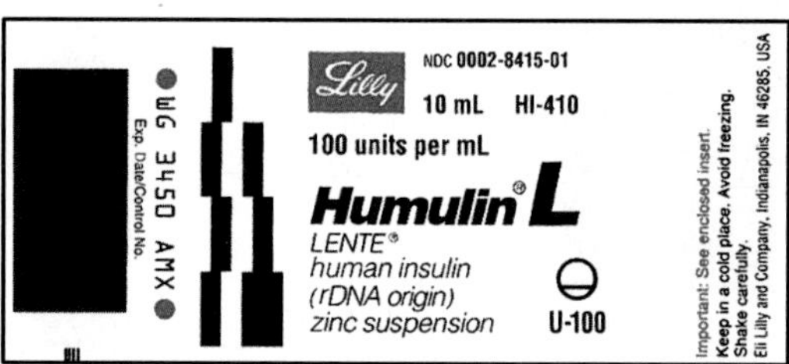

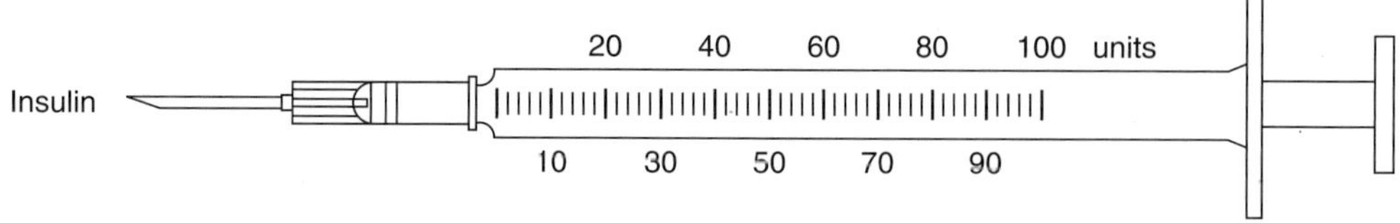

7. The licensed prescriber orders NPH insulin 16 units and regular insulin 8 units subcutaneous daily at 0800. You have NPH insulin U-100, regular insulin U-100, and a U-100 Lo-Dose syringe. Draw a vertical line through the syringe to indicate the amount of regular insulin to be given and a second line to indicate the total dose.

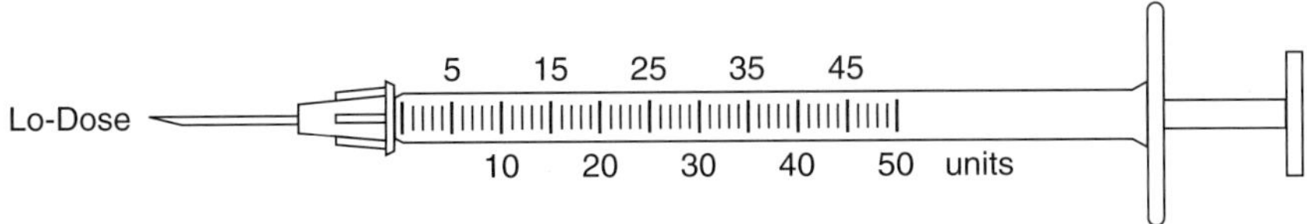

8. Your patient with chronic sinusitis receives penicillin V 300,000 units po four times a day. You have penicillin V oral solution 400,000 units/5 mL. How many milliliters will you administer? ______

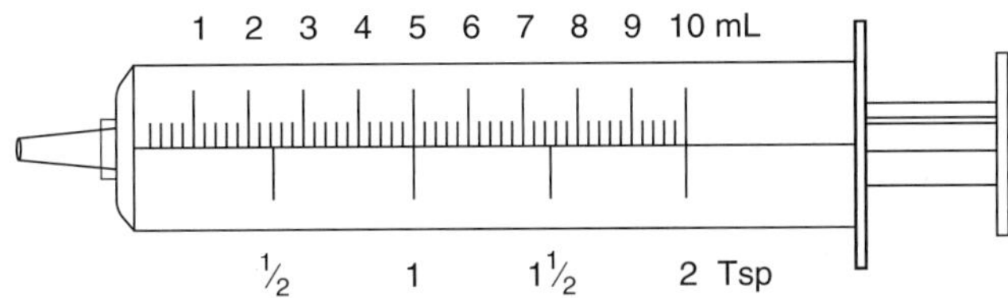

9. Your patient with insulin-dependent diabetes receives Lente insulin 25 units subcutaneous daily at 0800. Draw a vertical line through the syringe to indicate the amount of Lente insulin to be given.

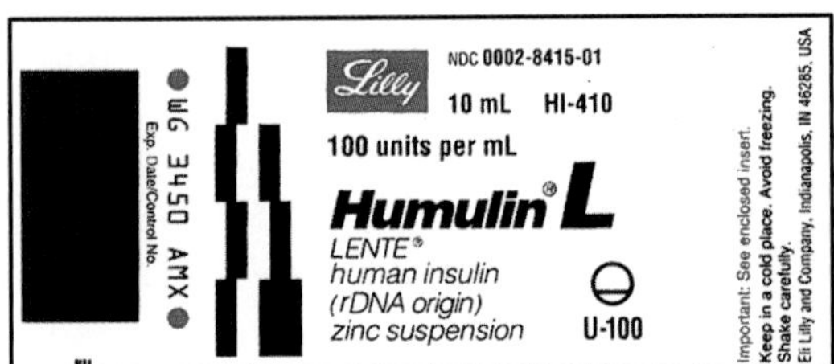

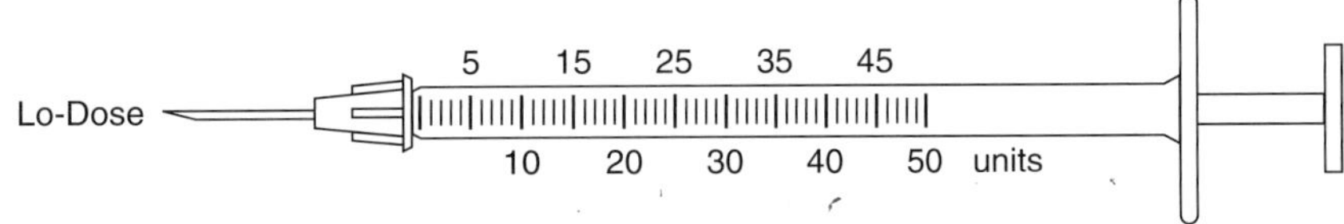

10. Mrs. Star has Epogen 16,000 units subcutaneous injection three times a week for anemia as a result of her chemotherapy. How many milliliters will you administer for each dose? ______

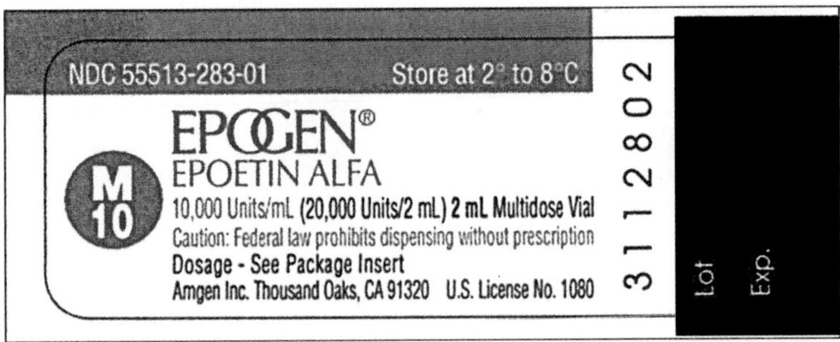

11. The licensed prescriber orders 50 units Lantus U-100 subcutaneous injection daily at bedtime. Draw a vertical line through the syringe to indicate the dose.

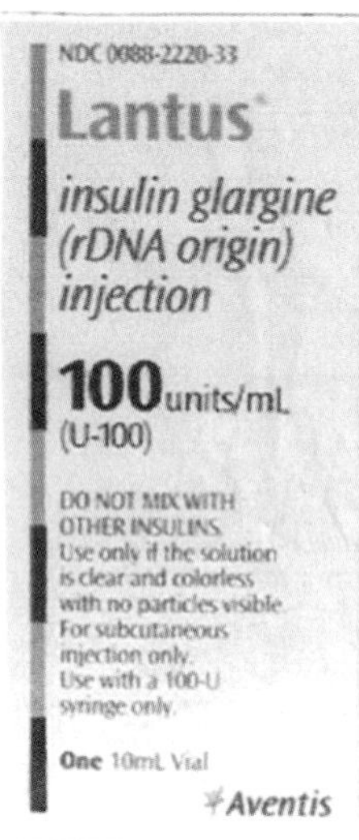

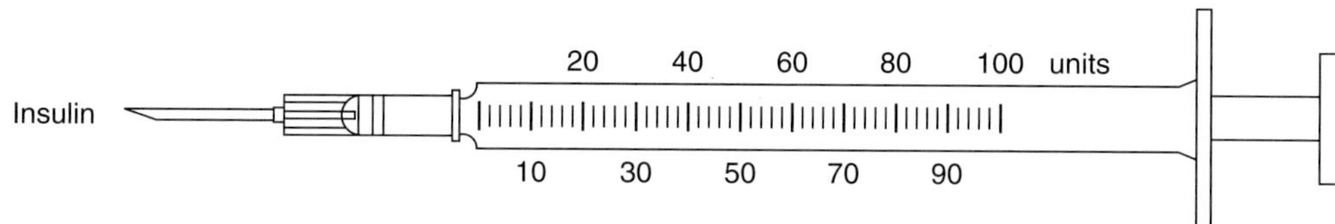

12. The licensed prescriber orders 12 units NovoLog U-100 subcutaneous injection daily at bedtime. Draw a vertical line through the syringe to indicate the dose.

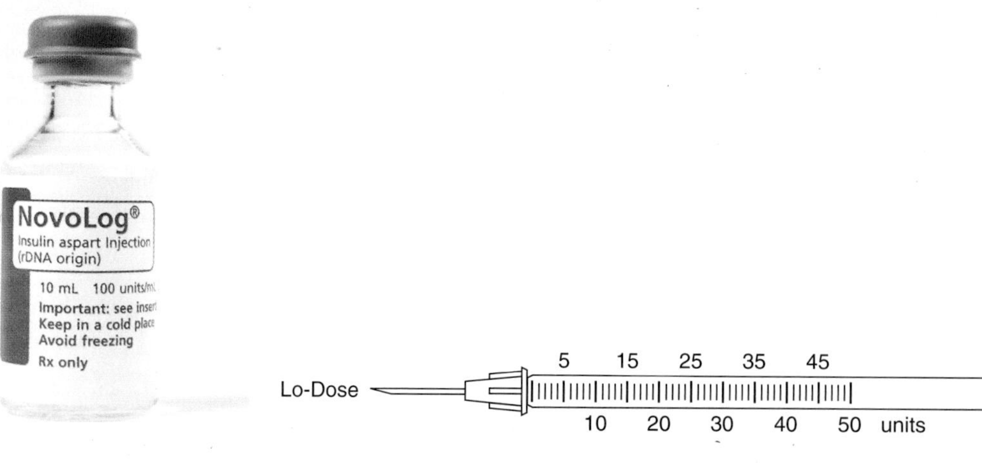

Used with permission from Novo Nordisk Inc.

13. An order for Lovenox 20 mg subcutaneous q 12 h is received. Draw a vertical line through the syringe to indicate the milliliters to administer to the patient.

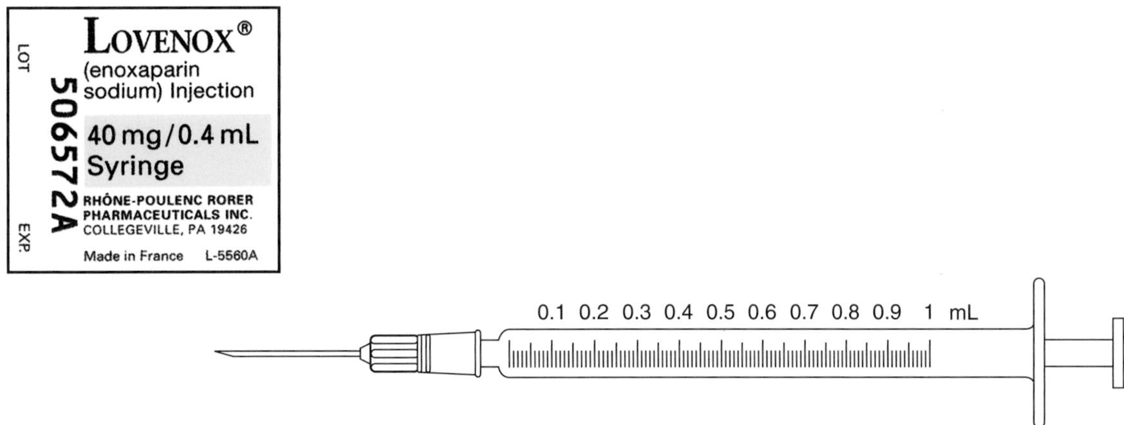

14. An order for Levimir 28 units subcutaneous daily is received. Draw a vertical line through the syringe to indicate the dose.

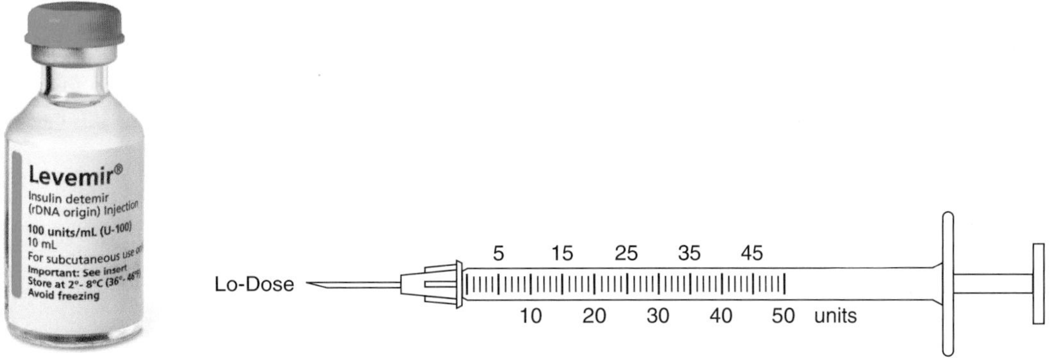

15. A postoperative patient has heparin 2500 units subcutaneous q 8 h ordered to prevent deep vein thrombosis. How many milliliters will the nurse administer?

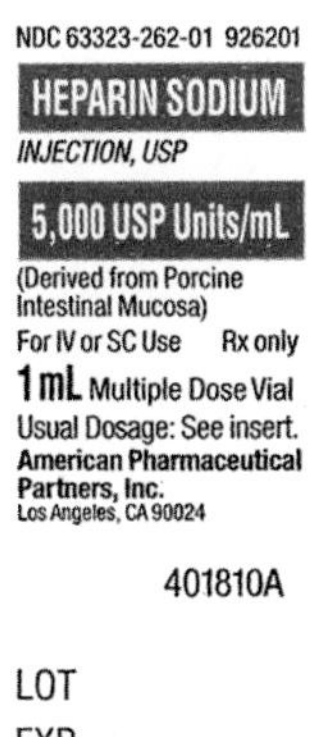

NDC 63323-262-01 926201
HEPARIN SODIUM
INJECTION, USP
5,000 USP Units/mL
(Derived from Porcine Intestinal Mucosa)
For IV or SC Use Rx only
1 mL Multiple Dose Vial
Usual Dosage: See insert.
American Pharmaceutical Partners, Inc.
Los Angeles, CA 90024
401810A
LOT
EXP

ANSWERS ON PP. 399–400 AND 406–407.

evolve For additional practice problems, refer to the Dosages Measured in Units section of *Elsevier's Interactive Drug Calculation Application*, version 1.

ANSWERS

CHAPTER 13 Dimensional Analysis—Work Sheet, pp. 379–384

1. $x \text{ mL} = \dfrac{1 \text{ mL}}{10{,}000 \text{ units}} \times \dfrac{12{,}000 \text{ units}}{1} = 1.2 \text{ mL}$

2. Lo-Dose

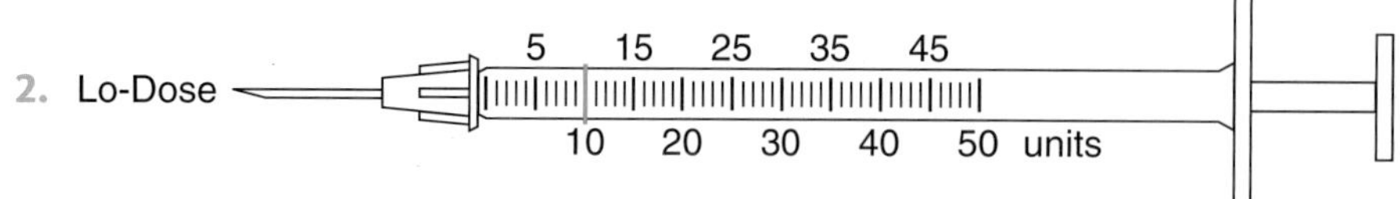

3. $x \text{ mL} = 0.2 \text{ mL}$ (the label reads 5000 units, and the order is for 5000 units)

4. Lo-Dose

5. $x \text{ mL} = \dfrac{1 \text{ mL}}{5000 \text{ units}} \times \dfrac{3000 \text{ units}}{1} = 0.6 \text{ mL}$

6. Lo-Dose

7. $x \text{ mL} = \dfrac{1 \text{ mL}}{10{,}000 \text{ units}} \times \dfrac{4500 \text{ units}}{1} = 0.45 \text{ mL}$

8. Lo-Dose

9. Lo-Dose

10. $x \text{ mL} = \dfrac{5 \text{ mL}}{200{,}000 \text{ units}} \times \dfrac{300{,}000 \text{ units}}{1} = 7.5 \text{ mL}$

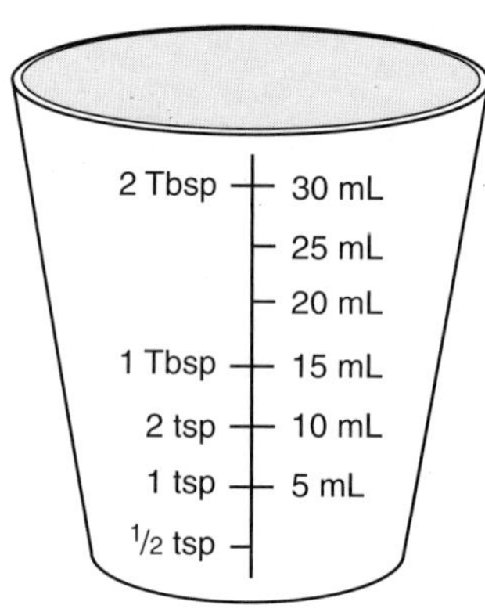

11. Lo-Dose

12. $x \text{ mL} = \dfrac{1 \text{ mL}}{5000 \text{ units}} \times \dfrac{4000 \text{ units}}{1} = 0.8 \text{ mL}$

13. $x \text{ mL} = \dfrac{1 \text{ mL}}{250{,}000 \text{ units}} \times \dfrac{200{,}000 \text{ units}}{1} = 0.8 \text{ mL}$

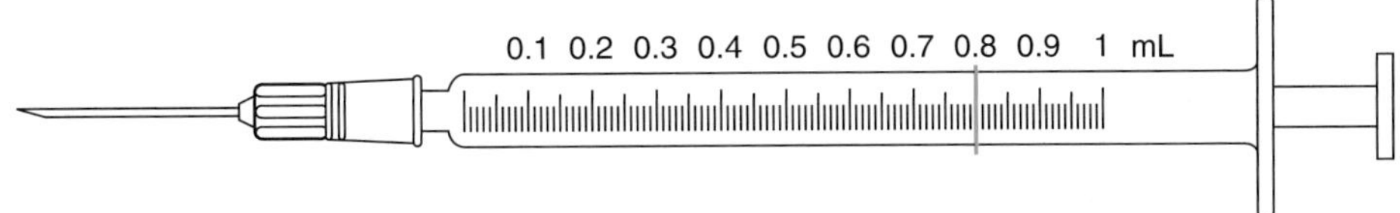

14. $x \text{ mL} = \dfrac{1 \text{ mL}}{10{,}000 \text{ IU}} \times \dfrac{5500 \text{ IU}}{1} = 0.55 \text{ mL}$

15. Insulin

16. $x \text{ mL} = \dfrac{1 \text{ mL}}{5000 \text{ units}} \times \dfrac{2500 \text{ units}}{1} = 0.5 \text{ mL}$

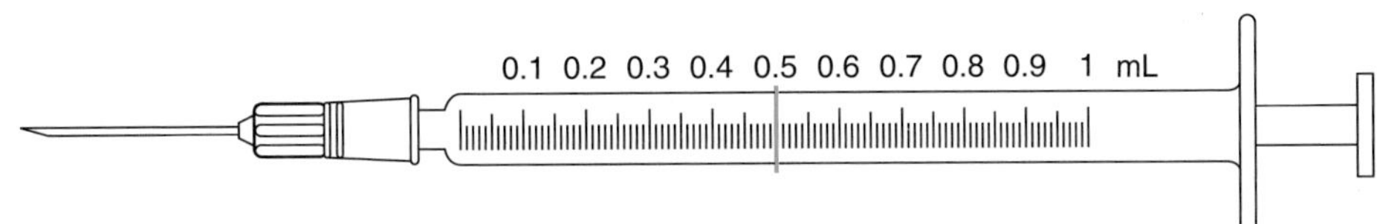

17. Lo-Dose

18. Insulin

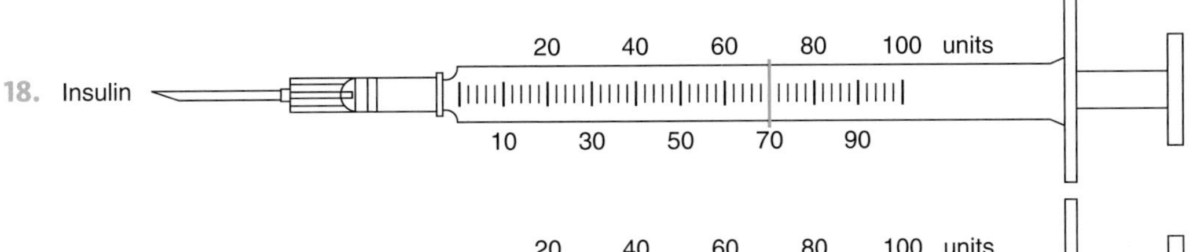

19. Insulin

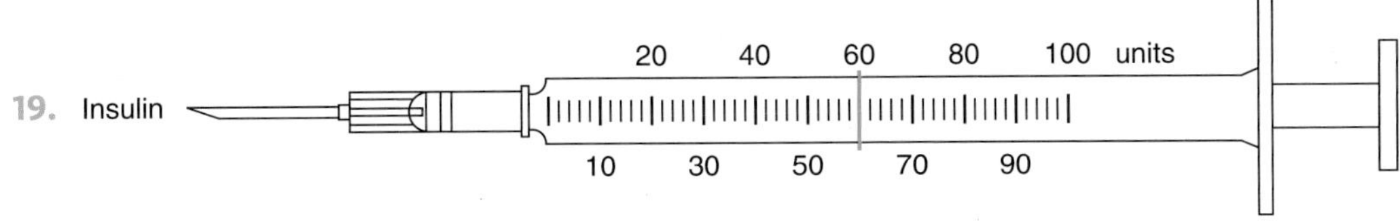

20. Lo-Dose

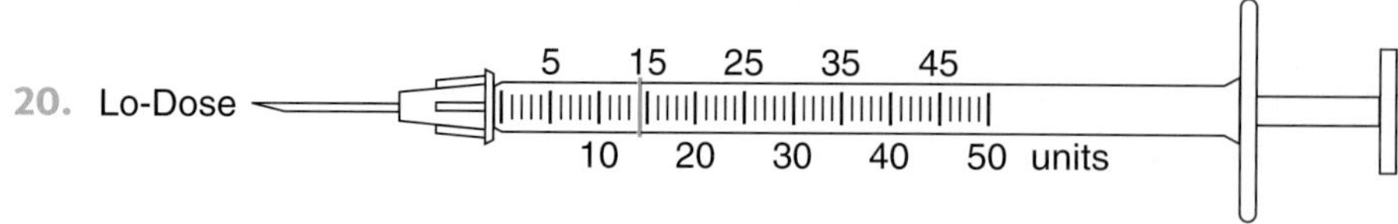

CHAPTER 13 Dimensional Analysis—Posttest 1, pp. 385–389

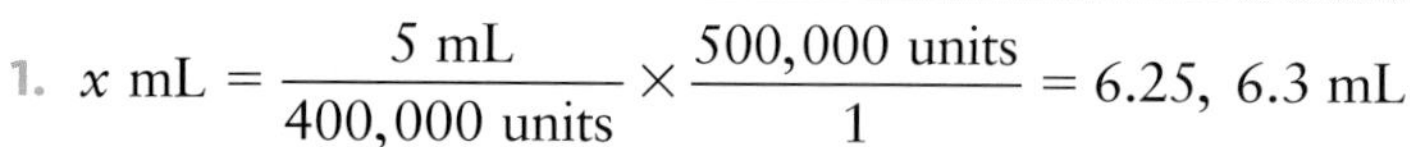

1. $x \text{ mL} = \dfrac{5 \text{ mL}}{400{,}000 \text{ units}} \times \dfrac{500{,}000 \text{ units}}{1} = 6.25,\ 6.3 \text{ mL}$

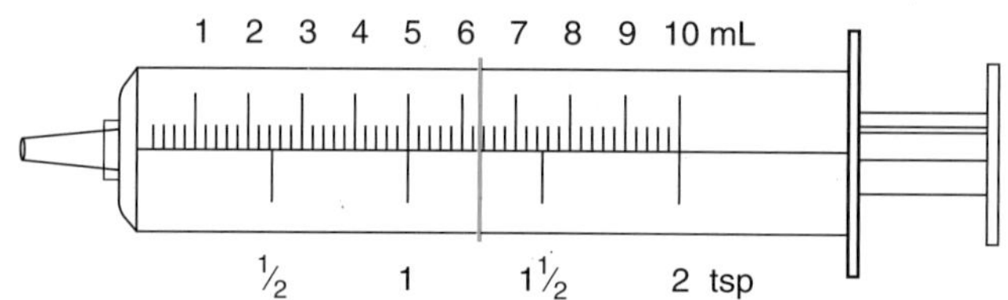

2. Insulin

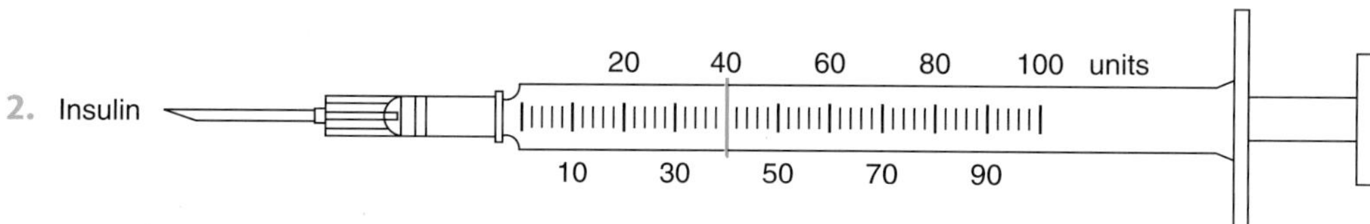

3. $x \text{ mL} = \dfrac{1 \text{ mL}}{40{,}000 \text{ units}} \times \dfrac{36{,}000 \text{ units}}{1} = 0.9 \text{ mL}$

4. Lo-Dose

5 15 25 35 45
10 20 30 40 50 units

5. Insulin

20 40 60 80 100 units
10 30 50 70 90

6. Insulin

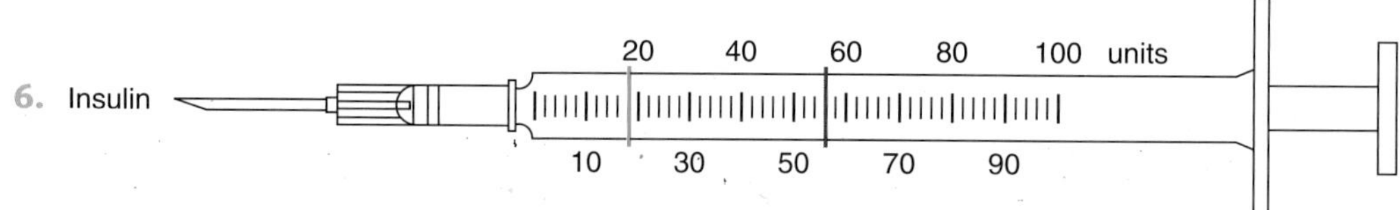

7. $x \text{ mL} = \dfrac{5 \text{ mL}}{200{,}000 \text{ units}} \times \dfrac{300{,}000 \text{ units}}{1} = 7.5 \text{ mL}$

8. $x \text{ mL} = \dfrac{5 \text{ mL}}{400{,}000 \text{ units}} \times \dfrac{200{,}000 \text{ units}}{1} = 2.5 \text{ mL}$

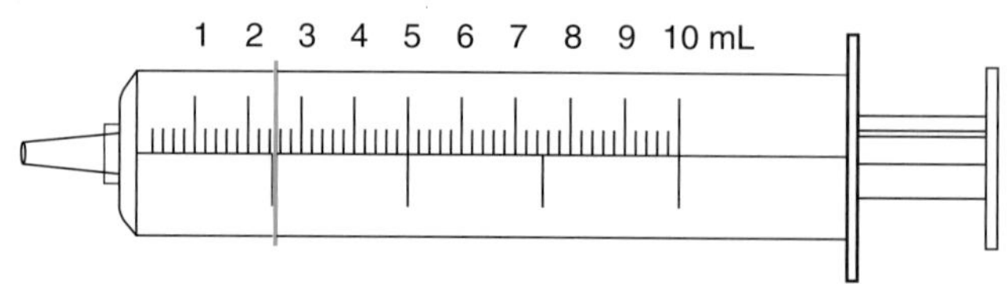

9. $x \text{ mL} = \dfrac{1 \text{ mL}}{2500 \text{ units}} \times \dfrac{5000 \text{ units}}{1} = 2 \text{ mL}$

10. $x \text{ mL} = \dfrac{0.2 \text{ mL}}{5000 \text{ units}} \times \dfrac{8700 \text{ units}}{1} = 0.348 \text{ or } 0.35 \text{ mL}$

11. $x \text{ mL} = \dfrac{1 \text{ mL}}{100{,}000 \text{ units}} \times \dfrac{600{,}000 \text{ units}}{1} = 6 \text{ mL}$

12. $x \text{ mL} = \dfrac{1 \text{ mL}}{3000 \text{ units}} \times \dfrac{2200 \text{ units}}{1} = 0.73 \text{ or } 0.7 \text{ mL}$

13. Insulin

14. Lo-Dose

15. Lo-Dose

CHAPTER 13 Dimensional Analysis—Posttest 2, pp. 391–395

1. Lo-Dose

2. $x \text{ mL} = \dfrac{1 \text{ mL}}{10{,}000 \text{ units}} \times \dfrac{14{,}000 \text{ units}}{1} = 1.4 \text{ mL}$

3. $x \text{ mL} = \dfrac{5 \text{ mL}}{200{,}000 \text{ units}} \times \dfrac{500{,}000 \text{ units}}{1} = 12.5 \text{ mL}$

4. Lo-Dose

5. $x \text{ mL} = \dfrac{0.2 \text{ mL}}{5000 \text{ units}} \times \dfrac{2500 \text{ units}}{1} = 0.1 \text{ mL}$

6. Insulin

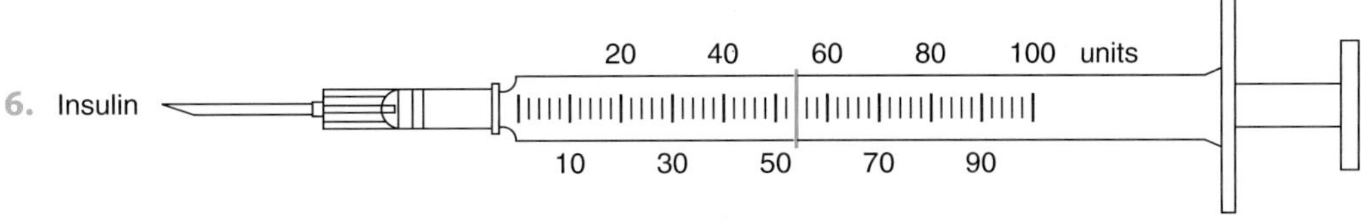

7. Lo-Dose

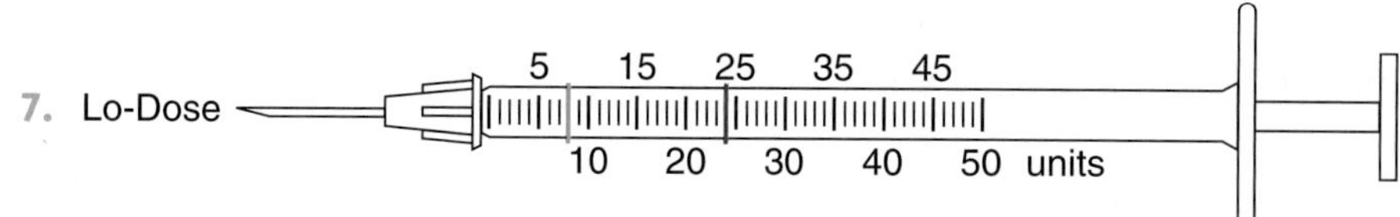

8. $x \text{ mL} = \dfrac{5 \text{ mL}}{400{,}000 \text{ units}} \times \dfrac{300{,}000 \text{ units}}{1} = 3.75,\ 3.8 \text{ mL}$

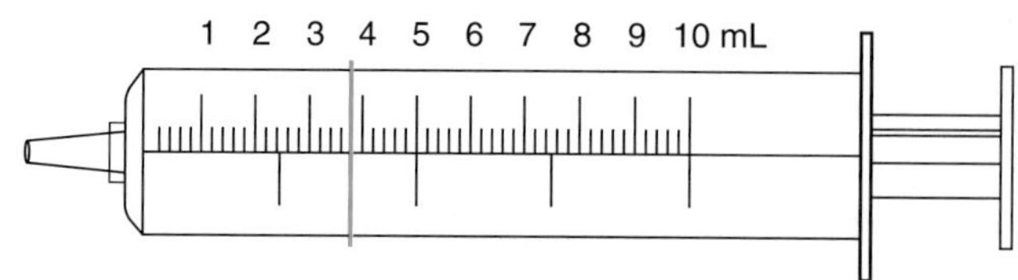

9. Lo-Dose

10. $x \text{ mL} = \dfrac{1 \text{ mL}}{10{,}000 \text{ units}} \times \dfrac{16{,}000 \text{ units}}{1} = 1.6 \text{ mL}$

11. Insulin

12. Lo-Dose

13. $x \text{ mL} = \dfrac{0.4 \text{ mL}}{40 \text{ mg}} \times \dfrac{20 \text{ mg}}{1} = 0.2 \text{ mL}$

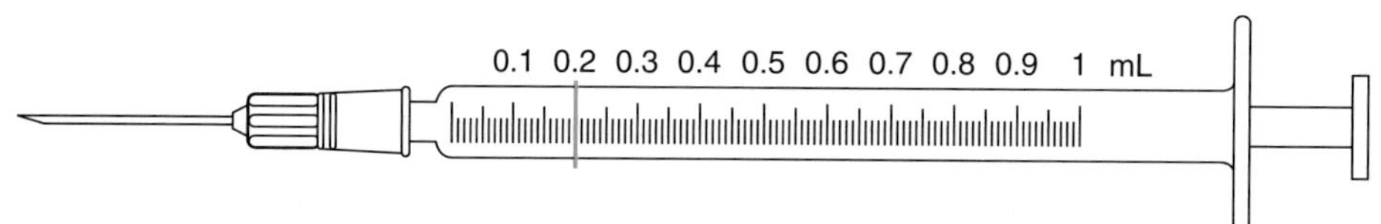

14. Lo-Dose

15. $x \text{ mL} = \dfrac{1 \text{ mL}}{5000 \text{ units}} \times \dfrac{2500 \text{ units}}{1} = 0.5 \text{ mL}$

ANSWERS

CHAPTER 13 Proportion/Formula Method—Work Sheet, pp. 379–384

Proportion	Formula
1. 10,000 units : 1 mL :: 12,000 units : x mL $10{,}000x = 12{,}000$ $x = \dfrac{12{,}000}{10{,}000}$ $x = 1.2$ mL	$\dfrac{12{,}000 \text{ units}}{10{,}000 \text{ units}} \times 1 \text{ mL} = 1.2 \text{ mL}$

2. Lo-Dose

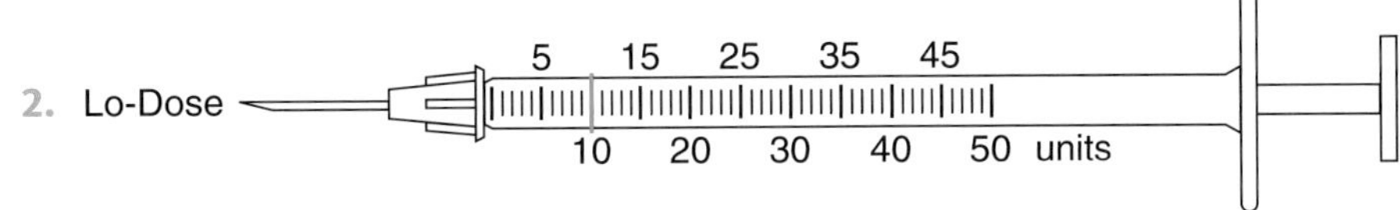

3. 0.2 mL (the label reads 5000 units and the order is for 5000 units)

4. Lo-Dose

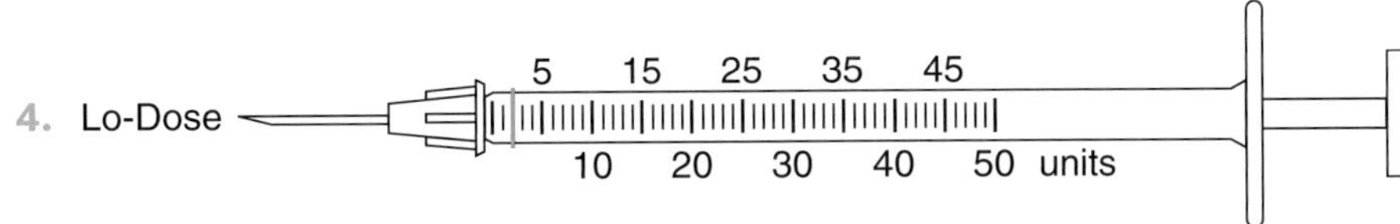

Proportion	Formula
5. 5000 units : 1 mL :: 3000 units : x mL $5000x = 3000$ $x = \dfrac{3000}{5000}$ $x = 0.6$ mL	$\dfrac{3000 \text{ units}}{5000 \text{ units}} \times 1 \text{ mL} = 0.6 \text{ mL}$

6. Lo-Dose

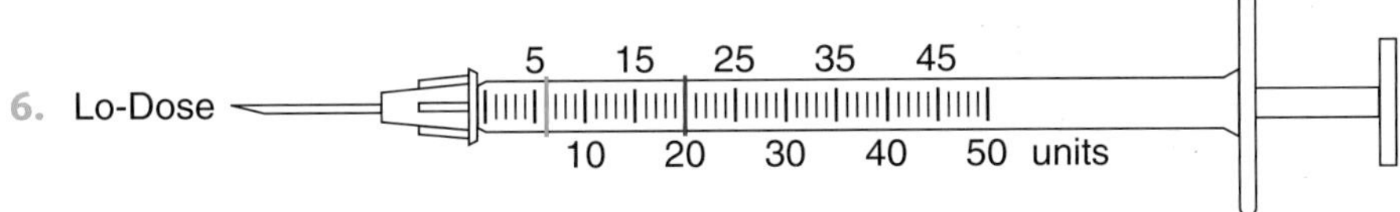

Proportion	Formula
7. 10,000 units : 1 mL :: 4500 units : x mL $10{,}000x = 4500$ $x = \dfrac{4500}{10{,}000}$ $x = 0.45$ mL	$\dfrac{4500 \text{ units}}{10{,}000 \text{ units}} \times 1 \text{ mL} = 0.45 \text{ mL}$

8. Lo-Dose

9. Lo-Dose

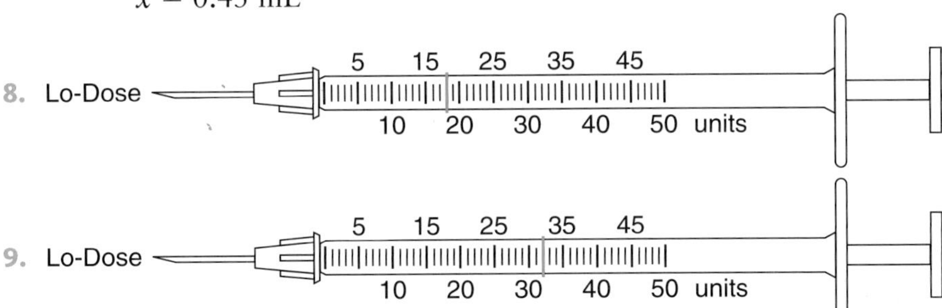

Proportion	Formula

10. 200,000 units : 5 mL :: 300,000 units : x mL

$$200{,}000x = 1{,}500{,}000$$
$$x = \frac{1{,}500{,}000}{200{,}000}$$
$$x = 7.5 \text{ mL}$$

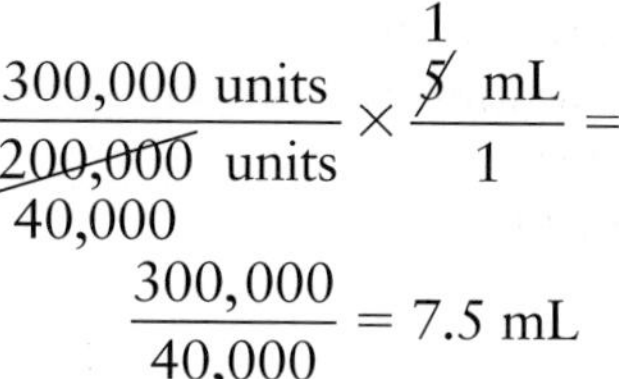

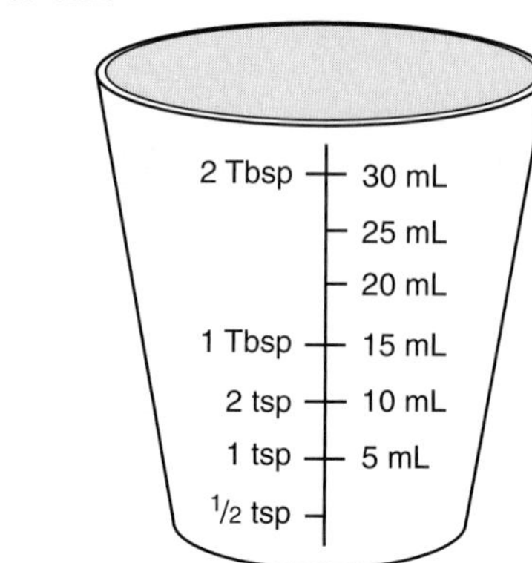

11. Lo-Dose

5 15 25 35 45

10 20 30 40 50 units

12. 5000 units : 1 mL :: 4000 units : x mL

$$5000x = 4000$$
$$x = \frac{4000}{5000}$$
$$x = 0.8 \text{ mL}$$

$$\frac{4000 \text{ units}}{5000 \text{ units}} \times 1 \text{ mL} = 0.8 \text{ mL}$$

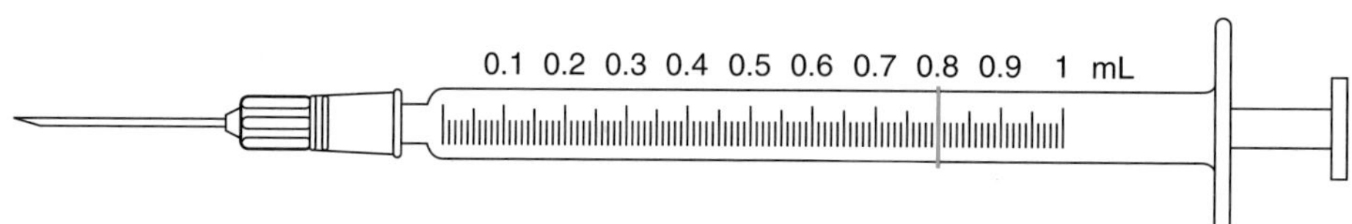

13. 250,000 units : 1 mL :: 200,000 units : x mL

$$250{,}000x = 200{,}000$$
$$x = \frac{200{,}000}{250{,}000}$$
$$x = 0.8 \text{ mL}$$

$$\frac{\overset{4}{\cancel{200{,}000}} \text{ units}}{\underset{5}{\cancel{250{,}000}} \text{ units}} \times 1 \text{ mL} = 0.8 \text{ mL}$$

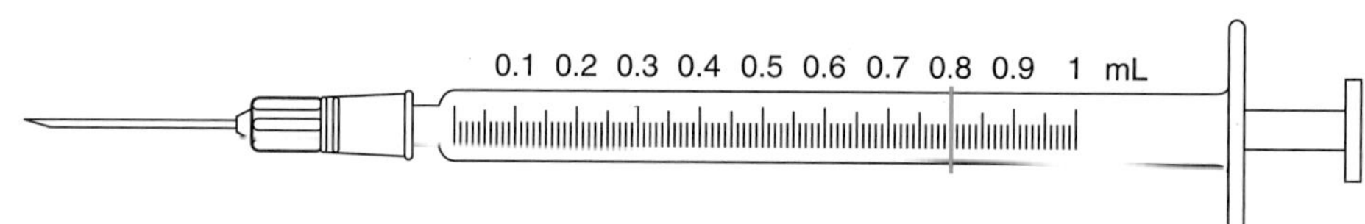

Proportion	**Formula**
14. 10,000 international units : 1 mL :: 5500 international units : x mL $10{,}000x = 5500$ $x = \dfrac{5500}{10{,}000}$ $x = 0.55$ mL	$\dfrac{5500 \text{ international units}}{10{,}000 \text{ international units}} \times 1 \text{ mL} = 0.55 \text{ mL}$

15. 40 units, then add the 35 for a total mark at 75.

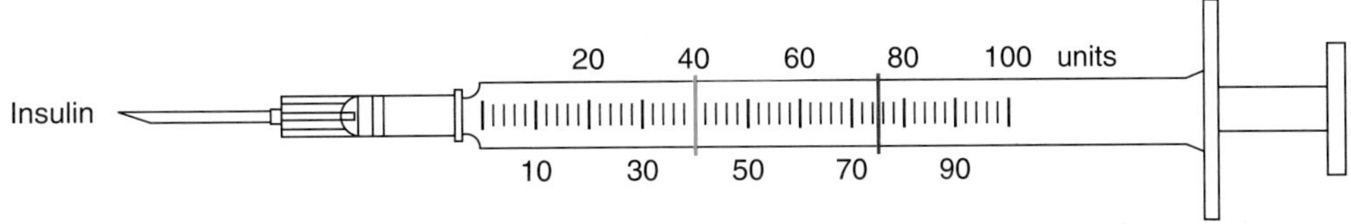

16. 5000 units : 1 mL :: 2500 units : x mL $5000x = 2500$ $x = \dfrac{2500}{5000}$ $x = 0.5$ mL	$\dfrac{2500 \text{ units}}{5000 \text{ units}} \times 1 \text{ mL} = 0.5 \text{ mL}$

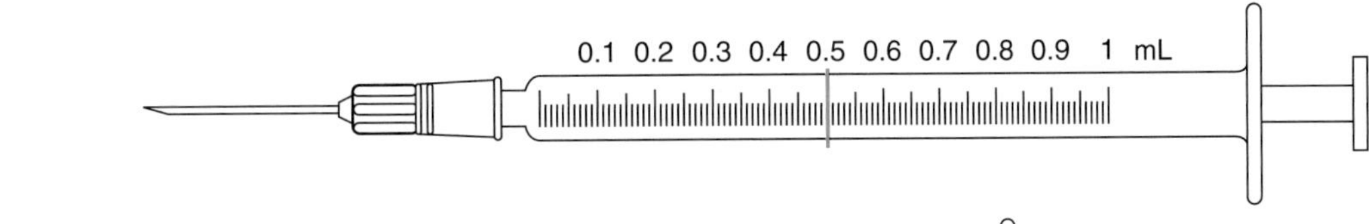

17.
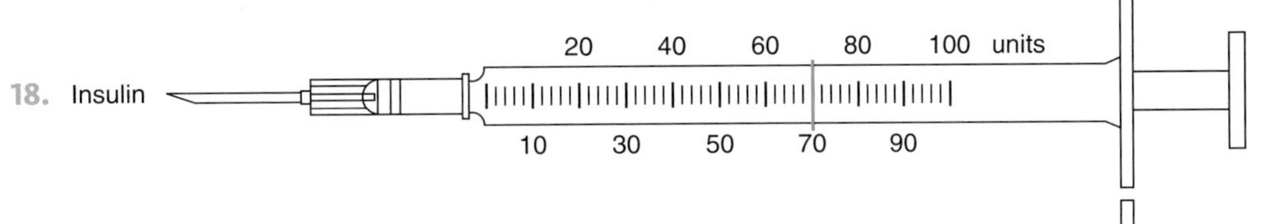

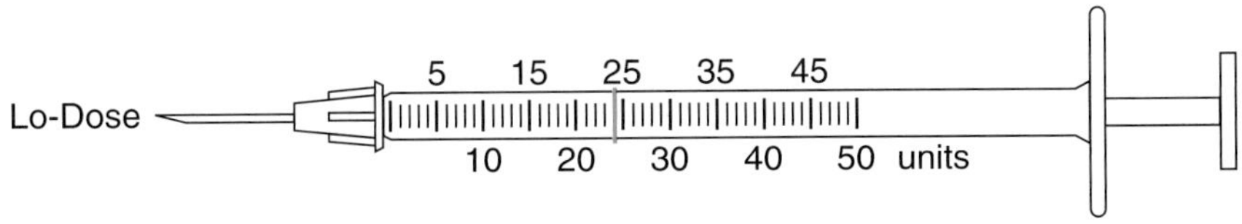

18.
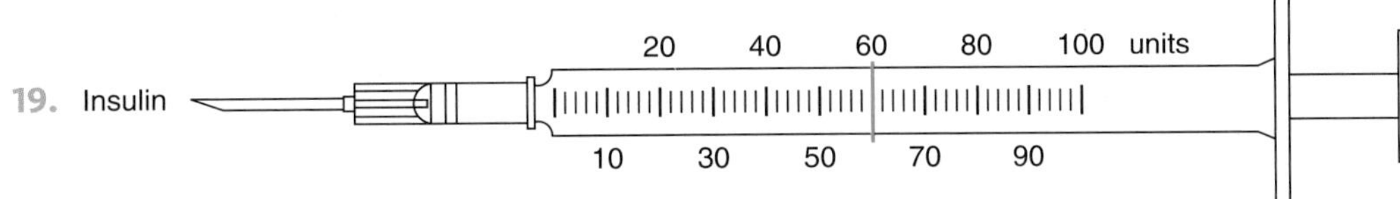

19.
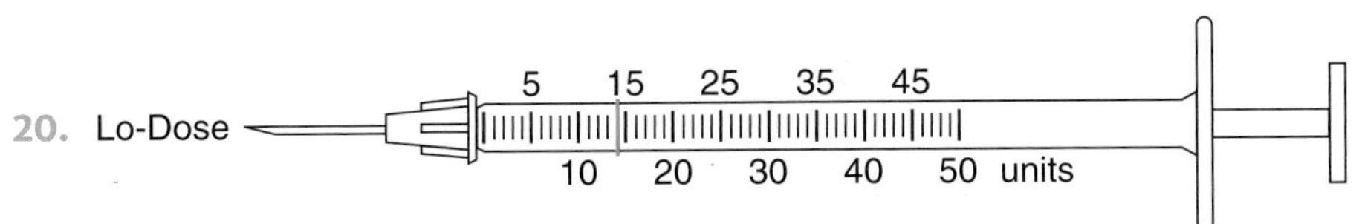

20. Lo-Dose

5 15 25 35 45

10 20 30 40 50 units

ANSWERS

CHAPTER 13 Proportion/Formula Method—Posttest 1, pp. 385–389

Proportion	Formula
1. 400,000 units : 5 mL :: 500,000 units : x mL $400{,}000x = 2{,}500{,}000$ $x = \frac{2{,}500{,}000}{400{,}000}$ $x = 6.25$, 6.3 mL	$\frac{500{,}000 \text{ units}}{400{,}000 \text{ units}} \times 5 \text{ mL} =$ $\frac{25}{4} = 6.25$, 6.3 mL

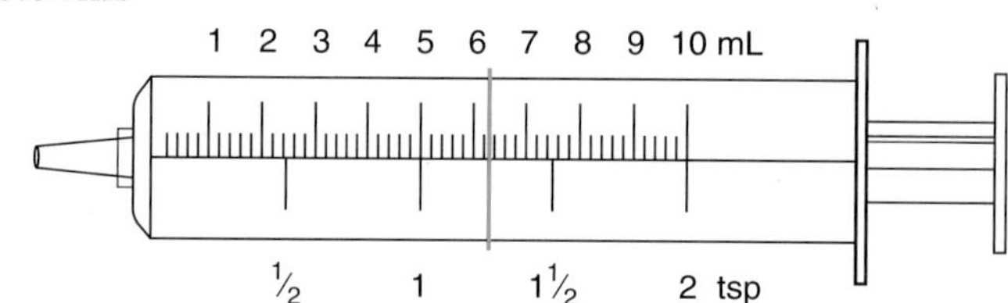

2. Insulin

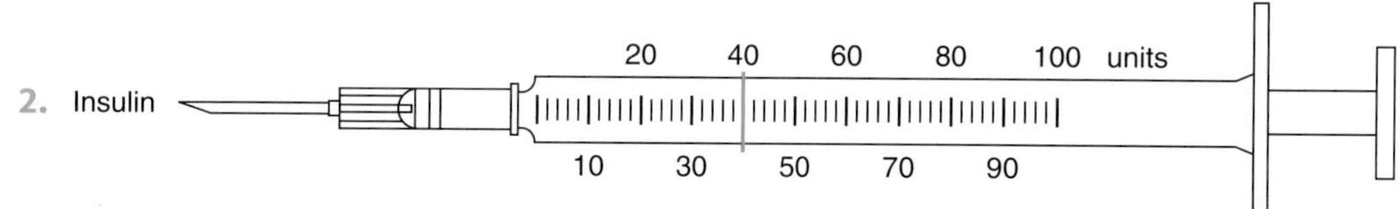

Proportion	Formula
3. 40,000 units : 1 mL :: 36,000 units : x mL $40{,}000x = 36{,}000$ $x = \frac{36{,}000}{40{,}000}$ $x = 0.9$ mL	$\frac{36{,}000 \text{ units}}{40{,}000 \text{ units}} \times 1 \text{ mL} = 0.9 \text{ mL}$

4. Lo-Dose

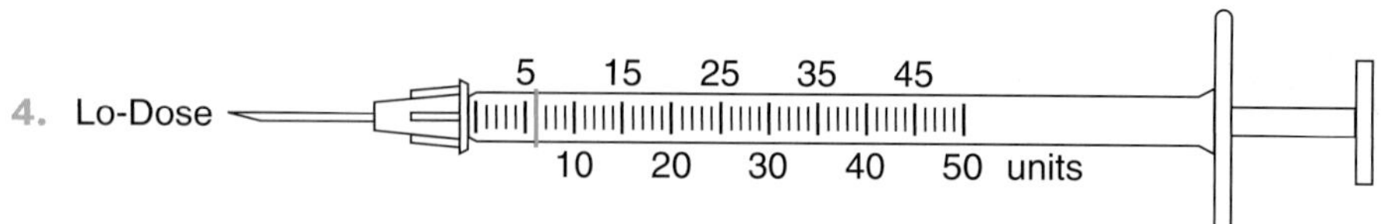

5. Insulin

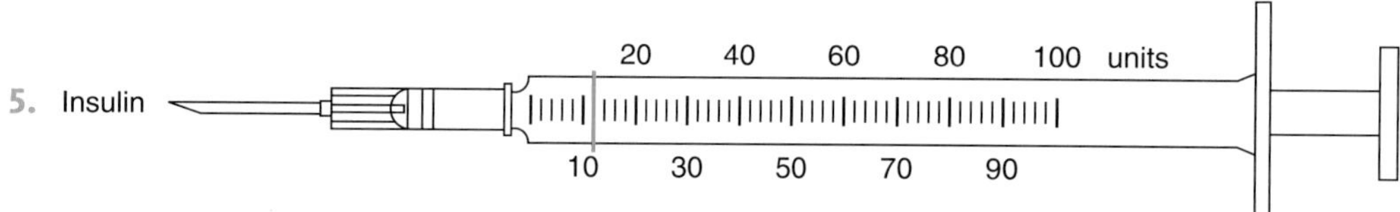

6. Insulin

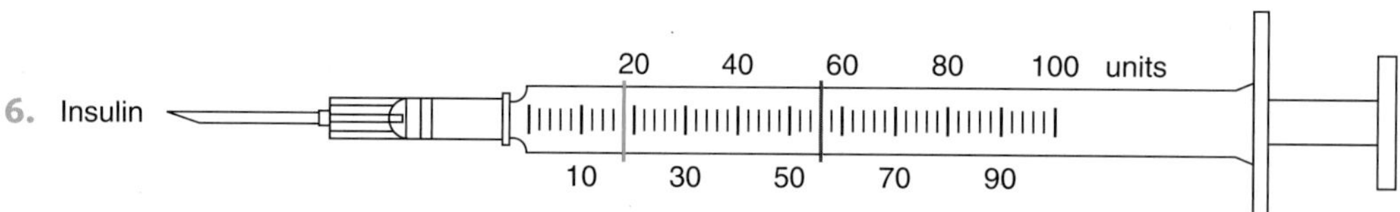

Proportion	Formula
7. 200,000 units : 5 mL :: 300,000 units : x mL $200{,}000x = 1{,}500{,}000$ $x = \frac{1{,}500{,}000}{200{,}000}$ $x = 7.5$ mL	$\frac{300{,}000 \text{ units}}{200{,}000 \text{ units}} \times 5 \text{ mL} =$ $\frac{15}{2} = 7.5$ mL

Proportion	Formula
8. 400,000 units : 5 mL :: 200,000 units : x mL $400{,}000x = 1{,}000{,}000$ $x = \frac{1{,}000{,}000}{400{,}000}$ $x = 2.5$ mL	$\frac{200{,}000 \text{ units}}{400{,}000 \text{ units}} \times 5 \text{ mL} =$ $\frac{1{,}000{,}000}{400{,}000} = 2.5 \text{ mL}$

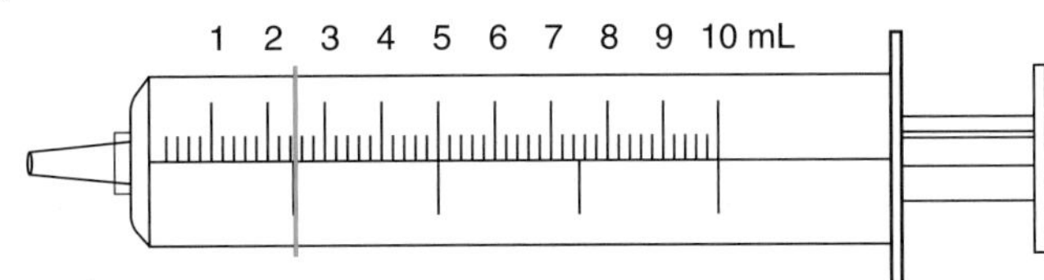

Proportion	Formula
9. 2500 units : 1 mL :: 5000 units : x mL $2500x = 5000$ $x = \frac{5000}{2500}$ $x = 2$ mL	$\frac{5000 \text{ units}}{2500 \text{ units}} \times 1 \text{ mL} = 2 \text{ mL}$
10. 5000 units : 0.2 mL :: 8700 units : x mL $5000x = 0.2 \times 8700$ $x = \frac{1740}{5000}$ $x = 0.35$ mL	$\frac{8700 \text{ units}}{5000 \text{ units}} \times 0.2 \text{ mL} = 0.348 \text{ or } 0.35 \text{ mL}$
11. 100,000 units : 1 mL :: 600,000 units : x mL $100{,}000x = 600{,}000$ $x = \frac{600{,}000}{100{,}000}$ $x = 6$ mL	$\frac{600{,}000 \text{ units}}{100{,}000 \text{ units}} \times 1 \text{ mL} = 6 \text{ mL}$
12. 3000 units : 1 mL :: 2200 units : x mL $3000x = 2200$ $x = \frac{2200}{3000}$ $x = 0.73, 0.7$ mL	$\frac{2200 \text{ units}}{3000 \text{ units}} \times 1 \text{ mL} = 0.73,\ 0.7 \text{ mL}$

13. Insulin

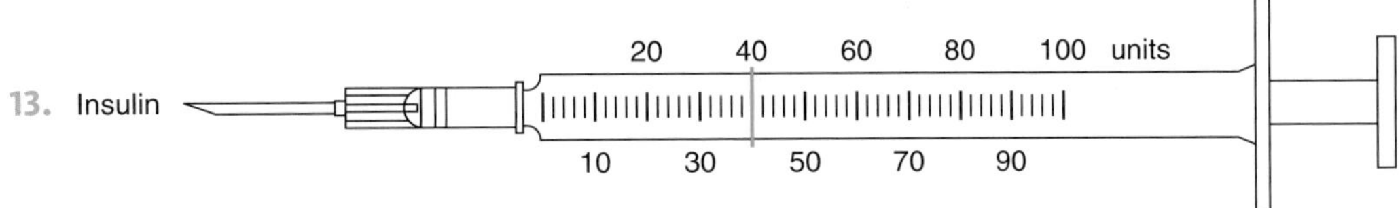

14. Lo-Dose

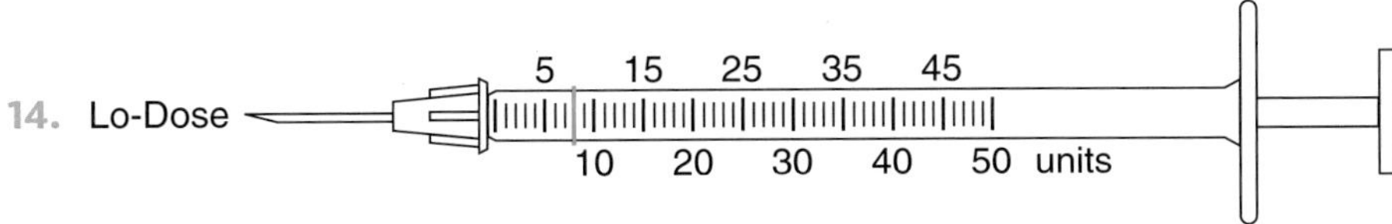

15. Lo-Dose

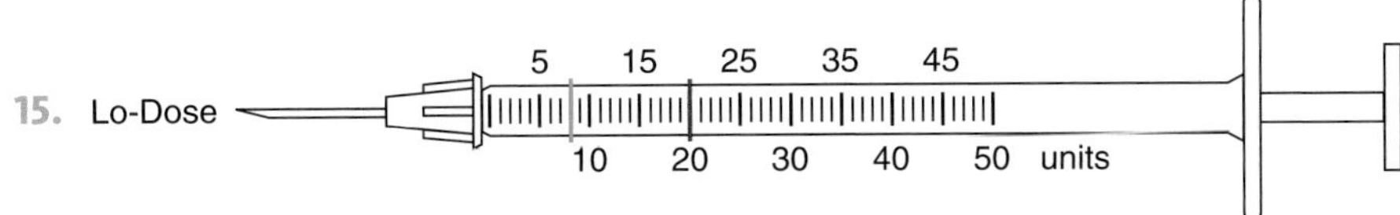

CHAPTER 13 Proportion/Formula Method—Posttest 2, pp. 391–395

Proportion | **Formula**

1. Lo-Dose

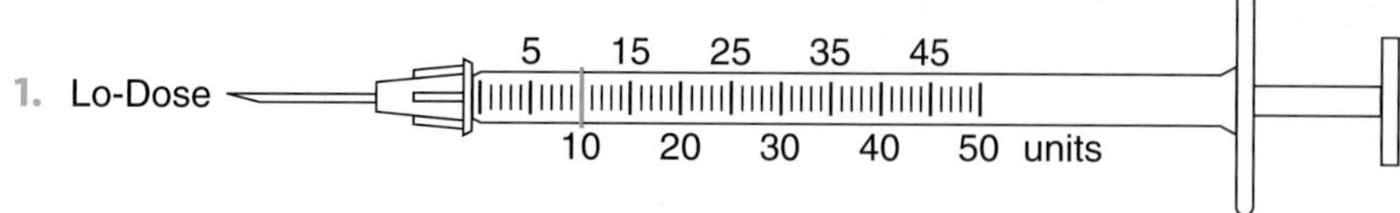

2. 10,000 units : 1 mL :: 14,000 units : x mL

$$10{,}000x = 14{,}000$$
$$x = \frac{14{,}000}{10{,}000}$$
$$x = 1.4 \text{ mL}$$

$$\frac{14{,}000 \text{ units}}{10{,}000 \text{ units}} \times 1 \text{ mL} = 1.4 \text{ mL}$$

3. 200,000 units : 5 mL :: 500,000 units : x mL

$$200{,}000x = 2{,}500{,}000$$
$$x = \frac{2{,}500{,}000}{200{,}000}$$
$$x = 12.5 \text{ mL}$$

$$\frac{500{,}000 \text{ units}}{\cancel{200{,}000}\ \text{units}\ _{40{,}000}} \times \frac{\overset{1}{\cancel{5}} \text{ mL}}{1} = 12.5 \text{ mL}$$

4. Lo-Dose

5. 5000 units : 0.2 mL :: 2500 units : x mL

$$5000x = 0.2 \times 2500$$
$$x = \frac{500}{2500}$$
$$x = 0.1 \text{ mL}$$

$$\frac{2500 \text{ units}}{5000 \text{ units}} \times 0.2 \text{ mL} = 0.1 \text{ mL}$$

6. Insulin

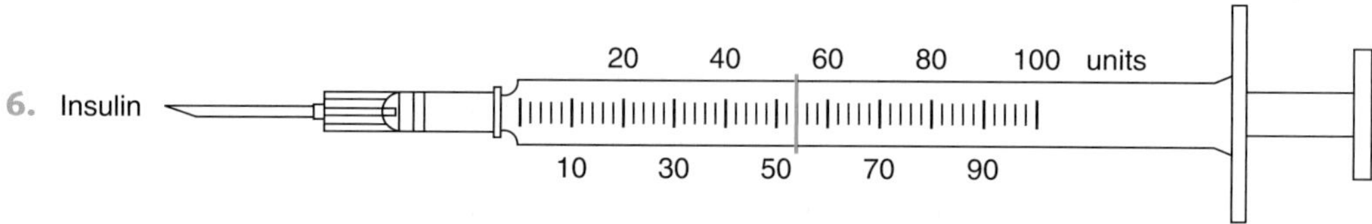

7. Lo-Dose

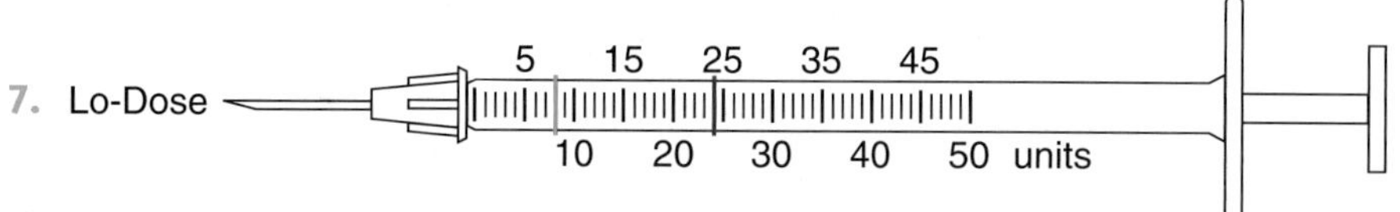

8. 400,000 units : 5 mL :: 300,000 units : x mL

$$400{,}000x = 1{,}500{,}000$$
$$x - \frac{1{,}500{,}000}{400{,}000}$$
$$x = 3.75, 3.8 \text{ mL}$$

$$\frac{300{,}000 \text{ units}}{400{,}000 \text{ units}} \times 5 \text{ mL} =$$
$$\frac{1{,}500{,}000}{400{,}000} = 3.75,\ 3.8 \text{ mL}$$

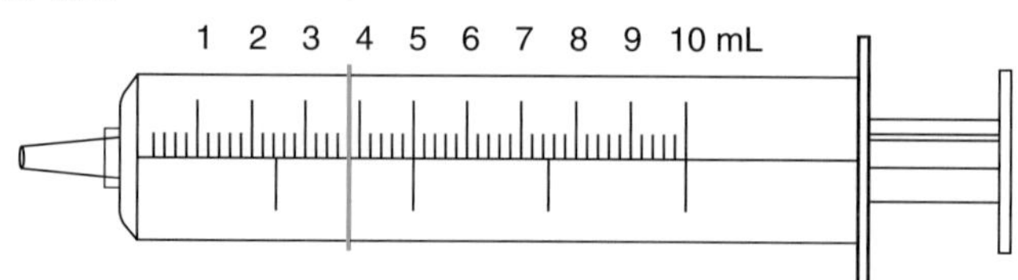

Proportion **Formula**

9. Lo-Dose

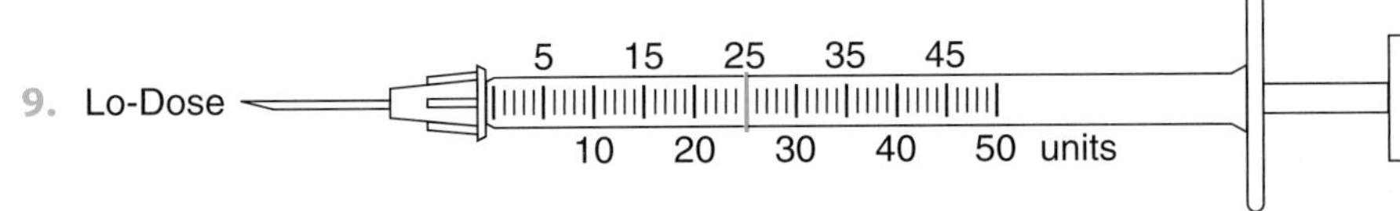

10. 10,000 units : 1 mL :: 16,000 units : x mL

$$10{,}000x = 16{,}000$$

$$x = \frac{16{,}000}{10{,}000}$$

$$x = 1.6 \text{ mL}$$

$$\frac{16{,}000 \text{ units}}{10{,}000 \text{ units}} \times 1 \text{ mL} = 1.6 \text{ mL}$$

11. Insulin

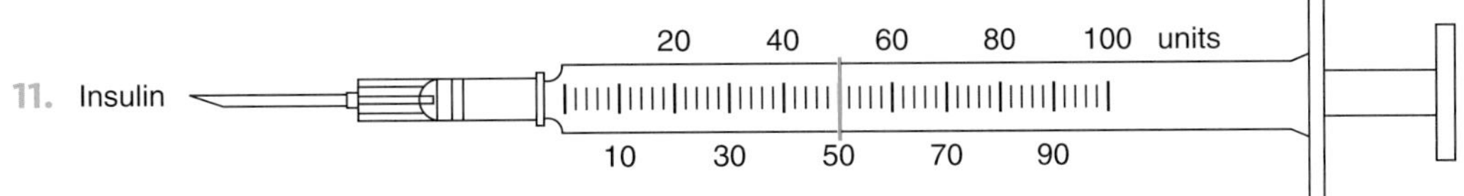

12. Lo-Dose

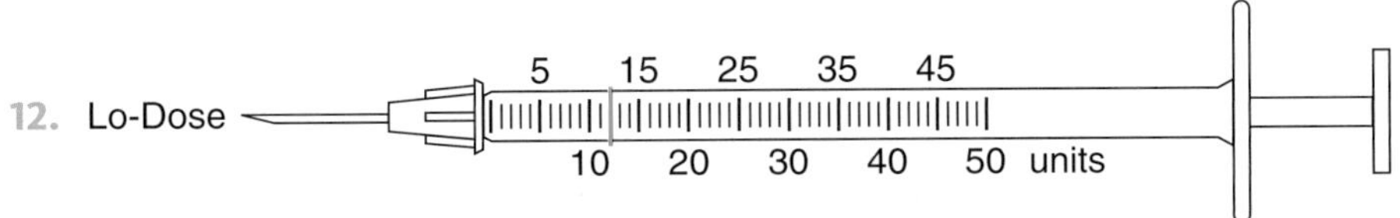

13. 40 mg : 0.4 mL :: 20 mg : x mL

$$40x = 8$$

$$x = \frac{8}{40}$$

$$x = 0.2 \text{ mL}$$

$$\frac{20 \text{ mg}}{40 \text{ mg}} \times 0.4 \text{ mL} = 0.2 \text{ mL}$$

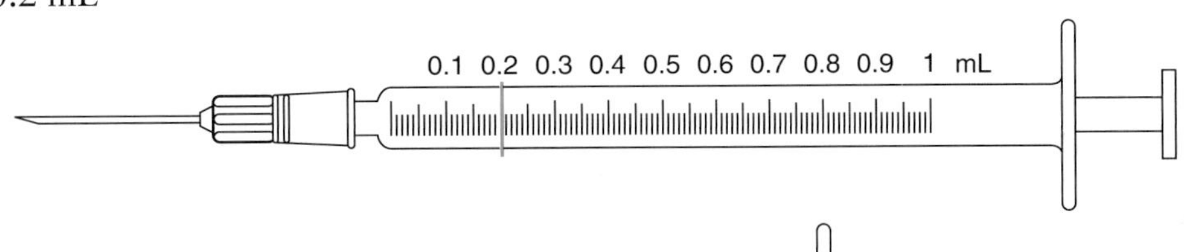

14. Lo-Dose

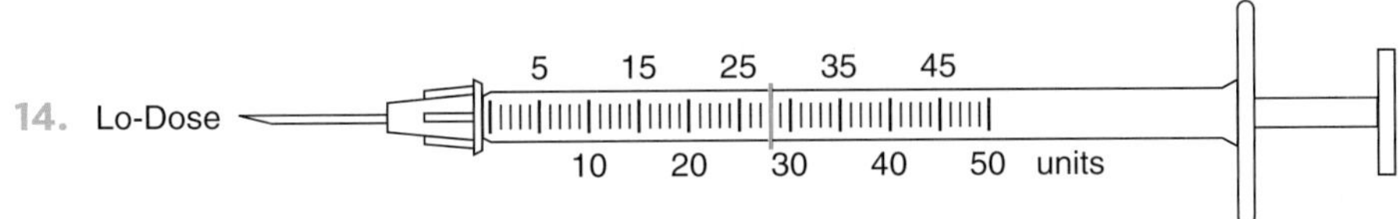

15. 5000 units : 1 mL :: 2500 units : x mL

$$5000x = 2500$$

$$x = \frac{2500}{5000} = 0.5 \text{ mL}$$

$$\frac{2500 \text{ units}}{5000 \text{ units}} \times 1 \text{ mL} = 0.5 \text{ mL}$$

ANSWERS

CHAPTER **14**

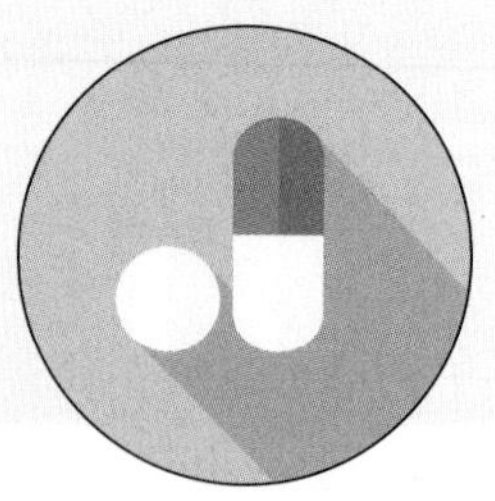

Reconstitution of Medications

LEARNING OBJECTIVES

Upon completion of the materials provided in this chapter, you will be able to perform computations accurately by mastering the following mathematical concepts:

1. Calculating drug dosage problems that first require reconstitution of a powdered drug into a liquid form
2. Using dimensional analysis, proportion, or formula methods to solve problems involving drugs measured in unit dosages

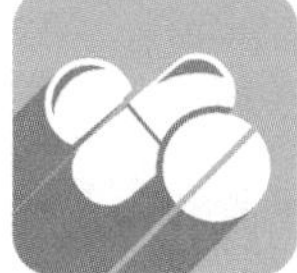

POWDER RECONSTITUTION

A drug in powdered form is necessary when a medication is unstable as a liquid form for a long period. This powdered drug must be reconstituted—dissolved with a sterile diluent—before administration. A **diluent** is a liquid used to dissolve a medication to be ingested (orally), injected (parenterally), or inhaled. The diluents commonly used include sterile water, sterile normal saline solution, 5% dextrose solution (D_5W), and bacteriostatic normal saline.

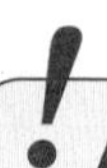

ALERT

Remember to always check the route of the administration for *all* reconstituted medications. Some will be oral and some will be parenteral.

Before reconstituting the medication, the nurse must follow several principles:

1. Carefully read the information and directions on the vial or package insert for reconstitution of the medication.
2. If no directions are available with the medication, consult the *Physicians' Desk Reference,* hospital drug formulary, pharmacology text, or hospital pharmacy.
3. Identify the type and amount of diluent and the route of administration.
4. Note the drug strength or concentration after reconstitution and circle or place this on the label, if not already written, when you use a multidose vial.
5. Note the length of time for which the medication is good once reconstituted and the directions for storage.
6. Be aware that the total reconstitution amount may be greater than the amount of diluent because of the volume of the powder.
7. After reconstitution of a multidose vial, place your initials, date of preparation, time of preparation, date of expiration, and time of expiration on the label.

In Figure 14-1, please review the steps required to reconstitute a medication.

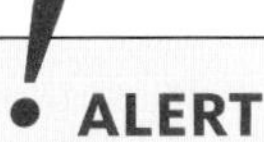

ALERT

A label must be placed on all multidose vials after reconstitution. The label must include the preparer's initials, the date and time of preparation, and the date and time of expiration.

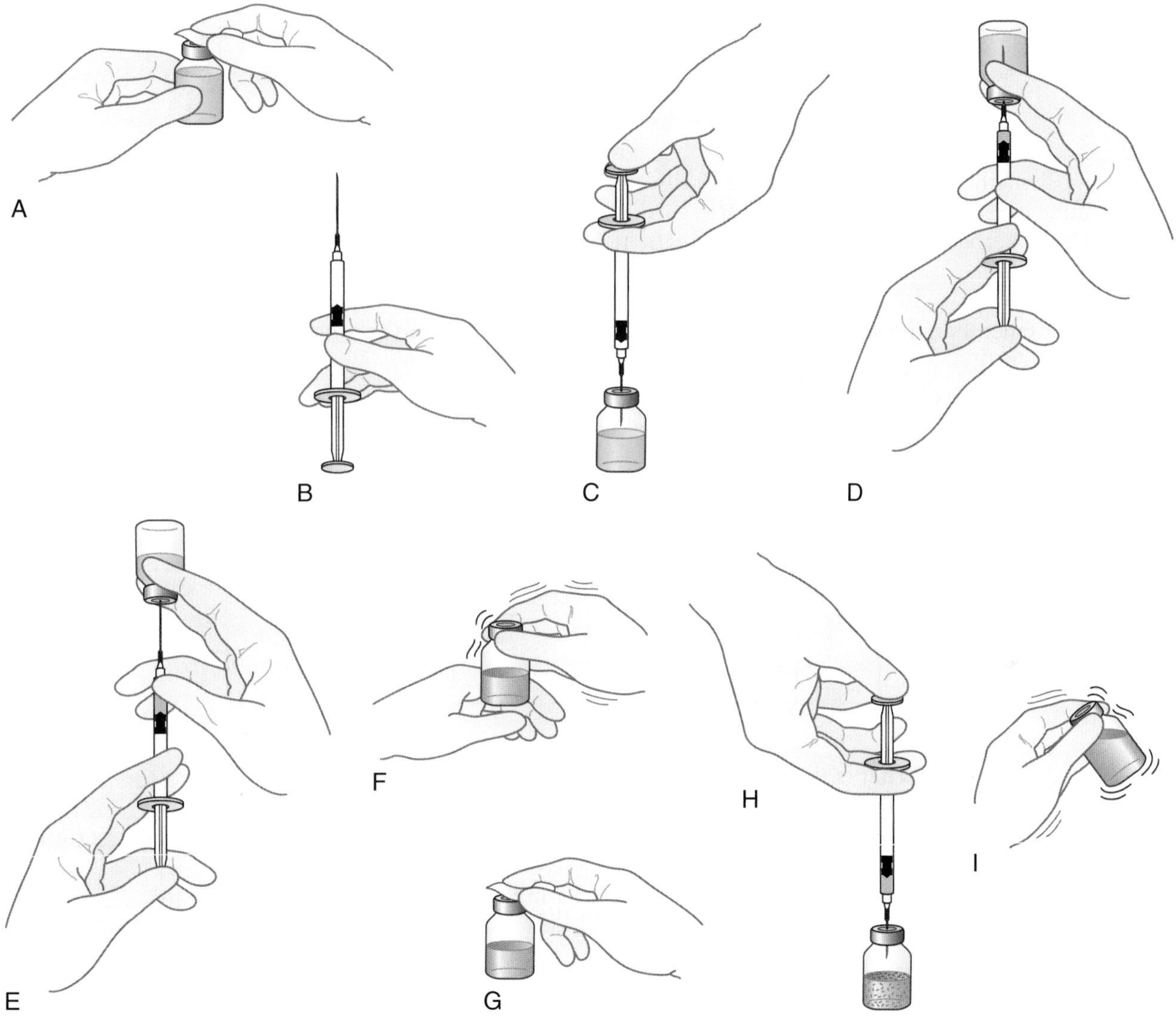

FIGURE 14-1 Removal of a volume of liquid from a vial: reconstitution of a powder. **A,** Cleanse the rubber diaphragm of the vial. **B,** Pull back on the plunger of the syringe to fill with an amount of air that is equal to the volume of the solution to be withdrawn. **C,** Insert the needle through the rubber diaphragm; inject the air with the vial sitting in a downward position. **D,** Withdraw the volume of diluent required to reconstitute the drug. **E,** Move the needle downward to facilitate the removal of all of the diluent. **F,** Tap the container with the powdered drug to break up the caked powder. **G,** Wipe the rubber diaphragm of the vial of the powdered drug with a new antiseptic alcohol wipe. **H,** Insert the needle with the diluent in the syringe into the rubber diaphragm, and inject the diluent into the powdered drug. **I,** Mix thoroughly to ensure that the powdered drug is dissolved before withdrawing the prescribed dose. **Note specific directions. Some medications should be rolled to mix—not shaken.** (From Clayton BD, Willihnganz MJ: *Basic pharmacology for nurses*, ed. 17, St Louis, 2017, Elsevier.)

Medications may also be supplied in a Mix-O-Vial container. This container supplies both the powdered medication for reconstitution and the diluent. See Figure 14-2.

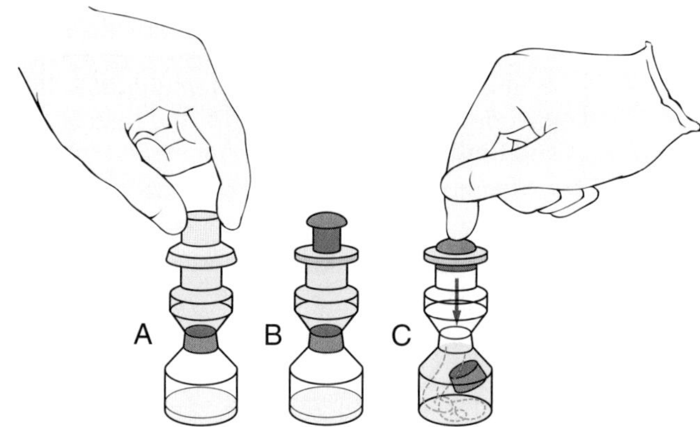

FIGURE 14-2 Using a Mix-O-Vial. **A,** Remove the plastic lid protector. **B,** The powdered drug is in the lower half; the diluent is in the upper half. **C,** Push firmly on the diaphragm plunger; downward pressure dislodges the divider between the two chambers. (From Clayton BD, Willihnganz MJ: *Basic pharmacology for nurses*, ed. 17, St Louis, 2017, Elsevier.)

Penicillin can be administered orally or parenterally. Before administering penicillin, the nurse must confer with the patient regarding previous allergies to the drug. After administering the drug, the nurse must observe the patient for signs of an allergic reaction, as with any other medication.

Remember, the strength of the medication is dependent on the amount of diluent added.

Reconstitution of Oral Medication

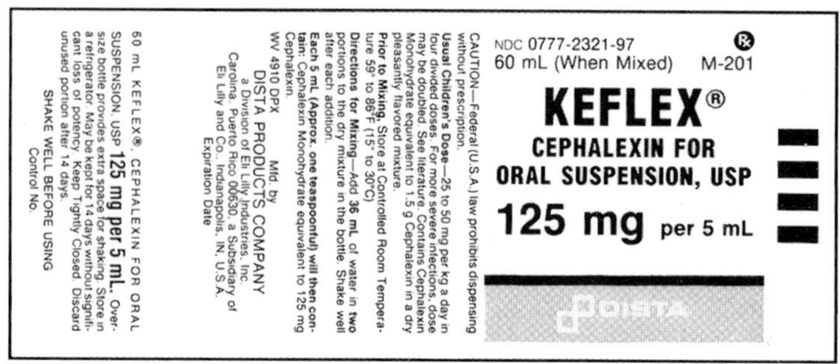

EXAMPLE:

Step 1. What is the route of administration? oral

Step 2. What type of diluent can be used? water

Step 3. If 36 mL of diluent is added, what is the medication concentration? 125 mg per mL

Step 4. The licensed prescriber orders 75 mg po q 6 h. How many milliliters will you give for each dose? 3 mL

Dimensional Analysis

$$x \text{ mL} = \frac{5 \text{ mL}}{125 \text{ mg}} \times \frac{75 \text{ mg}}{1} = \frac{15}{5} = 3 \text{ mL}$$

Proportion Method

Step 1. 125 mg : 5 mL ::

Step 2. 125 mg : 5 mL :: _____ mg : _____ mL

Step 3. 125 mg : 5 mL :: 75 mg : x mL

Step 4. $125x = 375$

$$x = \frac{375}{125}$$

Step 5. $x = 3$ mL

Reconstitution of Parenteral Medication

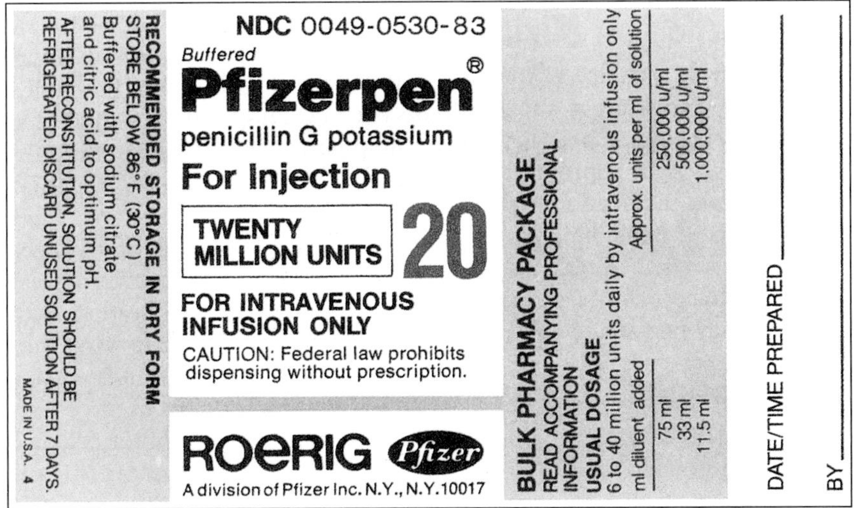

EXAMPLE:

Step 1.	What is the route of administration?	IV
Step 2.	What type of diluent can be used?	Check insert
Step 3.	How much diluent must be added?	75 mL, 33 mL, or 11.5 mL
Step 4.	If 75 mL of diluent is added, what is the medication concentration?	250,000 units/mL
Step 5.	How long will the medication maintain its potency after refrigeration?	7 days
Step 6.	The licensed prescriber orders 2,000,000 units IV q 4 h. How many milliliters will you give? Shade the syringe.	8 mL

Dimensional Analysis

$$x \text{ mL} = \frac{1 \text{ mL}}{250{,}000 \cancel{\text{units}}} \times \frac{2{,}000{,}000 \cancel{\text{units}}}{1} = \frac{2{,}000{,}000}{250{,}000} = 8 \text{ mL}$$

Proportion Method

Step 1. 250,000 units : 1 mL ::

Step 2. 250,000 units : 1 mL :: ______ units : ______ mL

Step 3. 250,000 units : 1 mL :: 2,000,000 units : x mL

Step 4. $250{,}000x = 2{,}000{,}000$

$$x = \frac{2{,}000{,}000}{250{,}000}$$

$$x = 8$$

Step 5. $x = 8$ mL

Formula

$$\frac{2{,}000{,}000}{250{,}000} \times 1 = 8 \text{ mL}$$

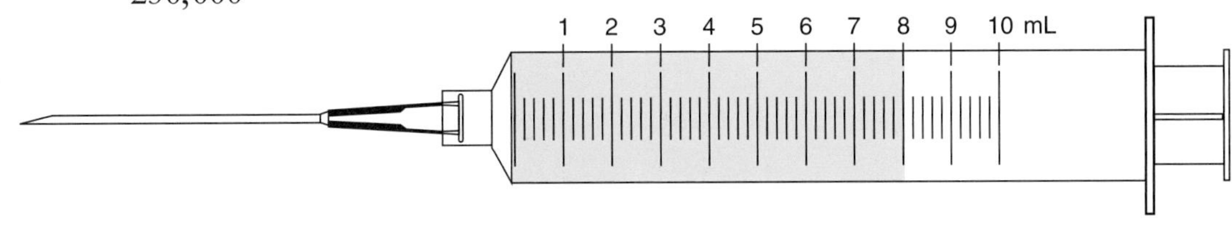

Once a medication has been reconstituted, you will solve the calculation dosage problems exactly as you have learned in previous chapters. The known strength, or what you have on hand, is just determined by the amount of diluent you added to the powdered medication.

Complete the following work sheet, which provides for extensive practice in the calculation of dosages measured in units. Check your answers. If you have difficulties, go back and review the necessary material. When you feel ready to evaluate your learning, take the first posttest. Check your answers. An acceptable score as indicated on the posttest signifies that you have successfully completed this chapter. An unacceptable score signifies a need for further study before taking the second posttest.

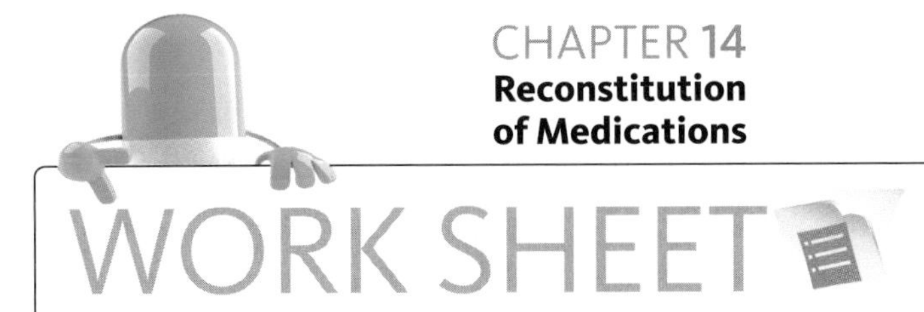

CHAPTER 14
Reconstitution of Medications

WORK SHEET

DIRECTIONS: Answer the questions. Calculate the doses. Show your work. Mark the medicine cup or syringe when provided to indicate the correct dose.

1. Your patient who has had a craniotomy has Ceclor suspension 250 mg po four times a day ordered. What should be used as the diluent? ______ How many milliliters of diluent should be added? ______ How many milligrams are in the bottle? ______ How many milliliters will you administer each dose? ______ How many doses are in the bottle? ______

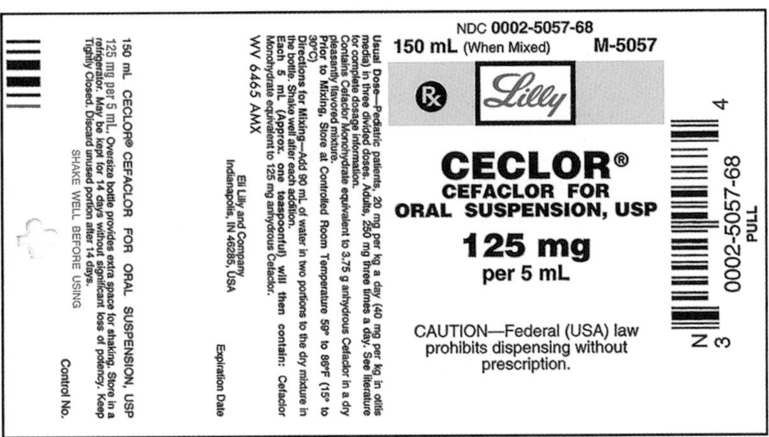

2. The licensed prescriber has ordered Keflex 275 mg po q 6 h for Mr. Smith after his thyroidectomy. What should be used as the diluent? ______ How many milliliters of diluent should be added? ______ How many milligrams are in the bottle? ______ How many milliliters will the nurse administer per dose? ______ How many doses are in the bottle? ______

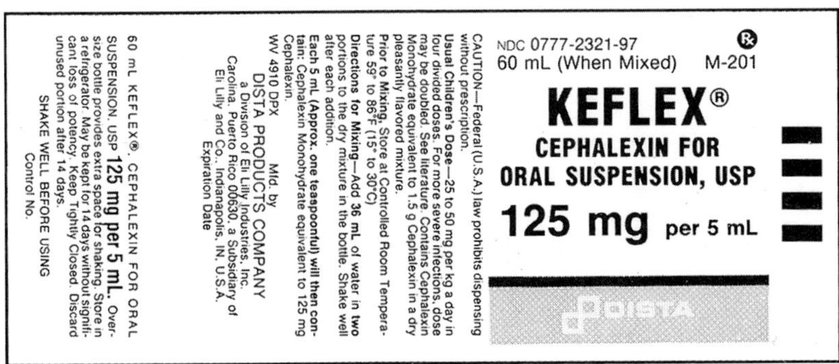

3. Mr. Davis receives cefaclor 600 mg po q 8 h for the treatment of acute bronchitis. What should be used as the diluent? ______ How many milliliters of diluent should be added? ______ How many milligrams are in the bottle? ______ How many milliliters will the nurse administer per dose? ______ How many doses are in the bottle? ______

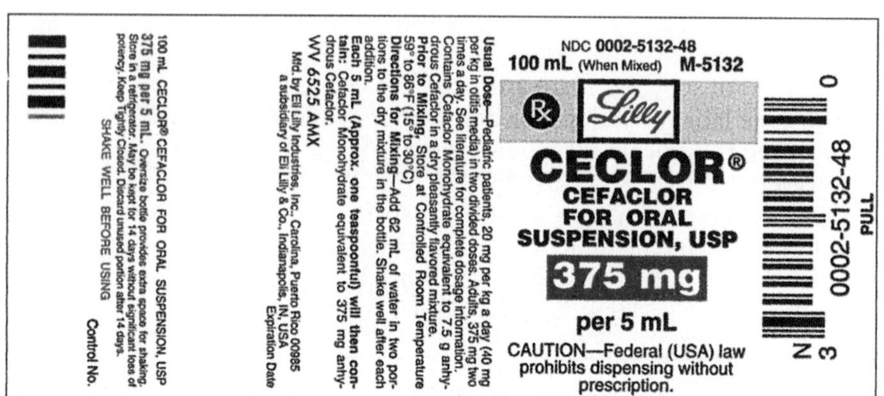

4. A patient with a temporal bone infection receives penicillin G 500,000 units IM q 6 h. How much diluent should be added? ______ What is the medication concentration? ______ How many milliliters will you administer? ______ What would you circle on the label to indicate concentration? ______

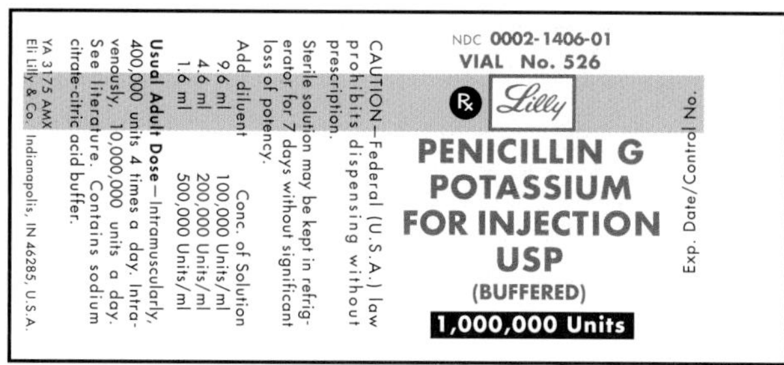

5. Your patient with a thoracotomy receives penicillin G 600,000 units IM twice a day. How much diluent should be added? ______ What is the medication concentration? ______ How many milliliters will you administer? ______ What is the best choice for the amount of dilution and why? ______

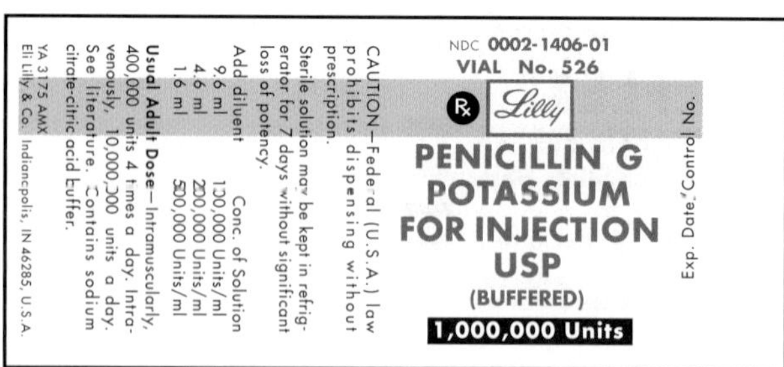

6. Mr. Rose has Pfizerpen 250,000 units IM now ordered. How many milliliters will the nurse administer if 8.2 mL of diluent is added? ______

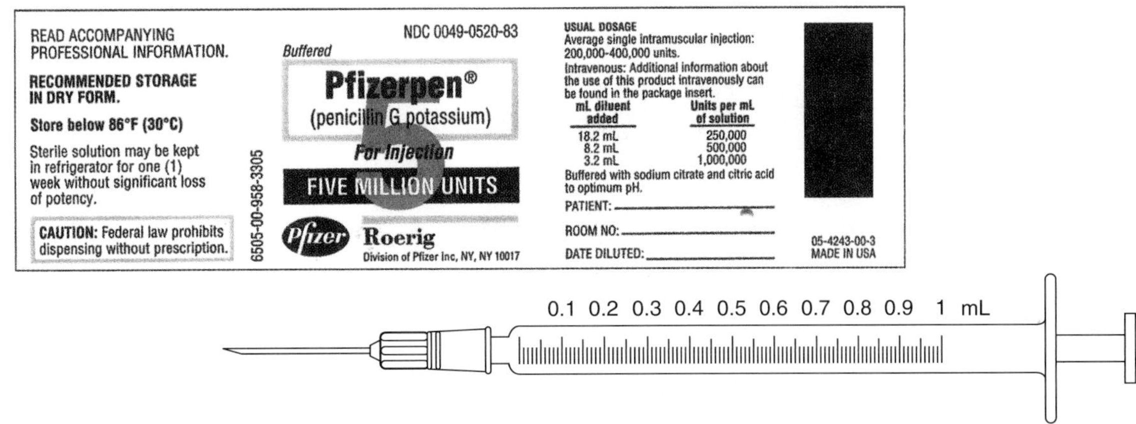

7. Mrs. Garden has penicillin G potassium 175,000 units IM now ordered. If 18.2 mL of diluent are added, how many milliliters will the nurse administer? ______

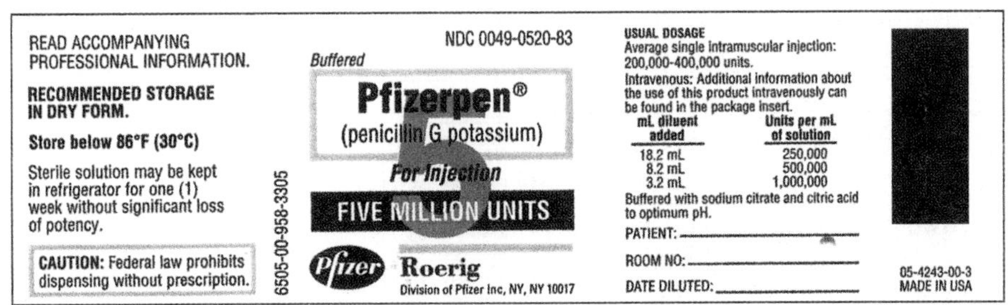

8. Lorabid 500 mg oral every 12 hours has been ordered for a patient with pneumonia. How much diluent will be added to the bottle? ______ What is the concentration after reconstitution? ______ How many milliliters will the nurse administer? ______

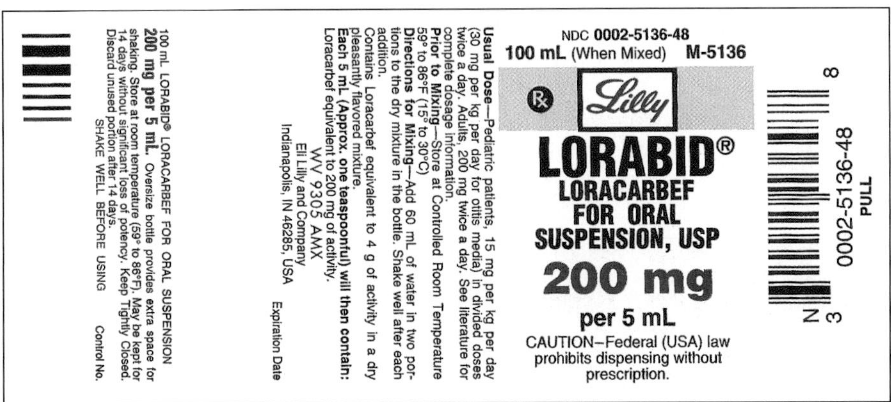

9. The licensed prescriber orders oxacillin 250 mg IM every 6 hours for a patient with a skin infection. How much diluent will be added to the bottle? ______ What is the concentration after reconstitution? ______ How many milliliters will the nurse administer? ______

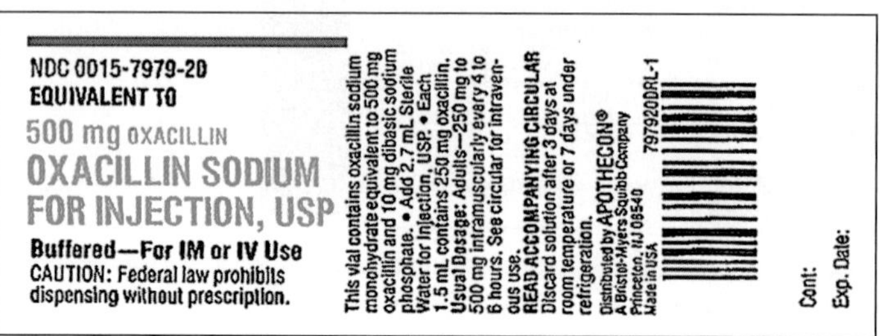

10. The licensed prescriber orders Vancocin 500 mg oral every 12 hours for a patient with pseudomembranous colitis. How much diluent will be added to the bottle? ______ What is the concentration after reconstitution? ______ How many milliliters will the nurse administer? ______

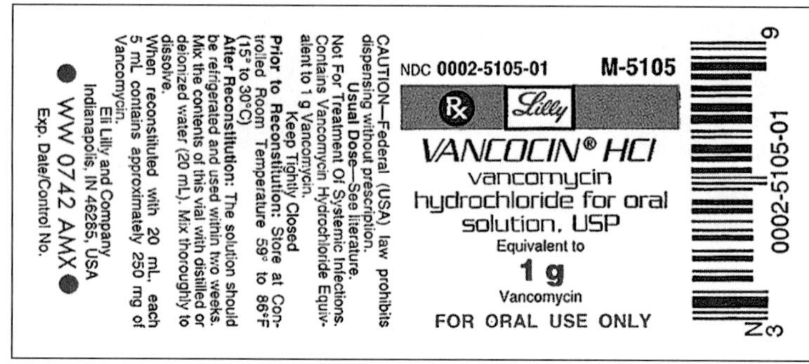

ANSWERS ON PP. 425–426 AND 428–430.

NAME ____________________

DATE ____________________

ACCEPTABLE SCORE 9

YOUR SCORE ______

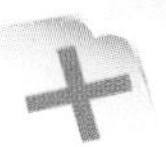

POSTTEST 1

DIRECTIONS: Answer the questions. Calculate the doses. Show your work. Mark the medicine cup or syringe when provided to indicate the correct dose.

1. Miss Kate has chronic sinusitis. Her licensed prescriber orders amoxicillin 375 mg po q 8 h. What should be used as the diluent? ______ How many milliliters of diluent should be added? ______ How many milligrams are in the bottle? ______ How many milliliters will you administer each dose? ______ How many doses are in the bottle? ______

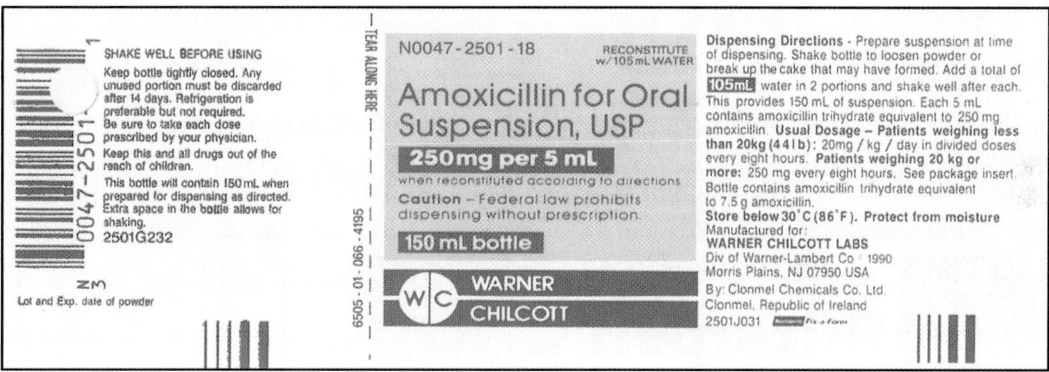

2. The licensed prescriber has ordered Amoxil suspension 250 po mg q 6 h. What should be used as the diluent? ______ How many milliliters of diluent should be added? ______ How many milligrams are in the bottle? ______ How many milliliters will the nurse administer per dose? ______ How many doses are in the bottle? ______

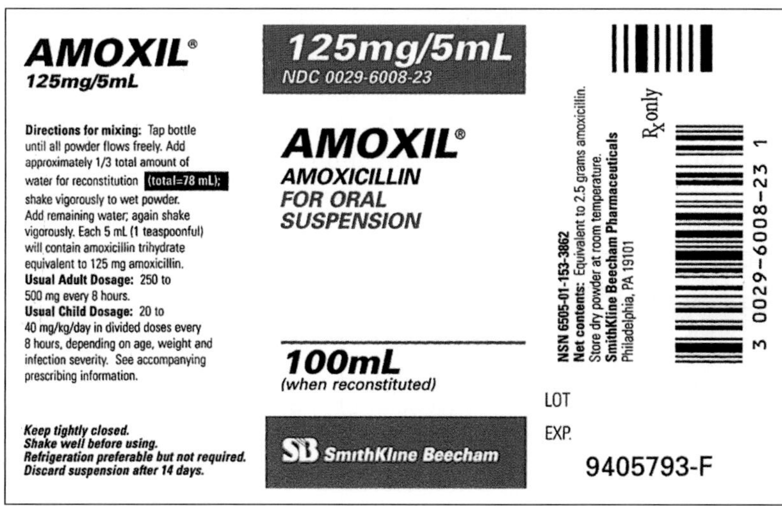

3. Mrs. Hall has acute bronchitis and has cefaclor 450 mg po q 12 h ordered. What should be used as the diluent? ______ How many milliliters of diluent should be added? ______ How many milligrams are in the bottle? ______ How many milliliters will the nurse administer per dose? ______ How many doses are in the bottle? ______

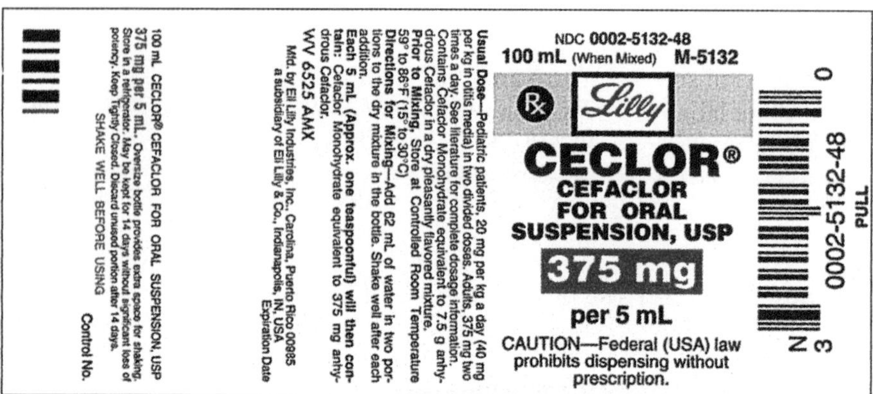

4. The licensed prescriber orders penicillin G potassium 3,000,000 units IV q 6 h for your patient with an ethmoidectomy. What is the medication concentration if 11.5 mL of diluent is added? ______ How many milliliters will you administer? ______

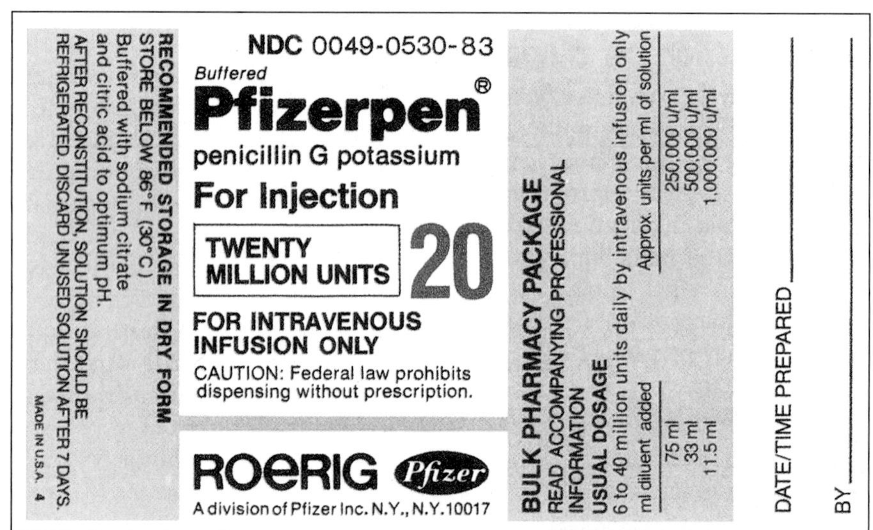

5. Mr. Cory has orders for Pfizerpen 600,000 units IM q 6 h for a serious pneumococcal infection. Select the most appropriate dilution. How many milliliters of diluent will you add? ______ How many milliliters will you administer? ______

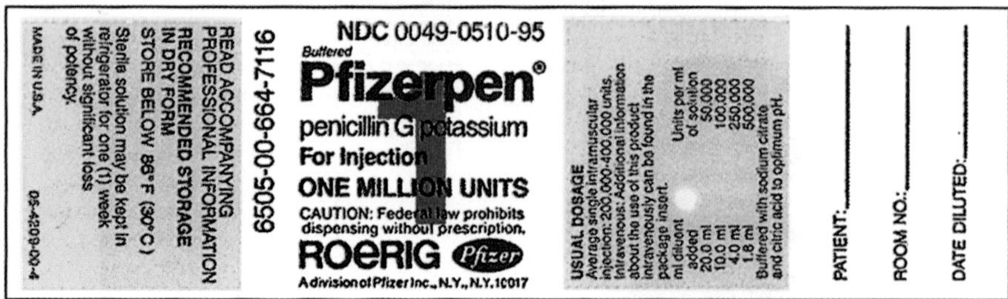

6. The licensed prescriber orders Pfizerpen 1.2 million units IV in a single dose today. What is the medication concentration if 11.5 mL of diluent is added? ______ How many milliliters will the nurse administer? ______

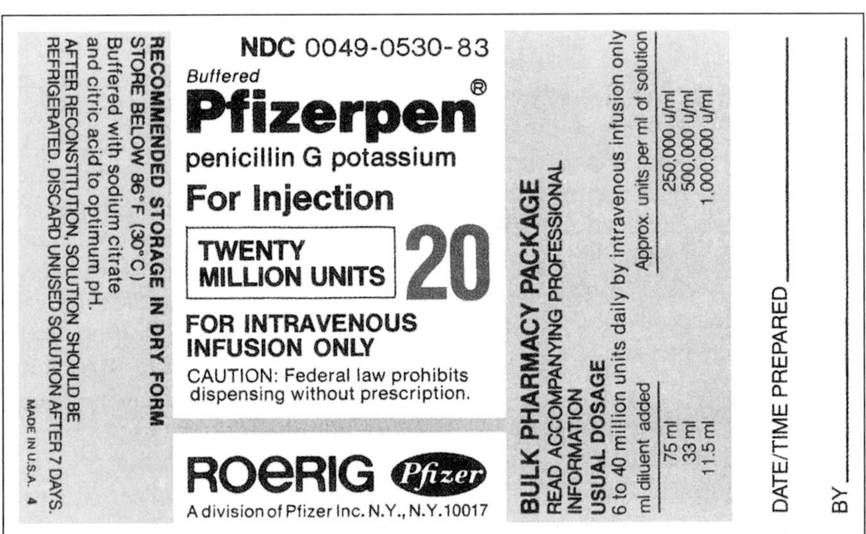

7. Mrs. Daisy receives nystatin oral suspension 600,000 units po four times a day. How many milliliters will the nurse administer? ______

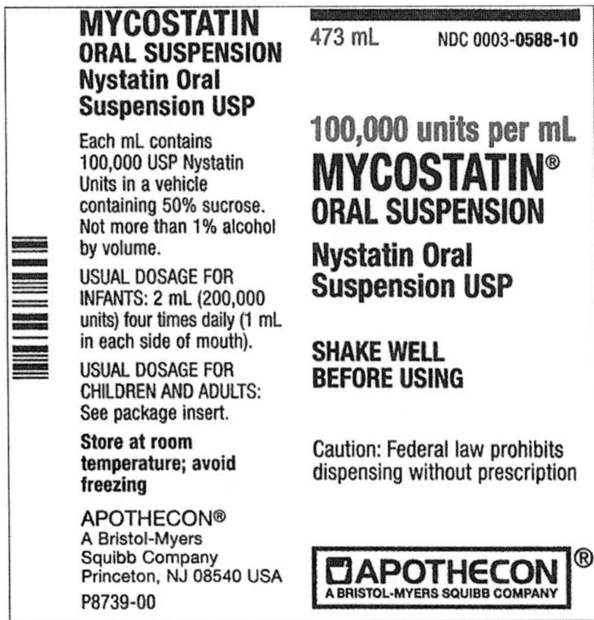

8. The licensed prescriber orders ampicillin 500 mg IM every 6 hours for a patient with pneumonia. How much diluent will be added to the bottle? ______ What is the concentration after reconstitution? ______ How many milliliters will the nurse administer? ______

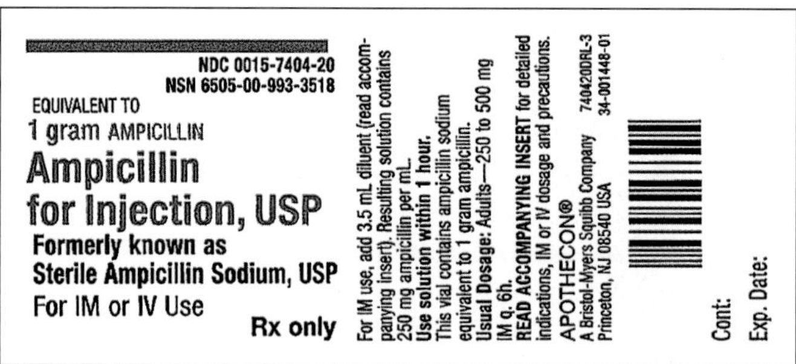

9. The licensed prescriber orders Ancef 500 mg IM every 12 hours for a patient with cellulitis. How much diluent will be added to the bottle? ______ What is the concentration after reconstitution? ______ How many milliliters will the nurse administer? ______

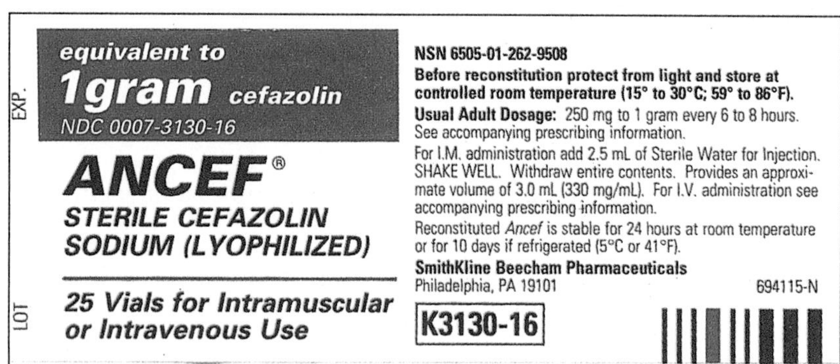

10. Vancocin 1000 mg oral every 6 hours has been ordered for a patient with colitis. How much diluent will be added to the bottle? ______ What is the concentration after reconstitution? ______ How many milliliters will the nurse administer? ______

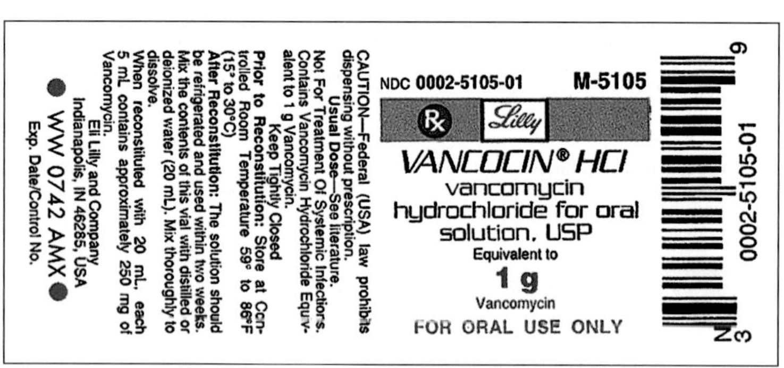

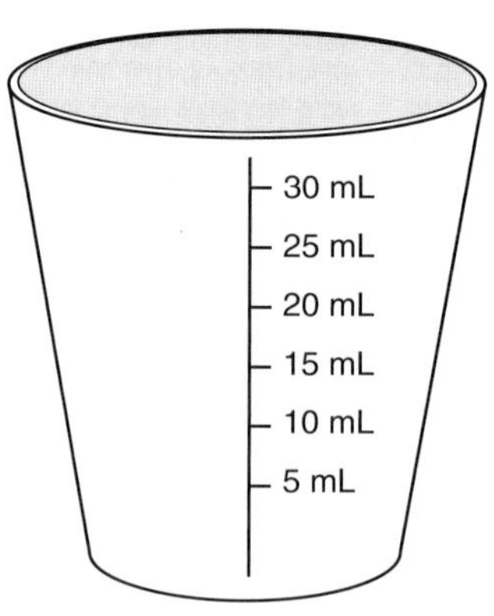

ANSWERS ON PP. 426–427 AND 430–432.

NAME ______________________

DATE ______________________

ACCEPTABLE SCORE **9**

YOUR SCORE ______

POSTTEST 2

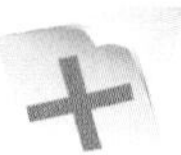

DIRECTIONS: Answer the questions. Calculate the doses. Show your work. Mark the medicine cup or syringe when provided to indicate the correct dose.

1. The licensed prescriber orders Keflin 400 mg IV q 6 h for your patient with an infection. Add 10 mL of 0.9% sodium chloride for diluent. How many milligrams are in the vial? ______ How many milliliters will you administer? ______ How many doses are in the vial? ______

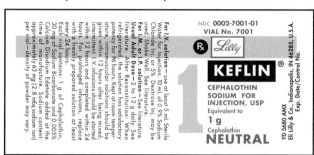

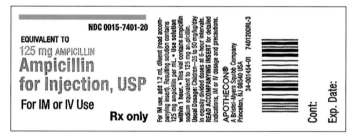

2. Your patient with an infection receives ampicillin 500 mg IV q 12 h. How many milliliters of diluent should be added? ______ How many milligrams are in the vial? ______ How many milliliters will you administer for each dose? ______ How many doses are in the vial? ______

3. The licensed prescriber orders penicillin G potassium 1.2 million units IV q 4 h for your patient after dental extraction. You have a vial containing 1,000,000 units/mL. How many milliliters will you prepare? ______

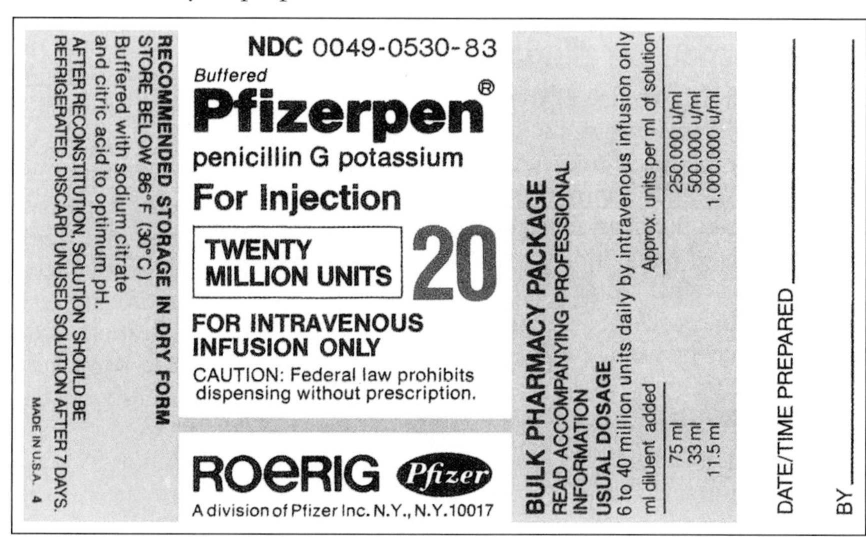

4. Ms. Martinez has 2 million units IV Pfizerpen q 4 h ordered for a severe pneumococcal infection. How much diluent will you add for a concentration of 1,000,000 units/mL? ______ How many milliliters will you administer? ______

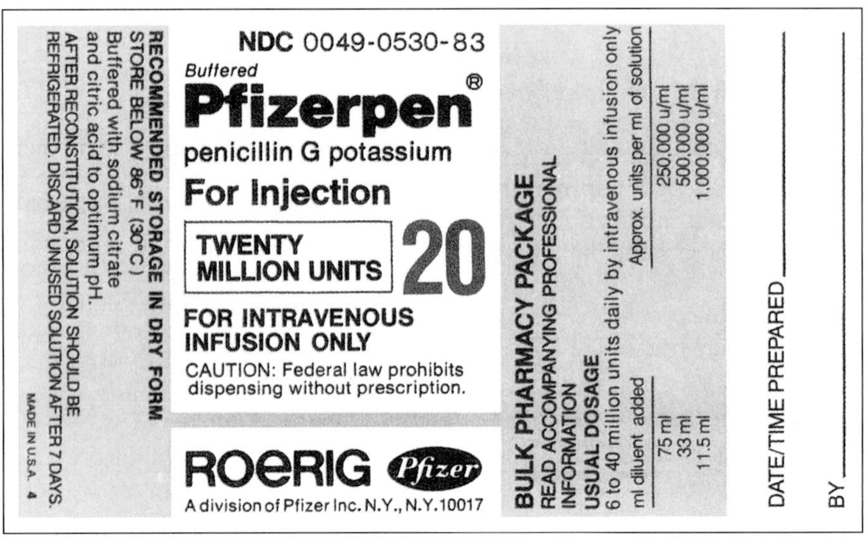

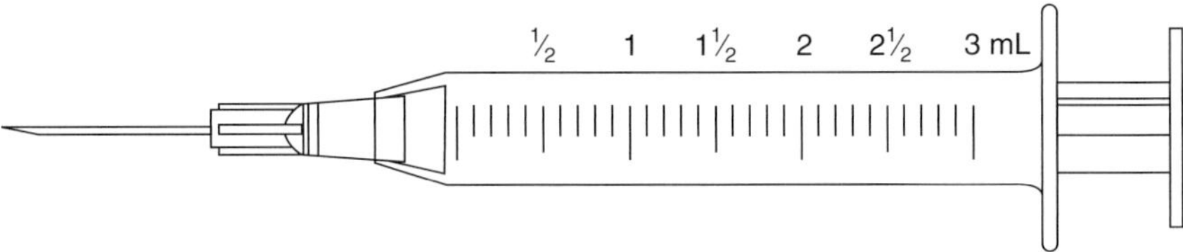

5. Your patient with osteomyelitis receives penicillin G 600,000 units IM twice daily. How much diluent should be added? ______ What is the medication concentration? ______ How many milliliters will you administer? ______

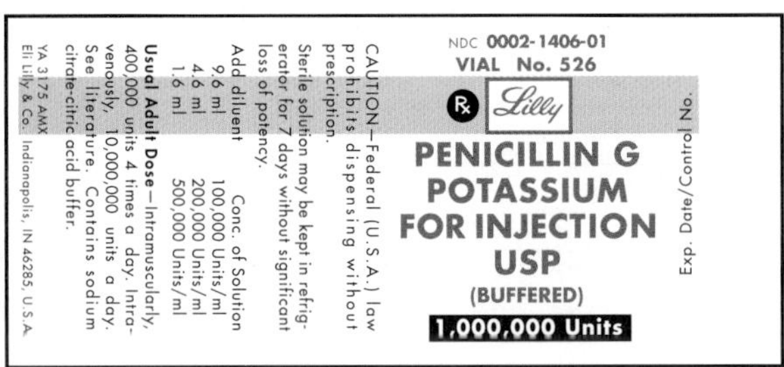

6. Miss Garrett has Pfizerpen 400,000 units IV q 4 h ordered for a severe streptococcal infection. You add 75 mL of diluent. How many milliliters will you administer? ______

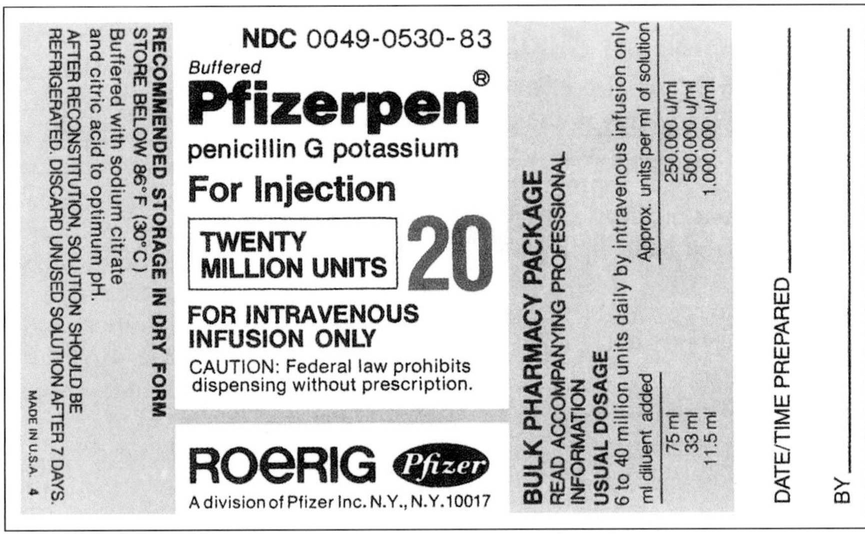

7. Mrs. Roy has Pfizerpen (penicillin G potassium) 300,000 units IM q 4 h ordered for a serious streptococcal infection. How much diluent will you add for a concentration of 250,000 units/mL? ______ How many milliliters will you administer? ______

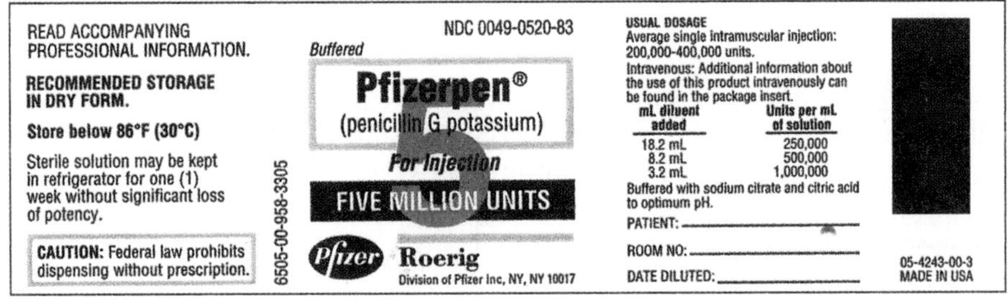

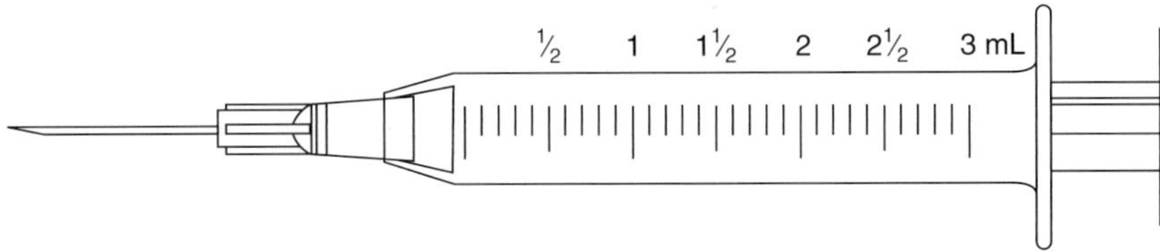

8. The licensed prescriber orders erythromycin 500 mg oral, one time, as a bowel preparation. How much diluent will be added to the bottle? ______ What is the concentration after reconstitution? ______ How many milliliters will the nurse administer? ______

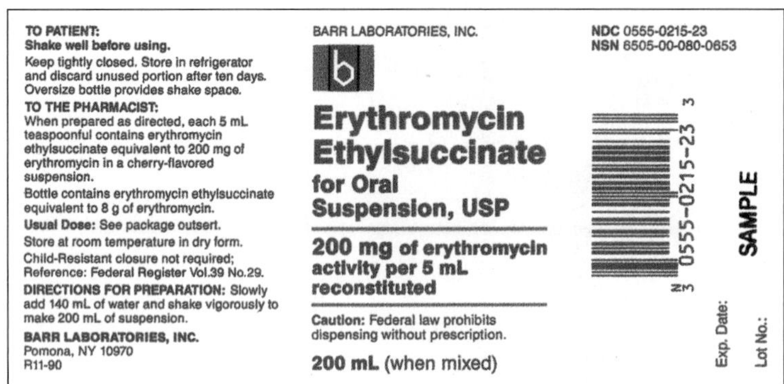

9. The licensed prescriber orders Cefobid 1000 mg IV every 12 hours for a patient with an infection. How much diluent will first be added to the bottle? ______ What is the concentration after this reconstitution? ______ How many milliliters will the nurse administer? ______

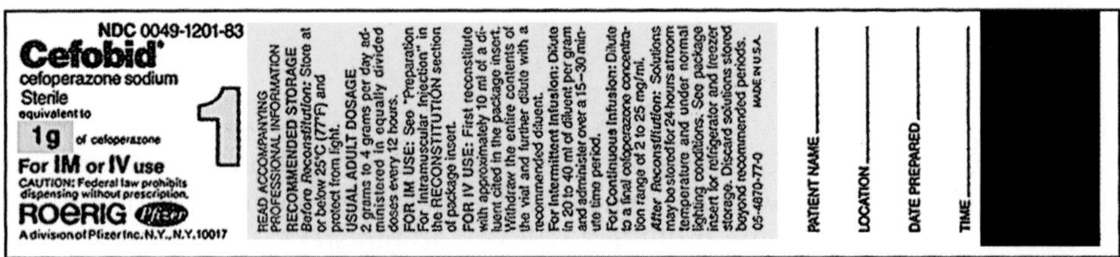

10. The licensed prescriber orders Amoxil 500 mg oral every 6 hours for tonsilitis. How much diluent will be added to the bottle? ______ What is the concentration after reconstitution? ______ How many milliliters will the nurse administer? ______

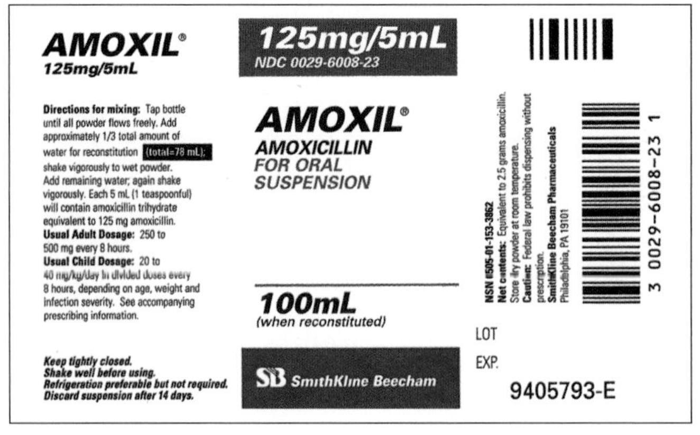

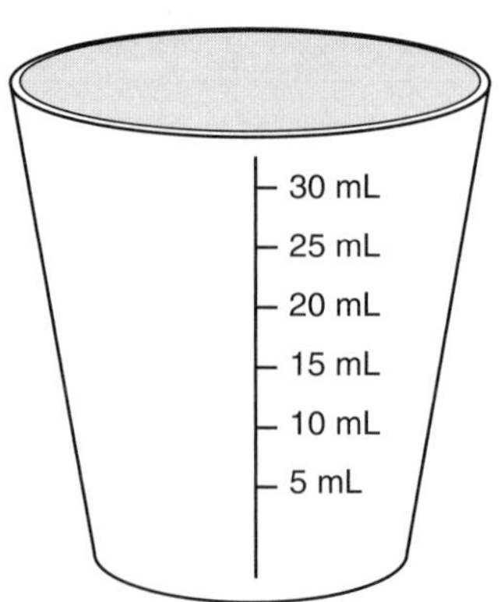

ANSWERS ON PP. 427–428 AND 432–434.

ANSWERS

CHAPTER 14 Dimensional Analysis—Work Sheet, pp. 413–416

pp. 413–416

1. Water, 90 mL, 3750 mg, 15 doses in bottle

$$x \text{ mL} = \frac{5 \text{ mL}}{125 \text{ mg}} \times \frac{250 \text{ mg}}{1} = \frac{1250}{125} = 10 \text{ mL}$$

2. Water, 36 mL, 1500 mg, 5.45, or 5 full doses in bottle

$$x \text{ mL} = \frac{5 \text{ mL}}{125 \text{ mg}} \times \frac{275 \text{ mg}}{1} = \frac{1375}{125} = 11 \text{ mL}$$

3. Water, 62 mL, 7500 mg, 8 mL, 12.5 doses

$$x \text{ mL} = \frac{5 \text{ mL}}{375 \text{ mg}} \times \frac{600 \text{ mg}}{1} = \frac{3000}{375} = 8 \text{ mL}$$

4. Diluent 4.6 mL, 200,000 units/mL

$$x \text{ mL} = \frac{1 \text{ mL}}{200{,}000 \text{ units}} \times \frac{500{,}000 \text{ units}}{1} = 2.5 \text{ mL}$$

Diluent 1.6 mL, 500,000 units/mL

$$x \text{ mL} = \frac{1 \text{ mL}}{500{,}000 \text{ units}} \times \frac{500{,}000 \text{ units}}{1} = 1 \text{ mL}$$

Circle the strength mixed.

5. Diluent 4.6 mL, 200,000 units/mL

$$x \text{ mL} = \frac{1 \text{ mL}}{200{,}000 \text{ units}} \times \frac{600{,}000 \text{ units}}{1} = 3 \text{ mL}$$

Diluent 1.6 mL, 500,000 units/mL

$$x \text{ mL} = \frac{1 \text{ mL}}{500{,}000 \text{ units}} \times \frac{600{,}000 \text{ units}}{1} = 1.2 \text{ mL}$$

Diluent 1.6 mL. The patient receives a smaller volume of medicine.

6. $$x \text{ mL} = \frac{1 \text{ mL}}{500{,}000 \text{ units}} \times \frac{250{,}000 \text{ units}}{1} = 0.5 \text{ mL}$$

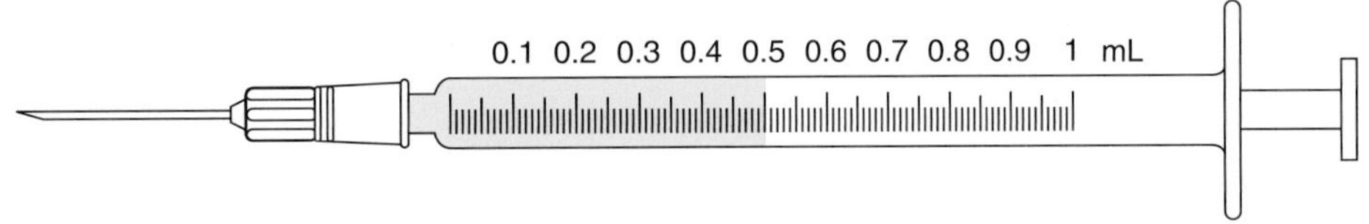

7. $$x \text{ mL} = \frac{1 \text{ mL}}{250{,}000 \text{ units}} \times \frac{175{,}000 \text{ units}}{1} = 0.7 \text{ mL}$$

8. Diluent 60 mL, 200 mg/5 mL

$$x \text{ mL} = \frac{5 \text{ mL}}{200 \text{ mg}} \times \frac{500 \text{ mg}}{1} = 12.5 \text{ mL}$$

9. Diluent 2.7 mL, 250 mg/1.5 mL

$$x \text{ mL} = \frac{1.5 \text{ mL}}{250 \text{ mg}} \times \frac{250 \text{ mg}}{1} = 1.5 \text{ mL}$$

10. Diluent 20 mL, 250 mg/5 mL

$$x \text{ mL} = \frac{5 \text{ mL}}{250 \text{ mg}} \times \frac{500 \text{ mg}}{1} = 10 \text{ mL}$$

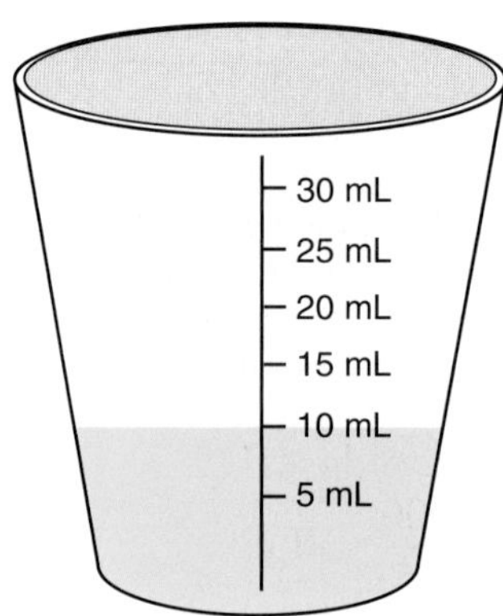

CHAPTER 14 Dimensional Analysis—Posttest 1, pp. 417–420

1. Water, 105 mL, 7500 mg, 20 doses per bottle

$$x \text{ mL} = \frac{5 \text{ mL}}{250 \text{ mg}} \times \frac{375 \text{ mg}}{1} = \frac{1875}{250} = 7.5 \text{ mL}$$

2. Water, 78 mL, 2500 mg, 10 doses per bottle

$$x \text{ mL} = \frac{5 \text{ mL}}{125 \text{ mg}} \times \frac{250 \text{ mg}}{1} = 10 \text{ mL}$$

3. Water, 62 mL, 4650 mg, 12.4, or 12 full doses in bottle

$$x \text{ mL} = \frac{5 \text{ mL}}{375 \text{ mg}} \times \frac{450 \text{ mg}}{1} = \frac{30}{5} = 6 \text{ mL}$$

4. 11.5 mL diluent, 1,000,000 units/mL

$$x \text{ mL} = \frac{1 \text{ mL}}{1{,}000{,}000 \text{ units}} \times \frac{3{,}000{,}000 \text{ units}}{1} = 3 \text{ mL}$$

5. Diluent 1.8 mL, 500,000 units/mL

$$x \text{ mL} = \frac{1 \text{ mL}}{500{,}000 \text{ units}} \times \frac{600{,}000 \text{ units}}{1} = 1.2 \text{ mL}$$

Diluent 4 mL, 250,000 units/mL

$$x \text{ mL} = \frac{1 \text{ mL}}{250{,}000 \text{ units}} \times \frac{600{,}000 \text{ units}}{1} = 2.4 \text{ mL}$$

6. If 11.5 mL diluent is added, concentration is 1,000,000 units per mL.

$$x \text{ mL} = \frac{1 \text{ mL}}{1{,}000{,}000 \text{ units}} \times \frac{1{,}200{,}000 \text{ units}}{1} = 1.2 \text{ mL}$$

7. $$x \text{ mL} = \frac{1 \text{ mL}}{100{,}000 \text{ units}} \times \frac{600{,}000 \text{ units}}{1} = 6 \text{ mL}$$

8. Diluent 3.5 mL, 250 mg/mL

$$x \text{ mL} = \frac{1 \text{ mL}}{250 \text{ mg}} \times \frac{500 \text{ mg}}{1} = 2 \text{ mL}$$

9. Diluent 2.5 mL, 330 mg/mL

$$x \text{ mL} = \frac{1 \text{ mL}}{330 \text{ mg}} \times \frac{500 \text{ mg}}{1} = 1.51,\ 1.5 \text{ mL}$$

10. Diluent 20 mL, 250 mg/5 mL

$$x \text{ mL} = \frac{5 \text{ mL}}{250 \text{ mg}} \times \frac{1000 \text{ mg}}{1} = 20 \text{ mL}$$

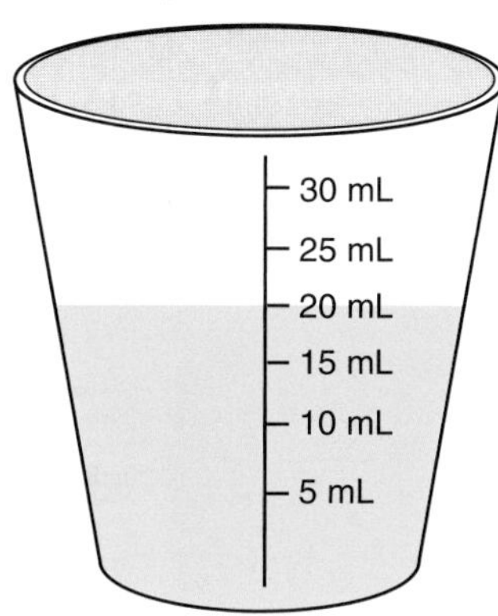

CHAPTER 14 Dimensional Analysis—Posttest 2, pp. 421–424

1. 1000 mg, 2.5, or 2 full doses in vial

$$x \text{ mL} = \frac{10 \text{ mL}}{1000 \text{ mg}} \times \frac{400 \text{ mg}}{1} = \frac{40}{10} = 4 \text{ mL}$$

2. Diluent added is 1.2 mL to each vial

125 mg are in each vial

4 vials would be needed for each dose

$$x \text{ mL} = \frac{1 \text{ mL}}{125 \text{ mg}} \times \frac{500 \text{ mg}}{1} = \frac{500}{125} = 4 \text{ mL each dose}$$

3. $$x \text{ mL} = \frac{1 \text{ mL}}{1{,}000{,}000 \text{ units}} \times \frac{1{,}200{,}000 \text{ units}}{1} = 1.2 \text{ mL}$$

4. $$x \text{ mL} = \frac{1 \text{ mL}}{1{,}000{,}000 \text{ units}} \times \frac{2{,}000{,}000 \text{ units}}{1} = 2 \text{ mL}$$

Add 11.5 mL of diluent.

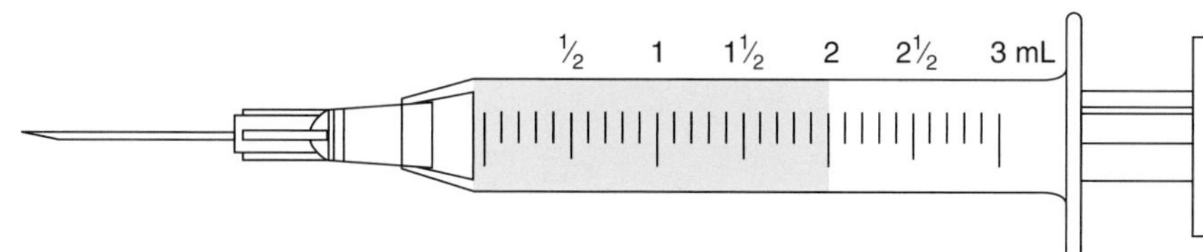

5. Diluent 4.6 mL, 200,000 units/mL

$$x \text{ mL} = \frac{1 \text{ mL}}{200{,}000 \text{ units}} \times \frac{600{,}000 \text{ units}}{1} = 3 \text{ mL}$$

Diluent 1.6 mL, 500,000 units/mL

$$x \text{ mL} = \frac{1 \text{ mL}}{500{,}000 \text{ units}} \times \frac{600{,}000 \text{ units}}{1} = 1.2 \text{ mL}$$

6. $$x \text{ mL} = \frac{1 \text{ mL}}{250{,}000 \text{ units}} \times \frac{400{,}000 \text{ units}}{1} = 1.6 \text{ mL}$$

7. $x \text{ mL} = \dfrac{1 \text{ mL}}{250{,}000 \text{ units}} \times \dfrac{300{,}000 \text{ units}}{1} = 1.2 \text{ mL}$

Add 18.2 mL of diluent.

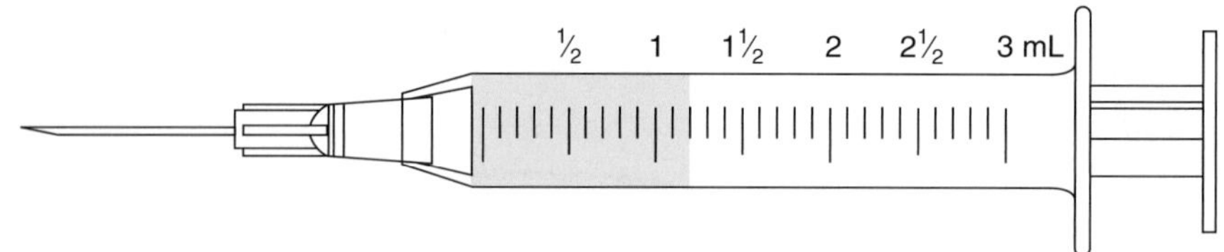

8. Diluent 140 mL, 200 mg/5 mL

$x \text{ mL} = \dfrac{5 \text{ mL}}{200 \text{ mg}} \times \dfrac{500 \text{ mg}}{1} = 12.5 \text{ mL}$

9. Diluent 10 mL, 1 g/10 mL

$x \text{ mL} = \dfrac{10 \text{ mL}}{1 \text{ g}} \times \dfrac{1 \text{ g}}{1000 \text{ mg}} \times \dfrac{1000 \text{ mg}}{1} = 10 \text{ mL}$

10. Diluent 78 mL, 125 mg/5 mL

$x \text{ mL} = \dfrac{5 \text{ mL}}{125 \text{ mg}} \times \dfrac{500 \text{ mg}}{1} = 20 \text{ mL}$

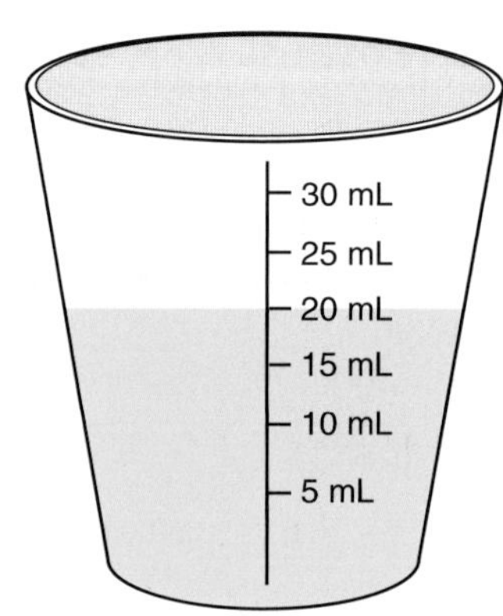

CHAPTER 14 Proportion/Formula Method—Work Sheet, pp. 413–416

Proportion | **Formula**

1. Water, 90 mL, 3750 mg, 15 doses in bottle

$125 \text{ mg} : 5 \text{ mL} :: 250 \text{ mg} : x \text{ mL}$

$125x = 1250$

$x = \dfrac{1250}{125}$

$x = 10 \text{ mL}$

Formula: $\dfrac{250}{125} \times \dfrac{5}{1} = \dfrac{1250}{125} = 10 \text{ mL}$

2. Water, 36 mL, 1500 mg, 5.45, or 5 full doses in bottle

$125 \text{ mg} : 5 \text{ mL} :: 275 \text{ mg} : x \text{ mL}$

$125x = 1375$

$x = \dfrac{1375}{125}$

$x = 11 \text{ mL}$

Formula: $\dfrac{275}{125} \times \dfrac{5}{1} = \dfrac{275}{25} = 11 \text{ mL}$

ANSWERS

Proportion	Formula

3. Water, 62 mL, 7500 mg, 8 mL, 12.5 doses

375 mg : 5 mL :: 600 mg : x mL
375 : 5 :: 600 : x
$375x = 3000$
$$x = \frac{3000}{375}$$
$x = 8$ mL

$$\frac{600 \text{ mg}}{375 \text{ mg}} \times \frac{5 \text{ mL}}{1} = \frac{3000}{375} = 8 \text{ mL}$$

4. There are two possible answers:

Diluent 4.6 mL, 200,000 units/mL
200,000 units : 1 mL :: 500,000 units : x mL
$200{,}000x = 500{,}000$
$$x = \frac{500{,}000}{200{,}000}$$
$x = 2.5$ mL

$$\frac{500{,}000 \text{ units}}{200{,}000 \text{ units}} \times 1 \text{ mL} = 2.5 \text{ mL}$$

Diluent 1.6 mL, 500,000 units/mL
500,000 units : 1 mL :: 500,000 units : x mL
$500{,}000x = 500{,}000$
$$x = \frac{500{,}000}{500{,}000}$$
$x = 1$ mL

$$\frac{500{,}000 \text{ units}}{500{,}000 \text{ units}} \times 1 \text{ mL} = 1 \text{ mL}$$

Circle the strength mixed.

5. There are two possible answers. However, the best choice for the amount of dilution is 1.6 mL because this would allow the least amount of fluid to be in the IM injection.

Diluent 4.6 mL, 200,000 units/mL
200,000 units : 1 mL :: 600,000 units : x mL
$200{,}000x = 600{,}000$
$$x = \frac{600{,}000}{200{,}000}$$
$x = 3$ mL

$$\frac{600{,}000 \text{ units}}{200{,}000 \text{ units}} \times 1 \text{ mL} = 3 \text{ mL}$$

Diluent 1.6 mL, 500,000 units/mL
500,000 units : 1 mL :: 600,000 : x mL
$500{,}000x = 600{,}000$
$$x = \frac{600{,}000}{500{,}000}$$
$x = 1.2$ mL

$$\frac{600{,}000 \text{ units}}{500{,}000 \text{ units}} \times 1 \text{ mL} = 1.2 \text{ mL}$$

Diluent 1.6 mL. The patient receives a smaller volume of medicine.

6. 8.2 mL of diluent

500,000 units : 1 mL :: 250,000 units : x mL
$500{,}000x = 250{,}000$
$$x = \frac{250{,}000}{500{,}000}$$
$x = 0.5$ mL

$$\frac{250{,}000 \text{ units}}{500{,}000 \text{ units}} \times 1 \text{ mL} = 0.5 \text{ mL}$$

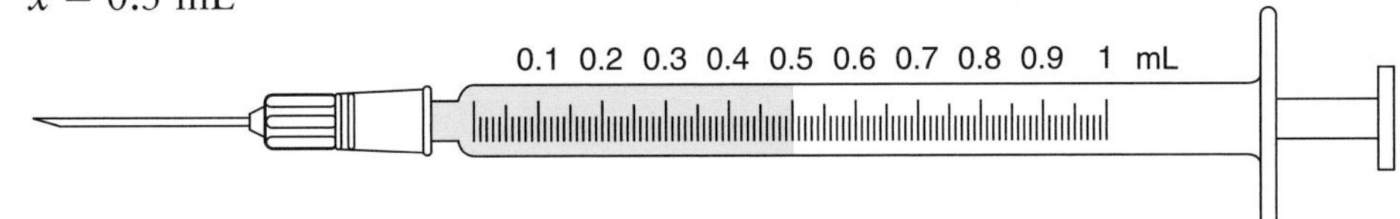

7. 250,000 units : 1 mL :: 175,000 units : x mL

$250{,}000x = 175{,}000$
$$x = \frac{175{,}000}{250{,}000}$$
$x = 0.7$ mL

$$\frac{175{,}000 \text{ units}}{250{,}000 \text{ units}} \times 1 \text{ mL} = 0.7 \text{ mL}$$

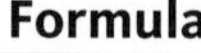

Proportion	Formula
8. Diluent 60 mL, 200 mg/5 mL 200 mg : 5 mL :: 500 mg : x mL $200x = 2500$ $x = \frac{2500}{200}$ $x = 12.5$ mL	$\frac{500}{200} \times 5 \text{ mL} = 12.5 \text{ mL}$
9. Diluent 2.7 mL, 250 mg/1.5 mL 250 mg : 1.5 mL :: 250 mg : x mL $250x = 375$ $x = \frac{375}{250}$ $x = 1.5$ mL	$\frac{250}{250} \times 1.5 \text{ mL} = 1.5 \text{ mL}$
10. Diluent 20 mL, 250 mg/5 mL 250 mg : 5 mL :: 500 mg : x mL $250x = 2500$ $x = \frac{2500}{250}$ $x = 10$ mL	$\frac{500}{250} \times 5 \text{ mL} = 10 \text{ mL}$

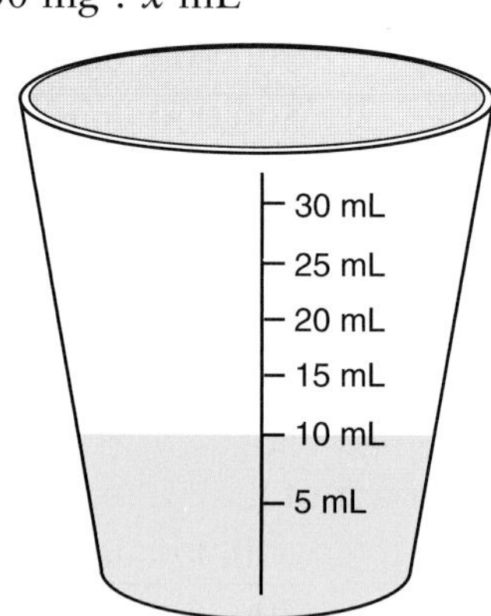

CHAPTER 14 Proportion/Formula Method—Posttest 1, pp. 417–420

Proportion	Formula
1. Water, 105 mL, 7500 mg, 20 doses per bottle 250 mg : 5 mL :: 375 mg : x mL $250x = 1875$ $x = \frac{1875}{250}$ $x = 7.5$ mL	$\frac{375}{250} \times \frac{5}{1} = \frac{1875}{250} = 7.5 \text{ mL}$
2. Water, 78 mL, 2500 mg, 10 doses per bottle 125 mg : 5 mL :: 250 mg : x mL $125x = 1250$ $x = \frac{1250}{125}$ $x = 10$ mL	$\frac{250}{125} \times \frac{5}{1} = 10 \text{ mL}$
3. Water, 62 mL, 4650 mg, 12.4, or 12 full doses in bottle 375 mg : 5 mL :: 450 mg : x mL $375x = 2250$ $x = \frac{2250}{375}$ $x = 6$ mL	$\frac{450}{375} \times \frac{5}{1} = \frac{450}{75} = 6 \text{ mL}$

ANSWERS

Proportion	Formula
4. 11.5 mL diluent, 1,000,000 units/mL 11.5 mL 1,000,000 units/mL 1,000,000 units : 1 mL :: 3,000,000 units : x mL $1{,}000{,}000x = 3{,}000{,}000$ $x = \frac{3{,}000{,}000}{1{,}000{,}000}$ $x = 3$ mL	$\frac{3{,}000{,}000 \text{ units}}{1{,}000{,}000 \text{ units}} \times 1 \text{ mL} = 3 \text{ mL}$
5. Diluent added = 1.8 mL 500,000 units : 1 mL :: 600,000 units : x mL $500{,}000x = 600{,}000$ $x = \frac{600{,}000}{500{,}000}$ $x = 1.2$ mL	$\frac{600{,}000 \text{ units}}{500{,}000 \text{ units}} \times 1 \text{ mL} = 1.2 \text{ mL}$
Diluent 4 mL, 250,000 units/mL 250,000 units : 1 mL :: 600,000 units : x mL $250{,}000x = 600{,}000$ $x = \frac{600{,}000}{250{,}000}$ $x = 2.4$ mL	$\frac{600{,}000 \text{ units}}{250{,}000 \text{ units}} \times 1 \text{ mL} = 2.4 \text{ mL}$
6. Concentration is 1,000,000 units/mL 1,000,000 units : 1 mL :: 1,200,000 units : x $1{,}000{,}000x = 1{,}200{,}000$ $x = \frac{1{,}200{,}000}{1{,}000{,}000}$ $x = 1.2$ mL	$\frac{1{,}200{,}000 \text{ units}}{1{,}000{,}000 \text{ units}} \times 1 \text{ mL} = 1.2 \text{ mL}$
7. 100,000 units : 1 mL :: 600,000 units : x mL $100{,}000x = 600{,}000$ $x = \frac{600{,}000}{100{,}000}$ $x = 6$ mL	$\frac{600{,}000 \text{ units}}{100{,}000 \text{ units}} \times 1 \text{ mL} = 6 \text{ mL}$
8. Diluent 3.5 mL, 250 mg/mL 250 mg : 1 mL :: 500 mg : x mL $250x = 500$ $x = \frac{500}{250}$ $x = 2$ mL	$\frac{500}{250} \times 1 \text{ mL} = 2 \text{ mL}$
9. Diluent 2.5 mL, 330 mg/mL 330 mg : 1 mL :: 500 mg : x mL $330x = 500$ $x = \frac{500}{330}$ $x = 1.51$, 1.5 mL	$\frac{500}{330} \times 1 \text{ mL} = 1.51,\ 1.5 \text{ mL}$

Proportion	Formula
10. Diluent 20 mL, 250 mg/5 mL 250 mg : 5 mL :: 1000 mg : x mL $250x = 5000$ $x = \frac{5000}{250}$ $x = 20$ mL	$\frac{1000}{250} \times 5 \text{ mL} = 20 \text{ mL}$

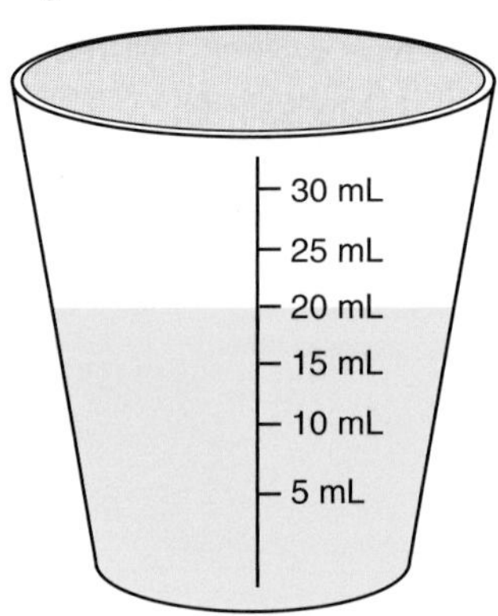

CHAPTER 14 Proportion/Formula Method—Posttest 2, pp. 421–424

Proportion	Formula
1. 1000 mg, 2.5, or 2 full doses in vial 1000 mg : 10 mL :: 400 mg : x mL $1000x = 4000$ $x = \frac{4000}{1000} = 4$ mL	$\frac{400}{1000} \times \frac{10}{1} = \frac{4000}{1000} = 4 \text{ mL}$
2. Diluent added is 1.2 mL to each vial 125 mg are in each vial 4 vials would be needed for each dose 125 mg : 1 mL :: 500 mg : x mL $125x = 500$ $x = \frac{500}{125} = 4$ mL	$\frac{500 \text{ mg}}{125 \text{ mg}} \times \frac{1 \text{ mL}}{1} = \frac{500}{125} = 4 \text{ mL}$
3. 1,000,000 units : 1 mL :: 1,200,000 units : x mL $1{,}000{,}000x = 1{,}200{,}000$ $x = \frac{1{,}200{,}000}{1{,}000{,}000}$ $x = 1.2$ mL	$\frac{1{,}200{,}000 \text{ units}}{1{,}000{,}000 \text{ units}} \times 1 \text{ mL} = 1.2 \text{ mL}$
4. Diluent = 11.5 mL 1,000,000 units : 1 mL :: 2,000,000 units : x mL $1{,}000{,}000x = 2{,}000{,}000$ $x = \frac{2{,}000{,}000}{1{,}000{,}000}$ $x = 2$ mL	$\frac{2{,}000{,}000 \text{ units}}{1{,}000{,}000 \text{ units}} \times 1 \text{ mL} = 2 \text{ mL}$

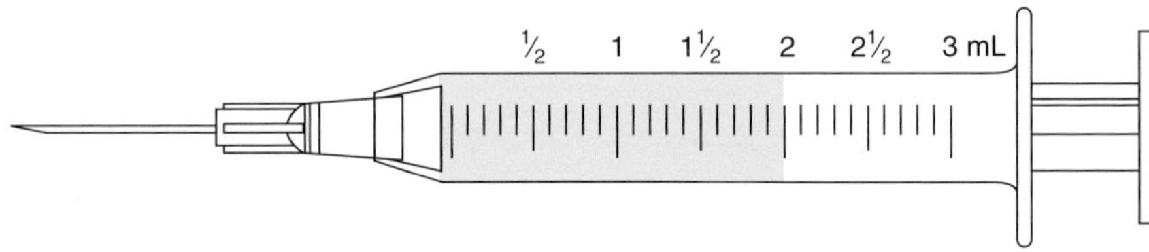

Proportion	Formula
5. 4.6 mL diluent, 200,000 units/mL 200,000 units : 1 mL :: 600,000 units : x mL $200{,}000x = 600{,}000$ $x = \frac{600{,}000}{200{,}000}$ $x = 3$ mL	$\frac{600{,}000 \text{ units}}{200{,}000 \text{ units}} \times 1 \text{ mL} = 3 \text{ mL}$
1.6 mL diluent, 500,000 units/mL 500,000 units : 1 mL :: 600,000 units : x mL $500{,}000x = 600{,}000$ $x = \frac{600{,}000}{500{,}000}$ $x = 1.2$ mL	$\frac{600{,}000 \text{ units}}{500{,}000 \text{ units}} \times 1 \text{ mL} = 1.2 \text{ mL}$
6. 250,000 units : 1 mL :: 400,000 units : x mL $250{,}000x = 400{,}000$ $x = \frac{400{,}000}{250{,}000}$ $x = 1.6$ mL	$\frac{400{,}000 \text{ units}}{250{,}000 \text{ units}} \times 1 \text{ mL} = 1.6 \text{ mL}$
7. Diluent = 18.2 mL 250,000 units : 1 mL :: 300,000 units : x mL $250{,}000x = 300{,}000$ $x = \frac{300{,}000}{250{,}000}$ $x = 1.2$ mL	$\frac{300{,}000 \text{ units}}{250{,}000 \text{ units}} \times 1 \text{ mL} = 1.2 \text{ mL}$

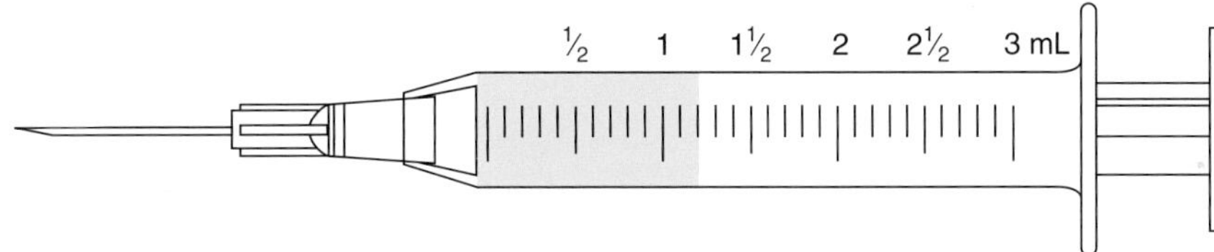

Proportion	Formula
8. Diluent 140 mL, 200 mg/5 mL 200 mg : 5 mL :: 500 mg : x mL $200x = 2500$ $x = \frac{2500}{200}$ $x = 12.5$ mL	$\frac{500}{200} \times 5 \text{ mL} = 12.5 \text{ mL}$
9. Diluent 10 mL, 1 g/10 mL 1000 mg : 10 mL :: 1000 mg : x mL $1000x = 10{,}000$ $x = \frac{10{,}000}{1000}$ $x = 10$ mL	$\frac{1000}{1000} \times 10 \text{ mL} = 10 \text{ mL}$

Proportion	Formula
10. Diluent 78 mL, 125 mg/5 mL 125 mg : 5 mL :: 500 mg : x mL $125x = 2500$ $x = \frac{2500}{125}$ $x = 20$ mL	$\frac{500}{125} \times 5 \text{ mL} = 20 \text{ mL}$

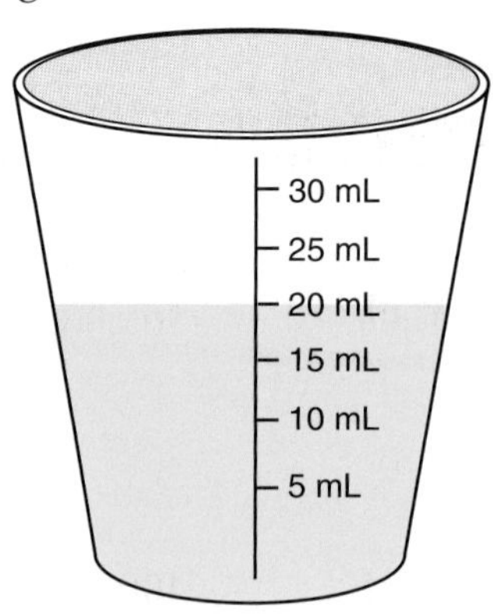

CHAPTER 15

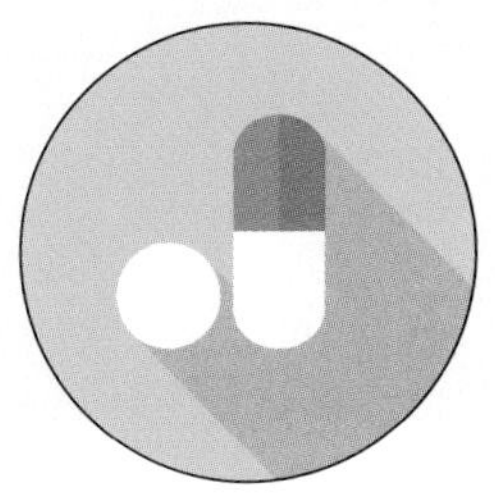

Intravenous Flow Rates

LEARNING OBJECTIVES

Upon completion of the materials provided in this chapter, you will be able to perform computations accurately by mastering the following mathematical concepts:

1. Calculating drops per minute (gtt/min) when given the total volume and time over which an IV solution or intravenous piggyback is to be infused
2. Calculating milliliters per hour (mL/h) when given the total volume and time over which an IV solution or intravenous piggyback is to be infused

It is sometimes necessary to deliver fluids and medications to a patient intravenously. Intravenous (IV) solutions and medications are placed directly into a vein. Infusions are injections of moderate to large quantities of fluids and nutrients into the patient's venous system. An IV medication or infusion may be prepared and administered by a licensed prescriber, nurse, or technician as regulated by state law and the policies of the particular health care agency. Medications and electrolyte milliequivalents are commonly ordered as additives to IV fluids. Medications may also be diluted and given in conjunction with IV solutions.

Intravenous fluids are available in a variety of volumes and solutions. Figures 15-1 and 15-2 show examples of two commonly used IV fluids: 5% dextrose and normal saline, respectively. These examples show 1000-mL IV bags, but IV fluids are also available in 50-mL, 100-mL, 250-mL, and 500-mL bags.

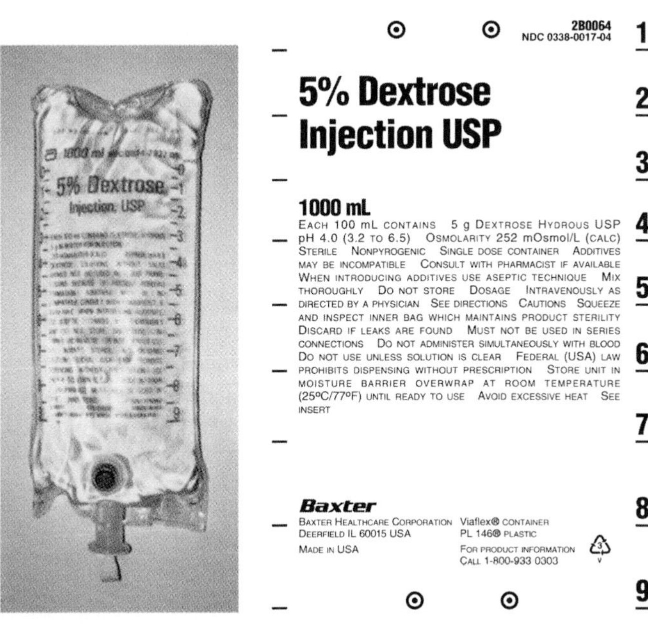

LOT
EXP
2B0064
NDC 0338-0017-04
5% Dextrose
Injection USP
1000 mL
EACH 100 mL CONTAINS 5 g DEXTROSE HYDROUS USP pH 4.0 (3.2 TO 6.5) OSMOLARITY 252 mOsmol/L (CALC) STERILE NONPYROGENIC SINGLE DOSE CONTAINER ADDITIVES MAY BE INCOMPATIBLE CONSULT WITH PHARMACIST IF AVAILABLE WHEN INTRODUCING ADDITIVES USE ASEPTIC TECHNIQUE MIX THOROUGHLY DO NOT STORE DOSAGE INTRAVENOUSLY AS DIRECTED BY A PHYSICIAN SEE DIRECTIONS CAUTIONS SQUEEZE AND INSPECT INNER BAG WHICH MAINTAINS PRODUCT STERILITY DISCARD IF LEAKS ARE FOUND MUST NOT BE USED IN SERIES CONNECTIONS DO NOT ADMINISTER SIMULTANEOUSLY WITH BLOOD DO NOT USE UNLESS SOLUTION IS CLEAR FEDERAL (USA) LAW PROHIBITS DISPENSING WITHOUT PRESCRIPTION STORE UNIT IN MOISTURE BARRIER OVERWRAP AT ROOM TEMPERATURE (25ºC/77ºF) UNTIL READY TO USE AVOID EXCESSIVE HEAT SEE INSERT
Baxter
BAXTER HEALTHCARE CORPORATION
DEERFIELD IL 60015 USA
MADE IN USA
Viaflex® CONTAINER
PL 146® PLASTIC
FOR PRODUCT INFORMATION
CALL 1-800-933 0303
1
2
3
4
5
6
7
8
9

FIGURE 15-1 5% dextrose. (From Brown M, Mulholland J: *Drug calculations: Ratio and proportion problems for clinical practice,* ed 10, St Louis, 2016, Elsevier.)

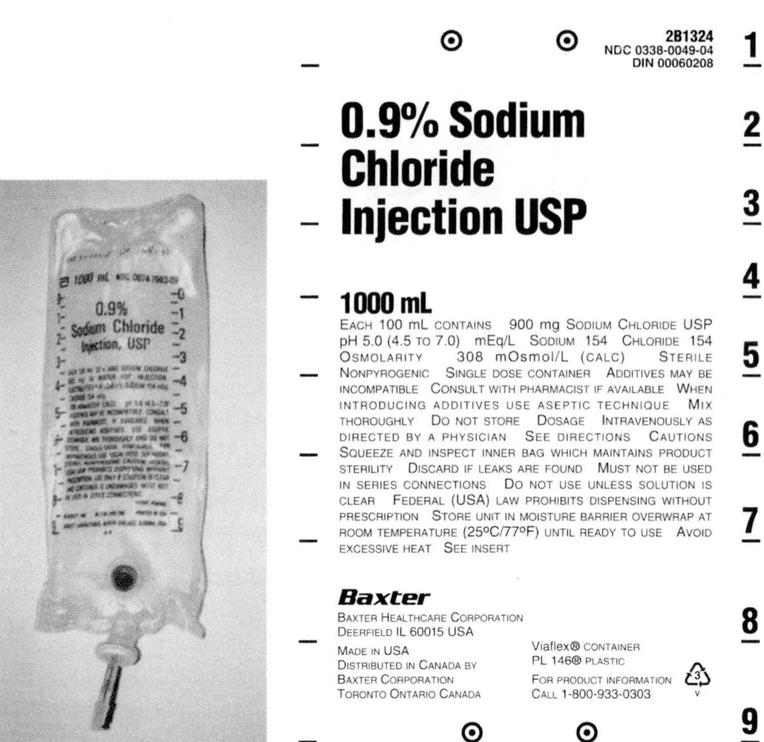
LOT
EXP
2B1324
NDC 0338-0049-04
DIN 00060208
0.9% Sodium Chloride Injection USP
1000 mL
EACH 100 mL CONTAINS 900 mg SODIUM CHLORIDE USP pH 5.0 (4.5 TO 7.0) mEq/L SODIUM 154 CHLORIDE 154 OSMOLARITY 308 mOsmol/L (CALC) STERILE NONPYROGENIC SINGLE DOSE CONTAINER ADDITIVES MAY BE INCOMPATIBLE CONSULT WITH PHARMACIST IF AVAILABLE WHEN INTRODUCING ADDITIVES USE ASEPTIC TECHNIQUE MIX THOROUGHLY DO NOT STORE DOSAGE INTRAVENOUSLY AS DIRECTED BY A PHYSICIAN SEE DIRECTIONS CAUTIONS SQUEEZE AND INSPECT INNER BAG WHICH MAINTAINS PRODUCT STERILITY DISCARD IF LEAKS ARE FOUND MUST NOT BE USED IN SERIES CONNECTIONS DO NOT USE UNLESS SOLUTION IS CLEAR FEDERAL (USA) LAW PROHIBITS DISPENSING WITHOUT PRESCRIPTION STORE UNIT IN MOISTURE BARRIER OVERWRAP AT ROOM TEMPERATURE (25°C/77°F) UNTIL READY TO USE AVOID EXCESSIVE HEAT SEE INSERT
Baxter
BAXTER HEALTHCARE CORPORATION
DEERFIELD IL 60015 USA
MADE IN USA
DISTRIBUTED IN CANADA BY
BAXTER CORPORATION
TORONTO ONTARIO CANADA
Viaflex® CONTAINER
PL 146® PLASTIC
FOR PRODUCT INFORMATION
CALL 1-800-933-0303
1
2
3
4
5
6
7
8
9

FIGURE 15-2 0.9% sodium chloride normal saline. (From Brown M, Mulholland J: *Drug calculations: ratio and proportion problems for clinical practice,* ed 10, St Louis, 2016, Elsevier.)

IV fluids are administered via an IV infusion set. This set includes two parts: the sealed bottle or bag containing the fluids and the tubing. The tubing is made up of the following parts: a drip chamber connected to the bottle or bag by a small tube or spike, and tubing that leads from the drip chamber down to and connecting with the needle or catheter at the site of insertion into the patient. The flow rate is adjusted to the desired drops per minute by a clamp placed around the tubing or by an IV pump or electronic device. The nurse must be knowledgeable about the equipment being used and, in particular, about the flow rate, or drops per milliliter, that a particular set of tubing will deliver.

IV ADMINISTRATION OF FLUIDS AND MEDICATIONS BY GRAVITY

IV fluids or medications may be administered by gravity (Figure 15-3). When gravity is used, infusion sets are used that allow the health care provider to count the drops per minute to regulate the flow.

Infusion sets come in a variety of sizes. The larger the diameter of the tubing where it enters the drip chamber, the bigger the drop will be. The **drop factor** of an infusion set is the number of drops contained in 1 mL. This equivalent may vary with different manufacturers. The most common drop factors are 10, 15, 20, and 60 drops/mL. Sets that deliver 10, 15, or 20 drops/mL are called *macrodrip sets.* A set that delivers 60 drops/mL is called *a microdrip set.* Macrodrip sets are larger than microdrip sets.

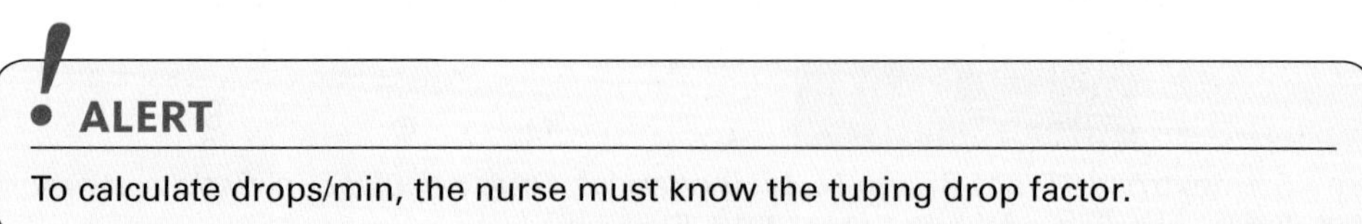

ALERT

To calculate drops/min, the nurse must know the tubing drop factor.

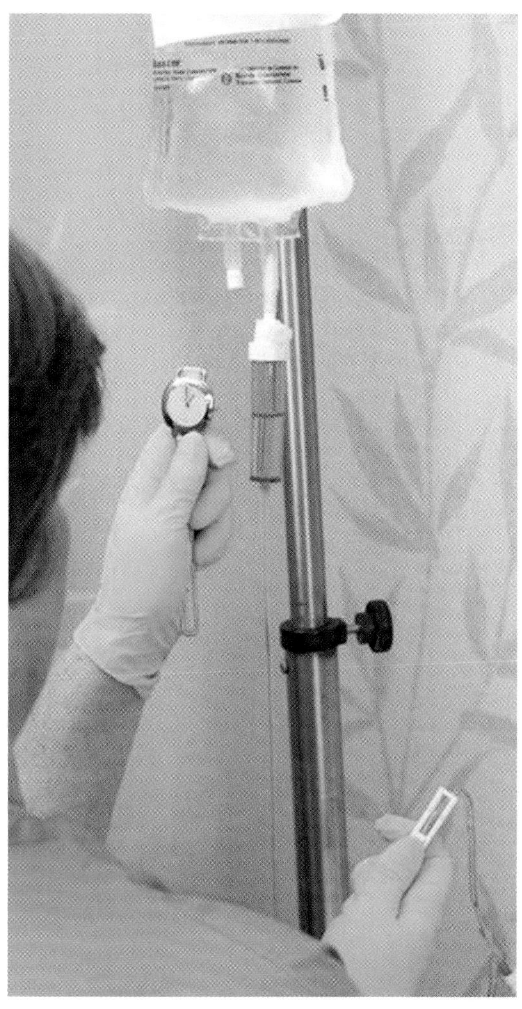

FIGURE 15-3 Count drops per minute by watching the drip chamber for 1 minute and adjusting the roller clamp as needed to deliver the desired number of drops per minute. (From Potter PA, Perry AG, Stockert PA, Hall AM: *Fundamentals of nursing,* ed 9, St Louis, 2017, Elsevier.)

If large volumes of fluid must be administered (125 mL/h or more), a macrodrip set is required. Microdrip sets are unable to deliver large volumes per hour because their drop size is so small. When an IV solution is to run at a rate of 50 mL/h or less, a microdrip set should be used. Some hospitals may even require a microdrip set for rates of 60 to 80 mL/h, for accuracy of flow rate and to help maintain the patency of the line. The number of drops per milliliter for the IV administration set is written on the outside of the box. This information is essential for solving problems related to the regulation of IV flow rates (Figure 15-4).

The licensed prescriber is responsible for writing the order for the type and amount of IV or hyperalimentation fluids. The number of hours the IV fluid will run or the rate of infusion is also ordered by the licensed prescriber.

Examples of Licensed Prescriber's Orders for IV fluids:

10/20/2023 *1300*	*Infuse 500 mL of 0.9% NS over 2 hours*
10/20/2023 *1600*	*Infuse D_5W ½ NS with 20 mEq of KCl at 125 mL/h continuous*

Sometimes the licensed prescriber will order medications to be administered in a small amount of IV fluid. This medication will need to be infused in addition to the regular IV fluids; it is called an *IV piggyback* (IVPB) because it is attached to the main IV tubing with shorter tubing of its own (Figure 15-5). The medication for the IVPB may be received premixed by the pharmacy or may need to be prepared by the nurse. The time frame for the IVPB infusion is usually 60 minutes or less.

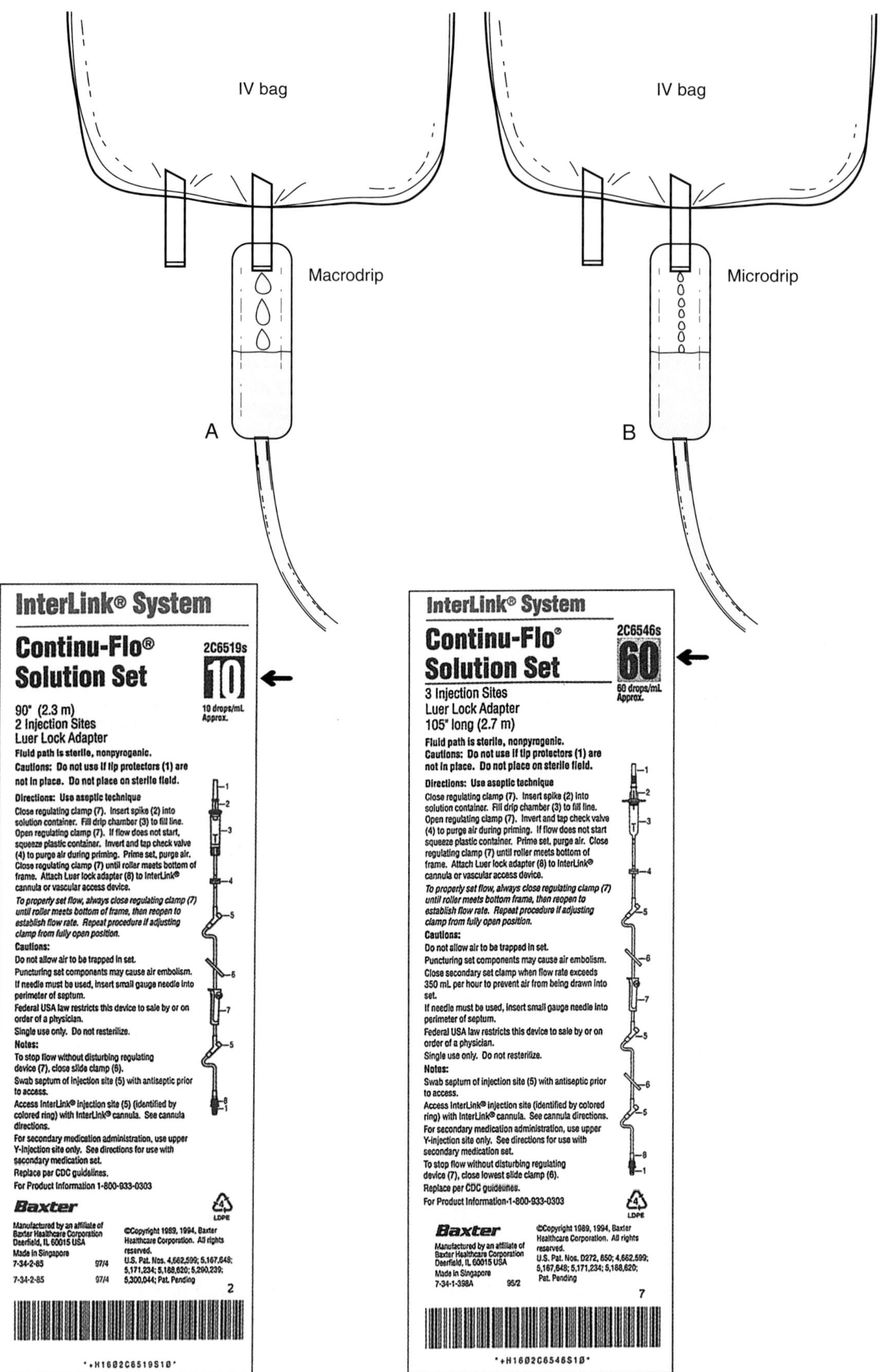

FIGURE 15-4 Administration sets. **A,** Set delivers 10 gtt/mL. **B,** Set delivers 60 gtt/mL.

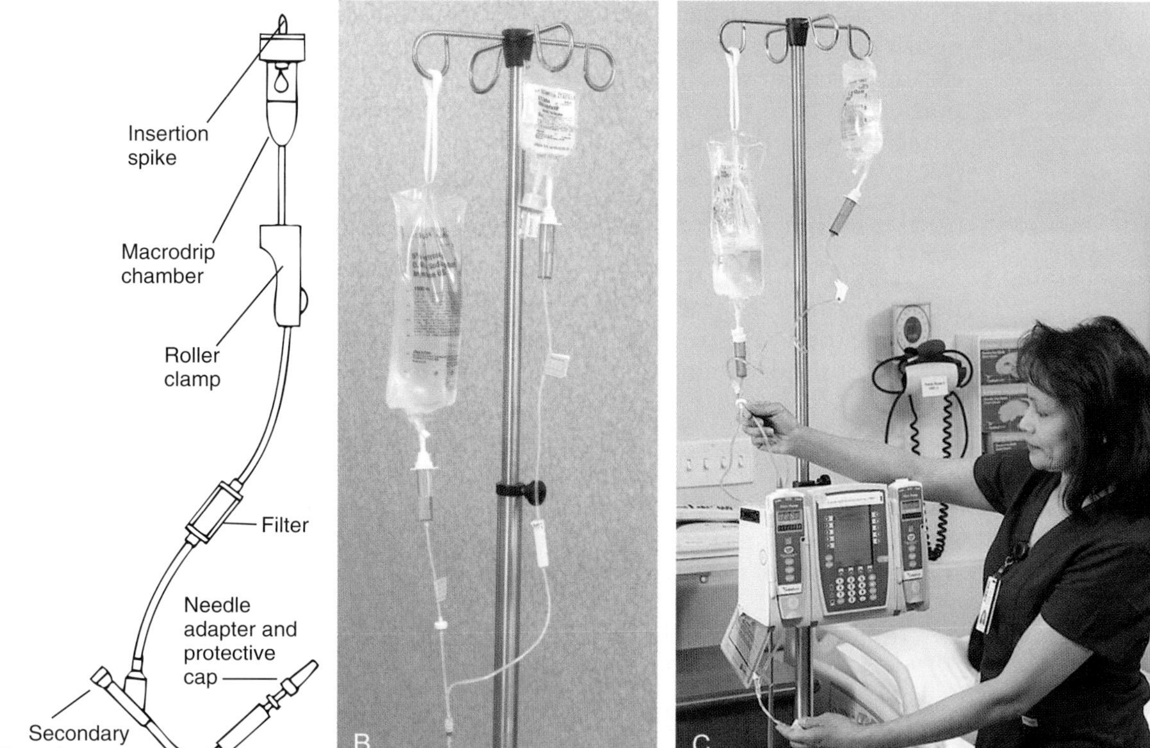

FIGURE 15-5 **A,** Infusion set. **B,** Gravity-flow IVPB. The IVPB is elevated above the existing IV solution, allowing it to infuse by gravity. **C,** IVPB infusion using an IV controller. (**A** from Clayton BD, Willihnganz M: *Basic pharmacology for nurses,* ed 17, St Louis, 2017, Elsevier. **B** from Lilley LL, Collins SR, Snyder JS: *Pharmacology and nursing process,* ed 8, St Louis, 2016, Elsevier. **C** from Perry AG, Potter PA, Ostendorf WR: *Clinical nursing skills and techniques,* ed 9, St Louis, 2018, Elsevier.)

If the licensed prescriber does not include an infusion time or rate, it is the nurse's responsibility to follow the manufacturer's guidelines. The hospital pharmacy and drug books such as the *Hospital Formulary* and *Intravenous Medications: A Handbook for Nurses and Health Professionals* are known resources for fluid rates. The nurse should always refer to recommended fluid limits and rates before IVPB administration.

It is usually the nurse's responsibility to regulate and maintain the infusion flow rate. It is the nurse's goal to ensure that the IV flow is regular. If the rate is irregular, too much or too little fluid may be infused. This may lead to complications such as fluid overload, dehydration, or medication overdose. Sometimes the flow rate must be adjusted because of interruptions caused by needle placement, condition of the vein, infiltration, or by a patient leaving the unit for a procedure.

The nurse must be able to determine the number of drops per minute (gtt/min) the patient must receive for the infusion to be completed within the specified time.

When the volume, time, or length of the infusion, and the constant drop factor are known, dimensional analysis or a simple formula can be used to calculate the desired drops per minute (gtt/min).

Calculating the Infusion of IV Fluids and Medications by Gravity: Dimensional Analysis Method

EXAMPLE 1: Hespan 500 mL is ordered to be infused over 3 hours. The drop factor is 15 gtt/mL. How many drops per minute should be given to infuse the total amount of Hespan over 3 hours?

Step 1. On the left side of the equation, place what you are solving for:

$$\frac{x \text{ gtt}}{\text{min}} =$$

Step 2. On the right side of the equation, place the available information related to the measurement or abbreviation that was placed on the left side. In this example the measurement we are solving for is *gtt/min*. We will deal with the numerator portion of our answer first, the *gtt*. This information is placed in the equation as a fraction, with the numerators matching.

$$\frac{x\ \textbf{gtt}}{\text{min}} = \frac{15\ \textbf{gtt}}{1\ \text{mL}}$$

Step 3. Next, find the information that matches the measurement used in the denominator of the fraction you created. In this example, *mL* is in the denominator, so Hespan 500 mL over 3 hours is used. Continue this process until all of the denominators except for *minute* can be canceled.

$$\frac{x\ \text{gtt}}{\text{min}} = \frac{15\ \text{gtt}}{1\ \text{mL}} \times \frac{500\ \text{mL}}{3\ \text{h}} \times \frac{1\ \text{h}}{60\ \text{min}}$$

Step 4. Then cancel out the abbreviations on the right side of the equation. If you have set up the problem correctly, the remaining measurements should match the measurements on the left side of the equation. Now solve for x.

$$\frac{x\ \text{gtt}}{\text{min}} = \frac{15\ \text{gtt}}{1\ \cancel{\text{mL}}} \times \frac{500\ \cancel{\text{mL}}}{3\ \cancel{\text{h}}} \times \frac{1\ \cancel{\text{h}}}{60\ \text{min}}$$

$$\frac{x\ \text{gtt}}{\text{min}} = \frac{15 \times 500}{3 \times 60}$$

$$x = 41.6 \text{ rounded to } 42 \text{ gtt/min}$$

Therefore the nurse will regulate the IV to drip at 42 drops/min, and the 500 mL of Hespan will be infused over 3 hours (Figure 15-3). Because the nurse cannot count a fraction of a drop, drops per minute are always rounded to the nearest whole number.

EXAMPLE 2: Cefuroxime 1 g in 50 mL of normal saline solution (NS) is ordered to be infused over 30 minutes. The tubing drop factor is 60 gtt/mL. How many drops per minute should be given to infuse the total amount of cefuroxime over 30 minutes?

Step 1. On the left side of the equation, place what you are solving for:

$$\frac{x\ \text{gtt}}{\text{min}} =$$

Step 2. On the right side of the equation, place the available information related to the measurement or abbreviation that was placed on the left side. In this example the measurement we are solving for is *gtt/min*. We will deal with the numerator portion of our answer first, the *gtt*. This information is placed in the equation as a fraction, with the numerators matching.

$$\frac{x\ \textbf{gtt}}{\text{min}} = \frac{60\ \textbf{gtt}}{1\ \text{mL}}$$

Step 3. Next, find the information that matches the measurement used in the denominator of the fraction you created. In this example, *mL* is in the denominator, so cefuroxime 50 mL over 30 minutes is used.

$$\frac{x\ \text{gtt}}{\text{min}} = \frac{60\ \text{gtt}}{1\ \text{mL}} \times \frac{50\ \text{mL}}{30\ \text{min}}$$

Step 4. Then cancel out the abbreviations on the right side of the equation. If you have set up the problem correctly, the remaining measurements should match the measurements on the left side of the equation. Now solve for *x*.

$$\frac{x \text{ gtt}}{\text{min}} = \frac{60 \text{ gtt}}{1 \not{\text{mL}}} \times \frac{50 \not{\text{mL}}}{30 \text{ min}}$$

$$\frac{x \text{ gtt}}{\text{min}} = \frac{60 \times 50}{30}$$

$$x = 100 \text{ gtt/min}$$

Therefore the nurse will regulate the IV to drip at 100 drops/min, and the 50 mL of cefuroxime will be infused over 30 minutes.

Calculating the Infusion of IV Fluids and Medications by Gravity: Formula Method

EXAMPLE 1: Hespan 500 mL is ordered to be infused over 3 hours. The drop factor is 15 gtt/mL. How many drops per minute should be given to infuse the total amount of Hespan over 3 hours?

$$\text{The formula: } \frac{\text{Total volume to be infused}}{\text{Total amount of time in minutes}} \times \text{Drop factor} = x \text{ gtt/min}$$

Step 1. Convert total hours to minutes.

1 h : 60 min :: 3 h : *x* min

$x = 180$

Therefore 3 hours equals 180 minutes.

Step 2. Calculate gtt/min.

This calculation depends on the drop factor of the tubing being used. Remember, this information is found on the package. For the problems in this work text, the drop factor is indicated. The drop factor for this problem is 15.

$$\text{(Formula setup)} \quad \frac{500 \text{ mL}}{180 \text{ min}} \times \frac{15 \text{ gtt/mL}}{} = x \text{ gtt/min}$$

$$\text{(Cancel)} \quad \frac{500 \not{\text{mL}}}{\overset{}{\underset{12}{\not{180}}} \text{ min}} \times \frac{\overset{1}{\not{15}} \text{ gtt/} \not{\text{mL}}}{} = x \text{ gtt/min}$$

$$\text{(Calculate)} \quad \frac{500}{12 \text{ min}} \times \frac{1 \text{ gtt}}{} = \frac{500}{12} = 41.6 \text{ rounded to } 42 \text{ gtt/min}$$

Therefore the nurse will regulate the IV to drip at 42 drops/min, and the 500 mL of Hespan will be infused over 3 hours (see Figure 15-3). Because the nurse cannot count a fraction of a drop, drops per minute are always rounded to a whole number.

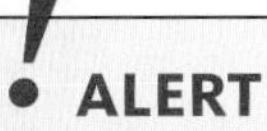

ALERT

When administering an IV fluid or medication by gravity, the nurse solves for gtt/min.

EXAMPLE 2: Cefuroxime 1 g in 50 mL of normal saline solution (NS) is ordered to be infused over 30 minutes. The tubing drop factor is 60 gtt/mL. How many drops per minute should be given to infuse the total amount of cefuroxime over 30 minutes?

$$\text{The formula: } \frac{\text{Total volume to be infused}}{\text{Total amount of time in minutes}} \times \text{Drop factor} = x \text{ gtt/min}$$

Calculate gtt/min.

$$\text{(Formula setup)} \quad \frac{50 \text{ mL}}{30 \text{ min}} \times \frac{60 \text{ gtt/mL}}{} = x \text{ gtt/min}$$

$$\text{(Cancel)} \quad \frac{50 \cancel{\text{mL}}}{\underset{1}{\cancel{30}} \text{ min}} \times \frac{\overset{2}{\cancel{60}} \text{ gtt/} \cancel{\text{mL}}}{} = x \text{ gtt/min}$$

$$\text{(Calculate)} \quad \frac{50}{1} \times 2 = 100 \text{ gtt/min}$$

Therefore the nurse will regulate the IVPB to drip at 100 gtt/min, and the cefuroxime will be infused over 30 minutes.

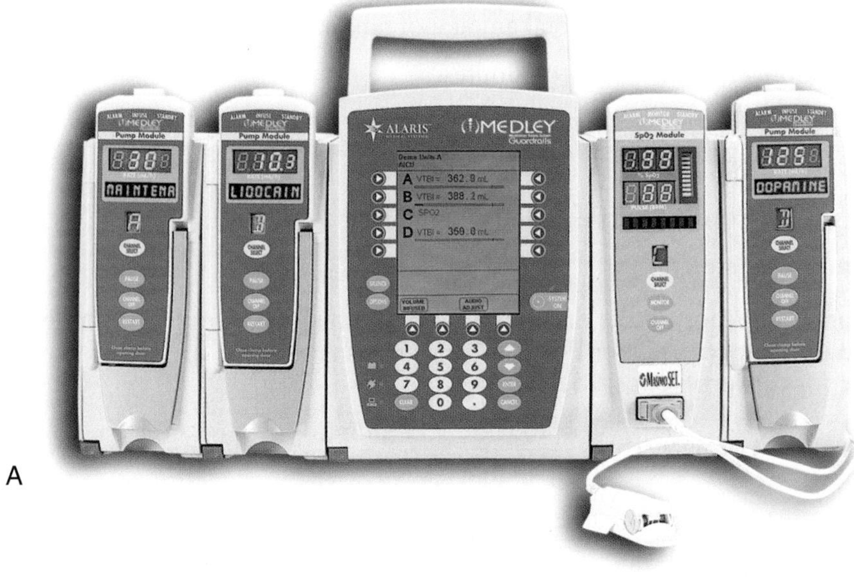

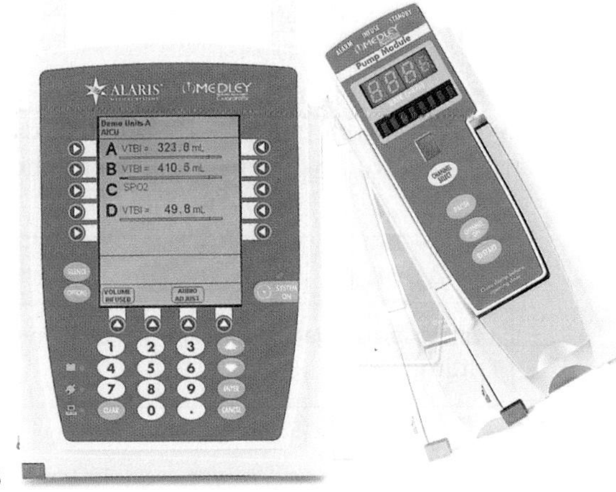

FIGURE 15-6 **A,** Medley™ Medication Safety System. **B,** Example of the Medley™ pump module attached to the Medley programming module. (Courtesy Becton, Dickinson and Company.)

INFUSION OF IV FLUIDS AND MEDICATIONS BY AN IV PUMP

IV flow rates are often controlled by an electronic device or pump. The IV pumps are programmed to deliver a set amount of fluid per hour. Safety for the patient is an advantage of electronic IV pumps. The pumps are used for patients in regular medical-surgical units, critical care areas, pediatrics, the operating room, and ambulatory care settings.

Many electronic pumps are on the market today. These vary from simple one-channel models to four multichannel pumps. Many of the newer models actually calculate flow rates and automatically start infusions at a later time. Convenience, safety, accuracy, and time-saving options are driving forces in the innovations currently available.

Some examples of equipment are pictured in Figures 15-6 and 15-7; in Figure 15-6 the Medley Medication Safety System and the Medley pump module (attached to the programming module) are shown. In Figure 15-7 the Medley Medication Safety System is being used on a patient in a critical care setting. Each company offers tubing for use with its pumps.

Newer IV pumps, as pictured in Figure 15-6, contain software that allows each facility to program safeguard information for medications into the IV pump. If a health care professional programs a rate, dose, or duration that is considered to be unsafe, a visual or audible alert will occur. The safeguards are determined by the facility to prevent IV medication errors. In some situations the health care professional will be required to infuse medications using an IV pump. Whether the medication is an electrolyte replacement, an antiinfective agent, or another type of medication to be infused by IVPB, the health care professional needs to calculate the rate, in milliliters per hour, for which the IV pump should be programmed.

! ALERT

When administering a medication or IV fluid by an IV pump, the nurse solves for mL/h.

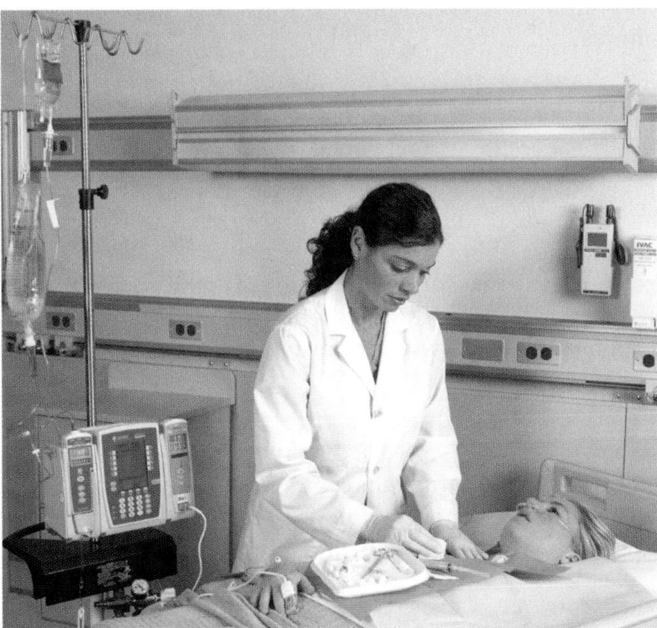

FIGURE 15-7 Medley™ Medication Safety System being used on a patient in a critical care setting. (Courtesy Becton, Dickinson and Company.)

Calculating the Infusion of IV Fluids and Medications by a Pump: Dimensional Analysis Method

EXAMPLE 1: Infuse 1000 mL of lactated Ringer's solution (LR) over 12 hours. How many mL/h should the IV pump be programmed for?

Step 1. On the left side of the equation, place what you are solving for:

$$\frac{x \text{ mL}}{\text{h}} =$$

Step 2. On the right side of the equation, place the available information related to the measurement or abbreviation that was placed on the left side. In this example the measurement we are solving for is *mL/h*. We will deal with the numerator portion of our answer first, the *mL*. This information is placed in the equation as a fraction, with the numerators matching.

$$\frac{x \textbf{ mL}}{\text{h}} = \frac{1000 \textbf{ mL}}{12 \text{ h}}$$

Step 3. Now solve for x.

$$\frac{x \text{ mL}}{\text{h}} = \frac{1000 \text{ mL}}{12 \text{ h}}$$

$$\frac{x \text{ mL}}{\text{h}} = \frac{1000}{12}$$

$$x = 83.3 \text{ or } 83 \text{ mL/h}$$

Therefore the nurse will program the IV pump for 83 mL/h and the 1000 mL of LR will be infused over 12 hours.

EXAMPLE 2: Cefazolin 1 g dissolved in 50 mL of D5W is ordered to be infused over 30 minutes. The IVPB may be given using an IV pump. How many milliliters per hour should the IV pump be programmed for to infuse the Kefzol over 30 minutes?

Step 1. On the left side of the equation, place what you are solving for:

$$\frac{x \text{ mL}}{\text{h}} =$$

Step 2. On the right side of the equation, place the available information related to the measurement or abbreviation that was placed on the left side of the equation. In this example, the measurement we are solving for is *mL/h*. We will deal with the numerator portion of our answer first, the *mL*. This information is placed in the equation as a fraction, with the numerators matching.

$$\frac{x \textbf{ mL}}{\text{h}} = \frac{50 \textbf{ mL}}{30 \text{ min}}$$

Step 3. Next, find the information that matches the measurement used in the denominator of the fraction you created. In this example, *min* is in the denominator, so 60 minutes over 1 hour is used.

$$\frac{x \text{ mL}}{\text{h}} = \frac{50 \text{ mL}}{30 \text{ min}} \times \frac{60 \text{ min}}{1 \text{ h}}$$

Step 4. Then cancel out the abbreviations on the right side of the equation. If you have set up the problem correctly, the remaining measurements should match the measurements on the left side of the equation. Now solve for x.

$$\frac{x \text{ mL}}{\text{h}} = \frac{50 \text{ mL}}{30 \cancel{\text{min}}} \times \frac{60 \cancel{\text{min}}}{1 \text{ h}}$$

$$\frac{x \text{ mL}}{\text{h}} = \frac{50 \times 60}{30}$$

$$x = 100 \text{ mL/h}$$

Therefore the nurse will program the IV pump for 100 mL/h, and the cefazolin will be infused over 30 minutes.

EXAMPLE 3: Dilute potassium 40 mEq in 250 mL of D5W and administer IV now. The facility's policy states to infuse potassium at a rate of 10 mEq/h. How many milliliters per hour should the IV pump be programmed for to infuse the potassium at a rate of 10 mEq/h?

Step 1. On the left side of the equation, place what you are solving for:

$$\frac{x \text{ mL}}{\text{h}} =$$

Step 2. On the right side of the equation, place the available information related to the measurement or abbreviation that was placed on the left side of the equation. In this example, the measurement we are solving for is *mL/h*. We will deal with the numerator portion of our answer first, the *mL*. This information is placed in the equation as a fraction, with the numerators matching.

$$\frac{x \textbf{ mL}}{\text{h}} = \frac{250 \textbf{ mL}}{40 \text{ mEq}}$$

Step 3. Next, find the information that matches the measurement used in the denominator of the fraction you created. In this example, *mEq* is in the denominator, so the policy of 10 mEq/h is used.

$$\frac{x \text{ mL}}{\text{h}} = \frac{250 \text{ mL}}{40 \text{ mEq}} \times \frac{10 \text{ mEq}}{1 \text{ h}}$$

Step 4. Then cancel out the abbreviations on the right side of the equation. If you have set up the problem correctly, the remaining measurements should match the measurements on the left side of the equation. Now solve for x.

$$\frac{x \text{ mL}}{\text{h}} = \frac{250 \text{ mL}}{40 \cancel{\text{mEq}}} \times \frac{10 \cancel{\text{mEq}}}{1 \text{ h}}$$

$$\frac{x \text{ mL}}{\text{h}} = \frac{250 \times 10}{40}$$

$$x = 62.5 \text{ or } 63 \text{ mL/h}$$

Therefore the nurse will program the IV pump for 63 mL/h, and the 40 mEq of potassium will infuse per the hospital policy.

Calculating the Infusion of IV Fluids and Medications by a Pump: Formula Method

In many facilities IV fluids are infused using an IV pump. IV pumps are programmed to infuse IV fluids by milliliters per hour (mL/h).

$$\text{The formula: } \frac{\text{Total volume in milliliters}}{\text{Total time in hours}} = x \text{ mL/h}$$

EXAMPLE 1: Infuse 1000 mL of lactated Ringer's solution (LR) over 12 hours. How many mL/h should the IV pump be programmed for?

Calculate mL/h.

$$\text{(Formula setup) } \frac{1000 \text{ mL}}{12 \text{ h}} = 83.3 \text{ or } 83 \text{ mL/h}$$

Therefore the nurse will program the IV pump for 83 mL/h, and the 1000 mL of LR will be infused over 12 hours.

EXAMPLE 2: Cefazolin 1 g dissolved in 50 mL of D_5W is ordered to be infused over 30 minutes. The IVPB may be given using an IV pump. How many milliliters per hour should the IV pump be programmed for to infuse the Kefzol over 30 minutes?

Step 1. Convert minutes to hours.

$1 \text{ h} : 60 \text{ min} :: x \text{ h} : 30 \text{ min}$

$60x = 30$

$$x = \frac{30}{60} = 0.5 \text{ h}$$

Step 2. Calculate mL/h.

$$\text{(Formula setup) } \frac{50 \text{ mL}}{0.5 \text{ h}} = 100 \text{ mL/h}$$

EXAMPLE 3: Dilute potassium 40 mEq in 250 mL of D_5W and administer IV now. The facility's policy states to infuse potassium at a rate of 10 mEq/h. How many milliliters per hour should the IV pump be programmed for to infuse the potassium at a rate of 10 mEq/h?

Using the ratio-proportion method:

Calculate mL/h.

(Formula setup) $40 \text{ mEq} : 250 \text{ mL} :: 10 \text{ mEq} : x \text{ mL}$

(Calculate) $40x = 2500$

$$x = \frac{2500}{40}$$

$$x = 62.5 \text{ or } 63 \text{ mL}$$

Therefore the nurse will program the IV pump for 63 mL/h, and the potassium will be infused at 10 mEq/h as stated in the facility's policy. (NOTE: Follow your facility's policy when you calculate the rate for any electrolyte replacement.)

Using the $\frac{D}{A} \times Q = x$ mL/h method:

Calculate mL/h.

(Formula setup) $\frac{10 \text{ mEq}}{40 \text{ mEq}} \times 250 \text{ mL} = x \text{ mL}$

(Cancel) $\frac{\overset{1}{\cancel{10}} \ \cancel{\text{mEq}}}{\underset{4}{\cancel{40}} \ \cancel{\text{mEq}}} \times 250 \text{ mL} = x \text{ mL}$

(Calculate) $\frac{1}{4} \times 250 \text{ mL} = \frac{250}{4} = 62.5 \text{ or } 63 \text{ mL/h}$

SALINE AND HEPARIN LOCKS

Saline and heparin locks are commonly used in a variety of health care settings. A saline lock is an IV catheter that is inserted into a peripheral vein. It may be used for medications or fluids, usually on an intermittent basis. The use of a saline lock prevents the patient from having to endure numerous venipunctures. Also, when fluid is not being infused, the patient enjoys greater freedom of movement. Each institution will have its own policy concerning the use and care of saline locks. The locks may be flushed with 2 to 3 mL of normal saline solution (Figures 15-8 and 15-9). Central line ports that are not being used for fluid or medication administration are heparin locks. The locks will be flushed with a heparin flush solution of 10 units of heparin per 1 mL. This practice is called *heparinization,* and it prevents clotting of the heparin lock. Because of concerns regarding heparin overdose errors and heparin-induced thrombocytopenia (HIT), the routine use of heparin flushes is decreasing.

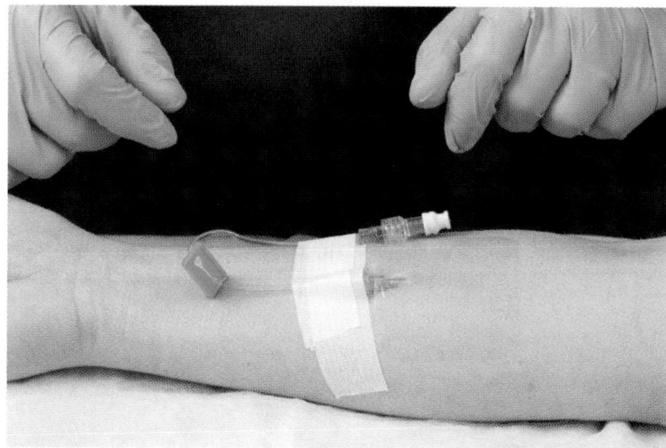

FIGURE 15-8 Example of a saline lock. (From Perry AG, Potter PA, Ostendorf WR: *Clinical nursing skills and techniques,* ed 9, St Louis, 2018, Elsevier.)

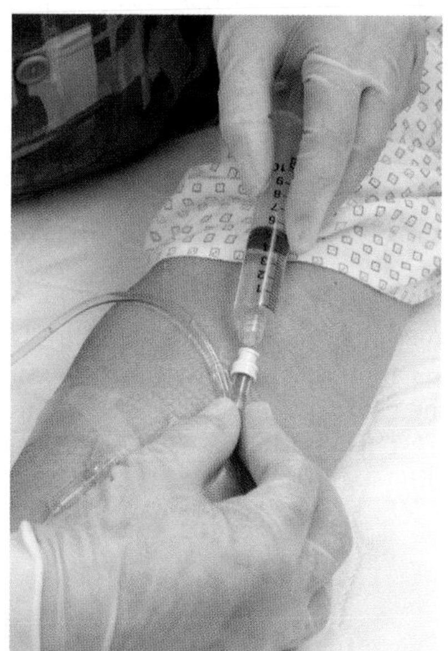

FIGURE 15-9 Example of a needleless system used within an intravenous line. (From Perry AG, Potter PA, Ostendorf WR: *Nursing interventions and clinical skills,* ed 6, St Louis, 2016, Elsevier.)

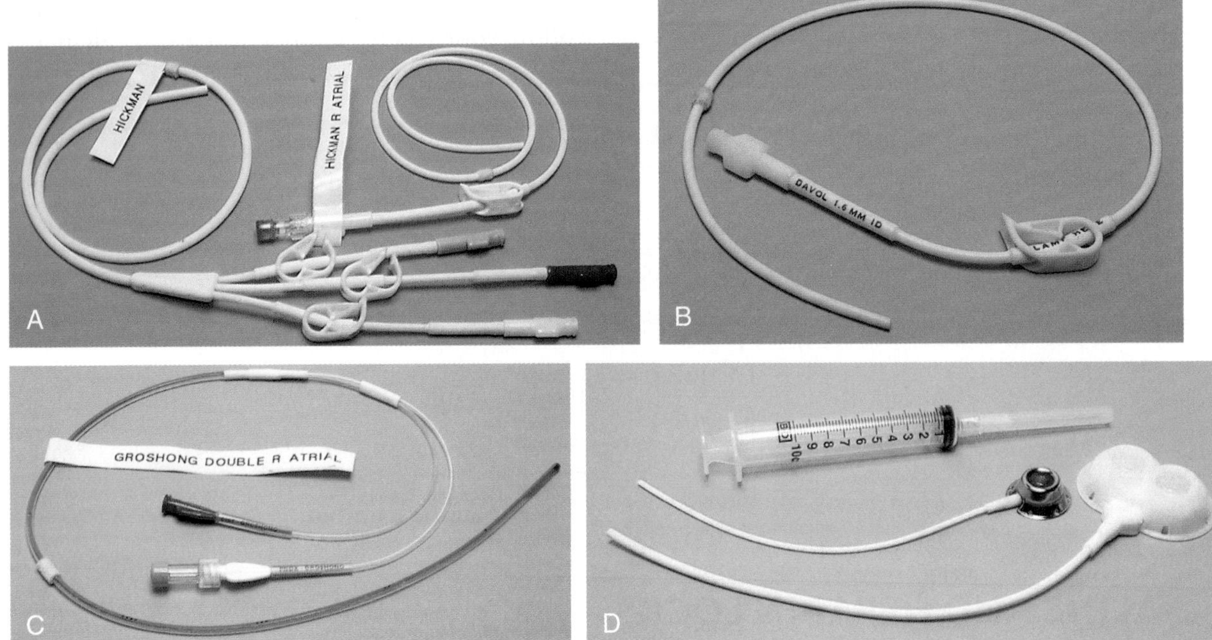

FIGURE 15-10 **A,** Hickman catheter. **B,** Broviac catheter. **C,** Groshong catheter. **D,** Silicone venous catherter. (From Clayton BD, Willihnganz M: *Basic pharmacology for nurses,* ed 16, St Louis, 2013, Elsevier.)

CENTRAL VENOUS CATHETERS

Occasionally, a patient will need a central venous catheter. Central venous catheters are indwelling, semipermanent central lines that are inserted into the right atrium of the heart via the cephalic, subclavian, or jugular vein (Figure 15-10).

This type of catheter may be required for clients who need frequent venipuncture, long-term IV infusions, hyperalimentation, chemotherapy, intermittent blood transfusions, or antibiotics. These catheters may be referred to as *triple-lumen catheters, Hickman lines, or peripherally inserted central catheters (PICCs).*

Central venous catheter management involves flushing the catheter with 5 to 10 mL of normal saline when the catheter access is routinely capped or clamped after blood draws. Please consult your institution's procedure or policy guidelines about central venous line flushes. If continuous fluids are ordered, these fluids **must** be regulated via an infusion pump. All central venous catheter management must be done under the supervision of a registered nurse.

The central venous catheter site must be assessed regularly. The catheter site should always remain sterile under an occlusive dressing that is changed according to the institution's procedure regarding central venous catheters.

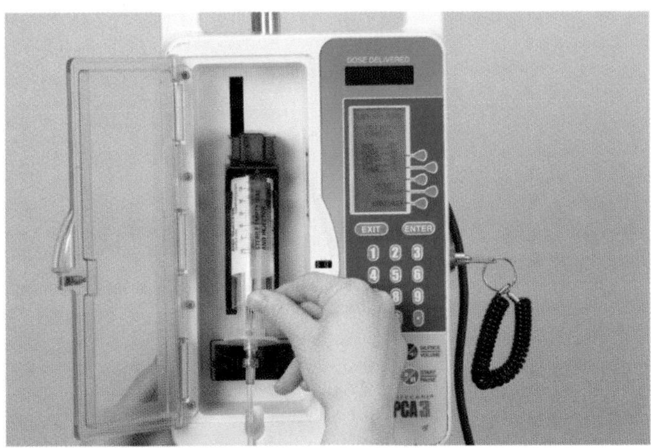

FIGURE 15-11 Patient-controlled analgesia device. (Perry PA, Potter AG, Ostendorf WR: *Nursing interventions and clinical skills*, ed 6, St. Louis, 2016, Elsevier.)

PATIENT-CONTROLLED ANALGESIA

Patient-controlled analgesia (PCA) or a PCA pump involves patients giving themselves an IV narcotic by pressing a button. This IV narcotic is given at intervals via an infusion pump (Figure 15-11). Only a registered nurse can be accountable for dispensing analgesia to be given in this manner. In addition, only a registered nurse can administer a PCA loading dose. For safety, most institutions now require that two registered nurses verify the PCA drug, dosage, and rate programmed into the machine.

Several considerations are crucial in the administration of PCA. IV narcotics may cause depressed respirations, hypotension, sedation, dizziness, and nausea or vomiting in the patient. The patient must be able to understand and comply with instructions and must have a desire to use the PCA because *only* the patient can press the button to dispense the dose. The materials needed for infusion include a PCA pump, PCA tubing, a PCA pump key, a narcotic injector vial, and maintenance IV fluids through which the IV narcotic will be infused.

EXAMPLE 1: The licensed prescriber orders morphine sulfate 1 mg every 10 minutes to a maximum of 30 mg in 4 hours. Morphine concentration is 1 mg/mL per 30-mL injector vial. What is the pump setting?

1 mg/10 min; 4-hour limit is 30 mg

EXAMPLE 2: The licensed prescriber orders hydromorphone 0.2 mg every 15 minutes to a maximum of 2 mg in 4 hours. Hydromorphone concentration is 1 mg/mL per 30-mL injector vial. What is the pump setting?

0.2 mg/15 min; 4-hour limit is 2 mg

Complete the following work sheet, which provides for practice in the calculation of IV solutions and IVPB by either the IV pump or gravity. Check your answers. If you have difficulties, go back and review the necessary material. When you feel ready to evaluate your learning, take the first posttest. Check your answers. An acceptable score as indicated on the posttest signifies that you have successfully completed the chapter. An unacceptable score signifies a need for further study before taking the second posttest.

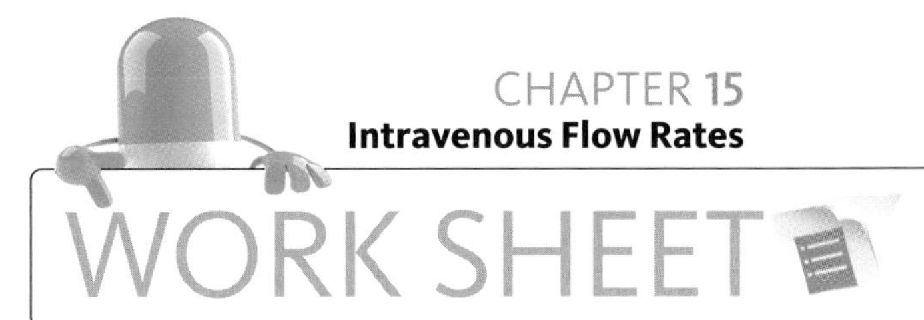

DIRECTIONS: The IV fluid or medication order is listed in each problem. Calculate the IV flow rates. Show your work. Follow your instructor's rules on rounding final answers.

1. The licensed prescriber orders 500 mL of dextran to be infused over 24 hours. How many milliliters per hour should the IV pump be programmed for? ______

2. A patient with genital herpes has an order for acyclovir 400 mg IVPB q 8 h. The acyclovir is dissolved in 100 mL 0.9% NS and is to be infused over 1 hour. How many milliliters per hour should the IV pump be programmed for? ______

3. Amikacin 80 mg is ordered IVPB q 12 h. The amikacin is dissolved in 100 mL D_5W and is to be infused over 30 minutes. With a tubing drop factor of 15 gtt/mL, how many drops per minute should be given? ______

4. The licensed prescriber orders 3000 mL of total parenteral nutrition (TPN) to be infused from 1900 to 0700. How many milliliters per hour should the IV pump be programmed for? ______

5. A patient with peptic ulcer disease has famotidine 20 mg in 100 mL D_5W ordered q 12 h. The famotidine is to be infused over 30 minutes. With a tubing drop factor of 10 gtt/mL, how many drops per minute should be given? ______

6. A malnourished patient has an order for 500 mL of fat emulsion 10% to be infused over 6 hours. How many milliliters per hour should the IV pump be programmed for? ______

7. An order is received to infuse penicillin G 4,000,000 units in 100 mL of D_5W q 12 h. The tubing drop factor is 10 gtt/mL. The penicillin should be infused over 60 minutes. How many drops per minute should be given? ______

8. A patient with hypokalemia has orders for potassium 60 mEq in 250 mL of D_5W. The facility's policy states to infuse the potassium at 20 mEq/h. How many milliliters per hour should the IV pump be programmed for? ______

9. A postoperative patient has ceftriaxone 1 g ordered q 8 h. The ceftriaxone is dissolved in 50 mL of D_5W and is to be infused over 30 minutes. The tubing drop factor is 60 gtt/mL. How many drops per minute should be given? ______

10. A postoperative patient has an order for 1000 mL of LR over 10 hours. How many milliliters per hour should the IV pump be programmed for? ______

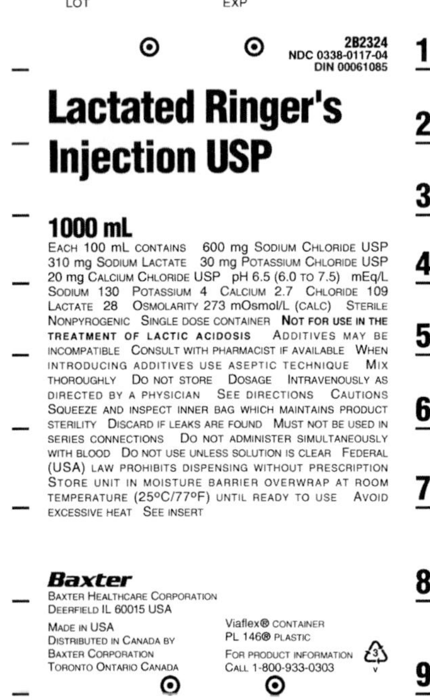
LOT
EXP
2B2324
NDC 0338-0117-04
DIN 00061085
Lactated Ringer's Injection USP
1000 mL
EACH 100 mL CONTAINS 600 mg SODIUM CHLORIDE USP 310 mg SODIUM LACTATE 30 mg POTASSIUM CHLORIDE USP 20 mg CALCIUM CHLORIDE USP pH 6.5 (6.0 TO 7.5) mEq/L SODIUM 130 POTASSIUM 4 CALCIUM 2.7 CHLORIDE 109 LACTATE 28 OSMOLARITY 273 mOsmol/L (CALC) STERILE NONPYROGENIC SINGLE DOSE CONTAINER NOT FOR USE IN THE TREATMENT OF LACTIC ACIDOSIS ADDITIVES MAY BE INCOMPATIBLE CONSULT WITH PHARMACIST IF AVAILABLE WHEN INTRODUCING ADDITIVES USE ASEPTIC TECHNIQUE MIX THOROUGHLY DO NOT STORE DOSAGE INTRAVENOUSLY AS DIRECTED BY A PHYSICIAN SEE DIRECTIONS CAUTIONS SQUEEZE AND INSPECT INNER BAG WHICH MAINTAINS PRODUCT STERILITY DISCARD IF LEAKS ARE FOUND MUST NOT BE USED IN SERIES CONNECTIONS DO NOT ADMINISTER SIMULTANEOUSLY WITH BLOOD DO NOT USE UNLESS SOLUTION IS CLEAR FEDERAL (USA) LAW PROHIBITS DISPENSING WITHOUT PRESCRIPTION STORE UNIT IN MOISTURE BARRIER OVERWRAP AT ROOM TEMPERATURE (25°C/77°F) UNTIL READY TO USE AVOID EXCESSIVE HEAT SEE INSERT
Baxter
BAXTER HEALTHCARE CORPORATION
DEERFIELD IL 60015 USA
MADE IN USA
DISTRIBUTED IN CANADA BY
BAXTER CORPORATION
TORONTO ONTARIO CANADA
Viaflex® CONTAINER
PL 146® PLASTIC
FOR PRODUCT INFORMATION
CALL 1-800-933-0303
1
2
3
4
5
6
7
8
9

11. A patient with sepsis has an order for cefazolin 1 g in 50 mL of D_5W IVPB over 15 minutes. The drop factor is 60 gtt/mL. How many drops per minute should be given? ______

12. A patient with a methicillin-resistant *Staphylococcus aureus* infection has ciprofloxacin 400 mg in 200 mL D_5W ordered. The pharmacy recommends that the ciprofloxacin be infused at a rate of 200 mg/h with an IV pump. How many milliliters per hour should the IV pump be programmed for? ______

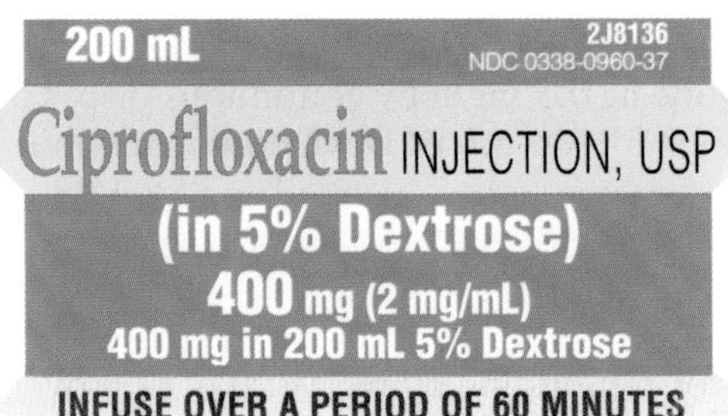

200 mL
2J8136
NDC 0338-0960-37
Ciprofloxacin INJECTION, USP
(in 5% Dextrose)
400 mg (2 mg/mL)
400 mg in 200 mL 5% Dextrose
INFUSE OVER A PERIOD OF 60 MINUTES

13. A patient with anuria has an order for 1000 mL of 0.9% NS to be infused over 1 hour. The tubing drop factor is 10 gtt/mL. How many drops per minute should be given? ______

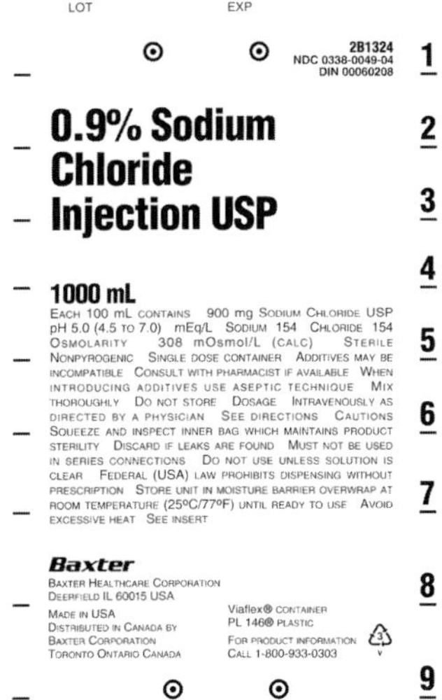

LOT
EXP
2B1324
NDC 0338-0049-04
DIN 00060208
0.9% Sodium Chloride Injection USP
1000 mL
Baxter
1
2
3
4
5
6
7
8
9

14. After surgery, a patient has an order for 500 mL of D_5W 0.45 NS to be infused over 4 hours. How many milliliters per hour should the IV pump be programmed for? ______

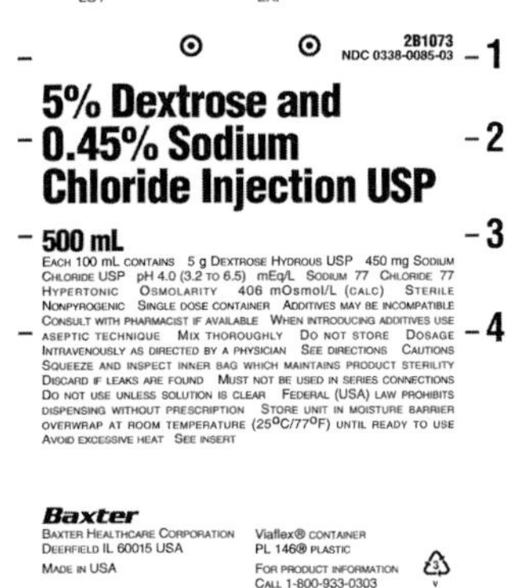

LOT
EXP
2B1073
NDC 0338-0085-03
5% Dextrose and 0.45% Sodium Chloride Injection USP
500 mL
Baxter
1
2
3
4

15. After a total hip replacement, a patient has an order for ketorolac 60 mg IVPB q 6 h over 15 minutes. The ketorolac is diluted in 25 mL of D_5W. The tubing drop factor is 15 gtt/mL. How many drops per minute should be given? ______

16. A terminal patient has an order for hydromorphone at 0.5 mg/h by continuous drip. Given a bag with a concentration of 20 mg hydromorphone in 100 mL of D_5W, how many milliliters per hour should the IV pump be programmed for? ______

17. A patient with peptic ulcer disease has an order for famotidine 20 mg IVPB q 12 h over 15 minutes. The famotidine is diluted in 25 mL of D_5W. The tubing drop factor is 20 gtt/mL. How many drops per minute should be given? ______

18. A patient with alcoholism has an order for magnesium sulfate 2 g in 100 mL of D_5W. The pharmacy recommends that the magnesium be infused at a rate of 1 g/h with an IV pump. How many milliliters per hour should the IV pump be programmed for? ______

19. A patient with aplastic anemia has an order for 1 unit of packed red blood cells (250 mL) to be infused. The facility's policy states to infuse the blood over 4 hours. The tubing drop factor is 20 gtt/mL. How many drops per minute should be given? ______

20. A patient has an order for Ofirmev 1000 mg in 100 mL of normal saline over 15 minutes for pain. How many milliliters per hour should be given? ______

21. A patient with hypokalemia has an order for 40 mEq of potassium to be infused intravenously now. The potassium is diluted in 200 mL of D_5W. The facility's policy states to infuse IV potassium at a rate of 10 mEq/h. How many milliliters per hour should the IV pump be programmed for? ______

22. A patient with Crohn's disease has an order for TPN from 2200 to 0800. The total volume of the TPN bag is 1350 mL. How many milliliters per hour should the IV pump be programmed for? ______

23. A patient with hypomagnesemia has an order for magnesium sulfate 2 g in 50 mL D_5W IV. The pharmacist recommends that the magnesium be infused at 1 g/h. How many milliliters per hour should the IV pump be programmed for? ______

24. A patient with herpes simplex virus 1 has acyclovir 700 mg in 200 mL of D_5W ordered to infuse over 1 hour. How many milliliters per hour should the IV pump be programmed for? ______

25. A patient with anasarca has albumin 25% 100 mL ordered over 30 minutes. The tubing drop factor is 20 gtt/mL. How many drops per minute should be given? ______

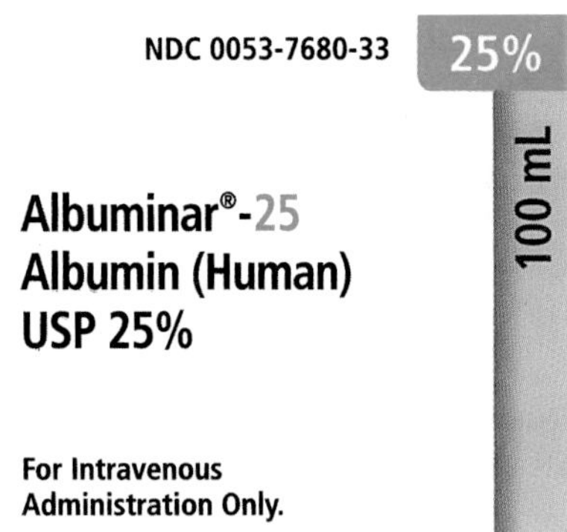

NDC 0053-7680-33
25%
100 mL
Albuminar®-25
Albumin (Human)
USP 25%
For Intravenous
Administration Only.

26. After the patient in question 25 receives her albumin, the licensed prescriber orders furosemide 100 mg in 50 mL of D_5W to be given over 30 minutes. How many milliliters per hour should the IV pump be set for? ______

27. A patient with multiple antibiotic allergies has a urinary tract infection. Amikacin 250 mg IVPB q 8 h is ordered over 1 hour. The amikacin is dissolved in 200 mL of D_5W. The drop factor is 20 gtt/mL. How many drops per minute should be given? ______

28. After surgery, a patient is hemorrhaging and has Amicar 8 g over 8 hours ordered. The Amicar is diluted in 500 mL of 0.9% NS. How many milliliters per hour should the IV pump be set for? ______

29. A patient with rapid atrial flutter has an order for diltiazem at 5 mg/h. The diltiazem concentration is 200 mg in 250 mL of 0.9% NS. How many milliliters per hour should the IV pump be set for? ______

30. A malnourished patient has folic acid 1 mg in 50 mL of 0.9% NS ordered to infuse over 30 minutes. An IV pump is not available. The nurse chooses a tubing with a 60 gtt/mL drop factor. How many drops per minute should be given? ______

31. Vancomycin 1250 mg in 250 mL of D_5W is ordered to infuse over 2 hours. How many milliliters per hour should the IV pump be set for? ______

32. A patient has a blood urea nitrogen level of 52 with oliguria and a blood pressure of 90/50 mm Hg. The licensed prescriber orders 1000 mL of 0.9% NS to be infused over 10 hours. How many milliliters per hour should the IV pump infuse? ______

33. Using the Parkland formula, the fluid requirements for a patient with severe burns reveal that 9600 mL should be infused over 8 hours. How many milliliters per hour should the IV pump be set for? ______

34. A patient has IV immunoglobulin G (IgG) 100 mL ordered over 3 hours. How many milliliters per hour should the IV pump be set for? ______

35. A patient with rapid atrial fibrillation has an order for diltiazem at 20 mg/h. The diltiazem concentration is 100 mg in 100 mL of 0.9% NS. How many milliliters per hour should the IV pump be set for? ______

36. A STAT dose of piperacillin/tazobactam 3.375 mg in 100 mL of 0.9% NS is ordered to be given over 15 minutes. How many milliliters per hour should the nurse program the IV pump for? ______

37. A patient with a vancomycin-resistant enterococci (VRE) has linezolid 600 mg intravenously ordered over 2 hours every 12 hours. How many milliliters per hour should the nurse program the IV pump for? ______

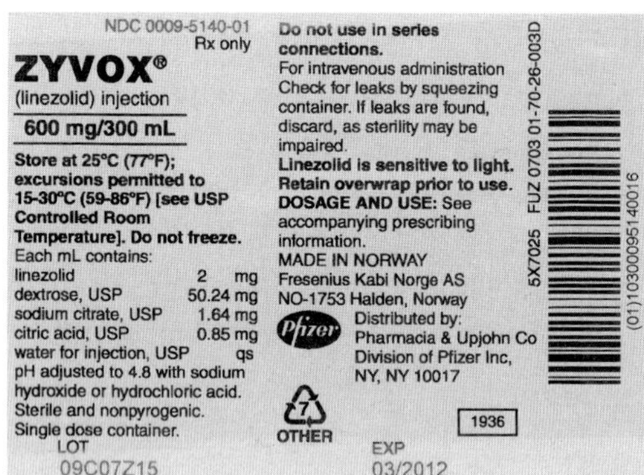

ANSWERS ON PP. 465 AND 467–469.

NAME ______________________

DATE ______________________

ACCEPTABLE SCORE **14**

YOUR SCORE ______

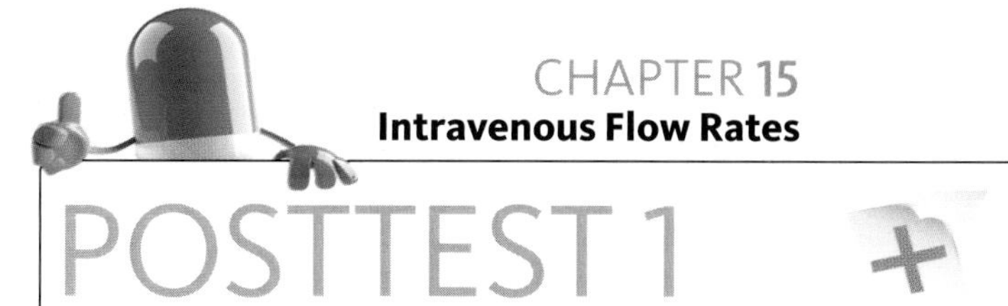

DIRECTIONS: The IV fluid order is listed in the problem. Calculate the appropriate infusion rate for each problem. Show your work. Follow your instructor's rules on rounding final answers.

1. A patient with hypotension has an order for 500 mL of plasma protein fraction to be infused over 2 hours. How many milliliters per hour should the IV pump be programmed for? ______

2. An order is received to infuse amphotericin B 240 mg in 500 mL D_5W over 4 hours. How many milliliters per hour should the IV pump be programmed for? ______

3. An NPO patient has an order for 0.9% NS at 120 mL/h. The drop factor is 12 gtt/mL. How many drops per minute should be given? ______

LOT EXP

2B1324
NDC 0338-0049-04
DIN 00060208

0.9% Sodium Chloride Injection USP

1000 mL

EACH 100 mL CONTAINS 900 mg SODIUM CHLORIDE USP pH 5.0 (4.5 TO 7.0) mEq/L SODIUM 154 CHLORIDE 154 OSMOLARITY 308 mOsmol/L (CALC) STERILE NONPYROGENIC SINGLE DOSE CONTAINER ADDITIVES MAY BE INCOMPATIBLE CONSULT WITH PHARMACIST IF AVAILABLE WHEN INTRODUCING ADDITIVES USE ASEPTIC TECHNIQUE MIX THOROUGHLY DO NOT STORE DOSAGE INTRAVENOUSLY AS DIRECTED BY A PHYSICIAN SEE DIRECTIONS CAUTIONS SQUEEZE AND INSPECT INNER BAG WHICH MAINTAINS PRODUCT STERILITY DISCARD IF LEAKS ARE FOUND MUST NOT BE USED IN SERIES CONNECTIONS DO NOT USE UNLESS SOLUTION IS CLEAR FEDERAL (USA) LAW PROHIBITS DISPENSING WITHOUT PRESCRIPTION STORE UNIT IN MOISTURE BARRIER OVERWRAP AT ROOM TEMPERATURE (25°C/77°F) UNTIL READY TO USE AVOID EXCESSIVE HEAT SEE INSERT

Baxter
BAXTER HEALTHCARE CORPORATION
DEERFIELD IL 60015 USA
MADE IN USA
DISTRIBUTED IN CANADA BY
BAXTER CORPORATION
TORONTO ONTARIO CANADA

Viaflex® CONTAINER
PL 146® PLASTIC
FOR PRODUCT INFORMATION
CALL 1-800-933-0303

1 2 3 4 5 6 7 8 9

4. After a burn injury Mr. Warren is to receive 500 mL of blood plasma over 4 hours. The tubing drop factor is 15 gtt/mL. How many drops per minute should be given? ______

5. A postpartum patient is to receive 1500 mL of LR over the next 8 hours. How many milliliters per hour should the IV pump be programmed for? ______

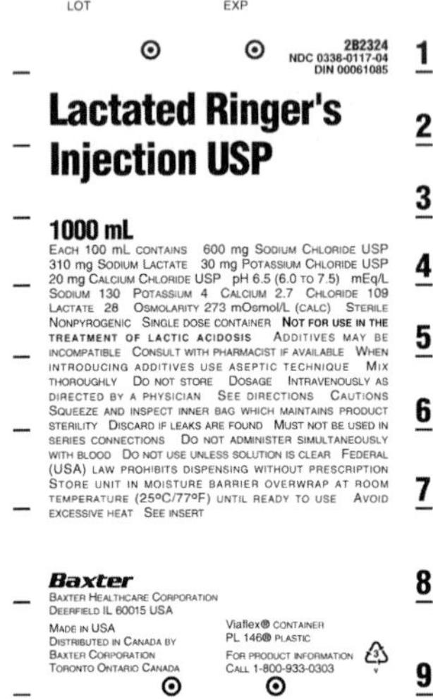

6. A patient is admitted with pernicious anemia. The licensed prescriber orders a unit of packed red blood cells (250 mL) to be infused over 3 hours. The tubing drop factor is 12 gtt/mL. How many drops per minute should be given? ______

7. An order for 1000 mL of LR over 12 hours is received. The tubing drop factor is 15 gtt/mL. How many drops per minute should be given? ______

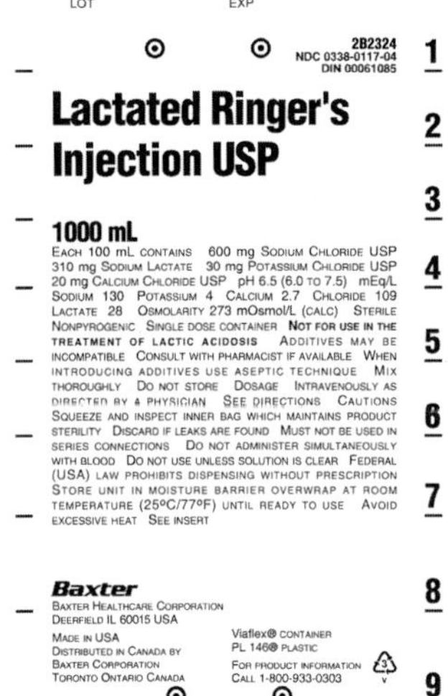

8. A patient with hypomagnesemia has an order for infusion of magnesium sulfate 2 g diluted in 50 mL D_5W. Policy states that the magnesium be infused at a rate of 1 g/h. How many milliliters per hour should the IV pump be programmed for? ______

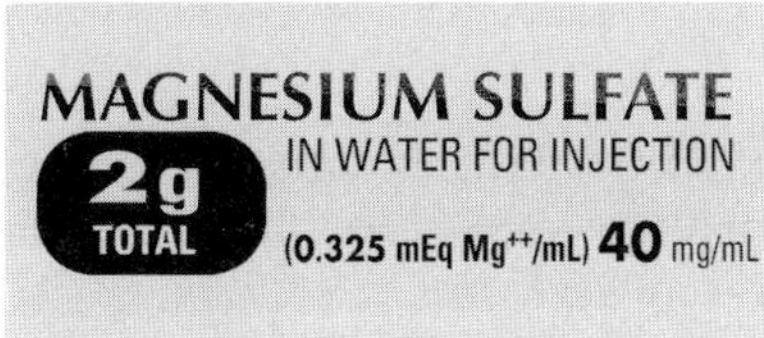
MAGNESIUM SULFATE
2g
TOTAL
IN WATER FOR INJECTION
(0.325 mEq Mg++/mL) 40 mg/mL

9. An order for NS to be infused at 150 mL/h after a transesophageal echocardiogram is received. The tubing drop factor is 60 gtt/mL. How many drops per minute should be given? ______

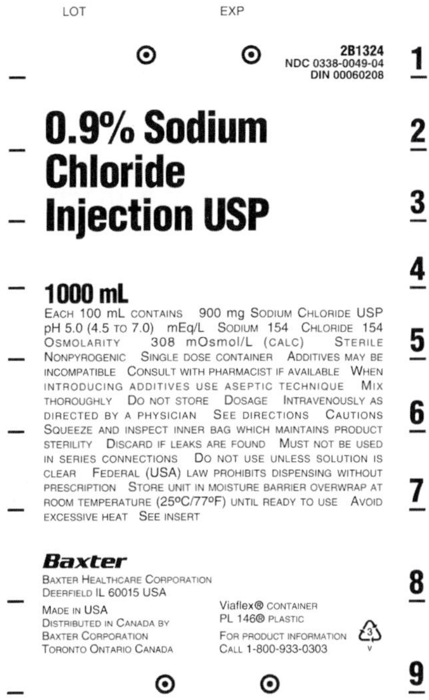
LOT
EXP
2B1324
NDC 0338-0049-04
DIN 00060208
0.9% Sodium Chloride Injection USP
1000 mL
EACH 100 mL CONTAINS 900 mg SODIUM CHLORIDE USP pH 5.0 (4.5 TO 7.0) mEq/L SODIUM 154 CHLORIDE 154 OSMOLARITY 308 mOsmol/L (CALC) STERILE NONPYROGENIC SINGLE DOSE CONTAINER ADDITIVES MAY BE INCOMPATIBLE CONSULT WITH PHARMACIST IF AVAILABLE WHEN INTRODUCING ADDITIVES USE ASEPTIC TECHNIQUE MIX THOROUGHLY DO NOT STORE DOSAGE INTRAVENOUSLY AS DIRECTED BY A PHYSICIAN SEE DIRECTIONS CAUTIONS SQUEEZE AND INSPECT INNER BAG WHICH MAINTAINS PRODUCT STERILITY DISCARD IF LEAKS ARE FOUND MUST NOT BE USED IN SERIES CONNECTIONS DO NOT USE UNLESS SOLUTION IS CLEAR FEDERAL (USA) LAW PROHIBITS DISPENSING WITHOUT PRESCRIPTION STORE UNIT IN MOISTURE BARRIER OVERWRAP AT ROOM TEMPERATURE (25°C/77°F) UNTIL READY TO USE AVOID EXCESSIVE HEAT SEE INSERT
Baxter
BAXTER HEALTHCARE CORPORATION
DEERFIELD IL 60015 USA
MADE IN USA
DISTRIBUTED IN CANADA BY
BAXTER CORPORATION
TORONTO ONTARIO CANADA
Viaflex® CONTAINER
PL 146® PLASTIC
FOR PRODUCT INFORMATION
CALL 1-800-933-0303
1
2
3
4
5
6
7
8
9

10. A patient has an order for 2500 mL of TPN to be infused over 24 hours. How many milliliters per hour should the IV pump be programmed for? ______

11. A patient with hypokalemia and hypophosphatemia has an order for potassium phosphate 30 milliosmole in 200 mL of 0.9% NS IV. The facility's policy states to infuse the potassium phosphate at 10 mOsm/h. How many milliliters per hour should the IV pump be programmed for? ______

12. A postoperative patient has an order for ceftazidime 1 g in 25 mL of D_5W over 15 minutes. The tubing drop factor is 60 gtt/mL. How many drops per minute should be given? ______

13. The licensed prescriber orders morphine sulfate 15 mg/h IV for a patient with metastatic cancer. Given a bag with a concentration of 100 mg of morphine sulfate in 200 mL of D_5W, how many milliliters per hour should the IV pump be programmed for? ______

14. A patient with an infection has an order for meropenem 1 g in 100 mL of D_5W IVPB q 8 h over 30 minutes. How many milliliters per hour should the IV pump be programmed for? ______

15. Timentin 3.1 g in 100 mL of D_5W IVPB over 1 hour is ordered for a patient with sepsis. The drop factor is 60 gtt/mL. How many drops per minute should be given?

ANSWERS ON PP. 466 AND 469–470.

NAME ____________________

DATE ____________________

ACCEPTABLE SCORE **14**

YOUR SCORE ______

POSTTEST 2

DIRECTIONS: The IV fluid order is listed in each problem. Calculate the appropriate infusion rate for each problem. Show your work. Follow your instructor's rules on rounding final answers.

1. A patient with poor wound healing has ascorbic acid 300 mg in 200 mL of 0.9% NS ordered to be infused over 6 hours. How many milliliters per hour should the IV pump be programmed for? ______

2. Moxifloxacin 400 mg daily IVPB is ordered for a patient with osteomyelitis. The moxifloxacin is to be infused over 60 minutes. The tubing drop factor is 10 gtt/mL. How many drops per minute should be given? ______

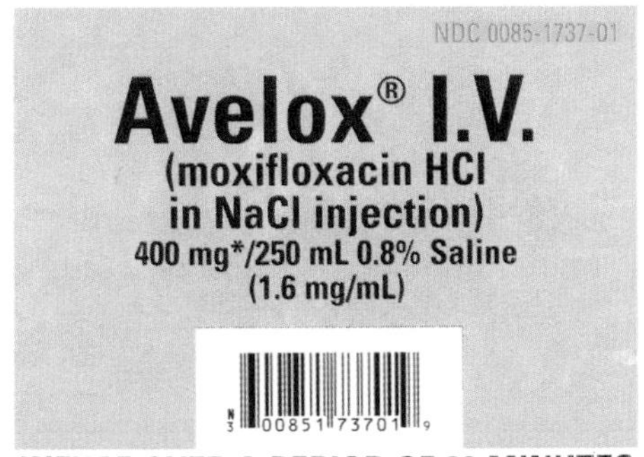

NDC 0085-1737-01
Avelox® I.V.
(moxifloxacin HCl
in NaCl injection)
400 mg*/250 mL 0.8% Saline
(1.6 mg/mL)
3 00851 73701 9
INFUSE OVER A PERIOD OF 60 MINUTES

3. A patient with iron-deficiency anemia has an order for iron dextran 100 mg in 200 mL of 0.9% NS over 6 hours. How many milliliters per hour should the IV pump be programmed for? ______

4. A patient with a gastrointestinal bleed has an order for 1 unit of whole blood (500 mL) to be given over 3 hours. The tubing drop factor is 15 gtt/mL. How many drops per minute should be given? ______

5. A patient with hypotension receives an order for 1000 mL of 0.9% NS over 6 hours. The tubing drop factor is 10 gtt/mL. How many drops per minute should be given? ______

LOT EXP

2B1324
NDC 0338-0049-04
DIN 00060208

0.9% Sodium Chloride Injection USP

1000 mL

EACH 100 mL CONTAINS 900 mg SODIUM CHLORIDE USP pH 5.0 (4.5 TO 7.0) mEq/L SODIUM 154 CHLORIDE 154 OSMOLARITY 308 mOsmol/L (CALC) STERILE NONPYROGENIC SINGLE DOSE CONTAINER ADDITIVES MAY BE INCOMPATIBLE CONSULT WITH PHARMACIST IF AVAILABLE WHEN INTRODUCING ADDITIVES USE ASEPTIC TECHNIQUE MIX THOROUGHLY DO NOT STORE DOSAGE INTRAVENOUSLY AS DIRECTED BY A PHYSICIAN SEE DIRECTIONS CAUTIONS SQUEEZE AND INSPECT INNER BAG WHICH MAINTAINS PRODUCT STERILITY DISCARD IF LEAKS ARE FOUND MUST NOT BE USED IN SERIES CONNECTIONS DO NOT USE UNLESS SOLUTION IS CLEAR FEDERAL (USA) LAW PROHIBITS DISPENSING WITHOUT PRESCRIPTION STORE UNIT IN MOISTURE BARRIER OVERWRAP AT ROOM TEMPERATURE (25°C/77°F) UNTIL READY TO USE AVOID EXCESSIVE HEAT SEE INSERT

Baxter
BAXTER HEALTHCARE CORPORATION
DEERFIELD IL 60015 USA
MADE IN USA
DISTRIBUTED IN CANADA BY
BAXTER CORPORATION
TORONTO ONTARIO CANADA

VIAFLEX® CONTAINER
PL 146® PLASTIC
FOR PRODUCT INFORMATION
CALL 1-800-933-0303

1 2 3 4 5 6 7 8 9

6. An order for a patient with hypocalcemia states to infuse 1 g of calcium chloride 10% over 30 minutes. The calcium chloride is diluted in 50 mL of 0.9% NS. How many milliliters per hour should the IV pump be programmed for? ______

7. A terminal patient has morphine sulfate ordered at 8 mg/h. The medication concentration is morphine 100 mg diluted in 100 mL of D_5W. How many milliliters per hour should the IV pump be programmed for? ______

8. A patient who has undergone hip replacement has an order for ketorolac 30 mg q 6 h. The ketorolac is diluted in 50 mL of 0.9% NS and is to be infused over 15 minutes. The tubing drop factor is 60 gtt/mL. How many drops per minute should be given? ______

9. A patient with severe nausea and vomiting has a one-time order for ondansetron 8 mg IVPB over 15 minutes. The ondansetron is diluted in 50 mL of D_5W. The tubing drop factor is 15 gtt/mL. How many drops per minute should be given? ______

10. A postoperative patient has an order for 1000 mL of LR over 6 hours. How many milliliters per hour should the IV pump be programmed for? _______

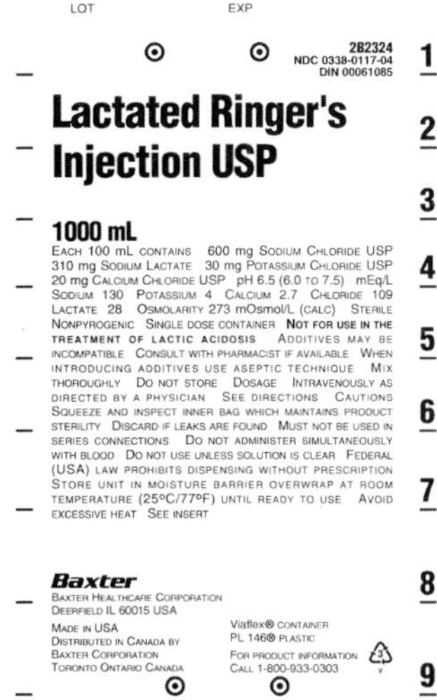
LOT
EXP
2B2324
NDC 0338-0117-04
DIN 00061085
1
Lactated Ringer's Injection USP
2
3
1000 mL
EACH 100 mL CONTAINS 600 mg SODIUM CHLORIDE USP 310 mg SODIUM LACTATE 30 mg POTASSIUM CHLORIDE USP 20 mg CALCIUM CHLORIDE USP pH 6.5 (6.0 TO 7.5) mEq/L SODIUM 130 POTASSIUM 4 CALCIUM 2.7 CHLORIDE 109 LACTATE 28 OSMOLARITY 273 mOsmol/L (CALC) STERILE NONPYROGENIC SINGLE DOSE CONTAINER NOT FOR USE IN THE TREATMENT OF LACTIC ACIDOSIS ADDITIVES MAY BE INCOMPATIBLE CONSULT WITH PHARMACIST IF AVAILABLE WHEN INTRODUCING ADDITIVES USE ASEPTIC TECHNIQUE MIX THOROUGHLY DO NOT STORE DOSAGE INTRAVENOUSLY AS DIRECTED BY A PHYSICIAN SEE DIRECTIONS CAUTIONS SQUEEZE AND INSPECT INNER BAG WHICH MAINTAINS PRODUCT STERILITY DISCARD IF LEAKS ARE FOUND MUST NOT BE USED IN SERIES CONNECTIONS DO NOT ADMINISTER SIMULTANEOUSLY WITH BLOOD DO NOT USE UNLESS SOLUTION IS CLEAR FEDERAL (USA) LAW PROHIBITS DISPENSING WITHOUT PRESCRIPTION STORE UNIT IN MOISTURE BARRIER OVERWRAP AT ROOM TEMPERATURE (25°C/77°F) UNTIL READY TO USE AVOID EXCESSIVE HEAT SEE INSERT
4
5
6
7
Baxter
BAXTER HEALTHCARE CORPORATION
DEERFIELD IL 60015 USA
MADE IN USA
DISTRIBUTED IN CANADA BY
BAXTER CORPORATION
TORONTO ONTARIO CANADA
Viaflex® CONTAINER
PL 146® PLASTIC
FOR PRODUCT INFORMATION
CALL 1-800-933-0303
8
9

11. A patient experiences bradypnea after intrathecal administration of anesthesia. An order for naloxone 0.4 mg/h is written. Given a bag with a concentration of 8 mg in 100 mL of 0.9% NS, how many milliliters per hour should the IV pump be programmed for? _______

12. A patient with a total gastrectomy has TPN ordered to be infused from 2200 to 0600. The total volume of the TPN bag is 1200 mL. How many milliliters per hour should the IV pump be programmed for? _______

13. Mannitol 10%, 200 mL is ordered to infuse over 90 minutes. How many milliliters per hour should the IV pump be programmed for? _______

14. A patient with oliguria receives an order for 1000 mL of 0.9% NS over 3 hours. The tubing drop factor is 10 gtt/mL. How many drops per minute should be given? ______

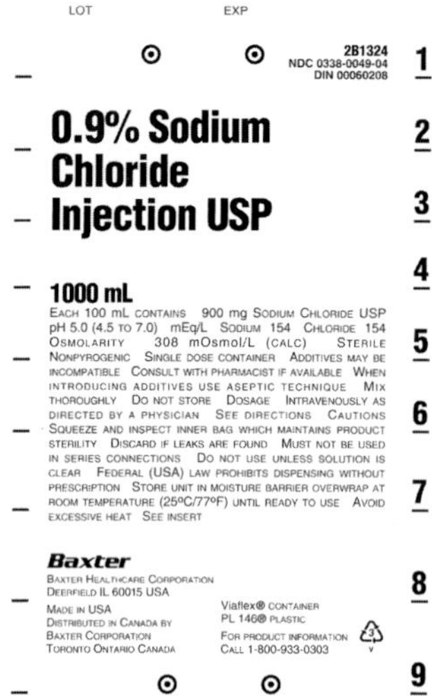
LOT
EXP
2B1324
NDC 0338-0049-04
DIN 00060208
0.9% Sodium
Chloride
Injection USP
1000 mL
Each 100 mL contains 900 mg Sodium Chloride USP pH 5.0 (4.5 to 7.0) mEq/L Sodium 154 Chloride 154 Osmolarity 308 mOsmol/L (calc) Sterile Nonpyrogenic Single dose container Additives may be incompatible Consult with pharmacist if available When introducing additives use aseptic technique Mix thoroughly Do not store Dosage Intravenously as directed by a physician See directions Cautions Squeeze and inspect inner bag which maintains product sterility Discard if leaks are found Must not be used in series connections Do not use unless solution is clear Federal (USA) law prohibits dispensing without prescription Store unit in moisture barrier overwrap at room temperature (25°C/77°F) until ready to use Avoid excessive heat See insert
Baxter
Baxter Healthcare Corporation
Deerfield IL 60015 USA
Made in USA
Distributed in Canada by
Baxter Corporation
Toronto Ontario Canada
Viaflex® container
PL 146® plastic
For product information
Call 1-800-933-0303
1
2
3
4
5
6
7
8
9

15. An NPO patient has an order for 500 mL of D_5W 0.45% NS over 6 hours. How many milliliters per hour should the IV pump be programmed for?

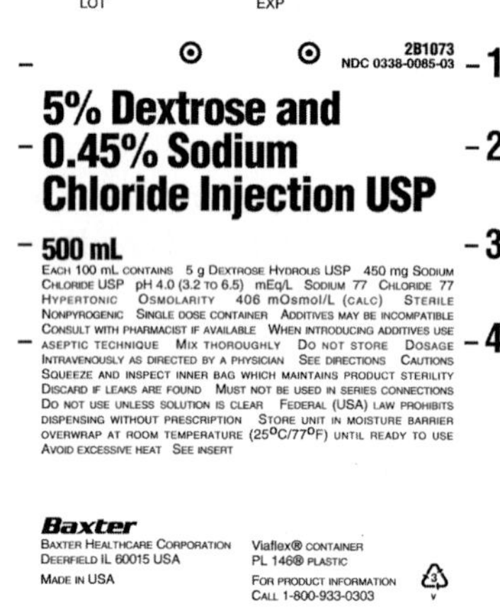
LOT
EXP
2B1073
NDC 0338-0085-03
5% Dextrose and
0.45% Sodium
Chloride Injection USP
500 mL
Each 100 mL contains 5 g Dextrose Hydrous USP 450 mg Sodium Chloride USP pH 4.0 (3.2 to 6.5) mEq/L Sodium 77 Chloride 77 Hypertonic Osmolarity 406 mOsmol/L (calc) Sterile Nonpyrogenic Single dose container Additives may be incompatible Consult with pharmacist if available When introducing additives use aseptic technique Mix thoroughly Do not store Dosage Intravenously as directed by a physician See directions Cautions Squeeze and inspect inner bag which maintains product sterility Discard if leaks are found Must not be used in series connections Do not use unless solution is clear Federal (USA) law prohibits dispensing without prescription Store unit in moisture barrier overwrap at room temperature (25°C/77°F) until ready to use Avoid excessive heat See insert
Baxter
Baxter Healthcare Corporation
Deerfield IL 60015 USA
Made in USA
Viaflex® container
PL 146® plastic
For product information
Call 1-800-933-0303
1
2
3
4

ANSWERS ON PP. 466 AND 471–472.

evolve For additional practice problems, refer to the Intravenous Flow Rates section of *Elsevier's Interactive Drug Calculation Application*, version 1.

ANSWERS

CHAPTER 15 Dimensional Analysis—Work Sheet, pp. 451–456

1. $\frac{x \text{ mL}}{\text{h}} = \frac{500 \text{ mL}}{24 \text{ h}} = 20.8$ or 21 mL/h

2. $\frac{x \text{ mL}}{\text{h}} = \frac{100 \text{ mL}}{1 \text{ h}} = 100$ mL/h

3. $\frac{x \text{ gtt}}{\text{min}} = \frac{15 \text{ gtt}}{1 \text{ mL}} \times \frac{100 \text{ mL}}{30 \text{ min}} = 50$ gtt/min

4. $\frac{x \text{ mL}}{\text{h}} = \frac{3000 \text{ mL}}{12 \text{ h}} = 250$ mL/h

5. $\frac{x \text{ gtt}}{\text{min}} = \frac{10 \text{ gtt}}{1 \text{ mL}} \times \frac{100 \text{ mL}}{30 \text{ min}}$
   = 33.3 rounded to 33 gtt/min

6. $\frac{x \text{ mL}}{\text{h}} = \frac{500 \text{ mL}}{6 \text{ h}} = 83.3$ or 83 mL/h

7. $\frac{x \text{ gtt}}{\text{min}} = \frac{10 \text{ gtt}}{1 \text{ mL}} \times \frac{100 \text{ mL}}{60 \text{ min}}$
   = 16.6 rounded to 17 gtt/min

8. $\frac{x \text{ mL}}{\text{h}} = \frac{250 \text{ mL}}{60 \text{ mEq}} \times \frac{20 \text{ mEq}}{1 \text{ h}}$
   = 83.3 or 83 mL/h

9. $\frac{x \text{ gtt}}{\text{min}} = \frac{60 \text{ gtt}}{1 \text{ mL}} \times \frac{50 \text{ mL}}{30 \text{ min}} = 100$ gtt/min

10. $\frac{x \text{ mL}}{\text{h}} = \frac{1000 \text{ mL}}{10 \text{ h}} = 100$ mL/h

11. $\frac{x \text{ gtt}}{\text{min}} = \frac{60 \text{ gtt}}{1 \text{ mL}} \times \frac{50 \text{ mL}}{15 \text{ min}} = 200$ gtt/min

12. $\frac{x \text{ mL}}{\text{h}} = \frac{200 \text{ mL}}{400 \text{ mg}} \times \frac{200 \text{ mg}}{1 \text{ h}} = 100$ mL/h

13. $\frac{x \text{ gtt}}{\text{min}} = \frac{10 \text{ gtt}}{1 \text{ mL}} \times \frac{1000 \text{ mL}}{1 \text{ h}} \times \frac{1 \text{ h}}{60 \text{ min}}$
    = 166.6 rounded to 167 gtt/min

14. $\frac{x \text{ mL}}{\text{h}} = \frac{500 \text{ mL}}{4 \text{ h}} = 125$ mL/h

15. $\frac{x \text{ gtt}}{\text{min}} = \frac{15 \text{ gtt}}{1 \text{ mL}} \times \frac{25 \text{ mL}}{15 \text{ min}} = 25$ gtt/min

16. $\frac{x \text{ mL}}{\text{h}} = \frac{100 \text{ mL}}{20 \text{ mg}} \times \frac{0.5 \text{ mg}}{1 \text{ h}}$
    = 2.5 or 3 mL/h

17. $\frac{x \text{ gtt}}{\text{min}} = \frac{20 \text{ gtt}}{1 \text{ mL}} \times \frac{25 \text{ mL}}{15 \text{ min}}$
    = 33.3 rounded to 33 gtt/min

18. $\frac{x \text{ mL}}{\text{h}} = \frac{100 \text{ mL}}{2 \text{ g}} \times \frac{1 \text{ g}}{1 \text{ h}} = 50$ mL/h

19. $\frac{x \text{ gtt}}{\text{min}} = \frac{20 \text{ gtt}}{1 \text{ mL}} \times \frac{250 \text{ mL}}{4 \text{ h}} \times \frac{1 \text{ h}}{60 \text{ min}}$
    = 20.8 rounded to 21 gtt/min

20. $\frac{x \text{ mL}}{\text{h}} = \frac{100 \text{ mL}}{15 \text{ min}} \times \frac{60 \text{ min}}{1 \text{ h}} = 400$ mL/h

21. $\frac{x \text{ mL}}{\text{h}} = \frac{200 \text{ mL}}{40 \text{ mEq}} \times \frac{10 \text{ mEq}}{1 \text{ h}} = 50$ mL/h

22. $\frac{x \text{ mL}}{\text{h}} = \frac{1350 \text{ mL}}{10 \text{ h}} = 135$ mL/h

23. $\frac{x \text{ mL}}{\text{h}} = \frac{50 \text{ mL}}{2 \text{ g}} \times \frac{1 \text{ g}}{1 \text{ h}} = 25$ mL/h

24. $\frac{x \text{ mL}}{\text{h}} = \frac{200 \text{ mL}}{1 \text{ h}} = 200$ mL/h

25. $\frac{x \text{ gtt}}{\text{min}} = \frac{20 \text{ gtt}}{1 \text{ mL}} \times \frac{100 \text{ mL}}{30 \text{ min}}$
    = 66.6 rounded to 67 gtt/min

26. $\frac{x \text{ mL}}{\text{h}} = \frac{50 \text{ mL}}{30 \text{ min}} \times \frac{60 \text{ min}}{1 \text{ h}} = 100$ mL/h

27. $\frac{x \text{ gtt}}{\text{min}} = \frac{20 \text{ gtt}}{1 \text{ mL}} \times \frac{200 \text{ mL}}{1 \text{ h}} \times \frac{1 \text{ h}}{60 \text{ min}}$
    = 66.6 rounded to 67 gtt/min

28. $\frac{x \text{ mL}}{\text{h}} = \frac{500 \text{ mL}}{8 \text{ h}} = 62.5$ or 63 mL/h

29. $\frac{x \text{ mL}}{\text{h}} = \frac{250 \text{ mL}}{200 \text{ mg}} \times \frac{5 \text{ mg}}{1 \text{ h}} = 6.3$ or 6 mL/h

30. $\frac{x \text{ gtt}}{\text{min}} = \frac{60 \text{ gtt}}{1 \text{ mL}} \times \frac{50 \text{ mL}}{30 \text{ min}} = 100$ gtt/min

31. $\frac{x \text{ mL}}{\text{h}} = \frac{250 \text{ mL}}{2 \text{ h}} = 125$ mL/h

32. $\frac{x \text{ mL}}{\text{h}} = \frac{1000 \text{ mL}}{10 \text{ h}} = 100$ mL/h

33. $\frac{x \text{ mL}}{\text{h}} = \frac{9600 \text{ mL}}{8 \text{ h}} = 1200$ mL/h

34. $\frac{x \text{ mL}}{\text{h}} = \frac{100 \text{ mL}}{3 \text{ h}} = 33.3$ or 33 mL/h

35. $\frac{x \text{ mL}}{\text{h}} = \frac{100 \text{ mL}}{100 \text{ mg}} \times \frac{20 \text{ mg}}{1 \text{ h}} = 20$ mL/h

36. $\frac{x \text{ mL}}{\text{h}} = \frac{100 \text{ mL}}{15 \text{ min}} \times \frac{60 \text{ min}}{1 \text{ h}} = 400$ mL/h

37. $\frac{x \text{ mL}}{\text{h}} = \frac{300 \text{ mL}}{2 \text{ h}} = 150$ mL/h

CHAPTER 15 Dimensional Analysis—Posttest 1, pp. 457–460

1. $\frac{x \text{ mL}}{\text{h}} = \frac{500 \text{ mL}}{2 \text{ h}} = 250 \text{ mL/h}$

2. $\frac{x \text{ mL}}{\text{h}} = \frac{500 \text{ mL}}{4 \text{ h}} = 125 \text{ mL/h}$

3. $\frac{x \text{ gtt}}{\text{min}} = \frac{12 \text{ gtt}}{1 \text{ mL}} \times \frac{120 \text{ mL}}{1 \text{ h}} \times \frac{1 \text{ h}}{60 \text{ min}}$
$= 24 \text{ gtt/min}$

4. $\frac{x \text{ gtt}}{\text{min}} = \frac{15 \text{ gtt}}{1 \text{ mL}} \times \frac{500 \text{ mL}}{4 \text{ h}} \times \frac{1 \text{ h}}{60 \text{ min}}$
$= 31.2$ rounded to 31 gtt/min

5. $\frac{x \text{ mL}}{\text{h}} = \frac{1500 \text{ mL}}{8 \text{ h}} = 187.5$ or 188 mL/h

6. $\frac{x \text{ gtt}}{\text{min}} = \frac{12 \text{ gtt}}{1 \text{ mL}} \times \frac{250 \text{ mL}}{3 \text{ h}} \times \frac{1 \text{ h}}{60 \text{ min}}$
$= 16.6$ rounded to 17 gtt/min

7. $\frac{x \text{ gtt}}{\text{min}} = \frac{15 \text{ gtt}}{1 \text{ mL}} \times \frac{1000 \text{ mL}}{12 \text{ h}} \times \frac{1 \text{ h}}{60 \text{ min}}$
$= 20.8$ rounded to 21 gtt/min

8. $\frac{x \text{ mL}}{\text{h}} = \frac{50 \text{ mL}}{2 \text{ g}} \times \frac{1 \text{ g}}{1 \text{ h}} = 25 \text{ mL/h}$

9. $\frac{x \text{ gtt}}{\text{min}} = \frac{60 \text{ gtt}}{1 \text{ mL}} \times \frac{150 \text{ mL}}{1 \text{ h}} \times \frac{1 \text{ h}}{60 \text{ min}}$
$= 150 \text{ gtt/min}$

10. $\frac{x \text{ mL}}{\text{h}} = \frac{2500 \text{ mL}}{24 \text{ h}} = 104.1$ or 104 mL/h

11. $\frac{x \text{ mL}}{\text{h}} = \frac{200 \text{ mL}}{30 \text{ mOsm}} \times \frac{10 \text{ mOsm}}{1 \text{ h}}$
$= 66.7$ or 67 mL/h

12. $\frac{x \text{ gtt}}{\text{min}} = \frac{60 \text{ gtt}}{1 \text{ mL}} \times \frac{25 \text{ mL}}{15 \text{ min}} = 100 \text{ gtt/min}$

13. $\frac{x \text{ mL}}{\text{h}} = \frac{200 \text{ mL}}{100 \text{ mg}} \times \frac{15 \text{ mg}}{1 \text{ h}} = 30 \text{ mL/h}$

14. $\frac{x \text{ mL}}{\text{h}} = \frac{100 \text{ mL}}{30 \text{ min}} \times \frac{60 \text{ min}}{1 \text{ h}} = 200 \text{ mL/h}$

15. $\frac{x \text{ gtt}}{\text{min}} = \frac{60 \text{ gtt}}{1 \text{ mL}} \times \frac{100 \text{ mL}}{1 \text{ h}} \times \frac{1 \text{ h}}{60 \text{ min}}$
$= 100 \text{ gtt/min}$

CHAPTER 15 Dimensional Analysis—Posttest 2, pp. 461–464

1. $\frac{x \text{ mL}}{\text{h}} = \frac{200 \text{ mL}}{6 \text{ h}} = 33.3$ or 33 mL/h

2. $\frac{x \text{ gtt}}{\text{min}} = \frac{10 \text{ gtt}}{1 \text{ mL}} \times \frac{250 \text{ mL}}{60 \text{ min}}$
$= 41.6$ rounded to 42 gtt/min

3. $\frac{x \text{ mL}}{\text{h}} = \frac{200 \text{ mL}}{6 \text{ h}} = 133.3$ or 133 mL/h

4. $\frac{x \text{ gtt}}{\text{min}} = \frac{15 \text{ gtt}}{1 \text{ mL}} \times \frac{500 \text{ mL}}{3 \text{ h}} \times \frac{1 \text{ h}}{60 \text{ min}}$
$= 41.6$ rounded to 42 gtt/min

5. $\frac{x \text{ gtt}}{\text{min}} = \frac{10 \text{ gtt}}{1 \text{ mL}} \times \frac{1000 \text{ mL}}{6 \text{ h}} \times \frac{1 \text{ h}}{60 \text{ min}}$
$= 27.7$ rounded to 28 gtt/min

6. $\frac{x \text{ mL}}{\text{h}} = \frac{50 \text{ mL}}{30 \text{ min}} \times \frac{60 \text{ min}}{1 \text{ h}} = 100 \text{ mL/h}$

7. $\frac{x \text{ mL}}{\text{h}} = \frac{100 \text{ mL}}{100 \text{ mg}} \times \frac{8 \text{ mg}}{1 \text{ h}} = 8 \text{ mL/h}$

8. $\frac{x \text{ gtt}}{\text{min}} = \frac{60 \text{ gtt}}{1 \text{ mL}} \times \frac{50 \text{ mL}}{15 \text{ min}} = 200 \text{ gtt/min}$

9. $\frac{x \text{ gtt}}{\text{min}} = \frac{15 \text{ gtt}}{1 \text{ mL}} \times \frac{50 \text{ mL}}{15 \text{ min}} = 50 \text{ gtt/min}$

10. $\frac{x \text{ mL}}{\text{h}} = \frac{1000 \text{ mL}}{6 \text{ h}} = 166.7$ or 167 mL/h

11. $\frac{x \text{ mL}}{\text{h}} = \frac{100 \text{ mL}}{8 \text{ mg}} \times \frac{0.4 \text{ mg}}{1 \text{ h}} = 5 \text{ mL/h}$

12. $\frac{x \text{ mL}}{\text{h}} = \frac{1200 \text{ mL}}{8 \text{ h}} = 150 \text{ mL/h}$

13. $\frac{x \text{ mL}}{\text{h}} = \frac{200 \text{ mL}}{90 \text{ min}} \times \frac{60 \text{ min}}{1 \text{ h}} = 100 \text{ mL/h}$

14. $\frac{x \text{ gtt}}{\text{min}} = \frac{10 \text{ gtt}}{1 \text{ mL}} \times \frac{1000 \text{ mL}}{3 \text{ h}} \times \frac{1 \text{ h}}{60 \text{ min}}$
$= 55.5$ rounded to 56 gtt/min

15. $\frac{x \text{ mL}}{\text{h}} = \frac{500 \text{ mL}}{6 \text{ h}} = 83.3$ or 83 mL/h

CHAPTER 15 Proportion/Formula Method—Work Sheet, pp. 451–456

Proportion	Formula
1.	$\frac{500 \text{ mL}}{24 \text{ h}} = 20.8 \text{ or } 21 \text{ mL/h}$
2.	$\frac{100 \text{ mL}}{1 \text{ h}} = 100 \text{ mL/h}$
3.	$\frac{100 \text{ mL}}{\underset{2}{\cancel{30}} \text{ min}} \times \overset{1}{\cancel{15}} \text{ gtt/mL} = \frac{100}{2} = 50 \text{ gtt/min}$
4.	$\frac{3000 \text{ mL}}{12 \text{ h}} = 250 \text{ mL/h}$
5.	$\frac{100 \text{ mL}}{\underset{3}{\cancel{30}} \text{ min}} \times \overset{1}{\cancel{10}} \text{ gtt/mL} = \frac{100}{3}$ $= 33.3$ rounded to 33 gtt/min
6.	$\frac{500 \text{ mL}}{6 \text{ h}} = 83.3 \text{ or } 83 \text{ mL/h}$
7.	$\frac{100 \text{ mL}}{\underset{6}{\cancel{60}} \text{ min}} \times \overset{1}{\cancel{10}} \text{ gtt/mL} = \frac{100}{6}$ $= 16.6$ rounded to 17 gtt/min
8. 60 mEq : 250 mL :: 20 mEq : x mL $60x = 5000$ $x = \frac{5000}{60}$ $x = 83.3$ or 83 mL/h	$\frac{\overset{1}{\cancel{20}} \text{ mEq}}{\underset{3}{\cancel{60}} \text{ mEq}} \times 250 \text{ mL} =$ $\frac{500}{6} = 83.3 \text{ mL or } 83 \text{ mL/h}$
9.	$\frac{50 \text{ mL}}{\underset{1}{\cancel{30}} \text{ min}} \times \overset{2}{\cancel{60}} \text{ gtt/mL} = \frac{100}{1} = 100 \text{ gtt/min}$
10.	$\frac{1000 \text{ mL}}{10 \text{ h}} = 100 \text{ mL/h}$
11.	$\frac{50 \text{ mL}}{\underset{1}{\cancel{15}} \text{ min}} \times \overset{4}{\cancel{60}} \text{ gtt/mL} = 200 \text{ gtt/min}$
12. 400 mg : 200 mL :: 200 mg : x mL $400x = 40{,}000$ $x = \frac{40{,}000}{400}$ $x = 100$ mL/h	$\frac{200 \text{ mg}}{\underset{2}{\cancel{400}} \text{ mg}} \times \overset{1}{\cancel{200}} \text{ mL} =$ $\frac{200}{2} = 100 \text{ mL/h}$
13.	$\frac{1000 \text{ mL}}{\underset{6}{\cancel{60}} \text{ min}} \times \overset{1}{\cancel{10}} \text{ gtt/mL} = \frac{1000}{6}$ $= 166.6$ rounded to 167 gtt/min
14.	$\frac{500 \text{ mL}}{4 \text{ h}} = 125 \text{ mL/h}$

Proportion	Formula
15.	$\frac{25\text{ mL}}{\overset{}{\cancel{15}}_{1}\text{ min}} \times \overset{1}{\cancel{15}}\text{ gtt/mL} = 25\text{ gtt/min}$
16. 20 mg : 100 mL :: 0.5 mg : x mL $20x = 50$ $x = \frac{50}{20}$ $x = 2.5$ or 3 mL/h	$\frac{0.5\text{ mg}}{\cancel{20}_{1}\text{ mg}} \times \overset{5}{\cancel{100}}\text{ mL} =$ $\frac{0.5}{1} \times 5 = 2.5$ or 3 mL/h
17.	$\frac{25\text{ mL}}{\cancel{15}_{3}\text{ min}} \times \overset{4}{\cancel{20}}\text{ gtt/mL} = \frac{100}{3}$ $= 33.3$ rounded to 33 gtt/min
18. 2 g : 100 mL :: 1 g : x mL $2x = 100$ $x = \frac{100}{2}$ $x = 50$ mL/h	$\frac{1\text{ g}}{\cancel{2}_{1}\text{ g}} \times \overset{50}{\cancel{100}}\text{ mL} =$ $\frac{50}{1} = 50$ mL/h
19.	$\frac{250\text{ mL}}{\cancel{240}_{12}\text{ min}} \times \overset{1}{\cancel{20}}\text{ gtt/mL} = \frac{250}{12}$ $= 20.8$ rounded to 21 gtt/min
20.	$\frac{100\text{ mL}}{0.25\text{ h}} = 400$ mL/h
21. 40 mEq : 200 mL :: 10 mEq : x mL $40x = 2000$ $x = \frac{2000}{40}$ $x = 50$ mL/h	$\frac{10\text{ mEq}}{\cancel{40}_{1}\text{ mEq}} \times \overset{5}{\cancel{200}}\text{ mL} =$ $\frac{10}{1} \times 5 = 50$ mL/h
22.	$\frac{1350\text{ mL}}{10\text{ h}} = 135$ mL/h
23. 2 g : 50 mL :: 1 g : x mL $2x = 50$ $x = \frac{50}{2}$ $x = 25$ mL/h	$\frac{1\text{ g}}{\cancel{2}_{1}\text{ g}} \times \overset{25}{\cancel{50}}\text{ mL} =$ $\frac{25}{1} = 25$ mL/h
24.	$\frac{200\text{ mL}}{1\text{ h}} = 200$ mL/h
25.	$\frac{100\text{ mL}}{\cancel{30}_{3}\text{ min}} \times \overset{2}{\cancel{20}}\text{ gtt/mL} = \frac{200}{3}$ $= 66.6$ rounded to 67 gtt/min
26.	$\frac{50\text{ mL}}{0.5\text{ h}} = 100$ mL/h

Proportion	Formula
27.	$\dfrac{200\text{ mL}}{\overset{}{\underset{3}{\cancel{60}}}\text{ min}} \times \overset{1}{\cancel{20}}\text{ gtt/mL} = \dfrac{200}{3}$ $= 66.66$ rounded to 67 gtt/min
28.	$\dfrac{500\text{ mL}}{8\text{ h}} = 62.5$ or 63 mL/h
29. 200 mg : 250 mL :: 5 mg : x mL $200x = 1250$ $x = \dfrac{1250}{200}$ $x = 6.3$ or 6 mL/h	$\dfrac{5\text{ mg}}{\underset{4}{\cancel{200}}\text{ mg}} \times \overset{5}{\cancel{250}}\text{ mL} = 6.3$ or 6 mL/h
30.	$\dfrac{50\text{ mL}}{\underset{1}{\cancel{30}}\text{ min}} \times \overset{2}{\cancel{60}}\text{ gtt/mL} = 100$ gtt/min
31.	$\dfrac{250\text{ mL}}{2\text{ h}} = 125$ mL/h
32.	$\dfrac{1000\text{ mL}}{10\text{ h}} = 100$ mL/h
33.	$\dfrac{9600\text{ mL}}{8\text{ h}} = 1200$ mL/h
34.	$\dfrac{100\text{ mL}}{3\text{ h}} = 33.3$ or 33 mL/h
35. 100 mg : 100 mL :: 20 mg : x mL $100x = 2000$ $x = \dfrac{2000}{100}$ $x = 20$ mL/h	$\dfrac{20\text{ mg}}{\underset{1}{\cancel{100}}\text{ mg}} \times \overset{1}{\cancel{100}}\text{ mL} = 20$ mL/h
36.	$\dfrac{100\text{ mL}}{0.25\text{ h}} = 400$ mL/h
37.	$\dfrac{300\text{ mL}}{2\text{ h}} = 150$ mL/h

CHAPTER 15 Proportion/Formula Method—Posttest 1, pp. 457–460

Proportion	Formula
1.	$\dfrac{500\text{ mL}}{2\text{ h}} = 250$ mL/h
2.	$\dfrac{500\text{ mL}}{4\text{ h}} = 125$ mL/h
3.	$\dfrac{120\text{ mL}}{\underset{5}{\cancel{60}}\text{ min}} \times \overset{1}{\cancel{12}}\text{ gtt/mL} = \dfrac{120}{5} = 24$ gtt/min

Proportion	Formula
4.	$\dfrac{\overset{50}{\cancel{500}}\text{ mL}}{\underset{24}{\cancel{240}}\text{ min}} \times 15\text{ gtt/mL} = \dfrac{750}{24}$ $= 31.2$ rounded to 31 gtt/min
5.	$\dfrac{1500\text{ mL}}{8\text{ h}} = 187.5$ or 188 mL/h
6.	$\dfrac{250\text{ mL}}{\underset{15}{\cancel{180}}\text{ min}} \times \overset{1}{\cancel{12}}\text{ gtt/mL} = \dfrac{250}{15}$ $= 16.6$ rounded to 17 gtt/min
7.	$\dfrac{1000\text{ mL}}{\underset{48}{\cancel{720}}\text{ min}} \times \overset{1}{\cancel{15}}\text{ gtt/mL} = \dfrac{1000}{48}$ $= 20.8$ rounded to 21 gtt/min
8. $2\text{ g} : 50\text{ mL} :: 1\text{ g} : x\text{ mL}$ $2x = 50$ $x = \dfrac{50}{2}$ $x = 25$ mL/h	$\dfrac{1\text{ g}}{2\text{ g}} \times 50\text{ mL} =$ $\dfrac{50}{2} = 25$ mL/h
9.	$\dfrac{150\text{ mL}}{\underset{1}{\cancel{60}}\text{ min}} \times \overset{1}{\cancel{60}}\text{ gtt/mL} = \dfrac{150}{1} = 150$ gtt/min
10.	$\dfrac{2500\text{ mL}}{24\text{ h}} = 104.1$ or 104 mL/h
11. $30\text{ mOsm} : 200\text{ mL} :: 10\text{ mOsm} : x\text{ mL}$ $30x = 2000$ $x = \dfrac{2000}{30}$ $x = 66.7$ or 67 mL/h	$\dfrac{\overset{1}{\cancel{10}}\text{ mOsm}}{\underset{3}{\cancel{30}}\text{ mOsm}} \times 200\text{ mL} =$ $\dfrac{200}{3} = 66.7$ or 67 mL/h
12.	$\dfrac{25\text{ mL}}{\underset{1}{\cancel{15}}\text{ min}} \times \overset{4}{\cancel{60}}\text{ gtt/mL} = \dfrac{25}{1} \times 4 = 100$ gtt/min
13. $100\text{ mg} : 200\text{ mL} :: 15\text{ mg} : x\text{ mL}$ $100x = 3000$ $x = \dfrac{3000}{100}$ $x = 30$ mL/h	$\dfrac{15\text{ mg}}{\underset{1}{\cancel{100}}\text{ mg}} \times \overset{2}{\cancel{200}}\text{ mL} =$ $\dfrac{15}{1} \times 2 = 30$ mL/h
14.	$\dfrac{100\text{ mL}}{0.5\text{ h}} = 200$ mL/h
15.	$\dfrac{100\text{ mL}}{\underset{1}{\cancel{60}}\text{ min}} \times \overset{1}{\cancel{60}}\text{ gtt/mL} = 100$ gtt/min

CHAPTER 15 Proportion/Formula Method—Posttest 2, pp. 461–464

Proportion	Formula
1.	$\frac{200 \text{ mL}}{6 \text{ h}} = 33.3 \text{ or } 33 \text{ mL/h}$
2.	$\frac{250 \text{ mL}}{\cancel{60}\,6 \text{ min}} \times \cancel{10}\,1 \text{ gtt/mL} = \frac{250}{6}$ $= 41.6$ rounded to 42 gtt/min
3.	$\frac{200 \text{ mL}}{6 \text{ h}} = 33.3 \text{ or } 33 \text{ mL/h}$
4.	$\frac{500 \text{ mL}}{\cancel{180}\,12 \text{ min}} \times \cancel{15}\,1 \text{ gtt/mL} = \frac{500}{12}$ $= 41.6$ rounded to 42 gtt/min
5.	$\frac{1000 \text{ mL}}{\cancel{360}\,36 \text{ min}} \times \cancel{10}\,1 \text{ gtt/mL} = \frac{1000}{36}$ $= 27.7$ rounded to 28 gtt/min
6.	$\frac{50 \text{ mL}}{0.5 \text{ h}} = 100 \text{ mL/h}$
7. $100 \text{ mg} : 100 \text{ mL} :: 8 \text{ mg} : x$ $100x = 800$ $x = \frac{800}{100}$ $x = 8 \text{ mL/h}$	$\frac{8 \text{ mg}}{\cancel{100}\,1 \text{ mg}} \times \cancel{100}\,1 \text{ mL} =$ $\frac{8}{1} = 8 \text{ mL/h}$
8.	$\frac{50 \text{ mL}}{\cancel{15}\,1 \text{ min}} \times \cancel{60}\,4 \text{ gtt/mL} = \frac{200}{1} = 200 \text{ gtt/min}$
9.	$\frac{50 \text{ mL}}{\cancel{15}\,1 \text{ min}} \times \cancel{15}\,1 \text{ gtt/mL} = \frac{50}{1} = 50 \text{ gtt/min}$
10.	$\frac{1000 \text{ mL}}{6 \text{ h}} = 166.7 \text{ or } 167 \text{ mL/h}$
11. $8 \text{ mg} : 100 \text{ mL} :: 0.4 \text{ mg} : x \text{ mL}$ $8x = 40$ $x = \frac{40}{8}$ $x = 5 \text{ mL/h}$	$\frac{0.4 \text{ mg}}{\cancel{8}\,2 \text{ mg}} \times \cancel{100}\,25 \text{ mL} =$ $\frac{10}{2} = 5 \text{ mL/h}$
12.	$\frac{1200 \text{ mL}}{8 \text{ h}} = 150 \text{ mL/h}$
13.	$\frac{200 \text{ mL}}{1.5 \text{ h}} = 133.3 \text{ or } 133 \text{ mL/h}$

Proportion	Formula
14.	$\frac{1000 \text{ mL}}{\cancel{180}_{18} \text{ min}} \times \cancel{10}^{1} \text{ gtt/mL} = \frac{1000}{18}$ $= 55.5$ rounded to 56 gtt/min
15.	$\frac{500 \text{ mL}}{6 \text{ h}} = 83.3$ or 83 mL/h

CHAPTER 16

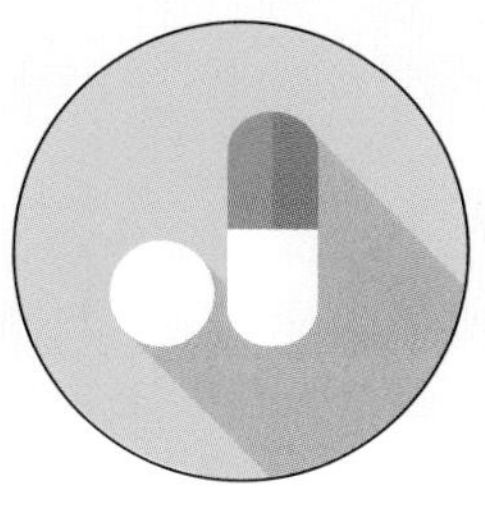

Intravenous Flow Rates for Dosages Measured in Units

LEARNING OBJECTIVES

Upon completion of the materials provided in this chapter, you will be able to perform computations accurately by mastering the following mathematical concepts:

1. Calculating the IV flow rate of medications in units per hour or international units per hour
2. Calculating the units per hour of medications from the IV flow rate
3. Calculating the IV flow rate of medications in units per kilogram per hour (weight-based heparin)

Some intravenous (IV) medications are ordered by units per hour, international units per hour, or units per kilogram per hour. IV heparin and IV insulin are among the medications ordered in this way. Medications ordered in this manner must be delivered with an IV controller or pump for safe administration. Because infusion pumps are set by milliliters per hour (mL/h), the health care provider needs to be familiar with the steps to convert the ordered drug dosage to milliliters per hour.

Calculating Milliliters/Hour from Units/Hour—Dimensional Analysis Method

EXAMPLE 1: A patient has an order for regular insulin IV at a rate of 5 units/h. The concentration is insulin 100 units/100 mL 0.9% NS. At what rate, in milliliters per hour, should the IV pump be programmed?

Step 1 On the left side of the equation, place what you are solving for.

$$x\ \frac{\text{mL}}{\text{h}} =$$

Step 2 Deal with the numerator portion of the answer first, the mL. We know that 100 units of insulin are diluted in the 100 mL. This information is placed in the equation as a fraction, with the numerator matching.

$$x\ \frac{\text{mL}}{\text{h}} = \frac{100\ \text{mL}}{100\ \text{units}}$$

Step 3 Next, find the information that matches the measurement used in the denominator *units*. The order is for 5 units/h. The equation now looks like

$$x\ \frac{\text{mL}}{\text{h}} = \frac{100\ \text{mL}}{100\ \textbf{units}} \times \frac{5\ \textbf{units}}{1\ \text{h}}$$

Step 4. Cancel the like abbreviations on the right side of the equation. Now solve for x.

$$\frac{x \text{ mL}}{\text{h}} = \frac{100 \text{ mL}}{100 \cancel{\text{units}}} \times \frac{5 \cancel{\text{units}}}{1 \text{ h}}$$

$$x = \frac{5 \text{ mL}}{100 \text{ h}}$$

$$x = 5 \text{ mL/h}$$

ALERT

Medications ordered by units per hour, international units per hour, or units per kilogram per hour must be delivered with an IV controller or pump for safe administration.

Therefore the nurse will program the IV pump for 5 mL/h, and the insulin will be infused at a rate of 5 units/h.

EXAMPLE 2: A patient with a femoral thrombus has an order for heparin IV at 1200 units/h. The concentration is heparin 20,000 units in 250 mL of D_5W. At what rate, in milliliters per hour, should the IV pump be programmed?

Step 1. On the left side of the equation, place what you are solving for.

$$\frac{x \text{ mL}}{\text{h}} =$$

Step 2. Deal with the numerator portion of the answer first, the mL. We know there are 20,000 units of heparin in 250 mL. This information is placed in the equation as a fraction, with the numerators matching.

$$\frac{x \text{ mL}}{\text{h}} = \frac{250 \text{ mL}}{20{,}000 \text{ units}}$$

Step 3. Next, find the information that matches the measurement used in the denominator *units*. The order is for 1200 units/h. The equation now looks like

$$\frac{x \text{ mL}}{\text{h}} = \frac{250 \text{ mL}}{20{,}000 \textbf{ units}} \times \frac{1200 \textbf{ units}}{1 \text{ h}}$$

Step 4. Cancel the like abbreviations on the right side of the equation. Now solve for x.

$$\frac{x \text{ mL}}{\text{h}} = \frac{250 \text{ mL}}{20{,}000 \cancel{\text{units}}} \times \frac{1200 \cancel{\text{units}}}{1 \text{ h}}$$

$$x = \frac{250 \text{ mL} \times 1200}{20{,}000 \text{ h}}$$

$$x = \frac{300{,}000 \text{ mL}}{20{,}000 \text{ h}}$$

$$x = 15 \text{ mL/h}$$

Therefore the nurse will program the IV pump for 15 mL/h, and the heparin will be infused at a rate of 1200 units/h.

Calculating Units/Hours from Milliliters/Hour—Dimensional Analysis Method

EXAMPLE 1: A patient has a continuous insulin infusion at 8 mL/h. The insulin concentration is regular insulin 100 units in 200 mL of 0.9% NS. The nurse needs to calculate how many units per hour of insulin the patient is receiving.

Step 1. On the left side of the equation, place what you are solving for:

$$\frac{x \text{ units}}{\text{h}} =$$

Step 2. Deal with the numerator portion of the answer first, the *units*. We know there are 100 units of regular insulin in 200 mL of 0.9% NS. This information is placed in the equation as a fraction, with the numerators matching.

$$\frac{x \textbf{ units}}{\text{h}} = \frac{100 \textbf{ units}}{200 \text{ mL}}$$

Step 3. Next, find the information that matches the measurement used in the denominator, *mL*. The equation now looks like

$$\frac{x \text{ units}}{\text{h}} = \frac{100 \text{ units}}{200 \textbf{ mL}} \times \frac{8 \textbf{ mL}}{\text{h}}$$

Step 4. Cancel the like abbreviations on the right side of the equation. Now solve for x.

$$\frac{x \text{ units}}{\text{h}} = \frac{100 \text{ units}}{200 \cancel{\text{mL}}} \times \frac{8 \cancel{\text{mL}}}{\text{h}}$$

$$\frac{x \text{ units}}{\text{h}} = \frac{100 \times 8}{200}$$

$$x = 4 \text{ units/h}$$

Therefore the patient is receiving 4 units/h of regular insulin.

EXAMPLE 2: A patient has a continuous heparin infusion at 14 mL/h. The heparin concentration is heparin 25,000 units/250 mL of 0.9% NS. The nurse needs to calculate how many units per hour of heparin the patient is receiving.

Step 1. On the left side of the equation, place what you are solving for:

$$\frac{x \text{ units}}{\text{h}} =$$

Step 2. Deal with the numerator portion of the answer first, the *units*. We know there are 25,000 units of heparin in 250 mL of 0.9% NS. This information is placed in the equation as a fraction, with the numerators matching.

$$\frac{x \textbf{ units}}{\text{h}} = \frac{25{,}000 \textbf{ units}}{250 \text{ mL}}$$

Step 3. Next, find the information that matches the measurement used in the denominator, *mL*. The equation now looks like

$$\frac{x \text{ units}}{\text{h}} = \frac{25{,}000 \text{ units}}{250 \textbf{ mL}} \times \frac{14 \textbf{ mL}}{\text{h}}$$

Step 4. Cancel out the like abbreviations on the right side of the equation. Now solve for x.

$$\frac{x \text{ units}}{\text{h}} = \frac{25{,}000 \text{ units}}{250 \cancel{\text{mL}}} \times \frac{14 \cancel{\text{mL}}}{\text{h}}$$

$$\frac{x \text{ units}}{\text{h}} = \frac{25{,}000 \times 14}{250}$$

$$x = 1400 \text{ units/h}$$

Therefore the patient is receiving heparin at 1400 units/h.

Calculating Weight-Based Heparin—Dimensional Analysis Method

EXAMPLE 1: The order is to start a heparin infusion using the heparin protocol. The patient's weight is 143 lb. Using the weight-based heparin protocol example below, the nurse needs to do two calculations: the heparin bolus and the rate, in milliliters per hour, at which to program the IV pump.

WEIGHT-BASED HEPARIN PROTOCOL (EXAMPLE)

1. Bolus dose of 70 units/kg, rounded to the nearest 100 units (e.g., 6850 units would be rounded to 6900 units).
2. Begin infusion of heparin at 17 units/kg/h (25,000 units/250 mL = 100 units/mL).
3. Obtain partial thromboplastin time (PTT) every 6 hours, and adjust the infusion using the following scale:

PTT Result	Heparin Dosing
<35	Bolus 70 units/kg and increase drip by 4 units/kg/h
35–54	Bolus 35 units/kg and increase drip by 3 units/kg/h
55–85	Therapeutic—no change
86–100	Decrease drip by 2 units/kg/h
>100	Hold infusion 1 hour; decrease drip by 3 units/kg/h, then restart drip

Bolus. The protocol calls for 70 units/kg, rounded to the nearest hundreds place.

Step 1. On the left side of the equation, place what you are solving for.

$$x \text{ units} =$$

Step 2. Deal with the numerator portion of the answer first, the *units*. We know from the protocol that 70 units/kg is needed; this information is placed in the equation, with the numerators matching.

$$x \textbf{ units} = \frac{70 \textbf{ units}}{1 \text{ kg}}$$

Step 3. Next, find the information that matches the measurement used in the denominator, *kg*. The conversion of 1 kg = 2.2 lb is used as the next fraction. The equation now looks like

$$x \text{ units} = \frac{70 \text{ units}}{\textbf{kg}} \times \frac{1 \textbf{ kg}}{2.2 \text{ lb}}$$

Step 4. Next, the *lb* in the denominator must be canceled out. We know from the problem that the patient weighs 143 lb.

$$x \text{ units} = \frac{70 \text{ units}}{1 \text{ kg}} \times \frac{1 \text{ kg}}{2.2 \textbf{ lb}} \times \frac{143 \textbf{ lb}}{1}$$

Step 5. Cancel the like abbreviations on the right side of the equation. Now solve for x.

$$x \text{ units} = \frac{70 \text{ units}}{\cancel{\text{kg}}} \times \frac{1 \cancel{\text{kg}}}{2.2 \cancel{\text{lb}}} \times \frac{143 \cancel{\text{lb}}}{1}$$

$$x \text{ units} = \frac{70 \times 143}{2.2}$$

$$x \text{ units} = \frac{10{,}010}{2.2}$$

$$x = 4550 \text{ or } 4600 \text{ units IV bolus}$$

IV Infusion. The health care provider needs to calculate how many milliliters are needed to deliver 17 units/kg (protocol states 17 units/kg/h, rounded to the nearest tenth).

Step 1. On the left side of the equation, place what you are solving for.

$$x \frac{\text{mL}}{\text{h}} =$$

Step 2. Deal with the numerator portion of the answer first, *mL*. We know from the protocol that there are 100 units of heparin in 1 mL. This information is placed in the equation with the numerators matching.

$$x \frac{\text{mL}}{\text{h}} = \frac{1 \text{ mL}}{100 \text{ units}}$$

Step 3. Next, find the information that matches the measurement used in the denominator, ***units***. The order is for 17 units/kg/h. The equation now looks like

$$x \frac{\text{mL}}{\text{h}} = \frac{1 \text{ mL}}{100 \textbf{ units}} \times \frac{17 \textbf{ units}}{\text{kg/h}}$$

Step 4. Now, the kg is the denominator that needs to be canceled. The conversion of 1 kg = 2.2 lb is used as the next fraction. Continue this process until all the denominators can be canceled.

$$x \frac{\text{mL}}{\text{h}} = \frac{1 \text{ mL}}{100 \text{ units}} \times \frac{17 \text{ units}}{\textbf{kg/h}} \times \frac{1 \textbf{ kg}}{2.2 \textbf{ lb}} \times \frac{143 \textbf{ lb}}{1}$$

Step 5. Cancel the like abbreviations on the right side of the equation. Now solve for x.

$$x\ \frac{\text{mL}}{\text{h}} = \frac{1\ \text{mL}}{100\ \cancel{\text{units}}} \times \frac{17\ \cancel{\text{units}}}{\cancel{\text{kg}}/\text{h}} \times \frac{1\ \cancel{\text{kg}}}{2.2\ \cancel{\text{lb}}} \times \frac{143\ \cancel{\text{lb}}}{1}$$

$$x\ \frac{\text{mL}}{\text{h}} = \frac{17 \times 143}{100 \times 2.2}$$

$$x\ \frac{\text{mL}}{\text{h}} = \frac{2431}{220}$$

$$x = 11.1 \text{ or } 11\ \text{mL/h}$$

Therefore the nurse will program the IV pump for 11.1 mL/h, and the heparin will be infused at a rate of 17 units/kg/h.

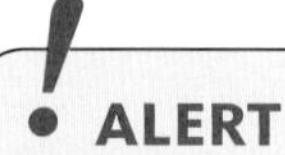

ALERT

An IV controller is required for medications that are titrated.

Facilities that administer high-risk medications have IV controllers that allow the health care professional to program medication rates with a decimal. Therefore answers should be **rounded to the nearest tenth decimal place unless otherwise directed.**

Calculating Milliliters/Hour from Units/Hour—Ratio-Proportion and Formula Methods

EXAMPLE 1: 200 units of regular insulin have been added to 500 mL of 0.9% normal saline (NS). The order states to infuse the regular insulin IV at 10 units/h. The nurse needs to calculate how many milliliters per hour the IV pump should be programmed for.

Using the Ratio-Proportion Method

(Formula setup) 200 units : 500 mL :: 10 units : x mL

$$200x = 5000$$

$$x = \frac{5000}{200}$$

$$x = 25\ \text{mL}$$

Therefore the nurse will program the IV pump for 25 mL/h to infuse the insulin at 10 units/h.

Using the $\frac{D}{A} \times Q$ Method

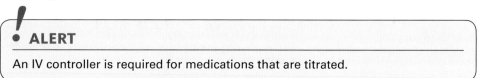

(Formula setup) $$\frac{10\ \text{units}}{200\ \text{units}} \times 500\ \text{mL} = x\ \text{mL}$$

(Cancel) $$\frac{10\ \cancel{\text{units}}}{\underset{2}{\cancel{200}}\ \cancel{\text{units}}} \times \overset{5}{\cancel{500}}\ \text{mL} = x\ \text{mL}$$

(Calculate) $$\frac{50}{2} = 25\ \text{mL}$$

EXAMPLE 2: 25,000 units of heparin have been added to 250 mL of dextrose 5% in water (D_5W). The order is to infuse the heparin drip at 2000 units/h. The health care provider needs to calculate how many milliliters per hour to program the IV pump for.

Using the Ratio-Proportion Method

(Formula setup) 25,000 units : 250 mL :: 2000 units : x mL

$$25{,}000x = 500{,}000$$

$$x = \frac{500{,}\cancel{000}}{25{,}\cancel{000}}$$

$$x = \frac{500}{25}$$

$$x = 20 \text{ mL}$$

Therefore the nurse will program the IV pump for 20 mL/h to deliver the heparin at 2000 units/h.

Using the $\frac{D}{A} \times Q$ Method

(Formula setup) $$\frac{2000 \text{ units}}{25{,}000 \text{ units}} \times 250 \text{ mL} = x \text{ mL}$$

(Cancel) $$\frac{2000 \cancel{\text{units}}}{\underset{100}{\cancel{25{,}000}} \cancel{\text{units}}} \times \overset{1}{\cancel{250}} \text{ mL} = x \text{ mL}$$

(Calculate) $$\frac{2000 \text{ mL}}{100} = 20 \text{ mL}$$

Calculating Units/Hour from Milliliter/Hour—Ratio-Proportion and Formula Methods

EXAMPLE 1: A patient has a continuous insulin drip infusing at 8 mL/h. The insulin concentration is regular insulin 100 units in 200 mL of 0.9% NS. The nurse needs to calculate how many units per hour of insulin the patient is receiving.

Using the Ratio-Proportion Method

(Formula setup) 100 units : 200 mL :: x units : 8 mL

$$200x = 800$$

$$x = \frac{800}{200}$$

$$x = 4 \text{ units}$$

Therefore the patient is receiving 4 units/h of regular insulin.

EXAMPLE 2: A patient has a continuous heparin drip infusing at 14 mL/h. The heparin concentration is heparin 25,000 units/250 mL of 0.9% NS. The nurse needs to calculate how many units per hour of heparin the patient is receiving.

Using the Ratio-Proportion Method

$$\text{(Formula setup)}\quad 25{,}000 \text{ units} : 250 \text{ mL} :: x \text{ units} : 14 \text{ mL}$$

$$250x = 350{,}000$$

$$x = \frac{350{,}000}{250}$$

$$x = 1400 \text{ units}$$

Therefore the patient is receiving 1400 units/h of heparin.

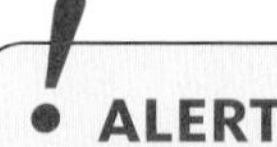

ALERT

Weight-based heparin requires 2 calculations: bolus and infusion.

Calculating Weight-Based Heparin—Ratio-Proportion and Formula Methods

WEIGHT-BASED HEPARIN PROTOCOL (EXAMPLE)

1. Bolus dose of 70 units/kg, rounded to the nearest 100 units (e.g., 6850 units would be rounded to 6900 units).
2. Begin infusion of heparin at 17 units/kg/h (25,000 units/250 mL = 100 units/mL).
3. Obtain partial thromboplastin time (PTT) every 6 hours, and adjust the infusion using the following scale:

PTT Result	Heparin Dosing
<35	Bolus 70 units/kg and increase drip by 4 units/kg/h
35–54	Bolus 35 units/kg and increase drip by 3 units/kg/h
55–85	Therapeutic—no change
86–100	Decrease drip by 2 units/kg/h
>100	Hold infusion 1 hour; decrease drip by 3 units/kg/h, then restart drip

EXAMPLE: The order is to start a heparin infusion using the heparin protocol. The patient's weight is 143 lb. The nurse needs to do two calculations: the heparin bolus and the rate, in milliliters per hour, at which to program the IV pump.

Bolus. The protocol calls for 70 units/kg, rounded to the nearest hundred.

Step 1. Convert pounds to kilograms.

$$\text{(Formula setup)}\quad 2.2 \text{ lb} : 1 \text{ kg} :: 143 \text{ lb} : x \text{ kg}$$

$$2.2x = 143$$

$$x = \frac{143}{2.2}$$

$$x = 65 \text{ kg}$$

Step 2. Calculate the units required for the IV bolus.

$$\text{(Formula setup)}\quad 1 \text{ kg} : 70 \text{ units} :: 65 \text{ kg} : x \text{ units}$$

$$x = 70 \times 65$$

$$x = 4550 \text{ or } 4600 \text{ units IV bolus}$$

IV Infusion. The protocol states 17 units/kg/h, rounded to the nearest tenth.

Step 1. Calculate how many units are needed for a patient weighing 65 kg.

(Formula setup) $1 \text{ kg} : 17 \text{ units/h} :: 65 \text{ kg} : x \text{ units/h}$

$$x = 17 \times 65$$

$$x = 1105$$

The formula shows that 1105 units/h are required for a 65-kg patient.

Step 2. Calculate mL/hr for the IV pump.

Using the Ratio-Proportion Method

(Formula setup) $100 \text{ units} : 1 \text{ mL} :: 1105 \text{ units} : x \text{ mL}$

$$100x = 1105$$

$$x = \frac{1105}{100}$$

$$x = 11.1 \text{ or } 11 \text{ mL/h}$$

Therefore the nurse will set the IV pump for 11.1 mL/h to infuse the heparin at 17 units/kg/h.

Using $\frac{D}{A} \times Q$ Method

(Formula setup) $\frac{1105 \text{ units}}{100 \text{ units}} \times 1 \text{ mL} = x \text{ mL}$

(Cancel) $\frac{1105 \cancel{\text{units}}}{100 \cancel{\text{units}}} \times 1 \text{ mL} = x \text{ mL}$

(Calculate) $\frac{1105}{100} = 11.1 \text{ or } 11 \text{ mL/h}$

Complete the following work sheet, which provides for practice of intravenous flow rates for dosages measured in units. Check your answers. If you have difficulties, go back and review the necessary material. An acceptable score as indicated on the posttest signifies that you have successfully completed the chapter. An unacceptable score signifies a need for further study before taking the second posttest.

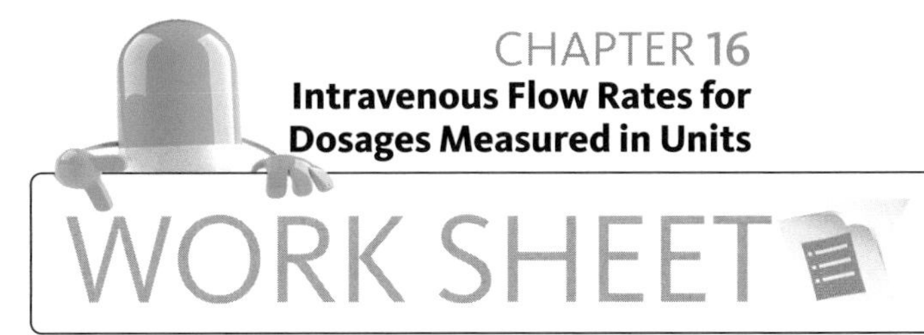

WORK SHEET

DIRECTIONS: The IV fluid order is listed in each problem. Calculate the IV flow rates using the appropriate formula required for the problem.

1. A patient has undergone aortic valve repair and has orders for heparin at 1000 units/h. The concentration is heparin 25,000 units in 250 mL of 0.9% NS. How many milliliters per hour should the IV pump be programmed for? ______

2. An order for regular insulin IV at 12 units/h is received for a patient with diabetic ketoacidosis. The concentration is insulin 100 units in 250 mL of 0.9% NS. How many milliliters per hour should the IV pump be programmed for? ______

3. The insulin order for the patient in problem 2 is reduced to 8 units/h. How many milliliters per hour should the IV pump be programmed for? ______

4. A patient who has undergone mitral valve repair has heparin ordered at 1000 units/h. The concentration is heparin 10,000 units in 500 mL of D_5W. How many milliliters per hour should the IV pump be programmed for? ______

5. A patient has a brachial thrombus and has streptokinase ordered at 100,000 international units/h. The concentration is 250,000 international units of streptokinase in 45 mL of 0.9% NS. How many milliliters per hour should the IV pump be programmed for? ______

6. A patient with deep vein thrombosis has a heparin infusion at 15 mL/h. The heparin concentration is 25,000 units in 500 mL of D_5W. How many units per hour is the patient receiving? ______

7. A patient with diabetic ketoacidosis has a continuous insulin drip at 10 mL/h. The insulin comes in a concentration of 100 units of regular insulin in 100 mL of 0.9% NS. How many units per hour is the patient receiving? ______

8. The licensed prescriber orders heparin per protocol (use protocol on p. 462). The patient's weight is 60 kg.

Bolus:

Infusion:

9. Six hours after the heparin protocol is begun (see question 8), the activated PTT (aPTT) returns at 98 seconds. Using the protocol on p. 462, does the heparin need to be changed? ______

Bolus:

Infusion:

10. The licensed prescriber orders heparin per protocol (use protocol on p. 462). The patient's weight is 80 kg. Calculate the heparin bolus and infusion.

Bolus:

Infusion:

11. Six hours after the heparin protocol is begun (see question 10), the aPTT returns at 48 seconds. Using the protocol on p. 462, does the heparin need to be changed? ______

Bolus:

Infusion:

ANSWERS ON PP. 488 AND 489–491.

CHAPTER 16
Intravenous Flow Rates for Dosages Measured in Units

NAME ______

DATE ______

ACCEPTABLE SCORE 4

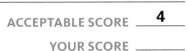

YOUR SCORE ______

POSTTEST 1

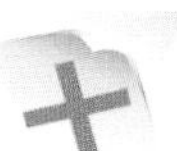

DIRECTIONS: The IV fluid order is listed in each problem. Calculate the appropriate rate for each problem.

1. A patient with diabetes has an order for regular insulin IV at 9 units/h. The concentration is insulin 500 units in 500 mL of 0.9% NS. How many milliliters per hour should the IV pump be programmed for? ______

2. A patient has a deep vein thrombosis and an order for heparin at 800 units/h. The concentration is heparin 50,000 units in 500 mL of D_5W. How many milliliters per hour should the IV pump be programmed for? ______

3. A patient with a thrombosis has a heparin infusion at 15 mL/h. The heparin concentration is 25,000 units in 250 mL of D_5W. How many units per hour is the patient receiving? ______

4. Begin heparin per protocol (use protocol example on p. 462). Patient's weight is 105 kg.

   Bolus:

   Infusion:

ANSWERS ON PP. 488 AND 491.

NAME ______________________

DATE ______________________

ACCEPTABLE SCORE 4

YOUR SCORE ______

POSTTEST 2

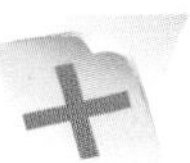

DIRECTIONS: The IV fluid order is listed in each problem. Calculate the rate needed in each problem to deliver the correct dose.

1. A patient with a pulmonary embolus has an order for streptokinase to be infused at 100,000 international units/h. The concentration is streptokinase 750,000 international units in 200 mL of 0.9% NS. How many milliliters per hour should the IV pump be programmed for? ______

2. A patient with diabetic ketoacidosis has a continuous insulin drip at 6 mL/h. The insulin comes in a concentration of 100 units of regular insulin in 200 mL of 0.9% NS. How many units per hour is the patient receiving? ______

3. A patient has a blood clot in his arm, and the licensed prescriber has ordered heparin to be infused at 1500 units/h. The concentration is heparin 20,000 units in 200 mL of D_5W. How many milliliters per hour should the IV pump be programmed for? ______

4. Begin heparin per protocol (use protocol example on p. 462). The patient's weight is 75 kg.

   Bolus:

   Infusion:

ANSWERS ON PP. 489 AND 492.

evolve For additional practice problems, refer to the Dosages Measured in Units section of *Elsevier's Interactive Drug Calculation Application*, version 1.

ANSWERS

CHAPTER 16 Dimensional Analysis—Work Sheet, pp. 483–484

1. $\frac{x\text{ mL}}{\text{h}} = \frac{250\text{ mL}}{25{,}000\text{ units}} \times \frac{1000\text{ units}}{1\text{ h}} = 10\text{ mL/h}$

2. $\frac{x\text{ mL}}{\text{h}} = \frac{250\text{ mL}}{100\text{ units}} \times \frac{12\text{ units}}{1\text{ h}} = 30\text{ mL/h}$

3. $\frac{x\text{ mL}}{\text{h}} = \frac{250\text{ mL}}{100\text{ units}} \times \frac{8\text{ units}}{1\text{ h}} = 20\text{ mL/h}$

4. $\frac{x\text{ mL}}{\text{h}} = \frac{500\text{ mL}}{10{,}000\text{ units}} \times \frac{1000\text{ units}}{1\text{ h}} = 50\text{ mL/h}$

5. $\frac{x\text{ mL}}{\text{h}} = \frac{45\text{ mL}}{250{,}000\text{ IU}} \times \frac{100{,}000\text{ IU}}{1\text{ h}} = 18\text{ mL/h}$

6. $\frac{x\text{ units}}{\text{h}} = \frac{25{,}000\text{ units}}{500\text{ mL}} \times \frac{15\text{ mL}}{1\text{ h}} = 750\text{ units/h}$

7. $\frac{x\text{ units}}{\text{h}} = \frac{100\text{ units}}{100\text{ mL}} \times \frac{10\text{ mL}}{1\text{ h}} = 10\text{ units/h}$

8. Bolus: $x\text{ units} = \frac{70\text{ units}}{1\text{ kg}} \times 60\text{ kg} = 4200\text{ units}$

   Infusion: $\frac{x\text{ mL}}{\text{h}} = \frac{1\text{ mL}}{100\text{ units}} \times \frac{17\text{ units}}{1\text{ kg/h}} \times \frac{60\text{ kg}}{1} = 10.2\text{ or }10\text{ mL/h}$

9. Yes, the heparin drip needs to be reduced by 2 units/kg/h.
   Bolus: No bolus is needed.

   Infusion: $\frac{x\text{ mL}}{\text{h}} = \frac{1\text{ mL}}{100\text{ units}} \times \frac{15\text{ units}}{1\text{ kg/h}} \times \frac{60\text{ kg}}{1} = 9\text{ mL/h}$

10. Bolus: $x\text{ units} = \frac{70\text{ units}}{1\text{ kg}} \times 80\text{ kg} = 5600\text{ units}$

    Infusion: $\frac{x\text{ mL}}{\text{h}} = \frac{1\text{ mL}}{100\text{ units}} \times \frac{17\text{ units}}{1\text{ kg/h}} \times \frac{80\text{ kg}}{1} = 13.6\text{ or }14\text{ mL/h}$

11. Yes, provide a bolus of 35 units/kg and increase the heparin drip by 3 units/kg/h.

    Bolus: $x\text{ units} = \frac{35\text{ units}}{1\text{ kg}} \times 80\text{ kg} = 2800\text{ units}$

    Infusion: $\frac{x\text{ mL}}{\text{h}} = \frac{1\text{ mL}}{100\text{ units}} \times \frac{20\text{ units}}{1\text{ kg/h}} \times \frac{80\text{ kg}}{1} = 16\text{ mL/h}$

CHAPTER 16 Dimensional Analysis—Posttest 1, p. 485

1. $\frac{x\text{ mL}}{\text{h}} = \frac{500\text{ mL}}{500\text{ units}} \times \frac{9\text{ units}}{1\text{ h}} = 9\text{ mL/h}$

2. $\frac{x\text{ mL}}{\text{h}} = \frac{500\text{ mL}}{50{,}000\text{ units}} \times \frac{800\text{ units}}{1\text{ h}} = 8\text{ mL/h}$

3. $\frac{x\text{ units}}{\text{h}} = \frac{25{,}000\text{ units}}{250\text{ mL}} \times \frac{15\text{ mL}}{1\text{ h}} = 1500\text{ units/h}$

4. Bolus: $x\text{ units} = \frac{70\text{ units}}{1\text{ kg}} \times 105\text{ kg} = 7350\text{ or }7400\text{ units}$

   Infusion: $\frac{x\text{ mL}}{\text{h}} = \frac{1\text{ mL}}{100\text{ units}} \times \frac{17\text{ units}}{1\text{ kg/h}} \times \frac{105\text{ kg}}{1} = 17.9\text{ or }18\text{ mL/h}$

CHAPTER 16 Dimensional Analysis—Posttest 2, p. 487

1. $\dfrac{x \text{ mL}}{\text{h}} = \dfrac{200 \text{ mL}}{750{,}000 \text{ units}} \times \dfrac{100{,}000 \text{ units}}{1 \text{ h}} = 26.7 \text{ or } 27 \text{ mL/h}$

2. $\dfrac{x \text{ units}}{\text{h}} = \dfrac{100 \text{ units}}{200 \text{ mL}} \times \dfrac{6 \text{ mL}}{1 \text{ h}} = 3 \text{ units/h}$

3. $\dfrac{x \text{ mL}}{\text{h}} = \dfrac{200 \text{ mL}}{20{,}000 \text{ units}} \times \dfrac{1500 \text{ units}}{1 \text{ h}} = 15 \text{ mL/h}$

4. Bolus: $x \text{ units} = \dfrac{70 \text{ units}}{1 \text{ kg}} \times \dfrac{75 \text{ kg}}{1} = 5250 \text{ or } 5300 \text{ units}$

   Infusion: $\dfrac{x \text{ mL}}{\text{h}} = \dfrac{1 \text{ mL}}{100 \text{ units}} \times \dfrac{17 \text{ units}}{1 \text{ kg/h}} \times \dfrac{75 \text{ kg}}{1} = 12.8 \text{ or } 13 \text{ mL/h}$

CHAPTER 16 Proportion/Formula Method—Work Sheet, pp. 483–484

Proportion

1. 25,000 units : 250 mL :: 1000 units : x mL
   $25{,}000x = 250{,}000$
   $x = \dfrac{250{,}000}{25{,}000}$
   $x = 10$ mL/h

2. 100 units : 250 mL :: 12 units : x mL
   $100x = 3000$
   $x = \dfrac{3000}{100}$
   $x = 30$ mL/h

3. 100 units : 250 mL :: 8 units : x mL
   $100x = 2000$
   $x = \dfrac{2000}{100}$
   $x = 20$ mL/h

4. 10,000 units : 500 mL :: 1000 units : x mL
   $10{,}000x = 500{,}000$
   $x = \dfrac{500{,}000}{10{,}000}$
   $x = 50$ mL/h

5. 250,000 IU : 45 mL :: 100,000 IU : x mL
   $250{,}000x = 4{,}500{,}000$
   $x = \dfrac{4{,}500{,}000}{250{,}000}$
   $x = 18$ mL/h

6. 25,000 units : 500 mL :: x units : 15 mL
   $500x = 375{,}000$
   $x = \dfrac{375{,}000}{500}$
   $x = 750$ units/h

Formula

1. $\dfrac{1000 \text{ units}}{\underset{100}{\cancel{25{,}000}} \text{ units}} \times \overset{1}{\cancel{250}} \text{ mL} =$
   $\dfrac{1000}{100} = 10 \text{ mL/h}$

2. $\dfrac{12 \text{ units}}{\underset{2}{\cancel{100}} \text{ units}} \times \overset{5}{\cancel{250}} \text{ mL} =$
   $\dfrac{60}{2} = 30 \text{ mL/h}$

3. $\dfrac{8 \text{ units}}{\underset{2}{\cancel{100}} \text{ units}} \times \overset{5}{\cancel{250}} \text{ mL} =$
   $\dfrac{40}{2} = 20 \text{ mL/h}$

4. $\dfrac{1000 \text{ units}}{\underset{20}{\cancel{10{,}000}} \text{ units}} \times \overset{1}{\cancel{500}} \text{ mL} =$
   $\dfrac{1000}{20} = 50 \text{ mL/h}$

5. $\dfrac{\overset{10}{\cancel{100{,}000}} \text{ IU}}{\underset{25}{\cancel{250{,}000}} \text{ IU}} \times 45 \text{ mL} =$
   $\dfrac{450}{25} = 18 \text{ mL/h}$

Proportion	Formula
7. 100 units : 100 mL :: x units : 10 mL $100x = 1000$ $x = \frac{1000}{100}$ $x = 10$ units/h	
8. Bolus: 1 kg : 70 units :: 60 kg : x units $x = 4200$ units IV bolus Infusion: *Step 1* 1 kg : 17 units/h :: 60 kg : x units/h $x = 17(60) = 1020$ units/h *Step 2* 100 units : 1 mL :: 1020 units : x mL $100x = 1020$ $x = \frac{1020}{100}$ $x = 10.2$ or 10 mL/h	$\frac{1020 \text{ units}}{100 \text{ units}} \times 1 \text{ mL} = 10.2$ or 10 mL/h
9. Yes, the heparin drip needs to be reduced by 2 units/kg/h. Bolus: No bolus is needed. Infusion: *Step 1* (17 units/kg/h − 2 units/kg/h = 15 units/kg/h) 1 kg : 15 units/h :: 60 kg : x units/h $x = 900$ units/h *Step 2* 100 units : 1 mL :: 900 units : x mL $100x = 900$ $x = \frac{900}{100}$ $x = 9$ mL/h	$\frac{900 \text{ units}}{100 \text{ units}} \times 1 \text{ mL} = 9$ mL/h
10. Bolus: 1 kg : 70 units :: 80 kg : x units $x = 5600$ units IV bolus Infusion: *Step 1* 1 kg : 17 units/h :: 80 kg : x units/h $x = 1360$ units/h *Step 2* 100 units : 1 mL :: 1360 units : x mL $100x = 1360$ $x = \frac{1360}{100}$ $x = 13.6$ or 14 mL/h	$\frac{1360 \text{ units}}{100 \text{ units}} \times 1 \text{ mL} = 13.6$ or 14 mL/h

Proportion | **Formula**

11. Yes, provide a bolus of 35 units/kg and increase the heparin drip by 3 units/kg/h.

Bolus: 1 kg : 35 units :: 80 kg : x units
x = 2800 units IV bolus

Infusion: *Step 1*
1 kg : 20 units/h :: 80 kg : x units/h
$x = 20(80) = 1600$ units/h

Step 2
100 units : 1 mL :: 1600 units : x mL
$100x = 1600$

$$x = \frac{1600}{100}$$

x = 16 mL/h

CHAPTER 16 Proportion/Formula Method—Posttest 1, p. 485

Proportion | **Formula**

1. 500 units : 500 mL :: 9 units : x mL
$500x = 4500$

$$x = \frac{4500}{500}$$

x = 9 mL/h

Formula:

$$\frac{9 \text{ units}}{\underset{1}{\cancel{500}} \text{ units}} \times \overset{1}{\cancel{500}} \text{ mL} =$$

$$\frac{9}{1} = 9 \text{ mL/h}$$

2. 50,000 units : 500 mL :: 800 units : x mL
$50{,}000x = 400{,}000$

$$x = \frac{400{,}000}{50{,}000}$$

x = 8 mL/h

Formula:

$$\frac{800 \text{ units}}{\underset{100}{\cancel{50{,}000}} \text{ units}} \times \overset{1}{\cancel{500}} \text{ mL} =$$

$$\frac{800}{100} = 8 \text{ mL/h}$$

3. 25,000 units : 250 mL :: x units : 15 mL
$250x = 375{,}000$

$$x = \frac{375{,}000}{250}$$

x = 1500 units/h

4. Bolus: 1 kg : 70 units :: 105 kg : x units
x = 7350 or 7400 units IV bolus

Infusion: *Step 1*
1 kg : 17 units/h :: 105 kg : x units/h
x = 1785 units/h

Step 2
100 units : 1 mL :: 1785 units : x mL
$100x = 1785$

$$x = \frac{1785}{100}$$

x = 17.9 or 18 mL/h

Formula:

$$\frac{1785 \text{ units}}{100 \text{ units}} \times 1 \text{ mL} = 17.9 \text{ or } 18 \text{ mL/h}$$

CHAPTER 16 Proportion/Formula Method—Posttest 2, p. 487

Proportion	Formula
1. 750,000 IU : 200 mL :: 100,000 IU : x mL $750{,}000x = 20{,}000{,}000$ $x = \dfrac{20{,}000{,}000}{750{,}000}$ $x = 26.7$ or 27 mL/h	$\dfrac{\overset{10}{\cancel{100{,}000}}\ \text{IU}}{\underset{75}{\cancel{750{,}000}}\ \text{IU}} \times 200\ \text{mL} =$ $\dfrac{2000}{75} = 26.7$ or 27 mL/h
2. 100 units : 200 mL :: x units : 6 mL $200x = 600$ $x = \dfrac{600}{200}$ $x = 3$ units/h	
3. 20,000 units : 200 mL :: 1500 units : x mL $20{,}000x = 300{,}000$ $x = \dfrac{300{,}000}{20{,}000}$ $x = 15$ mL/h	$\dfrac{1500\ \text{units}}{\underset{100}{\cancel{20{,}000}}\ \text{units}} \times \overset{1}{\cancel{200}}\ \text{mL} =$ $\dfrac{1500}{100} = 15$ mL/h
4. Bolus: 1 kg : 70 units :: 75 kg : x units $x = 5250$ or 5300 units IV bolus	
Infusion: *Step 1* 1 kg : 17 units/h :: 75 kg : x units/h $x = 1275$ units/h	
Step 2 100 units : 1 mL :: 1275 units : x mL $100x = 1275$ $x = \dfrac{1275}{100}$ $x = 12.8$ or 13 mL/h	$\dfrac{1275\ \text{units}}{100\ \text{units}} \times 1\ \text{mL} = 12.8$ or 13 mL/h

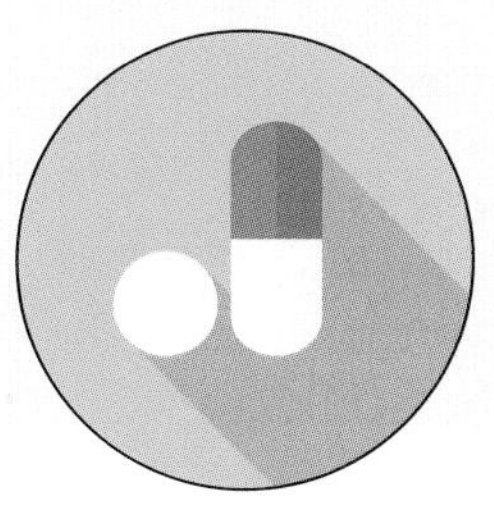

Critical Care Intravenous Flow Rates

LEARNING OBJECTIVES

Upon completion of the materials provided in this chapter, you will be able to perform computations accurately by mastering the following mathematical concepts:

1. Calculating the IV flow rate of medications in milligrams per minute
2. Calculating the IV flow rate of medications in micrograms per minute
3. Calculating the IV flow rate of medications in micrograms per kilogram per minute
4. Calculating the milligrams per minute of medications from the IV flow rate
5. Calculating the micrograms per minute of medications from the IV flow rate
6. Calculating the micrograms per kilogram per minute of medications from the IV flow rate

Critically ill patients in a hospital often receive special medications that are very potent and therefore need to be monitored closely. Some of these medications, such as regular insulin or heparin, may be ordered as a set amount of the drug measured in units to be infused over a given period. Other drugs used in the critical care setting may be ordered to be infused by amount of drug per kilogram of body weight per minute. These are called **titrations.** They are based on the manufacturer's provided recommended dosage and the patient's body weight measured in kilograms. In most health care institutions, these situations will occur in the emergency department, an intensive care unit, or a step-down unit. It is extremely important to accurately monitor the flow of these medications; therefore an intravenous (IV) machine is required. Because of the nature of these drugs, route of administration, and state of the patient, the importance of accuracy in calculating the drug dosage and IV flow rates cannot be overemphasized. It is truly a matter of life and death.

The following sections focus on medications that are ordered by micrograms per kilogram per minute (mcg/kg/min), micrograms per minute (mcg/min), and milligrams per minute (mg/min). All the following medications *must* be delivered with an IV controller or pump for safe administration. Because infusion pumps are set by milliliters per hour (mL/h), the health care provider needs to be familiar with the steps to convert the ordered drug dosage to milliliters per hour.

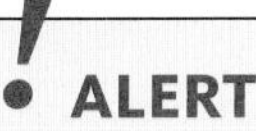

ALERT

An IV controller is required for medications that are titrated.

Facilities that administer medications with a hemodynamic effect usually have IV controllers that allow the health care professional to program medication rates with a decimal. Therefore answers should be **rounded to the nearest tenth decimal place.**

Calculating Milliliters/Hour from Milligrams/Minute—Dimensional Analysis Method

EXAMPLE: Lidocaine 1 g has been added to 500 mL of D_5W. The order states to infuse the lidocaine at 2 mg/min for a patient with ventricular tachycardia. The nurse needs to calculate the rate, in milliliters per hour, at which the IV pump should be set (rounded to the nearest tenth).

Step 1. On the left side of the equation, place what you are solving for.

$$\frac{x \text{ mL}}{\text{h}} =$$

Step 2. Deal with the numerator portion of the answer first, *mL*. We know there is 1 g of lidocaine in 500 mL of D_5W. This information is placed in the equation as a fraction with the numerators matching.

$$\frac{x \text{ mL}}{\text{h}} = \frac{500 \text{ mL}}{1 \text{ g}}$$

Step 3. Next, find the information that matches the measurement used in the denominator, *g*. The conversion of 1 g = 1000 mg is used. The equation now looks like

$$\frac{x \text{ mL}}{\text{h}} = \frac{500 \text{ mL}}{1 \text{ g}} \times \frac{1 \text{ g}}{1000 \text{ mg}}$$

Step 4. Now, the *mg* is the denominator that needs to be canceled. The order for 2 mg/min is used as the next fraction. Continue this process until all the denominators except *hour* can be canceled.

$$\frac{x \text{ mL}}{\text{h}} = \frac{500 \text{ mL}}{1 \text{ g}} \times \frac{1 \text{ g}}{1000 \textbf{ mg}} \times \frac{2 \textbf{ mg}}{1 \textbf{ min}} \times \frac{60 \textbf{ min}}{1 \text{ h}}$$

Step 5. Cancel the like abbreviations on the right side of the equation. Now solve for x.

$$\frac{x \text{ mL}}{\text{h}} = \frac{500 \text{ mL}}{1 \cancel{\text{g}}} \times \frac{1 \cancel{\text{g}}}{1000 \cancel{\text{mg}}} \times \frac{2 \cancel{\text{mg}}}{1 \cancel{\text{min}}} \times \frac{60 \cancel{\text{min}}}{1 \text{ h}}$$

$$\frac{x \text{ mL}}{\text{h}} = \frac{500 \times 2 \times 60}{1000}$$

$$\frac{x \text{ mL}}{\text{h}} = \frac{60{,}000}{1000}$$

$$x = 60 \text{ mL/h}$$

Therefore the nurse will program the IV pump for 60 mL/h, and the lidocaine will be infused at a rate of 2 mg/min.

Calculating Milliliters/Hour from Micrograms/Minute—Dimensional Analysis Method

EXAMPLE: The order is to infuse nitroglycerin at 5 mcg/min for a patient with chest pain; 50 mg of nitroglycerin has been added to 500 mL of 0.9% NS. The nurse needs to calculate the rate, in milliliters per hour, at which to set the IV pump.

Step 1. On the left side of the equation, place what you are solving for.

$$\frac{x \text{ mL}}{\text{h}} =$$

Step 2. Deal with the numerator portion of the answer first, *mL*. We know there are 50 mg of nitroglycerin in 500 mL of 0.9% NS. This information is placed in the equation as a fraction with the numerators matching.

$$\frac{x \text{ mL}}{\text{h}} = \frac{500 \text{ mL}}{50 \text{ mg}}$$

Step 3. Next, find the information that matches the measurement used in the denominator, *mg*. The conversion of 1 mg = 1000 mcg is used. The equation now looks like

$$\frac{x \text{ mL}}{\text{h}} = \frac{500 \text{ mL}}{50 \textbf{ mg}} \times \frac{1 \textbf{ mg}}{1000 \text{ mcg}}$$

Step 4. Now, *mcg* is the denominator that needs to be canceled. The order for 5 mcg/min is used as the next fraction. Continue this process until all the denominators except *hour* can be canceled.

$$\frac{x \text{ mL}}{\text{h}} = \frac{500 \text{ mL}}{50 \text{ mg}} \times \frac{1 \text{ mg}}{1000 \textbf{ mcg}} \times \frac{5 \textbf{ mcg}}{1 \textbf{ min}} \times \frac{60 \textbf{ min}}{1 \text{ h}}$$

Step 5. Cancel the like abbreviations on the right side of the equation. Now solve for x.

$$\frac{x \text{ mL}}{\text{h}} = \frac{500 \text{ mL}}{50 \cancel{\text{mg}}} \times \frac{1 \cancel{\text{mg}}}{1000 \cancel{\text{mcg}}} \times \frac{5 \cancel{\text{mcg}}}{1 \cancel{\text{min}}} \times \frac{60 \cancel{\text{min}}}{1 \text{ h}}$$

$$\frac{x \text{ mL}}{\text{h}} = \frac{500 \times 5 \times 60}{50 \times 1000}$$

$$\frac{x \text{ mL}}{\text{h}} = \frac{150{,}000}{50{,}000}$$

$$x = 3 \text{ mL/h}$$

Therefore the nurse will program the IV pump for 3 mL/h, and the nitroglycerin will be infused at a rate of 5 mcg/min.

Calculating Milliliters/Hour from Micrograms/Kilogram/Minute—Dimensional Analysis Method

EXAMPLE: The order is to begin a dopamine infusion at 3 mcg/kg/min for a patient with hypotension; 800 mg of dopamine is added to 250 mL of 0.9% NS. The patient's weight is 70 kg. The nurse needs to calculate the rate, in milliliters per hour, at which to set the IV pump.

Step 1. On the left side of the equation, place what you are solving for.

$$\frac{x \text{ mL}}{\text{h}} =$$

Step 2. Deal with the numerator portion of the answer first, *mL*. We know there are 800 mg of dopamine in 250 mL of 0.9% NS. This information is placed in the equation as a fraction with the numerators matching.

$$\frac{x \text{ mL}}{\text{h}} = \frac{250 \text{ mL}}{800 \text{ mg}}$$

Step 3. Next, find the information that matches the measurement used in the denominator, *mg*. The conversion of 1 mg = 1000 mcg is used. The equation now looks like

$$\frac{x \text{ mL}}{\text{h}} = \frac{250 \text{ mL}}{800 \textbf{ mg}} \times \frac{1 \textbf{ mg}}{1000 \text{ mcg}}$$

Step 4. Now, the mcg is the denominator that needs to be canceled. The order for 3 mcg/kg/min is used as the next fraction. Continue this process until all the denominators except *hour* can be canceled.

$$\frac{x \text{ mL}}{\text{h}} = \frac{250 \text{ mL}}{800 \text{ mg}} \times \frac{1 \text{ mg}}{1000 \textbf{ mcg}} \times \frac{3 \textbf{ mcg}}{\textbf{kg/min}} \times \frac{60 \textbf{ min}}{1 \text{ h}} \times \frac{70 \textbf{ kg}}{1}$$

Step 5. Cancel the like abbreviations on the right side of the equation. Now solve for x.

$$\frac{x \text{ mL}}{\text{h}} = \frac{250 \text{ mL}}{800 \cancel{\text{mg}}} \times \frac{1 \cancel{\text{mg}}}{1000 \cancel{\text{mcg}}} \times \frac{3 \cancel{\text{mcg}}}{\cancel{\text{kg}} \cancel{\text{min}}} \times \frac{60 \cancel{\text{min}}}{1 \text{ h}} \times \frac{70 \cancel{\text{kg}}}{1}$$

$$\frac{x \text{ mL}}{\text{h}} = \frac{250 \times 3 \times 60 \times 70}{800 \times 1000}$$

$$\frac{x \text{ mL}}{\text{h}} = \frac{3{,}150{,}000}{800{,}000}$$

$$x = 3.9 \text{ or } 4 \text{ mL/h}$$

Therefore the nurse will program the IV pump for 3.9 mL/h, and the dopamine will be infused at a rate of 3 mcg/kg/min.

Calculations for critical care medications do not stop with taking an order and calculating milliliters per hour. A nurse may receive in report, "Mr. Douglas is receiving dopamine at 15 mL/h, which is 10 mcg/kg/min." Because the nurse administering the medication during the upcoming shift is the final link in safety, this nurse needs to be able to take the milliliters per hour and calculate the exact dose of dopamine the patient is receiving. This situation also can be applied to medications that are ordered in milligrams per minute and micrograms per minute.

Calculating Milligrams/Minute from Milliliters/Hour—Dimensional Analysis Method

EXAMPLE: A patient is receiving lidocaine at 60 mL/h. The concentration of lidocaine is 1 g/500 mL of D_5W. The nurse needs to calculate the milligrams per minute the patient is receiving.

Step 1. On the left side of the equation, place what you are solving for:

$$\frac{x\ \text{mg}}{\text{min}} =$$

Step 2. Deal with the numerator portion of the answer first, *mg*. Milligrams are not in the problem, but grams are, so the first fraction created for the equation will be the conversion between milligrams and grams. This information is placed in the equation as a fraction with the numerators matching.

$$\frac{x\ \textbf{mg}}{\text{min}} = \frac{1000\ \textbf{mg}}{1\ \text{g}}$$

Step 3. Next, find the information that matches the measurement used in the denominator of the fraction you created. In this example, *g* is in the denominator, so 1 g of lidocaine in 500 mL D_5W is used. Continue this process until all of the denominators except *minute* can be canceled.

$$\frac{x\ \text{mg}}{\text{min}} = \frac{1000\ \text{mg}}{1\ \text{g}} \times \frac{1\ \text{g}}{500\ \textbf{mL}} \times \frac{60\ \textbf{mL}}{1\ \text{h}} \times \frac{1\ \text{h}}{60\ \text{min}}$$

Step 4. Cancel the abbreviations on the right side of the equation. Now solve for x.

$$\frac{x\ \text{mg}}{\text{min}} = \frac{1000\ \text{mg}}{1\ \cancel{\text{g}}} \times \frac{1\ \cancel{\text{g}}}{500\ \cancel{\text{mL}}} \times \frac{60\ \cancel{\text{mL}}}{1\ \cancel{\text{h}}} \times \frac{1\ \cancel{\text{h}}}{60\ \text{min}}$$

$$\frac{x\ \text{mg}}{\text{min}} = \frac{1000 \times 60}{500 \times 60}$$

$$x = 2\ \text{mg/min}$$

Therefore when the lidocaine is infusing at 60 mL/h, the patient is receiving a lidocaine dose of 2 mg/min.

Calculating Micrograms/Minute from Milliliters/Hour—Dimensional Analysis Method

EXAMPLE: A patient is receiving nitroglycerin at 3 mL/h. The concentration of nitroglycerin is 50 mg in 500 mL of 0.9% NS. The nurse needs to calculate the micrograms per minute the patient is receiving.

Step 1. On the left side of the equation, place what you are solving for:

$$\frac{x\ \text{mcg}}{\text{min}} =$$

Step 2. Deal with the numerator portion of the answer first, *mcg*. Micrograms are not in the problem, but milligrams are, so the first fraction will be the conversion between micrograms and milligrams. This information is placed in the equation as a fraction, with the numerators matching.

$$\frac{x\ \textbf{mcg}}{\text{min}} = \frac{1000\ \textbf{mcg}}{1\ \text{mg}}$$

Step 3. Next, find the information that matches the measurement used in the denominator of the fraction you created. In this example, *mg* is in the denominator, so 50 mg of nitroglycerin in 500 mL 0.9% NS is used. Continue this process until all of the denominators except for *minute* can be canceled.

$$\frac{x\ \text{mcg}}{\text{min}} = \frac{1000\ \text{mcg}}{1\ \textbf{mg}} \times \frac{50\ \textbf{mg}}{500\ \textbf{mL}} \times \frac{3\ \textbf{mL}}{1\ \textbf{h}} \times \frac{1\ \textbf{h}}{60\ \text{min}}$$

Step 4. Cancel the abbreviations on the right side of the equation. Now solve for x.

$$\frac{x\ \text{mcg}}{\text{min}} = \frac{1000\ \text{mcg}}{1\ \cancel{\text{mg}}} \times \frac{50\ \cancel{\text{mg}}}{500\ \cancel{\text{mL}}} \times \frac{3\ \cancel{\text{mL}}}{1\ \cancel{\text{h}}} \times \frac{1\ \cancel{\text{h}}}{60\ \text{min}}$$

$$\frac{x\ \text{mcg}}{\text{min}} = \frac{1000 \times 50 \times 3}{500 \times 60}$$

$$x = 5\ \text{mcg/min}$$

Therefore when the nitroglycerin is infusing at 3 mL/h, the patient is receiving a nitroglycerin dose of 5 mcg/min.

Calculating Micrograms/Kilogram/Minute from Milliliters/Hour—Dimensional Analysis Method

EXAMPLE: A patient is receiving dopamine at 12 mL/h. The concentration of dopamine is 200 mg in 250 mL of 0.9% NS. The nurse needs to calculate the micrograms per kilogram per minute the patient is receiving. The patient's weight is 70 kg.

Step 1. On the left side of the equation, place what you are solving for:

$$\frac{x\ \text{mcg}}{\text{kg/min}} =$$

Step 2. Deal with the numerator portion of the answer first, *mcg*. Micrograms are not in the problem, but milligrams are, so the first fraction will be the conversion between micrograms and milligrams. This information is placed in the equation as a fraction, with the numerators matching.

$$\frac{x\ \textbf{mcg}}{\text{kg/min}} = \frac{1000\ \textbf{mcg}}{1\ \text{mg}}$$

Step 3. Next, find the information that matches the measurement used in the denominator of the fraction you created. In this example, *mg* is in the denominator, so 200 mg of nitroglycerin in 250 mL 0.9% NS is used. Continue this process until all of the denominators except *minute* can be canceled.

$$\frac{x\text{ mcg}}{\text{kg/min}} = \frac{1000\text{ mcg}}{\mathbf{1\ mg}} \times \frac{\mathbf{200\ mg}}{\mathbf{250\ mL}} \times \frac{\mathbf{12\ mL}}{\mathbf{1\ h}} \times \frac{\mathbf{1\ h}}{60\text{ min}} \times \frac{}{70\text{ kg}}$$

Step 4. Cancel the abbreviations on the right side of the equation. Now solve for x.

$$\frac{x\text{ mcg}}{\text{kg/min}} = \frac{1000\text{ mcg}}{1\ \cancel{\text{mg}}} \times \frac{200\ \cancel{\text{mg}}}{250\ \cancel{\text{mL}}} \times \frac{12\ \cancel{\text{mL}}}{1\ \cancel{\text{h}}} \times \frac{1\ \cancel{\text{h}}}{60\text{ min}} \times \frac{}{70\text{ kg}}$$

$$\frac{x\text{ mcg}}{\text{kg/min}} = \frac{1000 \times 200 \times 12}{250 \times 60 \times 70}$$

$$x = 2.28\text{ rounded to }2.3\text{ mcg/kg/min}$$

Therefore when the dopamine is infusing at 12 mL/h, the patient is receiving a dopamine dose of 2.3 mcg/kg/min.

Calculating Milliliters/Hour from Milligrams/Minute—Formula Method

EXAMPLE: Lidocaine 1 g has been added to 500 mL of D_5W. The order states to infuse the lidocaine at 2 mg/min. The nurse needs to calculate the rate, in milliliters per hour, at which to set the IV pump.

$$\text{The formula: } \frac{\text{Desired mg/min} \times 60\text{ min/h}^*}{\text{Medication concentration (mg/mL)}}$$

*60 min/h is a constant fraction in the formula and represents the equivalency of 60 min = 1 h.

When this formula is used, the answer will always be expressed in milliliters per hour because the pair of values in milligrams will cancel each other, as will the pair of values in minutes.

Step 1. Convert total g in the IV bag to mg.

$$1\text{ g} = 1000\text{ mg}$$

Step 2. Calculate mL/h.

(Formula setup) $$\frac{2\text{ mg/min} \times 60\text{ min/h}}{2\text{ mg/mL}} = x\text{ mL/h}$$

(Cancel) $$\frac{\overset{1}{\cancel{2}}\text{ mg/min} \times 60\text{ min/h}}{\underset{1}{\cancel{2}}\text{ mg/mL}} = x\text{ mL/h}$$

(Calculate) $$\frac{1 \times 60}{1} = 60\text{ mL/h}$$

Calculating Milliliters/Hour from Micrograms/Minute—Formula Method

EXAMPLE: 50 mg of nitroglycerin has been added to 500 mL of 0.9% NS. The order is to infuse the nitroglycerin at 5 mcg/min. The nurse needs to calculate the rate, in milliliters per hour, at which to set the IV pump.

$$\text{The formula: } \frac{\text{Ordered mcg/min} \times 60 \text{ min/h}}{\text{Medication concentration (mcg/mL)}}$$

When this formula is used, the answer will always be expressed in milliliters per hour because the pair of values in milligrams will cancel each other, as will the pair of values in minutes.

Step 1. Convert total mg in the IV bag to mcg.

$$1 \text{ mg} : 1000 \text{ mcg} :: 50 \text{ mg} : x \text{ mcg}$$

$$x = 50{,}000 \text{ mcg}$$

Step 2. Calculate the concentration (mcg/mL) by dividing the total mcg by the total amount of fluid in the IV bag.

$$\frac{50{,}000 \text{ mcg}}{500 \text{ mL}} = 100 \text{ mcg/mL}$$

Step 3. Calculate the mL/h.

$$\text{(Formula setup)} \quad \frac{5 \text{ mcg/min} \times 60 \text{ min/h}}{100 \text{ mcg/mL}} = x \text{ mL/h}$$

$$\text{(Cancel)} \quad \frac{\overset{1}{\cancel{5}} \, \cancel{\text{mcg}}/\cancel{\text{min}} \times 60 \, \cancel{\text{min}}/\text{h}}{\underset{20}{\cancel{100}} \, \cancel{\text{mcg}}/\text{mL}} = x \text{ mL/h}$$

$$\text{(Calculate)} \quad \frac{1 \times 60}{20} = \frac{60}{20} = 3 \text{ mL/h}$$

Calculating Milliliters/Hour from Micrograms/Kilogram/Minute—Formula Method

EXAMPLE: 800 mg of dopamine is added to 250 mL of 0.9% NS. The order is to begin the infusion at 3 mcg/kg/min. The patient's weight is 70 kg. The nurse needs to calculate the rate, in milliliters per hour, at which to set the IV pump.

The formula for calculating the mL/h is:

$$\frac{\text{Ordered mcg/kg/min} \times \text{Patient's weight in kg} \times 60 \text{ min/h}}{\text{Medication concentration (mcg/mL)}}$$

When this formula is used, the result will always be expressed in milliliters per hour because the pair of values in micrograms cancel each other, as do the pair of values in kilograms and the pair of values in minutes.

Step 1. Before the medication concentration can be determined, the total mg in the IV bag must be converted to mcg.

$$1 \text{ mg} : 1000 \text{ mcg} :: 800 \text{ mg} : x \text{ mcg}$$

$$x = 800{,}000 \text{ mcg}$$

Step 2. Determine the concentration (mcg/mL) by dividing the total mcg in the IV bag by the total amount of fluid in the IV bag.

$$\frac{800{,}000 \text{ mcg}}{250 \text{ mL}} = \frac{3200 \text{ mcg}}{1 \text{ mL}} = 3200 \text{ mcg/mL}$$

Step 3. Calculate mL/h.

(Formula setup) $$\frac{3 \text{ mcg/kg/min} \times 70 \text{ kg} \times 60 \text{ min/h}}{3200 \text{ mcg/mL}} = x \text{ mL/h}$$

(Cancel) $$\frac{3 \cancel{\text{mcg}}/\cancel{\text{kg}}/\cancel{\text{min}} \times 70 \cancel{\text{kg}} \times 60 \cancel{\text{min}}/\text{h}}{3200 \cancel{\text{mcg}}/\text{mL}} = x \text{ mL/h}$$

(Calculate) $$\frac{3 \times 70 \times 60}{3200} = \frac{12{,}600}{3200} = 3.93 \text{ or } 3.9 \text{ mL/h}$$

Calculations for critical care medications do not stop with taking an order and calculating milliliters per hour. A nurse may receive in report, "Mr. Douglas is receiving dopamine at 15 mL/h, which is 10 mcg/kg/min." Because the nurse administering the medication during the upcoming shift is the final link in safety, this nurse needs to be able to take the milliliters per hour and calculate the exact dose of dopamine the patient is receiving. This situation can also be applied to medications that are ordered in milligrams per minute and micrograms per minute.

Calculating Milligrams/Minute from Milliliters/Hour—Formula Method

EXAMPLE: A patient is receiving lidocaine at 60 mL/h. The concentration of lidocaine is 1 g in 500 mL of D_5W. The nurse needs to calculate the milligrams per minute the patient is receiving.

The formula: $$\frac{\text{Concentration (mg/mL)} \times \text{Rate (mL/h)}}{60 \text{ min/h}}$$

When this formula is used, the answer will always be expressed in milligrams per minute because the pair of values in milliliters cancel each other, as do the pair of values in hours.

Step 1. Convert total g in the IV bag to mg.

$$1 \text{ g} = 1000 \text{ mg}$$

Step 2. Calculate the concentration (mg/mL).

$$\frac{1000 \text{ mg}}{500 \text{ mL}} = 2 \text{ mg/mL}$$

Step 3. Calculate the mg/min.

(Formula setup) $$\frac{2 \text{ mg/mL} \times 60 \text{ mL/h}}{60 \text{ min/h}}$$

(Cancel) $$\frac{2 \text{ mg}/\cancel{\text{mL}} \times \overset{1}{\cancel{60}} \cancel{\text{mL}}/\cancel{\text{h}}}{\underset{1}{\cancel{60}} \text{ min}/\cancel{\text{h}}}$$

(Calculate) 2 mg/min

Calculating Micrograms/Minute from Milliliters/Hour—Formula Method

EXAMPLE: A patient is receiving nitroglycerin at 3 mL/h. The concentration of nitroglycerin is 50 mg in 500 mL of 0.9% NS. The nurse needs to calculate the micrograms per minute the patient is receiving.

$$\text{The formula: } \frac{\text{Concentration (mcg/mL)} \times \text{Rate (mL/h)}}{\text{60 min/h}}$$

When this formula is used, the answer will always be expressed in micrograms per minute because the pair of values in milliliters cancel each other, as do the pair of values in hours.

Step 1. Convert total mg in the IV bag to mcg.

$$\text{(Formula setup)} \quad 1 \text{ mg} : 1000 \text{ mcg} :: 50 \text{ mg} : x \text{ mcg}$$

$$x = 1000 \times 50$$

$$x = 50{,}000 \text{ mcg}$$

Step 2. Calculate the concentration (mcg/mL).

$$\frac{50{,}000 \text{ mcg}}{500 \text{ mL}} = 100 \text{ mcg/mL}$$

Step 3. Calculate the mcg/min.

$$\text{(Formula setup)} \quad \frac{100 \text{ mcg/mL} \times 3 \text{ mL/h}}{60 \text{ min/h}}$$

$$\text{(Cancel)} \quad \frac{100 \text{ mcg}/\cancel{\text{mL}} \times \overset{1}{\cancel{3}} \ \cancel{\text{mL}}/\cancel{\text{h}}}{\underset{20}{\cancel{60}} \text{ min}/\cancel{\text{h}}}$$

$$\text{(Calculate)} \quad \frac{100}{20} = 5 \text{ mcg/min}$$

Calculating Micrograms/Kilogram/Minute from Milliliters/Hour—Formula Method

EXAMPLE: A patient is receiving dopamine at 12 mL/h. The concentration of dopamine is 200 mg in 250 mL of 0.9% NS. The nurse needs to calculate the micrograms per kilogram per minute the patient is receiving. The patient's weight is 70 kg.

$$\text{The formula: } \frac{\text{Concentration (mcg/mL)} \times \text{Rate (mL/h)}}{\text{60 min/h} \times \text{Weight (kg)}}$$

When this formula is used, the answer will always be expressed in micrograms per kilogram per minute because the pair of values in milliliters cancel each other, as do the pair of values in hours.

Step 1. Convert total mg in the IV bag to mcg.

$$\text{(Formula setup)} \quad 1 \text{ mg} : 1000 \text{ mcg} :: 200 \text{ mg} : x \text{ mcg}$$

$$x = 1000 \times 200$$

$$x = 200{,}000 \text{ mcg}$$

Step 2. Calculate the concentration (mcg/mL).

$$\frac{200{,}000\ \text{mcg}}{250\ \text{mL}} = 800\ \text{mcg/mL}$$

Step 3. Calculate the mcg/kg/min.

(Formula setup) $$\frac{800\ \text{mcg/mL} \times 12\ \text{mL/h}}{60\ \text{min/h} \times 70\ \text{kg}}$$

(Cancel) $$\frac{800\ \text{mcg}/\cancel{\text{mL}} \times \overset{1}{\cancel{12}}\ \cancel{\text{mL}}/\cancel{\text{h}}}{\underset{5}{\cancel{60}}\ \text{min}/\cancel{\text{h}} \times 70\ \text{kg}}$$

(Calculate) $$\frac{800}{5 \times 70} = \frac{800}{350} = 2.28 \text{ rounded to } 2.3\ \text{mcg/kg/min}$$

Some IV pumps have the capability of calculating the IV rate required for a specific drug. The nurse can select a drug from the IV pump "library," enter the desired dose, the concentration of the medication, and the patient's weight in kilograms. After all the information is entered, the IV pump will display the mL/h needed for the IV rate (Figure 17-1). Nurses should use this feature as a check of their own dosage calculation answer, not as the only means of dosage calculation.

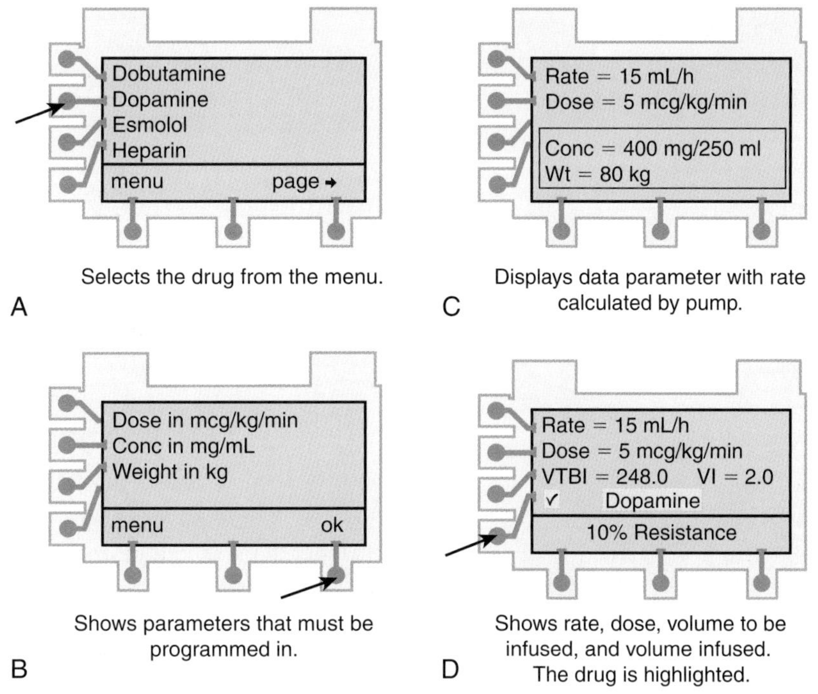

FIGURE 17-1 Using an IV pump library. (Courtesy Becton, Dickinson and Company.)

Complete the following work sheet, which provides for practice in the calculation of critical care IV flow rates. Check your answers. If you have difficulties, go back and review the necessary material. An acceptable score as indicated on the posttest signifies that you have successfully completed the chapter. An unacceptable score signifies a need for further study before taking the second posttest.

WORK SHEET

DIRECTIONS: The order is listed in each problem. Calculate the IV flow rates using the appropriate formula required for the problem.

1. The licensed prescriber orders dobutamine at 12 mcg/kg/min for Mrs. White, who weighs 75 kg. The concentration is dobutamine 1 g in 250 mL of D_5W. How many milliliters per hour should the IV pump be programmed for? ______

2. Mr. Baxter is having chest pain and has an order for nitroglycerin at 10 mcg/min. The concentration is nitroglycerin 100 mg in 500 mL of D_5W. How many milliliters per hour should the IV pump be programmed for? ______

3. The licensed prescriber orders dopamine at 5 mcg/kg/min. The concentration is dopamine 2 g in 250 mL of 0.9% NS. The patient's weight is 80 kg. How many milliliters per hour should the IV pump be programmed for? ______

4. The licensed prescriber has ordered amiodarone at 0.5 mg/min. The concentration is amiodarone 900 mg in 500 mL of D_5W. How many milliliters per hour should the IV pump be programmed for? ______

5. Your patient with malignant hypertension is ordered to have nitroprusside at 3 mcg/kg/min. The concentration is nitroprusside 50 mg in 250 mL of D_5W. The patient's weight is 70 kg. How many milliliters per hour should the IV pump be programmed for? ______

6. A patient with heart failure has dobutamine ordered at 10 mcg/kg/min. The patient weighs 100 kg. The concentration is dobutamine 2 g in 500 mL of D_5W. How many milliliters per hour should the IV pump be programmed for? ______

7. Mr. Nast has propofol ordered at 30 mcg/kg/min. The propofol concentration is 15 mg/mL. The patient's weight is 75 kg. How many milliliters per hour should the IV pump be programmed for? ______

8. A patient with a ventricular dysrhythmia has procainamide ordered at 4 mg/min. The concentration is procainamide 2 g in 250 mL of D_5W. How many milliliters per hour should the IV pump be programmed for? ______

9. Mrs. Waters, who has been resuscitated, has norepinephrine ordered at 10 mcg/min. The concentration is norepinephrine 2 mg in 250 mL of 0.9% NS. How many milliliters per hour should the IV pump be programmed for? ______

10. A patient with a dysrhythmia has an order for amiodarone 0.75 mg/min. The concentration is amiodarone 900 mg in 500 mL D_5W. How many milliliters per hour should the IV pump be programmed for? ______

11. A patient with hypotension has a vasopressor ordered at 15 mcg/min. The concentration is vasopressor 4 mg in 250 mL of D_5W. How many milliliters per hour should the IV pump be programmed for? ______

12. Mrs. Roberts has lidocaine ordered at 2 mg/min. The concentration is lidocaine 2 g in 250 mL of D_5W. How many milliliters per hour should the IV pump be programmed for? ______

13. The licensed prescriber orders dopamine at 10 mcg/kg/min. The concentration is dopamine 2 g in 250 mL of 0.9% NS. The patient's weight is 90 kg. How many milliliters per hour should the IV pump be programmed for? ______

14. Mr. Diaz is admitted to your ICU with dopamine infusing at 13.5 mL/h. His weight is 75 kg. The dopamine concentration is 1 g in 250 mL of D_5W. At what rate, in micrograms per kilogram per minute, is the dopamine infusing? ______

15. A patient with heart failure has nitroglycerin infusing at 3 mL/h. The nitroglycerin concentration is 100 mg in 500 mL of D_5W. At what rate, in micrograms per minute, is the nitroglycerin infusing? ______

16. A patient with supraventricular tachycardia has amiodarone infusing at 17 mL/h. The amiodarone concentration is 900 mg in 500 mL of D_5W. At what rate, in milligrams per minute, is the amiodarone infusing? ______

17. Ms. Hart requires mechanical ventilation and is agitated. Propofol is infusing at 9 mL/h. The patient's weight is 75 kg. The propofol concentration is 15 mg/mL. At what rate, in micrograms per kilogram per minute, is the propofol infusing? ______

18. Mr. Simon is admitted with angina. Nitroglycerin is infusing at 5 mL/h. The nitroglycerin concentration is 50 mg in 250 mL of D_5W. How many micrograms per minute is the patient receiving? ______

19. A patient with uncontrolled atrial fibrillation is receiving amiodarone at 20 mL/h. The amiodarone concentration is 900 mg in 500 mL of D_5W. How many milligrams per minute is the patient receiving? ______

20. Mr. McCormick is receiving dopamine at 15 mL/h by IV pump. The patient weighs 80 kg. The dopamine concentration is 2 g in 500 mL of D_5W. Calculate the micrograms per kilogram per minute. ______

21. A patient is receiving nitroglycerin at 10 mL/h by IV pump. The nitroglycerin concentration is 100 mg in 250 mL of D_5W. Calculate the micrograms per minute. ______

22. A patient is receiving amiodarone at 15 mL/h by IV pump. The amiodarone concentration is 900 mg in 250 mL of D_5W. Calculate the milligrams per minute. ______

23. Ms. Nesbitt is receiving lidocaine at 15 mL/h by IV pump. The lidocaine concentration is 1 g in 500 mL of 0.9% NS. Calculate the milligrams per minute. ______

24. Mr. Vargas has supraventricular tachycardia and has a maintenance infusion of esmolol 100 mcg/kg/min ordered. The esmolol concentration is 10 mg/mL. The patient's weight is 80 kg. At what rate, in milliliters per hour, should the IV pump be set?

ANSWERS ON PP. 513–514 AND 515–516.

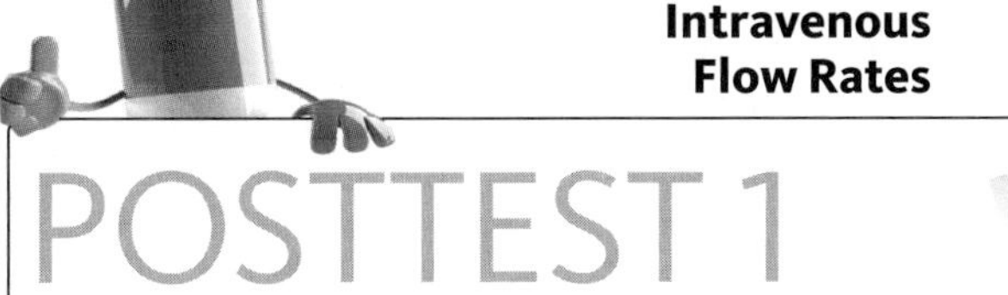

NAME ____________________

DATE ____________________

ACCEPTABLE SCORE **9**

YOUR SCORE ______

POSTTEST 1

DIRECTIONS: The order is listed in each problem. Calculate the appropriate rate for each problem.

1. A patient with hypertension has orders for nitroprusside at 5 mcg/kg/min. The concentration is nitroprusside 100 mg in 250 mL of D_5W. The patient weighs 62 kg. How many milliliters per hour should the IV pump be programmed for? ______

2. Mr. Marshall, who is admitted with pulmonary edema, has dobutamine ordered at 5 mcg/kg/min. The concentration is dobutamine 1 g in 250 mL of 0.9% NS. The patient's weight is 50 kg. How many milliliters per hour should the IV pump be programmed for? ______

3. A patient with an acute myocardial infarction has IV nitroglycerin ordered at 20 mcg/min. The concentration is nitroglycerin 50 mg in 250 mL of D_5W. How many milliliters per hour should the IV pump be programmed for? ______

4. A patient with a ventricular dysrhythmia has lidocaine ordered at 3 mg/min. The concentration is lidocaine 2 g in 500 mL of D_5W. How many milliliters per hour should the IV pump be programmed for? ______

5. Mrs. Morales has been resuscitated and now has norepinephrine ordered at 5 mcg/min. The concentration is norepinephrine 1 mg in 250 mL of 0.9% NS. How many milliliters per hour should the IV pump be programmed for? ______

6. An intubated patient has propofol ordered at 25 mcg/kg/min. The concentration of propofol is 10 mg/mL. The patient's weight is 50 kg. How many milliliters per hour should the IV pump be programmed for? ______

7. Mrs. Green, who has atrial fibrillation, has amiodarone ordered at 0.5 mg/min. The concentration is amiodarone 900 mg in 250 mL of D_5W. How many milliliters per hour should the IV pump be programmed for?

8. A patient with a blood pressure of 240/120 mm Hg is receiving nitroprusside at 63 mL/h. The patient's weight is 70 kg. The nitroprusside concentration is 50 mg in 250 mL of D_5W. How many micrograms per kilogram per minute of nitroprusside is infusing? ______

9. Mr. Messer is receiving vasopressin at 15 mL/h. The vasopressin concentration is 4 mg in 250 mL. How many micrograms per minute of vasopressin is the patient receiving? ______

10. A patient has hypotension after cardiac arrest. Dopamine is infusing at 15 mL/h. The patient's weight is 80 kg. The dopamine concentration is 2 g in 500 mL of D_5W. How many micrograms per kilogram per minute is the patient receiving? ______

ANSWERS ON PP. 514 AND 516.

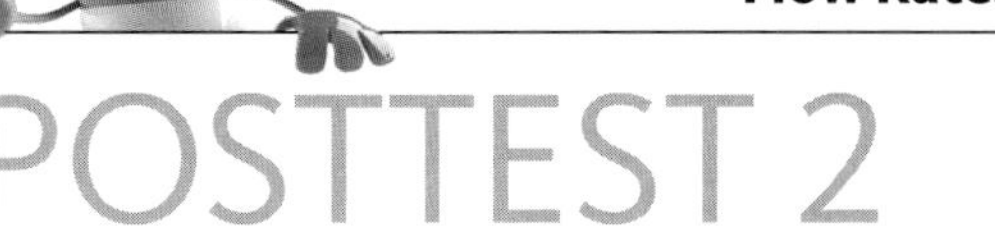

POSTTEST 2

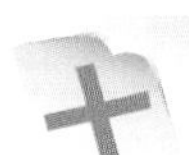

NAME ____________________

DATE ____________________

ACCEPTABLE SCORE **9**

YOUR SCORE ______

DIRECTIONS: The order is listed in each problem. Calculate the rate needed in each problem to deliver the correct dose.

1. A patient with hypotension has dopamine ordered at 3 mcg/kg/min. The patient weighs 85 kg. The concentration is dopamine 2 g in 500 mL of D_5W. How many milliliters per hour should the IV pump be programmed for? ______

2. Ms. Farmer, who has tachycardia, has an order for esmolol to be started at 50 mcg/kg/min. The concentration is esmolol 5 g in 500 mL of D_5W. The patient weighs 80 kg. How many milliliters per hour should the IV pump be programmed for? ______

3. A patient with a ventricular dysrhythmia has an order for amiodarone at 0.5 mg/min. The concentration is amiodarone 900 mg in 250 mL of D_5W. How many milliliters per hour should the IV pump be programmed for? ______

4. Mr. Wu has an order for a vasopressor at 10 mcg/min. The concentration is vasopressor 4 mg in 500 mL of D_5W. How many milliliters per hour should the IV pump be programmed for? ______

5. Mrs. Davis has an order for dobutamine at 7 mcg/kg/min. The concentration is dobutamine 1 g in 200 mL of 0.9% NS. The patient's weight is 55 kg. How many milliliters per hour should the IV pump be programmed for? ______

6. A patient in shock has an order for isoproterenol to be infused at 2 mcg/min. The concentration is isoproterenol 1 mg in 500 mL of D_5W. How many milliliters per hour should the IV pump be programmed for? ______

7. Ms. Shepard's blood pressure is 60/30 mm Hg. Norepinephrine is infusing at 75 mL/h. The norepinephrine concentration is 2 mg in 250 mL of 0.9% NS. How many micrograms per minute of norepinephrine is infusing? ______

8. A patient with ventricular tachycardia is receiving procainamide at 30 mL/h. The procainamide concentration is 2 g in 250 mL of D_5W. How many milligrams per minute of procainamide is infusing? ______

9. A hypotensive patient is receiving dopamine at 3 mL/h. The patient's weight is 80 kg. The dopamine concentration is 2 g in 250 mL of 0.9% NS. How many micrograms per kilogram per minute of dopamine is infusing? ______

10. Mr. Flores is receiving nitroprusside at 50 mL/h by IV pump. The patient's weight is 60 kg. The nitroprusside concentration is 50 mg in 250 mL of D_5W. Calculate the micrograms per kilogram per minute.

ANSWERS ON PP. 514–515 AND 516.

evolve For additional practice problems, refer to the Critical Care Dosages section of *Elsevier's Interactive Drug Calculation Application*, version 1.

ANSWERS

CHAPTER 17 Dimensional Analysis—Work Sheet, pp. 505–508

1. $\frac{x \text{ mL}}{\text{h}} = \frac{250 \text{ mL}}{1 \text{ g}} \times \frac{1 \text{ g}}{1{,}000{,}000 \text{ mcg}} \times \frac{12 \text{ mcg}}{\text{kg/min}} \times \frac{75 \text{ kg}}{1} \times \frac{60 \text{ min}}{1 \text{ h}} = 13.5 \text{ or } 14 \text{ mL/h}$

2. $\frac{x \text{ mL}}{\text{h}} = \frac{500 \text{ mL}}{100 \text{ mg}} \times \frac{1 \text{ mg}}{1000 \text{ mcg}} \times \frac{10 \text{ mcg}}{1 \text{ min}} \times \frac{60 \text{ min}}{1 \text{ h}} = 3 \text{ mL/h}$

3. $\frac{x \text{ mL}}{\text{h}} = \frac{250 \text{ mL}}{2 \text{ mg}} \times \frac{1 \text{ g}}{1{,}000{,}000 \text{ mcg}} \times \frac{5 \text{ mcg}}{\text{kg/min}} \times \frac{80 \text{ kg}}{1} \times \frac{60 \text{ min}}{1 \text{ h}} = 3 \text{ mL/h}$

4. $\frac{x \text{ mL}}{\text{h}} = \frac{500 \text{ mL}}{900 \text{ mg}} \times \frac{0.5 \text{ mg}}{1 \text{ min}} \times \frac{60 \text{ min}}{1 \text{ h}} = 16.7 \text{ or } 17 \text{ mL/h}$

5. $\frac{x \text{ mL}}{\text{h}} = \frac{250 \text{ mL}}{50 \text{ mg}} \times \frac{1 \text{ mg}}{1000 \text{ mcg}} \times \frac{3 \text{ mcg}}{\text{kg/min}} \times \frac{70 \text{ kg}}{1} \times \frac{60 \text{ min}}{1 \text{ h}} = 63 \text{ mL/h}$

6. $\frac{x \text{ mL}}{\text{h}} = \frac{500 \text{ mL}}{2 \text{ g}} \times \frac{1 \text{ g}}{1{,}000{,}000 \text{ mcg}} \times \frac{10 \text{ mcg}}{\text{kg/min}} \times \frac{100 \text{ kg}}{1} \times \frac{60 \text{ min}}{1 \text{ h}} = 15 \text{ mL/h}$

7. $\frac{x \text{ mL}}{\text{h}} = \frac{1 \text{ mL}}{15 \text{ mg}} \times \frac{1 \text{ mg}}{1000 \text{ mcg}} \times \frac{30 \text{ mcg}}{\text{kg/min}} \times \frac{75 \text{ kg}}{1} \times \frac{60 \text{ min}}{1 \text{ h}} = 9 \text{ mL/h}$

8. $\frac{x \text{ mL}}{\text{h}} = \frac{250 \text{ mL}}{2 \text{ g}} \times \frac{1 \text{ g}}{1000 \text{ mg}} \times \frac{4 \text{ mg}}{1 \text{ min}} \times \frac{60 \text{ min}}{1 \text{ h}} = 30 \text{ mL/h}$

9. $\frac{x \text{ mL}}{\text{h}} = \frac{250 \text{ mL}}{2 \text{ mg}} \times \frac{1 \text{ mg}}{1000 \text{ mcg}} \times \frac{10 \text{ mcg}}{1 \text{ min}} \times \frac{60 \text{ min}}{1 \text{ h}} = 75 \text{ mL/h}$

10. $\frac{x \text{ mL}}{\text{h}} = \frac{500 \text{ mL}}{900 \text{ mg}} \times \frac{0.75 \text{ mg}}{1 \text{ min}} \times \frac{60 \text{ min}}{1 \text{ h}} = 25 \text{ mL/h}$

11. $\frac{x \text{ mL}}{\text{h}} = \frac{250 \text{ mL}}{4 \text{ mg}} \times \frac{1 \text{ mg}}{1000 \text{ mcg}} \times \frac{15 \text{ mcg}}{1 \text{ min}} \times \frac{60 \text{ min}}{1 \text{ h}} = 56.3 \text{ or } 56 \text{ mL/h}$

12. $\frac{x \text{ mL}}{\text{h}} = \frac{250 \text{ mL}}{2 \text{ g}} \times \frac{1 \text{ g}}{1000 \text{ mg}} \times \frac{2 \text{ mg}}{1 \text{ min}} \times \frac{60 \text{ min}}{1 \text{ h}} = 15 \text{ mL/h}$

13. $\frac{x \text{ mL}}{\text{h}} = \frac{250 \text{ mL}}{2 \text{ g}} \times \frac{1 \text{ g}}{1{,}000{,}000 \text{ mcg}} \times \frac{10 \text{ mcg}}{\text{kg/min}} \times \frac{90 \text{ kg}}{1} \times \frac{60 \text{ min}}{1 \text{ h}} = 6.8 \text{ or } 7 \text{ mL/h}$

14. $\frac{x \text{ mcg}}{\text{kg/min}} = \frac{1{,}000{,}000 \text{ mcg}}{1 \text{ g}} \times \frac{1 \text{ g}}{250 \text{ mL}} \times \frac{13.5 \text{ mL}}{1 \text{ h}} \times \frac{1 \text{ h}}{60 \text{ min}} \times \frac{}{75 \text{ kg}} = 12 \text{ mcg/kg/min}$

15. $\frac{x \text{ mcg}}{\text{min}} = \frac{1000 \text{ mcg}}{1 \text{ mg}} \times \frac{100 \text{ mg}}{500 \text{ mL}} \times \frac{3 \text{ mL}}{1 \text{ h}} \times \frac{1 \text{ h}}{60 \text{ min}} = 10 \text{ mcg/min}$

16. $\frac{x \text{ mg}}{\text{min}} = \frac{900 \text{ mg}}{500 \text{ mL}} \times \frac{17 \text{ mL}}{1 \text{ h}} \times \frac{1 \text{ h}}{60 \text{ min}} = 0.51 \text{ rounded to } 0.5 \text{ mg/min}$

17. $\frac{x \text{ mcg}}{\text{kg/min}} = \frac{1000 \text{ mcg}}{1 \text{ mg}} \times \frac{15 \text{ mg}}{1 \text{ mL}} \times \frac{9 \text{ mL}}{1 \text{ h}} \times \frac{1 \text{ h}}{60 \text{ min}} \times \frac{}{75 \text{ kg}} = 30 \text{ mcg/kg/min}$

18. $\frac{x \text{ mcg}}{\text{min}} = \frac{1000 \text{ mcg}}{1 \text{ mg}} \times \frac{50 \text{ mg}}{250 \text{ mL}} \times \frac{5 \text{ mL}}{1 \text{ h}} \times \frac{1 \text{ h}}{60 \text{ min}} = 16.66 \text{ rounded to } 16.7 \text{ mcg/min}$

19. $\frac{x \text{ mg}}{\text{min}} = \frac{900 \text{ mg}}{500 \text{ mL}} \times \frac{20 \text{ mL}}{1 \text{ h}} \times \frac{1 \text{ h}}{60 \text{ min}} = 0.6 \text{ mg/min}$

20. $\frac{x \text{ mcg}}{\text{kg/min}} = \frac{1{,}000{,}000 \text{ mcg}}{1 \text{ g}} \times \frac{2 \text{ g}}{500 \text{ mL}} \times \frac{15 \text{ mL}}{1 \text{ h}} \times \frac{1 \text{ h}}{60 \text{ min}} \times \frac{}{80 \text{ kg}} = 12.5 \text{ mcg/kg/min}$

21. $\frac{x \text{ mcg}}{\text{min}} = \frac{1000 \text{ mcg}}{1 \text{ mg}} \times \frac{100 \text{ mg}}{250 \text{ mL}} \times \frac{10 \text{ mL}}{1 \text{ h}} \times \frac{1 \text{ h}}{60 \text{ min}} = 66.66 \text{ rounded to } 66.7 \text{ mcg/min}$

22. $\frac{x \text{ mg}}{\text{min}} = \frac{900 \text{ mg}}{250 \text{ mL}} \times \frac{15 \text{ mL}}{1 \text{ h}} \times \frac{1 \text{ h}}{60 \text{ min}} = 0.9 \text{ mg/min}$

23. $\frac{x \text{ mg}}{\text{min}} = \frac{1000 \text{ mg}}{1 \text{ g}} \times \frac{1 \text{ g}}{500 \text{ mL}} \times \frac{15 \text{ mL}}{1 \text{ h}} \times \frac{1 \text{ h}}{60 \text{ min}} = 0.5 \text{ mg/min}$

24. $\frac{x \text{ mL}}{\text{h}} = \frac{1 \text{ mL}}{10 \text{ mg}} \times \frac{1 \text{ mg}}{1000 \text{ mcg}} \times \frac{100 \text{ mcg}}{\text{kg/min}} \times \frac{80 \text{ kg}}{1} \times \frac{60 \text{ min}}{1 \text{ h}} = 48 \text{ mL/h}$

CHAPTER 17 Dimensional Analysis—Posttest 1, pp. 509–510

1. $\frac{x \text{ mL}}{\text{h}} = \frac{250 \text{ mL}}{100 \text{ mg}} \times \frac{1 \text{ mg}}{1000 \text{ mcg}} \times \frac{5 \text{ mcg}}{\text{kg/min}} \times \frac{62 \text{ kg}}{1} \times \frac{60 \text{ min}}{1 \text{ h}} = 46.5 \text{ or } 47 \text{ mL/h}$

2. $\frac{x \text{ mL}}{\text{h}} = \frac{250 \text{ mL}}{1 \text{ g}} \times \frac{1 \text{ g}}{1{,}000{,}000 \text{ mcg}} \times \frac{5 \text{ mcg}}{\text{kg/min}} \times \frac{50 \text{ kg}}{1} \times \frac{60 \text{ min}}{1 \text{ h}} = 3.8 \text{ or } 4 \text{ mL/h}$

3. $\frac{x \text{ mL}}{\text{h}} = \frac{250 \text{ mL}}{50 \text{ mg}} \times \frac{1 \text{ mg}}{1000 \text{ mcg}} \times \frac{20 \text{ mcg}}{1 \text{ min}} \times \frac{60 \text{ min}}{1 \text{ h}} = 6 \text{ mL/h}$

4. $\frac{x \text{ mL}}{\text{h}} = \frac{500 \text{ mL}}{2 \text{ g}} \times \frac{1 \text{ g}}{1000 \text{ mg}} \times \frac{3 \text{ mg}}{1 \text{ min}} \times \frac{60 \text{ min}}{1 \text{ h}} = 45 \text{ mL/h}$

5. $\frac{x \text{ mL}}{\text{h}} = \frac{250 \text{ mL}}{1 \text{ mg}} \times \frac{1 \text{ mg}}{1000 \text{ mcg}} \times \frac{5 \text{ mcg}}{1 \text{ min}} \times \frac{60 \text{ min}}{1 \text{ h}} = 75 \text{ mL/h}$

6. $\frac{x \text{ mL}}{\text{h}} = \frac{1 \text{ mL}}{10 \text{ mg}} \times \frac{1 \text{ mg}}{1000 \text{ mcg}} \times \frac{25 \text{ mcg}}{\text{kg/min}} \times \frac{50 \text{ kg}}{1} \times \frac{60 \text{ min}}{1 \text{ h}} = 7.5 \text{ or } 8 \text{ mL/h}$

7. $\frac{x \text{ mL}}{\text{h}} = \frac{250 \text{ mL}}{900 \text{ mg}} \times \frac{0.5 \text{ mg}}{1 \text{ min}} \times \frac{60 \text{ min}}{1 \text{ h}} = 8.3 \text{ or } 8 \text{ mL/h}$

8. $\frac{x \text{ mcg}}{\text{kg/min}} = \frac{1000 \text{ mcg}}{1 \text{ mg}} \times \frac{50 \text{ mg}}{250 \text{ mL}} \times \frac{63 \text{ mL}}{1 \text{ h}} \times \frac{1 \text{ h}}{60 \text{ min}} \times \frac{}{70 \text{ kg}} = 3 \text{ mcg/kg/min}$

9. $\frac{x \text{ mcg}}{\text{min}} = \frac{1000 \text{ mcg}}{1 \text{ mg}} \times \frac{4 \text{ mg}}{250 \text{ mL}} \times \frac{15 \text{ mL}}{1 \text{ h}} \times \frac{1 \text{ h}}{60 \text{ min}} = 4 \text{ mcg/min}$

10. $\frac{x \text{ mcg}}{\text{kg/min}} = \frac{1{,}000{,}000 \text{ mcg}}{1 \text{ g}} \times \frac{2 \text{ g}}{500 \text{ mL}} \times \frac{15 \text{ mL}}{1 \text{ h}} \times \frac{1 \text{ h}}{60 \text{ min}} \times \frac{}{80 \text{ kg}} = 12.5 \text{ mcg/kg/min}$

CHAPTER 17 Dimensional Analysis—Posttest 2, pp. 511–512

1. $\frac{x \text{ mL}}{\text{h}} = \frac{500 \text{ mL}}{2 \text{ g}} \times \frac{1 \text{ g}}{1{,}000{,}000 \text{ mcg}} \times \frac{3 \text{ mcg}}{\text{kg/min}} \times \frac{85 \text{ kg}}{1} \times \frac{60 \text{ min}}{1 \text{ h}} = 3.8 \text{ or } 4 \text{ mL/h}$

2. $\frac{x \text{ mL}}{\text{h}} = \frac{500 \text{ mL}}{5 \text{ g}} \times \frac{1 \text{ g}}{1{,}000{,}000 \text{ mcg}} \times \frac{50 \text{ mcg}}{\text{kg/min}} \times \frac{80 \text{ kg}}{1} \times \frac{60 \text{ min}}{1 \text{ h}} = 24 \text{ mL/h}$

3. $\frac{x \text{ mL}}{\text{h}} = \frac{250 \text{ mL}}{900 \text{ mg}} \times \frac{0.5 \text{ mg}}{1 \text{ min}} \times \frac{60 \text{ min}}{1 \text{ h}} = 8.3 \text{ or } 8 \text{ mL/h}$

4. $\frac{x \text{ mL}}{\text{h}} = \frac{500 \text{ mL}}{4 \text{ mg}} \times \frac{1 \text{ mg}}{1000 \text{ mcg}} \times \frac{10 \text{ mcg}}{1 \text{ min}} \times \frac{60 \text{ min}}{1 \text{ h}} = 75 \text{ mL/h}$

5. $\frac{x \text{ mL}}{\text{h}} = \frac{200 \text{ mL}}{1 \text{ g}} \times \frac{1 \text{ g}}{1{,}000{,}000 \text{ mcg}} \times \frac{7 \text{ mcg}}{\text{kg/min}} \times \frac{55 \text{ kg}}{1} \times \frac{60 \text{ min}}{1 \text{ h}} = 4.6 \text{ or } 5 \text{ mL/h}$

6. $\frac{x \text{ mL}}{\text{h}} = \frac{500 \text{ mL}}{1 \text{ mg}} \times \frac{1 \text{ mg}}{1000 \text{ mcg}} \times \frac{2 \text{ mcg}}{1 \text{ min}} \times \frac{60 \text{ min}}{1 \text{ h}} = 60 \text{ mL/h}$

7. $\frac{x \text{ mcg}}{\text{min}} = \frac{1000 \text{ mcg}}{1 \text{ mg}} \times \frac{2 \text{ mg}}{250 \text{ mL}} \times \frac{75 \text{ mL}}{1 \text{ h}} \times \frac{1 \text{ h}}{60 \text{ min}} = 10 \text{ mcg/min}$

8. $\frac{x \text{ mg}}{\text{min}} = \frac{1000 \text{ mg}}{1 \text{ g}} \times \frac{2 \text{ g}}{250 \text{ mL}} \times \frac{30 \text{ mL}}{1 \text{ h}} \times \frac{1 \text{ h}}{60 \text{ min}} = 4 \text{ mg/min}$

9. $\frac{x \text{ mcg}}{\text{kg/min}} = \frac{1{,}000{,}000 \text{ mcg}}{1 \text{ g}} \times \frac{2 \text{ g}}{250 \text{ mL}} \times \frac{3 \text{ mL}}{1 \text{ h}} \times \frac{1 \text{ h}}{60 \text{ min}} \times \frac{}{80 \text{ kg}} = 5 \text{ mcg/kg/min}$

10. $\frac{x \text{ mcg}}{\text{kg/min}} = \frac{1000 \text{ mcg}}{1 \text{ mg}} \times \frac{50 \text{ mg}}{250 \text{ mL}} \times \frac{50 \text{ mL}}{1 \text{ h}} \times \frac{1 \text{ h}}{60 \text{ min}} \times \frac{}{60 \text{ kg}} = 2.77 \text{ rounded to } 2.8 \text{ mcg/kg/min}$

CHAPTER 17 Formula Method—Work Sheet, pp. 505–508

1. $\frac{12 \text{ mcg} \times 75 \text{ kg} \times 60 \text{ min/h}}{4000 \text{ mcg/mL}} = \frac{54{,}000}{4000} = 13.5 \text{ or } 14 \text{ mL/h}$

2. $\frac{10 \text{ mcg/min} \times 60 \text{ min/h}}{200 \text{ mcg/mL}} = \frac{600}{200} = 3 \text{ mL/h}$

3. $\frac{5 \text{ mcg} \times 80 \text{ kg} \times 60 \text{ min/h}}{8000 \text{ mcg/mL}} = \frac{24{,}000}{8000} = 3 \text{ mL/h}$

4. $\frac{0.5 \text{ mg/min} \times 60 \text{ min/h}}{1.8 \text{ mg/mL}} = \frac{30}{1.8} = 16.7 \text{ or } 17 \text{ mL/h}$

5. $\frac{3 \text{ mcg} \times 70 \text{ kg} \times 60 \text{ min/h}}{200 \text{ mcg/mL}} = \frac{12{,}600}{200} = 63 \text{ mL/h}$

6. $\frac{10 \text{ mcg} \times 100 \text{ kg} \times 60 \text{ min/h}}{4000 \text{ mcg/mL}} = \frac{60{,}000}{4000} = 15 \text{ mL/h}$

7. $\frac{30 \text{ mcg} \times 75 \text{ kg} \times 60 \text{ min/h}}{15{,}000 \text{ mcg/mL}} = \frac{135{,}000}{15{,}000} = 9 \text{ mL/h}$

8. $\frac{4 \text{ mg/min} \times 60 \text{ min/h}}{8 \text{ mg/mL}} = \frac{240}{8} = 30 \text{ mL/h}$

9. $\frac{10 \text{ mcg/min} \times 60 \text{ min/h}}{8 \text{ mcg/mL}} = \frac{600}{8} = 75 \text{ mL/h}$

10. $\frac{0.75 \text{ mg/min} \times 60 \text{ min/h}}{1.8 \text{ mg/mL}} = \frac{45}{1.8} = 25 \text{ mL/h}$

11. $\frac{15 \text{ mcg/min} \times 60 \text{ min/h}}{16 \text{ mcg/mL}} = \frac{900}{16} = 56.3 \text{ or } 56 \text{ mL/h}$

12. $\frac{2 \text{ mg/min} \times 60 \text{ min/h}}{8 \text{ mg/mL}} = \frac{120}{8} = 15 \text{ mL/h}$

13. $\frac{10 \text{ mcg} \times 90 \text{ kg} \times 60 \text{ min/h}}{8000 \text{ mcg/mL}} = \frac{54{,}000}{8000} = 6.8 \text{ or } 7 \text{ mL/h}$

14. $\frac{4000 \text{ mcg/mL} \times 13.5 \text{ mL/h}}{60 \text{ min/h} \times 75 \text{ kg}} = \frac{54{,}000}{4500} = 12 \text{ mcg/kg/min}$

15. $\frac{200 \text{ mcg/mL} \times 3 \text{ mL/h}}{60 \text{ min/h}} = \frac{600}{60} = 10 \text{ mcg/min}$

16. $\frac{1.8 \text{ mg/mL} \times 17 \text{ mL/h}}{60 \text{ min/h}} = \frac{30.6}{60} = 0.51 \text{ rounded to } 0.5 \text{ mg/min}$

17. $\frac{15{,}000 \text{ mcg/mL} \times 9 \text{ mL/h}}{60 \text{ min/h} \times 75 \text{ kg}} = \frac{135{,}000}{4500} = 30 \text{ mcg/kg/min}$

18. $\frac{200 \text{ mcg/mL} \times 5 \text{ mL/h}}{60 \text{ min/h}} = \frac{1000}{60} = 16.66 \text{ rounded to } 16.7 \text{ mcg/min}$

19. $\frac{1.8 \text{ mg/mL} \times 20 \text{ mL/h}}{60 \text{ min/h}} = \frac{36}{60} = 0.6 \text{ mg/min}$

20. $\frac{4000 \text{ mcg/mL} \times 15 \text{ mL/h}}{60 \text{ min/h} \times 80 \text{ kg}} = \frac{60{,}000}{4800} = 12.5 \text{ mcg/kg/min}$

21. $\dfrac{400 \text{ mcg/mL} \times 10 \text{ mL/h}}{60 \text{ min/h}} = \dfrac{4000}{60}$
$= 66.66$ rounded to 66.7 mcg/min

22. $\dfrac{3.6 \text{ mg/mL} \times 15 \text{ mL/h}}{60 \text{ min/h}} = \dfrac{54}{60} = 0.9$ mg/min

23. $\dfrac{2 \text{ mg/mL} \times 15 \text{ mL/h}}{60 \text{ min/h}} = \dfrac{30}{60} = 0.5$ mg/min

24. $\dfrac{100 \text{ mcg} \times 80 \text{ kg} \times 60 \text{ min/h}}{10{,}000 \text{ mcg/mL}} = \dfrac{480{,}000}{10{,}000}$
$= 48$ mL/h

CHAPTER 17 Formula Method—Posttest 1, pp. 509–510

1. $\dfrac{5 \text{ mcg} \times 62 \text{ kg} \times 60 \text{ min/h}}{400 \text{ mcg/mL}} = \dfrac{18{,}600}{400}$
$= 46.5$ or 47 mL/h

2. $\dfrac{5 \text{ mcg} \times 50 \text{ kg} \times 60 \text{ min/h}}{4000 \text{ mcg/mL}} = \dfrac{15{,}000}{4000}$
$= 3.8$ or 4 mL/h

3. $\dfrac{20 \text{ mcg} \times 60 \text{ min/h}}{200 \text{ mcg/mL}} = \dfrac{1200}{200} = 6$ mL/h

4. $\dfrac{3 \text{ mg} \times 60 \text{ min/h}}{4 \text{ mg/mL}} = \dfrac{180}{4} = 45$ mL/h

5. $\dfrac{5 \text{ mcg} \times 60 \text{ min/h}}{4 \text{ mcg/mL}} = \dfrac{300}{4} = 75$ mL/h

6. $\dfrac{25 \text{ mcg} \times 50 \text{ kg} \times 60 \text{ min/h}}{10{,}000 \text{ mcg/mL}} = \dfrac{75{,}000}{10{,}000}$
$= 7.5$ or 8 mL/h

7. $\dfrac{0.5 \text{ mg} \times 60 \text{ min/h}}{3.6 \text{ mg/mL}} = \dfrac{30}{3.6} = 8.3$ or 8 mL/h

8. $\dfrac{200 \text{ mcg/mL} \times 63 \text{ mL/h}}{60 \text{ min/h} \times 70 \text{ kg}} = \dfrac{12{,}600}{4200}$
$= 3$ mcg/kg/min

9. $\dfrac{16 \text{ mcg/mL} \times 15 \text{ mL/h}}{60 \text{ min/h}} = \dfrac{240}{60} = 4$ mcg/min

10. $\dfrac{4000 \text{ mcg/mL} \times 15 \text{ mL/h}}{60 \text{ min/h} \times 80 \text{ kg}} = \dfrac{60{,}000}{4800}$
$= 12.5$ mcg/kg/min

CHAPTER 17 Formula Method—Posttest 2, pp. 511–512

1. $\dfrac{3 \text{ mcg} \times 85 \text{ kg} \times 60 \text{ min/h}}{4000 \text{ mcg/mL}} = \dfrac{15{,}300}{4000}$
$= 3.8$ or 4 mL/h

2. $\dfrac{50 \text{ mcg} \times 80 \text{ kg} \times 60 \text{ min/h}}{10{,}000 \text{ mcg/mL}} = \dfrac{240{,}000}{10{,}000}$
$= 24$ mL/h

3. $\dfrac{0.5 \text{ mg} \times 60 \text{ min/h}}{3.6 \text{ mg/mL}} = \dfrac{30}{3.6} = 8.3$ or 8 mL/h

4. $\dfrac{10 \text{ mcg} \times 60 \text{ min/h}}{8 \text{ mcg/mL}} = \dfrac{600}{8} = 75$ mL/h

5. $\dfrac{7 \text{ mcg} \times 55 \text{ kg} \times 60 \text{ min/h}}{5000 \text{ mcg/mL}} = \dfrac{23{,}100}{5000}$
$= 4.6$ or 5 mL/h

6. $\dfrac{2 \text{ mcg} \times 60 \text{ min/h}}{2 \text{ mcg/mL}} = \dfrac{120}{2} = 60$ mL/h

7. $\dfrac{8 \text{ mcg/mL} \times 75 \text{ mL/h}}{60 \text{ min/h}} = \dfrac{600}{60} = 10$ mcg/min

8. $\dfrac{8 \text{ mg/mL} \times 30 \text{ mL/h}}{60 \text{ min/h}} = \dfrac{240}{60} = 4$ mg/min

9. $\dfrac{8000 \text{ mcg/mL} \times 3 \text{ mL/h}}{60 \text{ min/h} \times 80 \text{ kg}} = \dfrac{24{,}000}{4800}$
$= 5$ mcg/kg/min

10. $\dfrac{200 \text{ mcg/mL} \times 50 \text{ mL/h}}{60 \text{ min/h} \times 60 \text{ kg}} = \dfrac{10{,}000}{3600}$
$= 2.77$ rounded to 2.8 mcg/kg/min

CHAPTER **18**

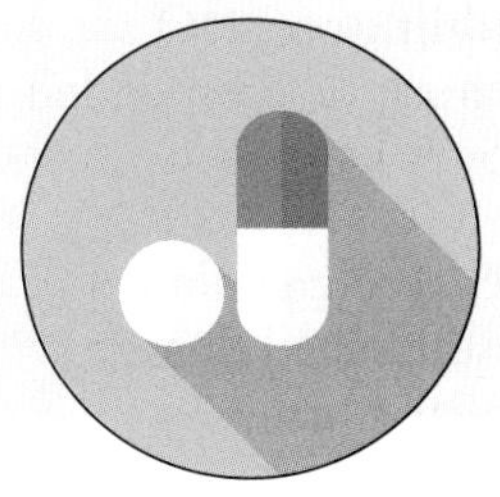

Pediatric Dosages

LEARNING OBJECTIVES

Upon completion of the materials provided in this chapter, you will be able to perform computations accurately by mastering the following mathematical concepts:

1. Converting the weight of a child from pounds to kilograms
2. Converting the neonate and infant weight from grams to kilograms
3. Performing pediatric dosage calculations
4. Calculating the single or individual dose of medications
5. Mathematically prove the prescribed dose is safe and therapeutic
6. Calculating a safe and therapeutic 24-hour dosage range
7. Calculating the single-dose range from a 24-hour dosage range
8. Determining whether the actual dosage (in milligrams per kilograms per 24 hours) is safe to administer
9. Calculating pediatric IV solutions
10. Administering IV medications to pediatric patients
11. Calculating the daily fluid requirements for infants and young children
12. Calculating the body surface area (BSA) for medication administration

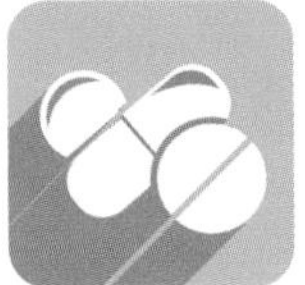

Children are more sensitive than adults to medications because of their weight, height, physical condition, immature systems, and metabolism. Nurses who administer medications to infants and children must be vigilant in determining whether the patient is receiving the correct medication. The correct dose is one of the six rights of drug administration: right patient, medication, route, time, dose, and documentation.

The licensed prescriber or provider will prescribe the medication to be delivered. However, the nurse is responsible for detecting any errors in calculation of dosage, as well as for preparing the medication and administering the drug. The nurse needs to be aware that pediatric dosages are often less than 1 mL; therefore a tuberculin syringe is used for accurate dosing.

Pediatric medications are calculated using the infant or child's kilogram weight. The dosages have been established by the drug companies. Safe and therapeutic dosages are readily available from a reliable source such as *The Harriet Lane Handbook*.

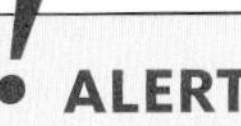

ALERT

Never exceed the adult dose or maximum dose recommended.

In general, pediatric dosages are rounded to the nearest tenth. For infants and young children, doses may be rounded to the nearest hundredth. The child who weighs more than 50 kg **may** receive adult dosages. If the calculated dose is greater than the recommended adult dose, DO NOT administer the medication. A child should not receive higher doses than those recommended for the adult, ever. Many drugs have a "do not exceed" or "max" dose in 24 hours listed; this must always be considered.

Additionally, the licensed prescriber may use the child's body surface area (BSA) to calculate a dosage of medication to administer. The BSA calculation may be used when an established dosage has not been determined by the drug company, as with some anticancer or specialized drugs.

KILOGRAM CONVERSIONS

Converting Pounds to Kilograms

The conversion: 2.2 lb = 1 kg

The weight of infants and young children must be converted from pounds to kilograms to accurately calculate medication doses and daily fluid requirements. Safe and therapeutic drug dosages have been established using kilogram weights.

Round the kilogram weight to the nearest tenth.

EXAMPLE 1: An infant weighs 24 lb. Convert the infant's weight to kilograms.

Dimensional Analysis

$$x \text{ kg} = \frac{1 \text{ kg}}{2.2 \text{ lb}} \times \frac{24 \text{ lb}}{1}$$

$$x \text{ kg} = \frac{24}{2.2}$$

$$x = 10.9 \text{ kg}$$

Proportion

$$2.2 \text{ lb} : 1 \text{ kg} :: 24 \text{ lb} : x \text{ kg}$$

$$2.2 : 1 :: 24 : x$$

$$2.2x = 24$$

$$x = \frac{24}{2.2}$$

$$x = 10.9 \text{ kg}$$

Formula Setup

$$\frac{2.2 \text{ lb}}{1 \text{ kg}} = \frac{24 \text{ lb}}{x \text{ kg}}$$

$$2.2x = 24$$

$$x = 10.9 \text{ kg}$$

EXAMPLE 2: A child weighs 47 lb. Convert the child's weight to kilograms.

Dimensional Analysis

$$x \text{ kg} = \frac{1 \text{ kg}}{2.2 \text{ lb}} \times \frac{47 \text{ lb}}{1}$$

$$x \text{ kg} = \frac{47}{2.2}$$

$$x = 21.36 \text{ or } 21.4 \text{ kg}$$

Proportion

$$2.2 \text{ lb} : 1 \text{ kg} :: 47 \text{ lb} : x \text{ kg}$$

$$2.2 : 1 :: 47 : x$$

$$2.2x = 47$$

$$x = \frac{47}{2.2}$$

$$x = 21.36 \text{ or } 21.4 \text{ kg}$$

Formula Setup

$$\frac{2.2 \text{ lb}}{1 \text{ kg}} = \frac{47 \text{ lb}}{x \text{ kg}}$$

$$2.2x = 47$$

$$x = 21.4 \text{ kg}$$

Converting Grams to Kilograms

The conversion: 1000 g = 1 kg

Newborn (neonate) and some infant weights are measured in grams. Converting grams to kilograms is done as shown below or by simply dividing the number of grams by 1000.

EXAMPLE 1: A neonate weighs 2300 g. Convert to kilograms.

Dimensional Analysis

$$x \text{ kg} = \frac{1 \text{ kg}}{1000 \text{ g}} \times \frac{2300 \text{ g}}{1}$$

$$x \text{ kg} = \frac{2300}{1000}$$

$$x = 2.3 \text{ kg}$$

Proportion

$$1000 \text{ g} : 1 \text{ kg} :: 2300 \text{ g} : x \text{ kg}$$

$$1000 : 1 :: 2300 : x$$

$$1000x = 2300$$

$$x = 2.3 \text{ kg}$$

EXAMPLE 2: A newborn weighs 4630 g at birth. Convert to kilograms.

Dimensional Analysis

$$x \text{ kg} = \frac{1 \text{ kg}}{1000 \text{ g}} \times \frac{4630 \text{ g}}{1}$$

$$x \text{ kg} = \frac{4630}{1000}$$

$x = 4.63$ or 4.6 kg

Proportion

1000 g : 1 kg :: 4630 g : x kg

1000 : 1 :: 4630 : x

$1000x = 4630$

$x = 4.63$ or 4.6 kg

Practice Problems. Convert pounds and grams to kilograms.

1. 27 lb ________ kg
2. 38 lb ________ kg
3. 52 lb ________ kg
4. 5220 g ________ kg
5. 3202 g ________ kg
6. 72 lb ________ kg
7. 16 lb ________ kg
8. 92 lb ________ kg

Answers

1. 12.3 kg
2. 17.3 kg
3. 23.6 kg
4. 5.2 kg
5. 3.2 kg
6. 32.7 kg
7. 7.3 kg
8. 41.8 kg

PEDIATRIC DOSAGE CALCULATIONS

In pediatric dosage calculations, you can use the dimensional analysis, proportion, or $\frac{D}{A} \times Q$ method.

EXAMPLE 1: The licensed prescriber orders diphenhydramine 12.5 mg po q 4–6 h prn for itching. The nurse has available diphenhydramine 25 mg/5 mL. How many milliliters would be needed to administer 12.5 mg? Show math.

Dimensional Analysis

$$x \text{ mL} = \frac{5 \text{ mL}}{25 \text{ mg}} \times \frac{12.5 \text{ mg}}{1}$$

$$x \text{ mL} = \frac{5 \times 12.5}{25}$$

$x = 2.5$ mL

Proportion

25 mg : 5 mL :: 12.5 mg : x mL

$x = 2.5$ mL

$\frac{\mathbf{D}}{\mathbf{A}} \times \mathbf{Q}$

$$\frac{12.5 \text{ mg}}{25 \text{ mg}} \times 5 \text{ mL} = x$$

$x = 2.5$ mL

EXAMPLE 2: The licensed prescriber orders morphine 15 mg by intravenous (IV) piggyback (IVPB) now. You have available morphine 10 mg/mL. How much would you give? Show math.

Dimensional Analysis

$$x \text{ mL} = \frac{1 \text{ mL}}{10 \text{ mg}} \times \frac{15 \text{ mg}}{1}$$

$$x \text{ mL} = \frac{15}{10}$$

$x = 1.5$ mL

Proportion

10 mg : 1 mL :: 15 mg : x mL

$x = 1.5$ mL

$\frac{\mathbf{D}}{\mathbf{A}} \times \mathbf{Q}$

$$\frac{15 \text{ mg}}{10 \text{ mg}} \times 1 \text{ mL} = x$$

$x = 1.5$ mL

CALCULATING THE SINGLE OR INDIVIDUAL DOSE (MILLIGRAMS/DOSE)

Medications such as acetaminophen and ibuprofen are administered as a single dose. This means that each time the infant or child receives the medication, it is calculated in a single or individual dose based on the kilogram weight.

Most of the medications prescribed in this manner are prn medications, which are given as needed for relief of symptoms such as pain, nausea, and fever. Again, the manufacturer of the drug has established a safe and therapeutic dosage or range. The nurse is responsible for administering the single dose that is safe and therapeutic. Therefore it is helpful for the nurse to know how the ordered dose is derived.

To **determine the correct single dose** for the child, you must **calculate the correct dose. A systematic approach is helpful in determining the safe and therapeutic dose range:**

- Change the child's weight in pounds to kilograms.
- Find the recommended dosage in a reliable source.
- Multiply the kilogram weight by the recommended dose(s).
- The answer is the individual or single dose *(mg/dose)* of medication to be given each time the child receives the medication.

EXAMPLE 1: A child weighs 22 lb. The child needs acetaminophen for pain and fever.

Step 1. Weight 22 lb = 10 kg

Step 2. Recommended 10 to 15 mg/kg/dose q 4–6 h

Step 3. Calculation

(Minimum Recommended Dose)

Dimensional Analysis

$$\frac{x \text{ mg}}{\text{dose}} = \frac{10 \text{ mg}}{\text{kg/dose}} \times \frac{1 \text{ kg}}{2.2 \text{ lb}} \times \frac{22 \text{ lb}}{1}$$

$$\frac{x \text{ mg}}{\text{dose}} = \frac{10 \times 22}{2.2}$$

$x = 100$ mg/dose

Proportion

$10 \text{ mg} : 1 \text{ kg} :: x \text{ mg} : 10 \text{ kg}$

$x = 10 \times 10$

$x = 100$ mg/dose

(Maximum Recommended Dose)

Dimensional Analysis

$$\frac{x \text{ mg}}{\text{dose}} = \frac{15 \text{ mg}}{\text{kg/dose}} \times \frac{1 \text{ kg}}{2.2 \text{ lb}} \times \frac{22 \text{ lb}}{1}$$

$$\frac{x \text{ mg}}{\text{dose}} = \frac{15 \times 22}{2.2}$$

$x = 150$ mg/dose

Proportion

$15 \text{ mg} : 1 \text{ kg} :: x \text{ mg} : 10 \text{ kg}$

$x = 15 \times 10$

$x = 150$ mg/dose

The child may receive 100 to 150 mg each time he or she is given acetaminophen. This is the single or individual dose. The dose is both safe and therapeutic for this child.

- A dose smaller than 100 mg is considered **safe but may not be therapeutic for the child's weight.**
- Doses larger than 150 mg are considered too much for the child's weight and may **exceed the therapeutic range.** There are exceptions—some dosages may be higher. Check *The Hariett Lane Handbook* or other pediatric dosing manuals.

! ALERT

Acetaminophen:
Never give more than 5 doses in 24 hours to the infant or young child.
Never exceed 4000 mg/day (4 grams) for the older child and adult.
Teach parents or caregivers.

EXAMPLE 2: Calculate a safe and therapeutic dose range of ibuprofen for a child who weighs 36 lb. Ibuprofen is available as 100 mg/5 mL. How many milliliters would you need to administer for the ordered dose to be safe and therapeutic?

Step 1. Weight 36 lb = 16.4 kg

Step 2. Recommended 5 to 10 mg/kg/dose q 6–8 h

Step 3. Calculations

(Minimum Recommended Dose)

Dimensional Analysis

$$\frac{x \text{ mg}}{\text{dose}} = \frac{5 \text{ mg}}{\text{kg/dose}} \times \frac{1 \text{ kg}}{2.2 \text{ lb}} \times \frac{36 \text{ lb}}{1}$$

$$\frac{x \text{ mg}}{\text{dose}} = \frac{5 \times 36}{2.2}$$

$x = 81.8$ mg

Proportion

5 mg : 1 kg :: x mg : 16.4 kg

$x = 5 \times 16.4$

$x = 82$ mg/dose

(Maximum Recommended Dose)

Dimensional Analysis

$$\frac{x \text{ mg}}{\text{dose}} = \frac{10 \text{ mg}}{\text{kg/dose}} \times \frac{1 \text{ kg}}{2.2 \text{ lb}} \times \frac{36 \text{ lb}}{1}$$

$$\frac{x \text{ mg}}{\text{dose}} = \frac{10 \times 36}{2.2}$$

$x = 163.6$ mg/dose

Proportion

10 mg : 1 kg :: x mg : 16.4 kg

$x = 10 \times 16.4$

$x = 164$ mg/dose

The safe and therapeutic single-dose range for this child is 81.8 to 163.6 mg when using the dimensional analysis method and 82 to 164 mg when using the proportion method.

Step 4. Now perform dosage calculations for the single-dose range using the 100 mg/5 mL strength:

(Minimum Recommended Dose)

Dimensional Analysis

x mL =

$$x \text{ mL} = \frac{5 \text{ mL}}{100 \text{ mg}}$$

$$x \text{ mL} = \frac{5 \text{ mL}}{100 \text{ mg}} \times \frac{81.8 \text{ mg}}{1}$$

$$x = \frac{5 \times 81.8}{100} = 4.09 \text{ mL}$$

Proportion

100 mg : 5 mL :: 82 mg : x mL

$100x = 5 \times 82$

$$x = \frac{410}{100}$$

$x = 4.1$ mL

(Maximum Recommended Dose)

Dimensional Analysis

x mL =

$$x \text{ mL} = \frac{5 \text{ mL}}{100 \text{ mg}}$$

$$x \text{ mL} = \frac{5 \text{ mL}}{100 \text{ mg}} \times \frac{163.6 \text{ mg}}{1}$$

$$x = \frac{5 \times 163.6}{100} = 8.18 \text{ mL}$$

Proportion

100 mg : 5 mL :: 164 mg : x mL

$100x = 5 \times 164$

$$x = \frac{820}{100}$$

$x = 8.2$ mL

MATHEMATICALLY PROVE WHETHER THE PRESCRIBED DOSE IS SAFE AND THERAPEUTIC (MILLIGRAMS/KILOGRAM/DOSE)

This method will **determine whether the child is receiving a safe and therapeutic dosage** of the drug that is prescribed by the licensed prescriber. The nurse must determine whether the ordered dose is within the recommended range.

Even though the licensed prescriber has prescribed the medication to be given, it is the nurse's responsibility to mathematically prove the prescribed dose is safe and therapeutic to administer to the child. This is done by **dividing the ordered dosage by the child's weight in kilograms (mg/kg/dose).** A systematic approach is needed.

- Obtain the child's weight in kilograms.
- Obtain the ordered dosage.
- Divide the ordered dose by the child's weight.
- The answer is the mg/kg/dose (for each dose administered).
- Check your drug book to determine whether the ordered dose is safe and therapeutic in the recommended dosage range.

EXAMPLE: The licensed prescriber has ordered 210 mg of acetaminophen q 4–6 h for pain and fever for a postoperative child. The child weighs 39 lb. The recommended dose range for acetaminophen is 10 to 15 mg/kg/dose q 4–6 h. Acetaminophen is supplied as 160 mg/5 mL.

Is the ordered dose safe and therapeutic to administer? If the dose ordered is safe and therapeutic to administer, how many milliliters will be needed?

Step 1. Weight 39 lb = 17.7 kg

Step 2. Ordered 210 mg q 4–6 h

Step 3. Calculation

Dimensional Analysis

$$\frac{x \text{ mg}}{\text{kg/dose}} = \frac{210 \text{ mg}}{\text{dose}} \times \frac{2.2 \text{ lb}}{1 \text{ kg}} \times \frac{}{39 \text{ lb}}$$

$$\frac{x \text{ mg}}{\text{kg/dose}} = \frac{210 \text{ mg}}{\text{dose}} \times \frac{2.2 \text{ lb}}{1 \text{ kg}} \times \frac{}{39 \text{ lb}}$$

$$\frac{x \text{ mg}}{\text{kg/dose}} = \frac{210 \times 2.2}{39}$$

$x = 11.84$ or 11.8 mg/kg/dose

Formula

$$\frac{210 \text{ mg}}{17.7 \text{ kg/dose}} = 11.86 \text{ or } 11.9 \text{ mg/kg/dose}$$

The dose for this child is 11.8 mg/kg/dose when using the dimensional analysis method and 11.9 mg/kg/dose when using the formula method.

Step 4. Recommended 10 to 15 mg/kg/dose

Yes, it is safe to administer the acetaminophen because it is within the safe and therapeutic dosage range of 10 to 15 mg/kg/dose.

Step 5. Perform dosage calculation using 160 mg/5 mL concentration:

Dimensional Analysis

$$x \text{ mL} = \frac{5 \text{ mL}}{160 \text{ mg}} \times \frac{210 \text{ mg}}{1}$$

$$x \text{ mL} = \frac{5 \times 210}{160} = 6.56 \text{ or } 6.6 \text{ mL}$$

Proportion

160 mg : 5 mL :: 210 mg : x mL

$160x = 5 \times 210$

$$x = \frac{1050}{160}$$

$x = 6.56$ or 6.6 mL

Remember to round all doses to the nearest tenth. Exceptions: Round all narcotics, antiepileptics, and cardiac medications to *nearest hundredth*. Medications that may be rounded to the nearest hundredth include phenobarbital, morphine, dilantin, digoxin, and anticancer drugs.

CALCULATE THE 24-HOUR DOSAGE (RANGES)

Many drugs are calculated based on the recommended 24-hour dose, then divided into single doses to be given every 12, 8, 6, or 4 hours or as recommended by the drug manufacturers. These divided time schedules vary, and the licensed prescriber, nurse practitioner, or licensed prescriber's assistant will order the medication based on the recommended schedules.

Antibiotics especially are given this way. Additionally, an antibiotic may be given in dosages or ranges that have been found to be effective for the child's diagnosis. The licensed prescriber chooses how often the medication is to be delivered. An example of an antibiotic with many dosing choices is ampicillin.

Recommended dosages for ampicillin may be any of the following:

<2 kg	50 to 100 mg/kg/24 h/q 12 h
>2 kg	75 to 150 mg/kg/24 h/q 8 h
Mild to moderate infection	25 to 200 mg/kg/24 h/q 6–8 h
Severe infection	200 to 400 mg/kg/24 h/q 4–6 h

The licensed prescriber must determine the dosage to be given to the infant or child. If an infant or child is diagnosed with otitis media (OM), then the licensed prescriber may choose the dosage of antibiotic in the mild to moderate range. However, if an infant is admitted with a diagnosis of fever of undetermined origin, sepsis, or meningitis, then the licensed prescriber may decide to prescribe a larger dosage of the antibiotic, as in the severe infection range.

Knowing the diagnosis is helpful in determining whether the infant or child will be receiving safe and therapeutic dosages of antibiotics. Nurses who administer antibiotics or antiinfectives can learn how to determine the doses needed for the patient. **However, only the licensed prescriber, advanced practice nurse, or licensed prescriber's assistant can prescribe and order the infant's or child's medications.**

EXAMPLE 1: An infant is admitted to the hospital to rule out sepsis. The infant weighs 8 lb. Ampicillin is prescribed. Calculate a safe and therapeutic 24-hour dosage range for this infant with a possible severe infection.

Step 1. Weight 8 lb = 3.6 kg

Step 2. Recommended 200 to 400 mg/kg/24 h q 4–6 h

Step 3. Calculation

(Minimum Recommended Dose)

Dimensional Analysis

$$\frac{x\text{ mg}}{\text{day}} = \frac{200\text{ mg}}{\text{kg/day}} \times \frac{1\text{ kg}}{2.2\text{ lb}} \times \frac{8\text{ lb}}{1}$$

$$\frac{x\text{ mg}}{\text{day}} = \frac{200\text{ mg}}{\cancel{\text{kg}}\text{/day}} \times \frac{1\ \cancel{\text{kg}}}{2.2\ \cancel{\text{lb}}} \times \frac{8\ \cancel{\text{lb}}}{1}$$

$$\frac{x\text{ mg}}{\text{day}} = \frac{200 \times 8}{2.2}$$

$x = 727.27$ or 727.3 mg/24 h

Formula

3.6 kg × 200 mg/kg/24 h =

$3.6\ \cancel{\text{kg}} \times 200\text{ mg}/\cancel{\text{kg}}/24\text{ h} = 720\text{ mg}/24\text{ h}$

(Maximum Recommended Dose)

Dimensional Analysis

$$\frac{x\text{ mg}}{\text{day}} = \frac{400\text{ mg}}{\text{kg/day}} \times \frac{1\text{ kg}}{2.2\text{ lb}} \times \frac{8\text{ lb}}{1}$$

$$\frac{x\text{ mg}}{\text{day}} = \frac{400\text{ mg}}{\cancel{\text{kg}}\text{/day}} \times \frac{1\ \cancel{\text{kg}}}{2.2\ \cancel{\text{lb}}} \times \frac{8\ \cancel{\text{lb}}}{1}$$

$$\frac{x\text{ mg}}{\text{day}} = \frac{400 \times 8}{2.2}$$

$x = 1454.54$ or 1454.5 mg/24 h

Formula

3.6 kg × 400 mg/kg/24 h =

$3.6\ \cancel{\text{kg}} \times 400\text{ mg}/\cancel{\text{kg}}/24\text{ h} = 1440\text{ mg}/24\text{ h}$

Step 4. 24-hour dosage range

Dimensional Analysis

727.3 to 1454.5 mg/24 h

Formula

720 to 1440 mg/24 h

This means that the infant can receive 727.3 to 1454.5 mg in a 24-hour period when the dimensional analysis method is used or 720 to 1440 mg in a 24-hour period when the formula method is used.

EXAMPLE 2: The child weighs 35 lb and is diagnosed with OM. The licensed prescriber prescribes amoxicillin. Calculate a safe and therapeutic 24-hour dosage range for this patient.

Step 1. Weight 35 lb = 15.9 kg

Step 2. Recommended 25 to 50 mg/kg/24 h two or three times a day

Adult dosage 250 to 500 mg/dose two times a day

Step 3. Calculation

(Minimum Recommended Dose)

Dimensional Analysis

$$\frac{x\text{ mg}}{\text{day}} = \frac{25\text{ mg}}{\text{kg/day}} \times \frac{1\text{ kg}}{2.2\text{ lb}} \times \frac{35\text{ lb}}{1}$$

$$\frac{x\text{ mg}}{\text{day}} = \frac{25\text{ mg}}{\cancel{\text{kg}}\text{/day}} \times \frac{1\ \cancel{\text{kg}}}{2.2\ \cancel{\text{lb}}} \times \frac{35\ \cancel{\text{lb}}}{1}$$

$$\frac{x\text{ mg}}{\text{day}} = \frac{25 \times 35}{2.2}$$

$x = 397.72$ or 397.7 mg/24 h

Formula

15.9 kg × 25 mg/kg/24 h =

$15.9\ \cancel{\text{kg}} \times 25\text{ mg}/\cancel{\text{kg}}/24\text{ h} = 397.5\text{ mg/24 h}$

(Maximum Recommended Dose)

Dimensional Analysis

$$\frac{x\text{ mg}}{\text{day}} = \frac{50\text{ mg}}{\text{kg/day}} \times \frac{1\text{ kg}}{2.2\text{ lb}} \times \frac{35\text{ lb}}{1}$$

$$\frac{x\text{ mg}}{\text{day}} = \frac{50\text{ mg}}{\cancel{\text{kg}}\text{/day}} \times \frac{1\ \cancel{\text{kg}}}{2.2\ \cancel{\text{lb}}} \times \frac{35\ \cancel{\text{lb}}}{1}$$

$$\frac{x\text{ mg}}{\text{day}} = \frac{50 \times 35}{2.2}$$

$x = 795.45$ or 795.5 mg/24 h

Formula

15.9 kg × 50 mg/kg/24 h =

$15.9\ \cancel{\text{kg}} \times 50\text{ mg}/\cancel{\text{kg}}/24\text{ h} = 795\text{ mg/24 h}$

Step 4. 24-hour dosage range

Dimensional Analysis
397.7 to 795.5 mg/24 h

Formula
397.5 to 795 mg/24 h

This means that the child can receive 397.7 to 795.5 mg in a 24-hour period when the dimensional analysis method is used or 397.5 to 795 mg in a 24-hour period when the formula method is used.

Remember not to exceed the adult dose or "max" dose. The licensed prescriber will now decide how often the child will receive the medication. This is called the individual or single dose, based on 24 hours.

CALCULATE THE INDIVIDUAL DOSE OR SINGLE DOSE (MILLIGRAMS/KILOGRAM/24 HOURS DIVIDED)

The licensed prescriber will now determine how often the antibiotic will be administered as a single or individual dose. First determine the 24-hour dosage range. Then divide the 24-hour dosage into single doses (the number of times per day the medication is to be given).

- This is the individual dose each time the patient receives the medication.
- These times are established by the drug companies (e.g., q 4 h, q 6 h, q 8 h, q 12 h, or every day).
- **As long as the dose does not exceed the maximum dose established in 24 hours and the dose does not exceed the adult dose, then it can be given safely.**
- The licensed prescriber will decide how often the medication is to be given.

EXAMPLE 1: A child weighs 22 lb. The licensed prescriber prescribes ampicillin 100 to 200 mg/kg/24 h divided q 6 h. Calculate the individual dose for ampicillin.

Step 1. Weight 22 lb = 10 kg

Step 2. Recommended 100 to 200 mg/kg/24 h divided q 6 h

Step 3. **Calculation**

(Minimum Recommended Dose)

Dimensional Analysis

$$\frac{x \text{ mg}}{\text{dose}} = \frac{100 \text{ mg}}{\text{kg/day}} \times \frac{1 \text{ kg}}{2.2 \text{ lb}} \times \frac{22 \text{ lb}}{1}$$

$$\frac{x \text{ mg}}{\text{dose}} = \frac{100 \text{ mg}}{\cancel{\text{kg}}\text{/day}} \times \frac{1 \cancel{\text{kg}}}{2.2 \cancel{\text{lb}}} \times \frac{22 \cancel{\text{lb}}}{1}$$

Formula

$10 \text{ kg} \times 100 \text{ mg/kg/24 h} =$

$10 \cancel{\text{kg}} \times 100 \text{ mg/}\cancel{\text{kg}}\text{/24 h} = 1000 \text{ mg/24 h}$

(Maximum Recommended Dose)

Dimensional Analysis

$$\frac{x \text{ mg}}{\text{dose}} = \frac{200 \text{ mg}}{\text{kg/day}} \times \frac{1 \text{ kg}}{2.2 \text{ lb}} \times \frac{22 \text{ lb}}{1}$$

$$\frac{x \text{ mg}}{\text{dose}} = \frac{200 \text{ mg}}{\cancel{\text{kg}}\text{/day}} \times \frac{1 \cancel{\text{kg}}}{2.2 \cancel{\text{lb}}} \times \frac{22 \cancel{\text{lb}}}{1}$$

Formula

$10 \text{ kg} \times 200 \text{ mg/kg/24 h} =$

$10 \cancel{\text{kg}} \times 200 \text{ mg/}\cancel{\text{kg}}\text{/24 h} = 2000 \text{ mg/24 h}$

Step 4. **Divided q 6 h (4 doses in 24 h)**

(Minimum Recommended Dose)

Dimensional Analysis

$$\frac{x \text{ mg}}{\text{dose}} = \frac{100 \text{ mg}}{\text{kg/day}} \times \frac{1 \text{ kg}}{2.2 \text{ lb}} \times \frac{22 \text{ lb}}{1} \times \frac{1 \text{ day}}{4 \text{ doses}}$$

$$\frac{x \text{ mg}}{\text{dose}} = \frac{100 \text{ mg}}{\cancel{\text{kg}}/\cancel{\text{day}}} \times \frac{1 \cancel{\text{kg}}}{2.2 \cancel{\text{lb}}} \times \frac{22 \cancel{\text{lb}}}{1} \times \frac{1 \cancel{\text{day}}}{4 \text{ doses}}$$

$$x = \frac{100 \times 22}{2.2 \times 4} = 250 \text{ mg/dose}$$

Formula

$$\frac{1000 \text{ mg/24 h}}{4 \text{ doses/24 h}} =$$

$$\frac{1000 \text{ mg/}\cancel{24 \text{ h}}}{4 \text{ doses/}\cancel{24 \text{ h}}} = 250 \text{ mg/dose}$$

(Maximum Recommended Dose)

Dimensional Analysis

$$\frac{x \text{ mg}}{\text{dose}} = \frac{200 \text{ mg}}{\text{kg/day}} \times \frac{1 \text{ kg}}{2.2 \text{ lb}} \times \frac{22 \text{ lb}}{1} \times \frac{1 \text{ day}}{4 \text{ doses}}$$

$$\frac{x \text{ mg}}{\text{dose}} = \frac{200 \text{ mg}}{\cancel{\text{kg}}/\cancel{\text{day}}} \times \frac{1 \cancel{\text{kg}}}{2.2 \cancel{\text{lb}}} \times \frac{22 \cancel{\text{lb}}}{1} \times \frac{1 \cancel{\text{day}}}{4 \text{ doses}}$$

$$x = \frac{200 \times 22}{2.2 \times 4} = 500 \text{ mg/dose}$$

Formula

$$\frac{2000 \text{ mg/24 h}}{4 \text{ doses/24 h}} =$$

$$\frac{2000 \text{ mg/}\cancel{24 \text{ h}}}{4 \text{ doses/}\cancel{24 \text{ h}}} = 500 \text{ mg/dose}$$

Step 5. **Single-dose range** 250 to 500 mg/dose

EXAMPLE 2: A child weighs 60 lb. The licensed prescriber orders cefuroxime. The recommended dosage is 75 to 100 mg/kg/24 h q 8 h. What is the safe and therapeutic dosage range for this child?

Step 1. **Weight** 60 lb = 27.3 kg

Step 2. **Recommended** 75 to 100 mg/kg/24 h q 8 h

Step 3. Calculation

(Minimum Recommended Dose)

Dimensional Analysis

$$\frac{x\text{ mg}}{\text{dose}} = \frac{75\text{ mg}}{\text{kg/day}} \times \frac{1\text{ kg}}{2.2\text{ lb}} \times \frac{60\text{ lb}}{1}$$

$$\frac{x\text{ mg}}{\text{dose}} = \frac{75\text{ mg}}{\cancel{\text{kg}}/\text{day}} \times \frac{1\ \cancel{\text{kg}}}{2.2\ \cancel{\text{lb}}} \times \frac{60\ \cancel{\text{lb}}}{1}$$

Formula

$27.3\text{ kg} \times 75\text{ mg/kg/24 h} =$

$27.3\ \cancel{\text{kg}} \times 75\text{ mg/}\cancel{\text{kg}}\text{/24 h} = 2047.5\text{ mg/24 h}$

(Maximum Recommended Dose)

Dimensional Analysis

$$\frac{x\text{ mg}}{\text{dose}} = \frac{100\text{ mg}}{\text{kg/day}} \times \frac{1\text{ kg}}{2.2\text{ lb}} \times \frac{60\text{ lb}}{1}$$

$$\frac{x\text{ mg}}{\text{dose}} = \frac{100\text{ mg}}{\cancel{\text{kg}}/\text{day}} \times \frac{1\ \cancel{\text{kg}}}{2.2\ \cancel{\text{lb}}} \times \frac{60\ \cancel{\text{lb}}}{1}$$

Formula

$27.3\text{ kg} \times 100\text{ mg/kg/24 h} =$

$27.3\ \cancel{\text{kg}} \times 100\text{ mg/}\cancel{\text{kg}}\text{/24 h} = 2730\text{ mg/24 h}$

Step 4. Divided q 8 h (3 doses in 24 h)

(Minimum Recommended Dose)

Dimensional Analysis

$$\frac{x\text{ mg}}{\text{dose}} = \frac{75\text{ mg}}{\text{kg/day}} \times \frac{1\text{ kg}}{2.2\text{ lb}} \times \frac{60\text{ lb}}{1} \times \frac{1\text{ day}}{3\text{ doses}}$$

$$\frac{x\text{ mg}}{\text{dose}} = \frac{75\text{ mg}}{\cancel{\text{kg}}/\cancel{\text{day}}} \times \frac{1\ \cancel{\text{kg}}}{2.2\ \cancel{\text{lb}}} \times \frac{60\ \cancel{\text{lb}}}{1} \times \frac{1\ \cancel{\text{day}}}{3\text{ doses}}$$

$$x = \frac{75 \times 60}{2.2 \times 3} = 681.81\text{ or }681.8\text{ mg/dose}$$

Formula

$$\frac{2047.5\text{ mg/24 h}}{3\text{ doses/24 h}} =$$

$$\frac{2047.5\text{ mg/}\cancel{24\text{ h}}}{3\text{ doses/}\cancel{24\text{ h}}} = 682.5\text{ mg/dose}$$

(Maximum Recommended Dose)

Dimensional Analysis

$$\frac{x\text{ mg}}{\text{dose}} = \frac{100\text{ mg}}{\text{kg/day}} \times \frac{1\text{ kg}}{2.2\text{ lb}} \times \frac{60\text{ lb}}{1} \times \frac{1\text{ day}}{3\text{ doses}}$$

$$\frac{x\text{ mg}}{\text{dose}} = \frac{100\text{ mg}}{\cancel{\text{kg}}/\cancel{\text{day}}} \times \frac{1\ \cancel{\text{kg}}}{2.2\ \cancel{\text{lb}}} \times \frac{60\ \cancel{\text{lb}}}{1} \times \frac{1\ \cancel{\text{day}}}{3\text{ doses}}$$

$$x = \frac{100 \times 60}{2.2 \times 3} = 909.09\text{ or }909.1\text{ mg/dose}$$

Formula

$$\frac{2730\text{ mg/24 h}}{3\text{ doses/24 h}} =$$

$$\frac{2730\text{ mg/}\cancel{24\text{ h}}}{3\text{ doses/}\cancel{24\text{ h}}} = 910\text{ mg/dose}$$

Step 5. Single-dose range

681.8 to 909.1 mg/dose (DA)
682.5 to 910 mg/dose (formula)

DETERMINE THE ACTUAL MILLIGRAMS/KILOGRAM/24 HOURS OR DOSE/KILOGRAM/24 HOURS

The nurse must understand how to *prove* that the patient is actually receiving a safe and therapeutic dosage or range. When a licensed prescriber prescribes a medication, he or she has a range from which to choose. As a nurse, you need to check to see whether the medication falls within the safe and therapeutic dosage or range. This is important because medication doses are patient–weight specific.

Determining the actual milligrams per kilogram per 24 hours that the patient is receiving is done simply by dividing the actual milligrams to be given in 24 hours by the patient's weight. Remember that the licensed prescriber has already prescribed the medication based on the recommended dose in milligrams per kilogram per 24 hours. **For nurses, knowing how to prove safe and therapeutic dosing is critical.**

To determine (prove) whether the patient is receiving a safe and therapeutic dosage, the nurse will need to:

- Obtain the infant's or child's kilogram weight.
- Obtain the medication order.
- Determine the amount of medication the child will receive in the 24-hour period (the 24-hour dosage).
- Divide the prescribed 24-hour dosage by the patient's weight.
- Compare the ordered dosage with the safe and therapeutic dosage range.

There is no need to calculate a dosage range because the licensed prescriber has already done this.

EXAMPLE 1: A 4-year-old child is receiving vancomycin 220 mg q 6 h IV via syringe pump. She weighs 48 lb. Safe and therapeutic dosage range is 40 to 60 mg/kg/24 h q 6 h.

How many milligrams per kilogram per 24 hours is this child receiving? Is the ordered dosage safe and therapeutic?

Step 1. **Weight** 48 lb = 21.8 kg

Step 2. **Ordered** Vancomycin 220 mg q 6 h

Step 3. **24-hour dosage**

(Minimum Recommended Dose)

Dimensional Analysis

$$\frac{x \text{ mg}}{\text{kg/24 h}} = \frac{220 \text{ mg}}{\text{dose}} \times \frac{4 \text{ doses}}{1 \text{ day}}$$

Formula

$$220 \text{ mg} \times 4 \text{ doses} = 880 \text{ mg/24 h}$$

Step 4. **mg/kg/24 h**

Dimensional Analysis

$$\frac{x \text{ mg}}{\text{kg/day}} = \frac{220 \text{ mg}}{\text{dose}} \times \frac{4 \text{ doses}}{1 \text{ day}} \times \frac{2.2 \text{ lb}}{1 \text{ kg}} \times \frac{}{48 \text{ lb}}$$

$$\frac{x \text{ mg}}{\text{kg/day}} = \frac{220 \text{ mg}}{\cancel{\text{dose}}} \times \frac{4 \cancel{\text{doses}}}{1 \text{ day}} \times \frac{2.2 \cancel{\text{lb}}}{1 \text{ kg}} \times \frac{}{48 \cancel{\text{lb}}}$$

$$x = \frac{220 \times 4 \times 2.2}{48} = 40.3 \text{ mg/kg/24 h (1 day)}$$

Formula

$$\frac{880 \text{ kg/24 h}}{21.8 \text{ kg}} =$$

40.36 or 40.4 mg/kg/24 h

Step 5. **Recommended** 40 to 60 mg/kg/24 h q 6-8 h

The patient is receiving 40.3 (DA) or 40.4 (formula) mg/kg/24 h, which is within the safe and therapeutic range.

EXAMPLE 2: A 75-lb patient is receiving 900 mg of ampicillin IVPB q 6 h. How many milligrams per kilogram per 24 hours is the patient receiving? Is the dosage safe and therapeutic?

Step 1. **Weight** 75 lb = 34.1 kg

Step 2. **Ordered** Ampicillin 900 mg IVPB q 6 h

Step 3. 24-hour dosage

Dimensional Analysis

$$\frac{x \text{ mg}}{\text{kg/24 h}} = \frac{900 \text{ mg}}{\text{dose}} \times \frac{4 \text{ doses}}{1 \text{ day}}$$

Formula

$$900 \text{ mg} \times 4 \text{ doses} = 3600 \text{ mg/24 h}$$

Step 4. mg/kg/24 h

Dimensional Analysis

$$\frac{x \text{ mg}}{\text{kg/day}} = \frac{900 \text{ mg}}{\text{dose}} \times \frac{4 \text{ doses}}{1 \text{ day}} \times \frac{2.2 \text{ lb}}{1 \text{ kg}} \times \frac{}{75 \text{ lb}}$$

$$\frac{x \text{ mg}}{\text{kg/day}} = \frac{900 \text{ mg}}{\cancel{\text{dose}}} \times \frac{4 \cancel{\text{doses}}}{1 \text{ day}} \times \frac{2.2 \cancel{\text{lb}}}{1 \text{ kg}} \times \frac{}{75 \cancel{\text{lb}}}$$

$$x = \frac{900 \times 4 \times 2.2}{75} = 105.6 \text{ mg/kg/24 h (1 day)}$$

Formula

$$\frac{3600 \text{ mg/24 h}}{34.1 \text{ kg}} =$$

105.6 mg/kg/24 h

Step 5. Recommended 100 to 200 mg/kg/24 h q 6–8 h

The patient is receiving a safe and therapeutic dose at 105.6 mg/kg/24 h. Between 100 and 200 mg/kg/24 h is safe.

CALCULATING PEDIATRIC IV SOLUTIONS

Pediatric patients require smaller volumes of IV fluids and medications than adults. An IV pump, a buretrol (soluset), or both may be used for the pediatric patient. Each facility has guidelines for preparing and administering IV solutions and medications to the pediatric patient. Also, for a pediatric patient, IV tubing with a drop factor of 60 gtt/mL is usually recommended.

The concentration of the IV medication is also an important factor in medication administration. Administering a medication with a higher concentration than recommended is avoided because of the vein irritation that can result.

EXAMPLE 1: Infuse 100 mL of 0.9% NS over 5 hours to a 6-month-old child. How many milliliters per hour should the IV pump be programmed for?

Dimensional Analysis

$$\frac{x \text{ mL}}{\text{h}} = \frac{100 \text{ mL}}{5 \text{ h}}$$

$$x = 20 \text{ mL/h}$$

Formula

$$\frac{\text{Total volume to be infused}}{\text{Total time in hours}} = x \text{ mL/h}$$

$$\frac{100 \text{ mL}}{5 \text{ h}} = 20 \text{ mL/h}$$

EXAMPLE 2: Infuse 150 mL of D_5LR over 3 hours to a 3-year-old child. How many milliliters per hour should the IV pump be programmed for?

Dimensional Analysis

$$\frac{x \text{ mL}}{\text{h}} = \frac{150 \text{ mL}}{3 \text{ h}}$$

$$x = 50 \text{ mL/h}$$

Formula

$$\frac{\text{Total volume to be infused}}{\text{Total time in hours}} = x \text{ mL/h}$$

$$\frac{150 \text{ mL}}{3 \text{ h}} = 50 \text{ mL/h}$$

If an IV pump is not used, IV fluids may be given by gravity.

EXAMPLE 3: Infuse 200 mL lactated Ringer's solution (LR) over 4 hours to an 8-year-old child. The tubing drop factor is 60 gtt/mL. How many drops per minute of LR should be infused?

Dimensional Analysis

$$\frac{x \text{ gtt}}{\text{min}} = \frac{60 \text{ gtt}}{1 \cancel{\text{mL}}} \times \frac{200 \cancel{\text{mL}}}{4 \cancel{\text{h}}} \times \frac{1 \cancel{\text{h}}}{60 \text{ min}}$$

$$\frac{x \text{ gtt}}{\text{min}} = \frac{60 \times 200}{4 \times 60}$$

$x = 50$ gtt/min

Formula

$$\frac{\text{Total volume to be infused}}{\text{Total time in hours}} \times \text{drop factor}$$

a. Convert hours to minutes

1 h : 60 min :: 4 h : x min

$x = 60 \times 4 = 240$ min

b. $\frac{200 \text{ mL}}{240 \text{ min}} \times 60 \text{ gtt/mL} = 50 \text{ gtt/min}$

EXAMPLE 4: Infuse 500 mL of D_5W over 8 hours to a 14-year-old child. The tubing drop factor is 60 gtt/mL. How many drops per minute of D_5W should be infused?

Dimensional Analysis

$$\frac{x \text{ gtt}}{\text{min}} = \frac{60 \text{ gtt}}{1 \text{ mL}} \times \frac{500 \text{ mL}}{8 \text{ h}} \times \frac{1 \text{ h}}{60 \text{ min}}$$

$$\frac{x \text{ gtt}}{\text{min}} = \frac{60 \times 500}{8 \times 60}$$

$x = 62.5$ rounded to 63 gtt/min

Formula

$$\frac{\text{Total volume to be infused}}{\text{Total time in minutes}} \times \text{drop factor}$$

a. Convert hours to minutes

1 h : 60 min :: 8 h : x min

$x = 60 \times 8 = 480$ min

b. $\frac{500 \text{ mL}}{480 \text{ min}} \times 60 \text{ gtt/mL}$

$= 62.5$ rounded to 63 gtt/min

ADMINISTRATION OF IV MEDICATIONS TO PEDIATRIC PATIENTS

The formulas to calculate the administration rate of IV medications to pediatric patients are not different from those used for adults. The difference in administration of medications to a pediatric patient lies in the volume of solution used. Pediatric patients require a smaller volume of IV solutions; therefore care must be taken to give the medication at the recommended infusion concentration. Using a concentration that is higher than recommended may result in vein irritation and phlebitis. Unit policies and IV drug books provide the guidelines needed for appropriate concentration of IV medications for the pediatric patient.

If the medication is to be infused with an IV pump, the formula would be

$$\frac{\text{Total volume to be infused}}{\text{Total time for infusion in hours}} = x \text{ mL/h}$$

If the medication is to be infused with a buretrol (soluset) by gravity (Figure 18-1), then the formula would be

$$\frac{\text{Total volume to be infused}}{\text{Total time for infusion in minutes}} \times \text{Drop factor} = x \text{ gtt/min}$$

EXAMPLE 1: An 18-month-old child has cefazolin 450 mg q 4 h IVPB over 15 minutes ordered. The child weighs 19 kg. The maximum recommended infusion concentration is 50 mg/mL. The vial of medication has a concentration of cefazolin 250 mg/mL. How many milliliters of medication will provide

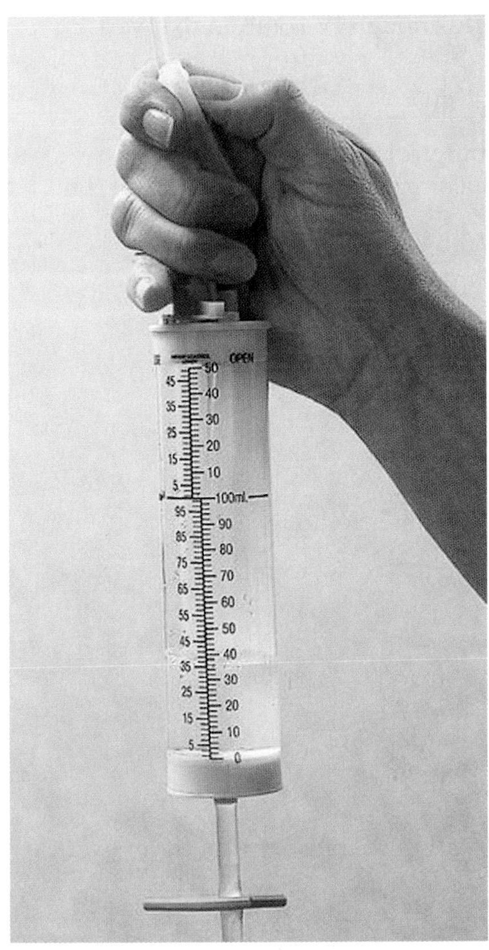

FIGURE 18-1 Using a buretrol to administer a medication. (Modified from Potter PA, Perry AG, Stockert PA, Hall AM: *Fundamentals of nursing,* ed 9, St Louis, 2018, Elsevier.)

450 mg? ______ How many milliliters of IV solution need to be added to the medication to equal the recommended final concentration? ______ How many milliliters per hour should the IV pump be programmed for? ______

Step 1. Calculate volume of medication to withdraw from the vial.

Dimensional Analysis

$$x \text{ mL} = \frac{1 \text{ mL}}{250 \text{ mg}} \times \frac{450 \text{ mg}}{1}$$

$$x = \frac{450}{250} = 1.8 \text{ mL}$$

Proportion

$$250 \text{ mg} : 1 \text{ mL} :: 450 \text{ mg} : x \text{ mL}$$

$$250x = 450$$

$$x = \frac{450}{250} = 1.8 \text{ mL}$$

Therefore the nurse would withdraw 1.8 mL from the vial to administer 450 mg of cefazolin.

Step 2. Calculate the volume of IV solution to provide the recommended final concentration.

Dimensional Analysis

$$x \text{ mL} = \frac{1 \text{ mL}}{50 \text{ mg}} \times \frac{450 \text{ mg}}{1}$$

$$x = \frac{450}{50} = 9 \text{ mL}$$

Formula

$$\text{Ordered dose} \times \frac{1 \text{ mL}}{\text{Recommended concentration}} = x \text{ mL}$$

$$450 \text{ mg} \times \frac{1 \text{ mL}}{50 \text{ mg}} = 9 \text{ mL}$$

Therefore to the 1.8 mL of cefazolin, the nurse must add enough IV solution to give a **TOTAL** of 9 mL.

$$9 \text{ mL} - 1.8 \text{ mL} = 7.2 \text{ mL}$$

1. Add 1.8 mL of cefazolin to an empty buretrol.
2. Add 7.2 mL of compatible IV fluid diluent to make a total volume of 9 mL.

$$\begin{array}{r} 1.8 \text{ mL} \\ +\ 7.2 \text{ mL} \\ \hline 9.0 \text{ mL} \end{array}$$

Final concentration: 50 mg/mL

Step 3. Calculate the milliliters per hour to program the IV pump.

Dimensional Analysis

$$\frac{x \text{ mL}}{\text{h}} = \frac{9 \text{ mL}}{15 \text{ min}} \times \frac{60 \text{ min}}{1 \text{ h}}$$

$$\frac{x \text{ mL}}{\text{h}} = \frac{9 \times 60}{15}$$

$$x = 36 \text{ mL/h}$$

Formula

a. Convert minutes to hours

$$1 \text{ h} : 60 \text{ min} :: x \text{ h} : 15 \text{ min}$$

$$60x = 15$$

$$x = \frac{15}{60} = 0.25 \text{ h}$$

b. $\frac{9 \text{ mL}}{0.25 \text{ h}} = 36 \text{ mL/h}$

Therefore the nurse would program the IV pump for 36 mL/h to infuse the cefazolin over 15 minutes.

EXAMPLE 2: A child weighing 30 kg has an order for nafcillin 850 mg IVPB q 6 h over 10 minutes. The nafcillin vial gives a concentration of 250 mg/mL. The recommended infusion concentration of nafcillin is 100 mg/mL. How many milliliters of medication will provide 850 mg of nafcillin? ______ How many milliliters of IV solution need to be added to the medication to equal the recommended final concentration? ______ How many drops per minute should the IVPB be programmed for? ______

Step 1. Calculate the volume of medication to withdraw from the vial.

Dimensional Analysis

$$x \text{ mL} = \frac{1 \text{ mL}}{250 \text{ mg}} \times \frac{850 \text{ mg}}{1}$$

$$x = \frac{850}{250} = 3.4 \text{ mL}$$

Proportion

$$250 \text{ mg} : 1 \text{ mL} :: 850 \text{ mg} : x \text{ mL}$$

$$250x = 850$$

$$x = \frac{850}{250} = 3.4 \text{ mL}$$

Therefore the nurse will withdraw 3.4 mL from the vial to administer 850 mg of nafcillin.

Step 2. Calculate the volume of IV solution to provide the recommended final concentration.

Dimensional Analysis

$$x \text{ mL} = \frac{1 \text{ mL}}{100 \text{ mg}} \times \frac{850 \text{ mg}}{1}$$

$$x = \frac{850}{100} = 8.5 \text{ mL}$$

Formula

$$\text{Ordered dose} \times \frac{1 \text{ mL}}{\text{Recommended concentration}} = x \text{ mL}$$

$$850 \text{ mg} \times \frac{1 \text{ mL}}{100 \text{ mg}} = 8.5 \text{ mL}$$

Therefore to the 3.4 mL of nafcillin, the nurse must add enough IV solution to give a **TOTAL** of 8.5 mL.

$$8.5 \text{ mL} - 3.4 \text{ mL} = 5.1 \text{ mL}$$

Therefore the nurse will add an additional 5.1 mL of IV solution to the 3.4 mL of nafcillin to give a total of 8.5 mL.

Step 3. Calculate gtt/min (a buretrol or soluset has a drop factor of 60 gtt/mL).

Dimensional Analysis

$$\frac{x \text{ gtt}}{\text{min}} = \frac{60 \text{ gtt}}{1 \text{ mL}} \times \frac{8.5 \text{ mL}}{10 \text{ min}}$$

$$\frac{x \text{ gtt}}{\text{min}} = \frac{60 \times 8.5}{10}$$

$$x = 51 \text{ gtt/min}$$

Formula

$$\frac{8.5 \text{ mL}}{10 \text{ min}} \times 60 \text{ gtt/mL} = 51 \text{ gtt/min}$$

CALCULATION OF DAILY FLUID REQUIREMENTS FOR THE PEDIATRIC PATIENT

Maintenance fluids are those fluids needed daily for bodily function. Overhydration or dehydration (underhydration) can pose a great danger to the infant or young child. Therefore understanding daily fluid requirements is essential for the pediatric nurse. Use the formula below to calculate daily requirements.

PEDIATRIC FLUID REQUIREMENTS (not appropriate for neonatal use)

Patient weight	Maintenance fluid requirements in 24 hours
0-10 kg	100 mL/kg
>10-20 kg	1000 mL + 50 mL/kg (for every kg >10 kg)
>20 kg	1500 mL + 20 mL/kg (for every kg >20 kg)

*Modified from Perry SE, et al: *Maternal child nursing care*, ed 5, St. Louis, 2014, Elsevier.

To calculate the milliliters per hour, as when the patient receives IV fluids, simply divide the calculated amount of fluids required in 24 hours by 24 to obtain the amount of fluids needed per hour (see formula in Example 1).

EXAMPLE 1: An infant weighs 20 pounds. Calculate the hourly IV fluid rate for this infant.

Step 1. Weight	20 lb = 9.1 kg
Step 2. Calculation	9.1 kg × 100 mL/kg/24 h = 910 mL/24 h
Step 3. Daily fluid requirement	910 mL/24 h
Step 4. Calculation	

Dimensional Analysis

$$\frac{x \text{ mL}}{\text{h}} = \frac{910 \text{ mL}}{24 \text{ h}}$$

$$x = 37.9 \text{ or } 38 \text{ mL/h}$$

Formula

$$\frac{\text{Total volume to be infused}}{\text{Total time in hours}} = x \text{ mL/h}$$

$$\frac{910 \text{ mL}}{24 \text{ h}} = 37.9 \text{ or } 38 \text{ mL/h}$$

Step 5. Fluid per hour 37.9 or 38 mL/h

EXAMPLE 2: A child weighs 19.3 kg. Calculate the hourly IV fluid rate for this child.

Step 1. Weight — 19.3 kg

Step 2. Calculation — First 10 kg = 1000 mL
Remaining 9.3 kg × 50 mL/kg = 465 mL
1000 mL + 465 mL = 1465 mL/24 h

Step 3. Daily fluid requirement — 1465 mL/24 h

Step 4. Calculation

Dimensional Analysis

$$\frac{x \text{ mL}}{\text{h}} = \frac{1465 \text{ mL}}{24 \text{ h}}$$

$x = 61$ mL/h

Formula

$$\frac{\text{Total volume to be infused}}{\text{Total time in hours}} = x \text{ mL/h}$$

$$\frac{1465 \text{ mL}}{24 \text{ h}} = 61 \text{ mL/h}$$

Step 5. Fluid per hour — 61 mL/hr

NOTE: These rules apply to infants and young children.

Fluid requirements are 2000 to 3000 mL/24 h for the adult and for the child who approaches adult weight. Never exceed adult fluid requirements in a 24-hour period.

BODY SURFACE AREA CALCULATIONS

Body surface area (BSA) is determined by using a child's height and weight along with the West nomogram. If the child has a normal height and weight for his or her age, the BSA may be ascertained by the weight alone. For example, in Figure 18-2 showing the West nomogram, you can see that a child who weighs 70 lb has a BSA of 1.10 m^2.

When using the West nomogram, take a few minutes to assess the markings of each column. Note that the markings are not at the same intervals throughout each column.

If the child is not of normal height and weight for his or her age, an extended use of the nomogram is required. The far right column is for weight measured in pounds and kilograms. The far left column is for height measured in centimeters and inches. Place a ruler on the nomogram and draw a line connecting the height and weight points. Where the line crosses the surface area (SA) column, the SA in square meters (m^2) will be indicated.

Practice Problems. Using the West nomogram, state the BSA in square meters for each child of normal height and weight listed below:

1. Child weighs 22 lb. BSA = ______
2. Child weighs 4 lb. BSA = ______
3. Child weighs 75 lb. BSA = ______
4. Child weighs 10 lb. BSA = ______
5. Child weighs 32 lb. BSA = ______

Answers

1. 0.46 m^2
2. 0.15 m^2
3. 1.15 m^2
4. 0.27 m^2
5. 0.62 m^2

Calculation of Dosage Based on Body Surface Area

The calculation of dosage may be based on BSA. The BSA method provides a means of converting an adult dosage to a safe pediatric dosage. There are three steps to the calculation with this method.

1. Determine the child's weight in kilograms.
2. Calculate the BSA in square meters. The formula for this calculation is as follows:

$$\frac{4\text{ W (Child's weight in kilograms)} + 7}{\text{W (Child's weight in kilograms)} + 90} = \text{BSA in square meters}$$

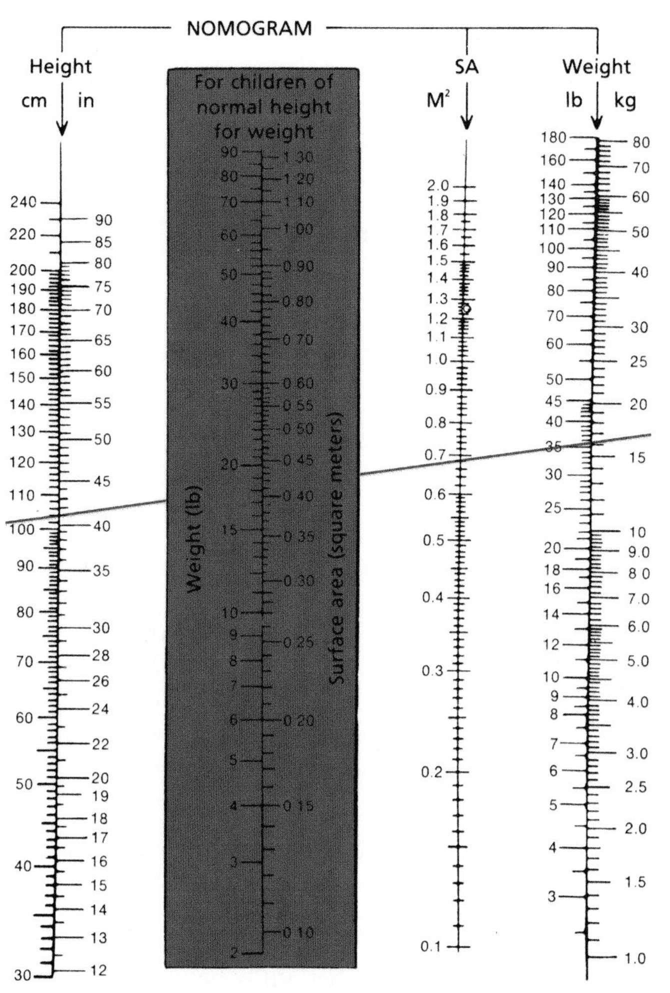

FIGURE 18-2 West nomogram for estimation of body surface areas in children. A straight line is drawn between height and weight. The point where the line crosses the surface area *(SA)* column is the estimated body surface. (Nomogram modified with data from Kliegman RM, Stanton BF, St Geme JW, Schor NF, Behrman RE: *Nelson textbook of pediatrics,* ed 20, Philadelphia, 2016, Elsevier.)

3. Calculate the pediatric dosage using the following formula. The formula is based on the premise that an adult who weighs 140 lb has a BSA of 1.7 m².

$$\frac{\text{BSA in square meters}}{1.7} \times \text{Adult dose} = \text{Child's dose}$$

EXAMPLE: The child weighs 24 lb and the adult dose is 100 mg.

Step 1. First, convert the child's weight to kilograms.

Dimensional Analysis

$$x \text{ kg} = \frac{1 \text{ kg}}{2.2 \text{ lb}} \times \frac{24 \text{ lb}}{1}$$

$$x = \frac{24}{2.2} = 10.9 \text{ kg}$$

Proportion

$$1 \text{ kg} : 2.2 \text{ lb} :: x \text{ kg} : 24 \text{ lb}$$

$$2.2x = 24$$

$$x = \frac{24}{2.2} = 10.9 \text{ kg}$$

Step 2. Next, calculate the child's BSA in m².

$$\frac{4(10.9)+7}{10.9+90} = \frac{43.6+7}{10.9+90} = \frac{50.6}{100.9} = 0.5$$

$$\text{Child's BSA} = 0.5 \text{ m}^2$$

Step 3. Finally, calculate the appropriate dosage for this child.

Dimensional Analysis

$$x \text{ mg} = \frac{100 \text{ mg}}{1.7 \text{ m}^2} = \frac{0.5 \text{ m}^2}{1}$$

$$x = \frac{100}{1.7} \times 0.5 = 29.41 \text{ or } 29.4 \text{ mg}$$

Proportion

$$\frac{0.5 \text{ m}^2}{1.7 \text{ m}^2} \times 100 \text{ mg} =$$

$$\frac{0.5 \text{ m}^2}{1.7 \text{ m}^2} \times 100 \text{ mg} = 29.41 \text{ or } 29.4 \text{ mg}$$

Practice Problems. Calculate the following children's dosages.

		Answers
1. Child weighs 40 lb, adult dose = 300 mg.	Child's dose = ______	**1.** 132 mg
2. Child weighs 65 lb, adult dose = 30 mL.	Child's dose = ______	**2.** 18.5 mL
3. Child weighs 20 lb, adult dose = 50 mg.	Child's dose = ______	**3.** 13 mg
4. Child weighs 90 lb, adult dose = 10 mL.	Child's dose = ______	**4.** 7.65 mL
5. Child weighs 14 lb, adult dose = 2 g.	Child's dose = ______	**5.** 0.4 g

Practice Problems. Using the West nomogram, calculate the BSA for each child with the following heights and weights:

		Answers
1. Child weighs 6 kg, height is 110 cm.	BSA = ______	**1.** 0.41 m^2
2. Child weighs 5 lb, height is 19 in.	BSA = ______	**2.** 0.18 m^2
3. Child weighs 25 kg, height is 70 cm.	BSA = ______	**3.** 0.74 m^2
4. Child weighs 30 lb, height is 90 cm.	BSA = ______	**4.** 0.58 m^2
5. Child weighs 160 lb, height is 200 cm.	BSA = ______	**5.** 2.0 m^2

Complete the following work sheet, which provides for extensive practice in the calculation of pediatric dosages. Check your answers. If you have difficulties, go back and review the necessary material. When you feel ready to evaluate your learning, take the first posttest. Check your answers. An acceptable score as indicated on the posttest signifies that you have successfully completed this chapter. An unacceptable score signifies a need for further study before taking the second posttest.

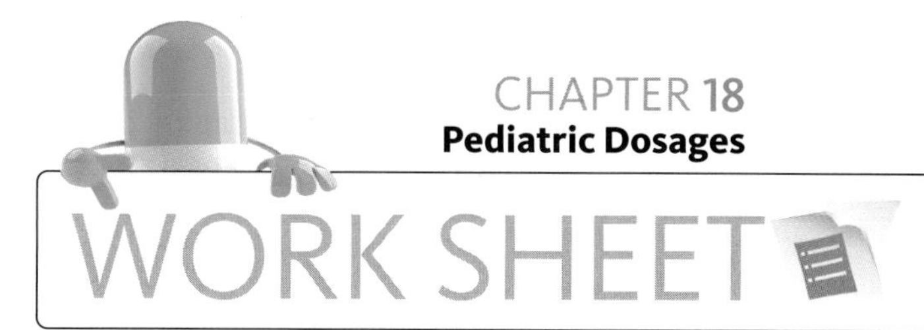

CHAPTER 18
Pediatric Dosages

WORK SHEET

DIRECTIONS: The medication order is listed at the beginning of each problem. Calculate the child's weight in kilograms, determine the safe and therapeutic dosage or range, determine the safety of the order, and calculate the drug dose. Show your work.

1. The licensed prescriber orders cephalexin 250 mg po four times a day for a child weighing 50 lb. You have cephalexin 250-mg capsules. The recommended daily po dosage for a child is 25 to 50 mg/kg/day in divided doses q 6 h. a. Child's weight is ______ kg. b. What is the safe and therapeutic range for this child? ______ c. Is the order safe? ______ d. If yes, how many capsules will you administer? ______

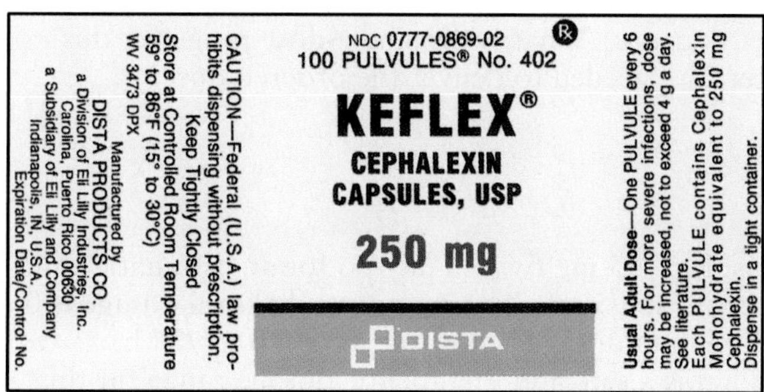

2. The licensed prescriber orders digoxin 12.5 mg po daily for an infant weighing 6 lb 8 oz. You have digoxin 0.05 mg/mL. The recommended daily dosage for an infant is 0.035 to 0.06 mg/kg/day in divided doses two times a day. a. Child's weight is ______ kg. b. What is the safe and therapeutic range for this child? ______ c. Is the order safe? ______ d. If yes, how many milliliters will you administer? ______

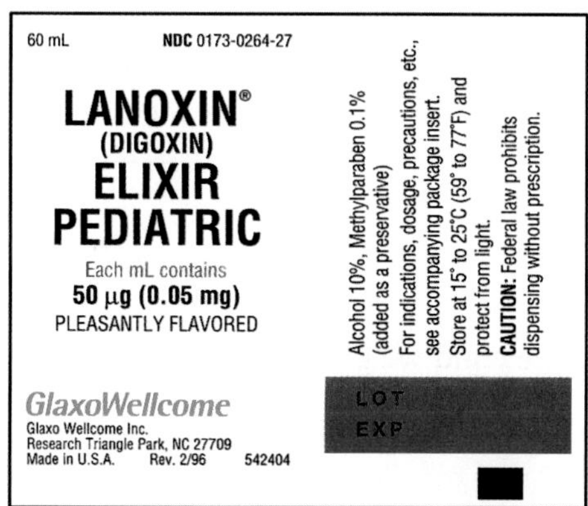

3. The licensed prescriber orders diphenhydramine 25 mg IV q 6 h for a child weighing 50 lb. You have available diphenhydramine 12.5 mg/mL. The recommended daily dosage for a child weighing more than 12 kg is 5 mg/kg/24 h in four divided doses. a. Child's weight is ______ kg. b. What is the safe and therapeutic dosage for this child? ______ c. Is the order safe? ______ d. If yes, how many milliliters will you prepare? ______

4. Calculate the 24-hour maintenance fluids for a child who weighs 28 lb. a. ________ b. How many milliliters per hour are needed to deliver the maintenance fluids? ______

5. The licensed prescriber orders cefdinir 70 mg po twice a day for a child weighing 22 lb. The recommended dosage for cefdinir is 14 mg/kg/24 h twice a day for 10 days for skin infections. It is available as 125 mg/5 mL. a. Child's weight is ______ kg. b. Is the order safe and therapeutic? Prove your answer. ________ c. If the dose is safe and therapeutic, how many milliliters are needed to deliver the ordered dose? ______

6. The licensed prescriber orders ciprofloxacin 300 mg q 12 h po for a child weighing 30.3 kg. You have ciprofloxacin 250 mg/5 mL. The recommended oral dosage is 20 to 30 mg/kg/24 h q 12 h. a. Child's weight is ______ kg. b. What is the safe and therapeutic 24-hour dosage range for this child? ______ c. What is the single-dose range for this child? ______ d. How many milliliters are needed to deliver the ordered dose? ______

7. The licensed prescriber orders prednisolone 45 mg twice a day po for an asthmatic child weighing 94 lb. You have prednisolone 15 mg/5 mL. The recommended oral dosage is 0.5 to 2 mg/kg/24 h divided twice a day. Maximum dosage is not to exceed 80 mg/24 h. a. Child's weight is ______ kg. b. What is a safe and therapeutic dosage range for this child? ______ c. Is the order safe? ______ d. Would you administer this medication as dosed? ________

8. The licensed prescriber orders phenytoin 60 mg po q 12 h for a child weighing 40 lb. You have phenytoin 30-mg chewable tablets available. The recommended oral dosage for a child is 5 to 7 mg/kg/24 h in divided doses q 12 h. a. Child's weight is ______ kg. b. What is the safe and therapeutic 24-hour dosage range for this child? ______ c. Is the order safe? ______ d. If yes, how many chewtabs will you administer per dose? ______

9. A child is to receive vancomycin 750 mg IVPB q 6 h. The child weighs 68 lb. The recommended dosage of vancomycin is 40 to 60 mg/kg/24 h. a. Child's weight is ______ kg. b. What dose per kilogram per 24 hours is the child receiving? ______ c. Is the order safe? ______

10. The licensed prescriber orders amoxicillin 300 mg po q 12 h for a child weighing 42 lb. You have amoxicillin 125 mg/5 mL. The recommended oral dosage is 25 to 50 mg/kg/24 h q 12 h. a. Child's weight is ______ kg. b. What is the safe and therapeutic single-dose range for this child? ______ c. How many milliliters are needed to deliver the ordered dose? ______

11. The licensed prescriber orders 100 mL D_5W bolus IV to run over 30 minutes to a 3-year-old child. The drop factor of the tubing is 60 gtt/mL (microdrip). How many drops per minute are needed to deliver the bolus of D_5W? ______

12. The licensed prescriber orders carbamazephine 150 mg po three times a day for a child weighing 58 lb. You have carbamazephine 100 mg/5 mL. The recommended oral dosage for a child is 10 to 20 mg/kg/24 h divided in doses three times a day. a. Child's weight is ______ kg. b. What is the safe and therapeutic single dose range for this child? ______ c. Is the order safe? ______ d. If yes, how many milliliters are needed? ______

NDC 58887-019-76 FSC 1841
6505-01-302-4467
Tegretol®
carbamazepine USP
Suspension
100 mg/5 ml
EXP
LOT
450 ml
BASEL
Pharmaceuticals

13. Calculate the 24-hour maintenance fluid requirements for a child who weighs 72 lb. a. Child's weight is ______ kg. b. The maintenance fluid requirements are ______. c. How many milliliters per hour are needed to deliver the maintenance fluids? ______

14. The licensed prescriber orders ibuprofen 100 mg for a child who weighs 52 lb. Recommended dose for ibuprofen is 5 to 10 mg/kg/dose q 6 h. It is available as 100 mg/5 mL. a. Child's weight is ______ kg. b. What is a safe and therapeutic single-dose range for this child? ______ c. How many milliliters are needed to deliver the ordered dose? ______

15. The licensed prescriber orders cefazolin 350 mg po q 6 h for a child weighing 81 lb. You have cefazolin 500 mg/5 mL. The recommended daily oral dosage is 25 to 50 mg/kg/24 h divided q 6 h. a. Child's weight is ______ kg. b. What is the safe and therapeutic single-dose range for this child? ______ c. Is the order safe? ______ d. If yes, how many milliliters will you prepare? ______

16. The licensed prescriber orders cimetidine 60 mg po q 8 h for an infant weighing 16 lb. Cimetidine 300 mg/5 mL is available. The recommended daily oral dosage is 15 to 20 mg/kg/24 h divided q 8 h. a. Child's weight is ______ kg. b. What is the safe and therapeutic dosage range for this child? ______ c. Is the order safe? ______ d. How many milligrams per kilogram per 24 hours is the child receiving? ______ e. If the ordered dosage is safe, how many milliliters will you administer? ______

17. The licensed prescriber orders prednisone 8 mg po q 12 h for a child weighing 19 lb. You have prednisone syrup 5 mg/5 mL. The recommended oral dosage is 0.5 to 2 mg/kg/24 h given once daily or divided and given in two doses per day. a. Child's weight is ______ kg. b. What is a safe and therapeutic single-dose range for this child? ______ c. Is the order safe? ______ d. If yes, how many milliliters will you draw up? ______

18. The licensed prescriber orders cefazolin 400 mg IV q 8 h for a child weighing 32 lb. You have cefazolin 330 mg/mL. The recommended daily IV dosage for a child is 100 mg/kg/24 h in divided doses q 6–8 h. a. Child's weight is ______ kg. b. What is the safe and therapeutic dose for this child? ______ c. Is the order safe? ______ d. If yes, how many milliliters will you prepare? ______

EXP.
LOT
equivalent to
1gram cefazolin
NDC 0007-3130-16
ANCEF®
CEFAZOLIN FOR INJECTION (LYOPHILIZED)
Formerly sterile cefazolin sodium (lyophilized)
25 Vials for Intramuscular or Intravenous Use

NSN 6505-01-262-9508
Before reconstitution protect from light and store between 15° and 30°C (59° and 86°F).
Usual Adult Dosage: 250 mg to 1 gram every 6 to 8 hours. See accompanying prescribing information.
For I.M. administration add 2.5 mL of Sterile Water for Injection. SHAKE WELL. Withdraw entire contents. Provides an approximate volume of 3.0 mL (330 mg/mL). For I.V. administration see accompanying prescribing information.
Reconstituted *Ancef* is stable for 24 hours at room temperature or for 10 days if refrigerated (5°C or 41°F).
SmithKline Beecham Pharmaceuticals
Philadelphia, PA 19101
694115-P
K3130-16
3 0007-3130-16 2

19. The order is to infuse 250 mL of D_5W over 3 hours to an 11-year-old child. How many milliliters per hour should the IV pump be programmed for? ______

20. A 25-kg child has an order for gentamicin 40 mg IVPB twice a day over 20 minutes. The concentration of the vial states 10 mg/mL. The recommended infusion concentration is 2 mg/mL. a. How many milliliters of medication will provide 40 mg of gentamicin? ______ b. How many milliliters of IV solution need to be added to the medication to equal the recommended final concentration? ______ c. How many drops per minute of gentamicin should be infused? ______

ANSWERS ON PP. 549–551 AND 555.

NAME ____________

DATE ____________

ACCEPTABLE SCORE **12**

YOUR SCORE ______

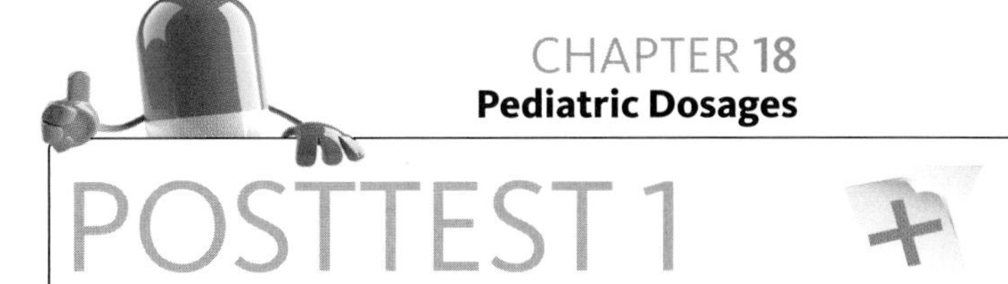

CHAPTER 18
Pediatric Dosages

POSTTEST 1

DIRECTIONS: The medication order is listed at the beginning of each problem. Calculate the child's weight in kilograms, determine the safe and therapeutic dosage or range, determine the safety of the order, and calculate the drug dosage. Show your work.

1. The licensed prescriber orders phenobarbital 60 mg po q 12 h for a child weighing 55 lb. Phenobarbital elixir is available as 20 mg/5 mL. The recommended daily dosage for a child is 4 to 6 mg/kg/24 h divided q 12 h. a. Child's weight is ______ kg. b. What is the safe and therapeutic single-dose range for this child? ______ c. Is the order safe? Explain. ______ d. If so, how many milliliters will the nurse administer? ______

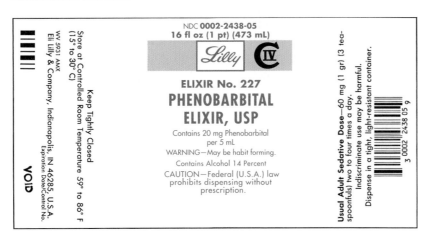

2. The licensed prescriber orders amoxicillin 500 mg po q 6 h for a child weighing 44 lb. Amoxicillin is supplied in 250-mg capsules. The recommended daily oral dosage is 25 to 50 mg/kg/24 h in divided doses q 6 h. a. Child's weight is ______ kg. b. What is the safe and therapeutic single-dose range for this child? ______ c. Is the order safe? Explain. ______ d. If the order is safe, how many capsules will the nurse administer? ______

3. The licensed prescriber orders cephalexin 300 mg po q 8 h for a child who weighs 34 lb. Cephalexin is supplied in an oral suspension of 125 mg/5 mL. The recommended daily oral dosage for a child is 50 to 100 mg/kg/24 h divided q 8 h. a. Child's weight is ______ kg. b. How many milligrams per kilogram per 24 hours is the child receiving? ______ c. If the dosage is safe and therapeutic, how many milliliters will you administer? ______

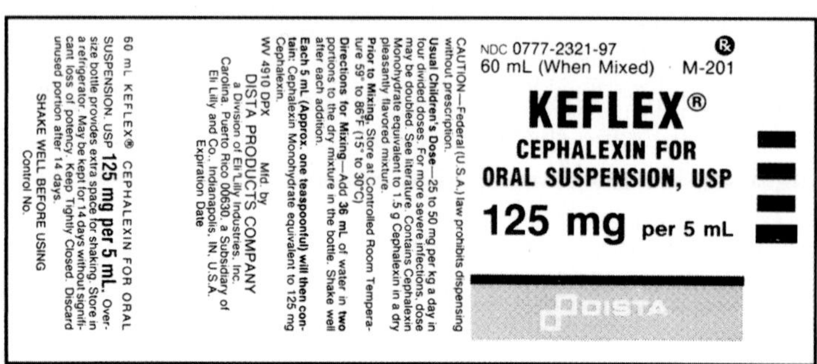

4. The licensed prescriber orders morphine sulfate 4 mg IM STAT for a child weighing 78 lb. Available is morphine sulfate 15 mg/mL. The recommended intramuscular (IM) dosage for a child is 0.1 to 0.2 mg/kg/dose q 2–4 h as needed. a. Child's weight is ______ kg. b. What is the safe and therapeutic dosage range? ______ c. Is the order safe? Prove. ______________ d. If yes, how many milliliters will you administer? ______

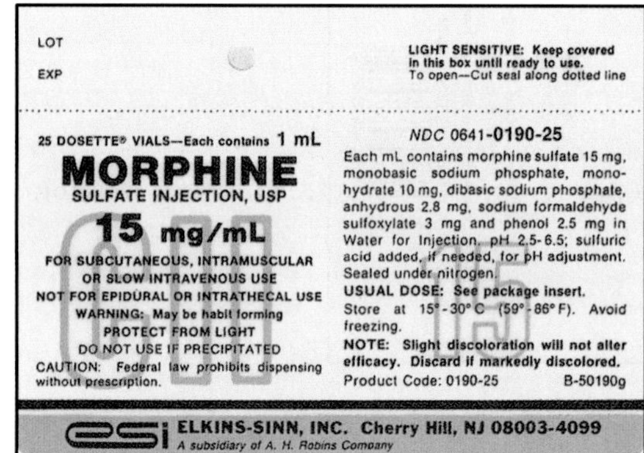

5. A child has a fever of 101.5° F orally and needs acetaminophen. Calculate a safe and therapeutic dosage or range of acetaminophen for this child, who weighs 62 lb. Recommended dosage range for acetaminophen is 10 to 15 mg/kg/dose q 4–6 h. It is available as an elixir 160 mg/5 mL. a. Child's weight is ______ kg. b. What is a safe and therapeutic dosage range for this child? ______ c. How many milliliters are needed for this range? ______

6. The licensed prescriber orders 1000 mL of 0.9% NS to run over 16 hours. What rate is needed to deliver the ordered fluids? ______

7. The licensed prescriber orders clarithromycin 300 mg po twice a day for a child who weighs 92 lb. Available is clarithromycin 125 mg/5 mL. The recommended dosage is 15 mg/kg/24 h divided q 12 h. a. Child's weight is ______ kg. b. What is the safe and therapeutic dosage for this child? ______ c. Is the order safe? Prove. ______________________ d. If yes, how many milliliters will you administer? ______

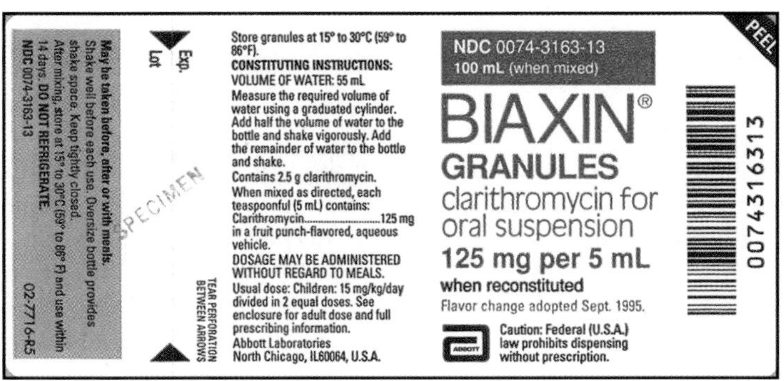

8. A child is to receive IV fluids at maintenance rate. She weighs 25 lb. a. Child's weight is ______ kg. b. Calculate her 24-hour fluid requirements ______ c. How many milliliters per hour are needed to deliver the maintenance fluids? ______

9. A patient is to receive vancomycin 650 mg IVPB q 6 h. The patient weighs 96 lb on admission. The recommended dosage is 40 to 60 mg/kg/24 h q 6 h. a. Child's weight is ______ kg. b. How many milligrams per kilogram per 24 hours is the patient receiving? ______ c. Is the written order safe and therapeutic? Explain. ______________________

10. The licensed prescriber orders cefaclor 300 mg po suspension q 8 h for treatment of otitis media. Recommended oral dosage for infant and child is 20 to 40 mg/kg/24 h q 8 h. Maximum dosage is 2 g/24 h. The patient weighs 95 lb. a. Child's weight is ______ kg. b. How many milligrams per kilogram per 24 hours is the patient receiving? ______ c. Is this a safe and therapeutic dosage for this patient? Prove. ______________________

11. A 10-month-old infant has an order for 100 mL of 0.9% NS to be infused over 6 hours. How many milliliters per hour should the IV pump be programmed for? ______

12. An infant weighing 15 kg has an order for ampicillin 400 mg IVPB over 30 minutes. The ampicillin vial gives a concentration of 250 mg/mL. The recommended infusion concentration is 50 mg/mL. a. How many milliliters of the medication will provide 400 mg of ampicillin? ______ b. How many milliliters of IV solution need to be added to the medication to equal the recommended final concentration? ______ c. How many drops per minute of ampicillin should be infused? ______

13. The licensed prescriber orders 60 mg of prednisone po twice a day for a patient who weighs 30 kg. It is available as 15 mg/5 mL. Recommended dosage is 0.5 to 2 mg/kg/24 h given in one or two doses. Maximum dose is 80 mg/24 h. a. What dose per kilogram per day is the patient receiving? ______ b. Is this a safe and therapeutic dose? ______ c. Would you administer this medication? ____________________

14. The licensed prescriber orders cefaclor 400 mg po q 12 h for a child who weighs 89 lb. Cefaclor is available as 375 mg/5 mL. The recommended dosage is 15 to 20 mg/kg/24 h divided q 12 h. a. Child's weight is ______ kg. b. What is the safe and therapeutic dosage range for this child? ______ c. Is the order safe and therapeutic? ______ d. If so, how many milliliters will you administer? ______

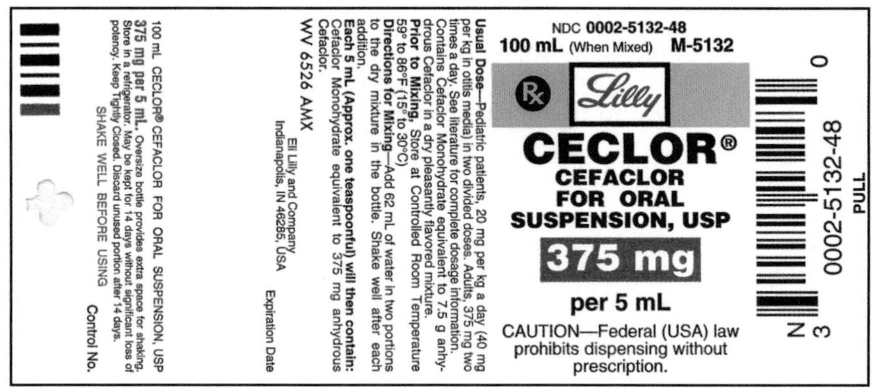
NDC 0002-5132-48
100 mL (When Mixed) M-5132
Lilly
CECLOR®
CEFACLOR FOR ORAL SUSPENSION, USP
375 mg
per 5 mL
CAUTION—Federal (USA) law prohibits dispensing without prescription.
Usual Dose—Pediatric patients, 20 mg per kg a day (40 mg per kg in otitis media) in two divided doses. Adults, 375 mg two times a day. See literature for complete dosage information.
Contains Cefaclor Monohydrate equivalent to 7.5 g anhydrous Cefaclor in a dry pleasantly flavored mixture.
Prior to Mixing, Store at Controlled Room Temperature 59° to 86°F (15° to 30°C).
Directions for Mixing—Add 62 mL of water in two portions to the dry mixture in the bottle. Shake well after each addition.
Each 5 mL (Approx. one teaspoonful) will then contain: Cefaclor Monohydrate equivalent to 375 mg anhydrous Cefaclor.
WV 6526 AMX
Eli Lilly and Company
Indianapolis, IN 46285, USA
Expiration Date
100 mL CECLOR® CEFACLOR FOR ORAL SUSPENSION, USP
375 mg per 5 mL. Oversize bottle provides extra space for shaking. Store in a refrigerator. May be kept for 14 days without significant loss of potency. Keep Tightly Closed. Discard unused portion after 14 days.
SHAKE WELL BEFORE USING
Control No.
0002-5132-48
PULL

15. Nafcillin 90 mg q 6 h IV is ordered for a child who weighs 11 lb. The recommended IM/IV dosage is 50 to 100 mg/kg/24 h q 6 h for mild to moderate infections and 100 to 200 mg/kg/24 h q 4–6 h for severe infections. a. Child's weight is ______ kg. b. How many milligrams per kilogram per 24 hours is the patient receiving? ______ c. Is the order safe and therapeutic? ______

ANSWERS ON PP. 551–553 AND 558–560.

NAME ______________________

DATE ______________________

ACCEPTABLE SCORE **12**

YOUR SCORE ______

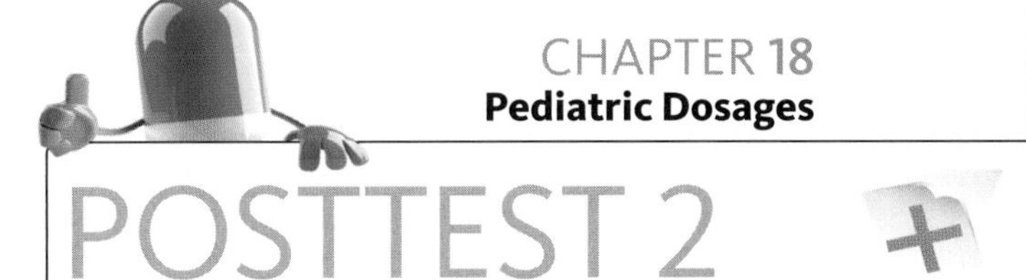

DIRECTIONS: The medication order is listed at the beginning of each problem. Calculate the child's weight in kilograms, determine the safe and therapeutic dosage or range, determine the safety of the order, and calculate the drug dosage. Show your work.

1. A child is to receive vancomycin 450 mg IVPB q 6 h. The patient weighs 70 lb on admission. The recommended dosage is 40 to 60 mg/kg/24 h q 6 h. a. Child's weight is ______ kg. b. How many milligrams per kilogram per 24 hours is the patient receiving? ______ c. Is the order safe and therapeutic? Prove. ______

2. The licensed prescriber orders phenytoin 100 mg po q 12 h for a child weighing 62 lb. You have phenytoin 125 mg/5 mL on hand. The recommended daily oral dosage for a child is 7 to 8 mg/kg/24 h in divided doses two or three times per day. a. Child's weight is ______ kg. b. What is a safe and therapeutic 24-hour dosage range for this child? ______ c. What is the single-dose range for this child? ______ d. Is the prescribed dose safe to administer? ______ e. If yes, how many milliliters will you administer? ______

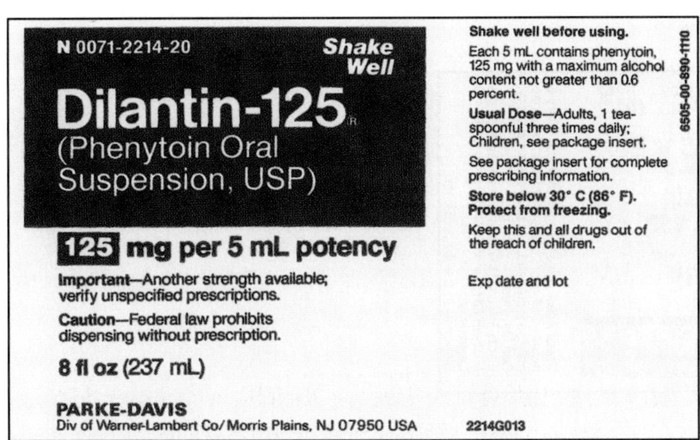

N 0071-2214-20
Shake Well
Dilantin-125®
(Phenytoin Oral Suspension, USP)
125 mg per 5 mL potency
Important—Another strength available; verify unspecified prescriptions.
Caution—Federal law prohibits dispensing without prescription.
8 fl oz (237 mL)
PARKE-DAVIS
Div of Warner-Lambert Co/Morris Plains, NJ 07950 USA
Shake well before using.
Each 5 mL contains phenytoin, 125 mg with a maximum alcohol content not greater than 0.6 percent.
Usual Dose—Adults, 1 teaspoonful three times daily; Children, see package insert.
See package insert for complete prescribing information.
Store below 30° C (86° F).
Protect from freezing.
Keep this and all drugs out of the reach of children.
Exp date and lot
2214G013
6505-00-890-1110

3. An infant is to receive 150 mL of whole blood over 3 hours. Using a microdrip (60 gtt/mL), how many drops per minute are needed? ______

4. The licensed prescriber orders amoxicillin 400 mg po q 12 h for a child weighing 58 lb. You have amoxicillin suspension 250 mg/5 mL. The recommended daily oral dosage for a child is 25 to 50 mg/kg/24 h in divided doses q 12 h. a. Child's weight is ______ kg. b. What is the safe and therapeutic 24-hour dosage range for this child? ______ c. What is the single-dose range for this child? ______ d. How many milligrams per kilogram per 24 hours is the patient receiving with this order? ______ e. How many milliliters are needed to deliver the ordered dose? ______

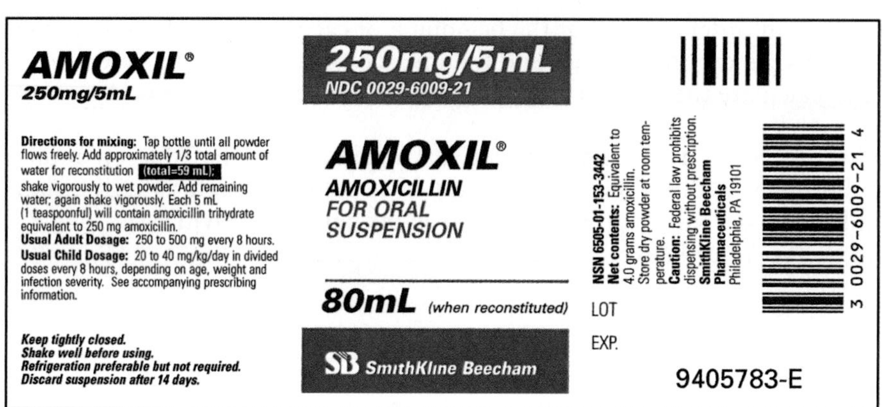

5. The licensed prescriber orders cephalexin 500 mg po q 6 h for a 99-lb school-age child. Available is cephalexin 250-mg capsules. The recommended daily oral dosage is 50 to 100 mg/kg/24 h divided q 6 h. Maximum dosage is not to exceed 2 g/24 h. a. Child's weight is ______ kg. b. How many milligrams per kilogram per 24 hours is this child receiving? ______ c. Is the order safe? ______ d. If yes, how many capsules will you administer? ______

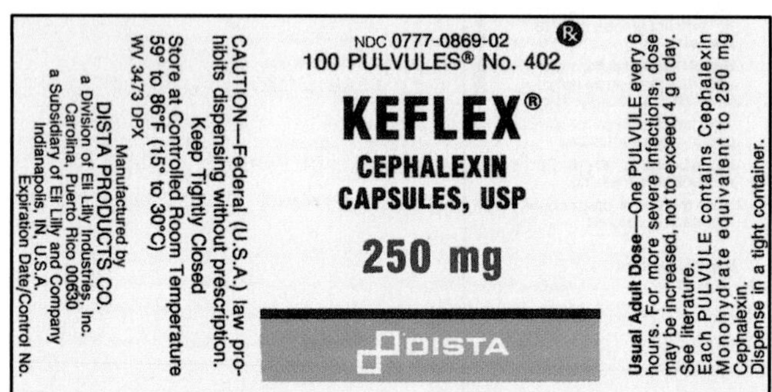

6. The licensed prescriber orders cefdinir 200 mg po q 12 h for a child weighing 66 lb. Cefdinir is available as 125 mg/5 mL. Recommended dosage is 14 mg/kg/24 h divided q 12 h. a. Child's weight is ______ kg. b. How many milligrams per kilogram per 24 hours is the child receiving? ______ c. Is the order safe? ______ d. If yes, how many milliliters are needed? ______

7. A neonate weighs 2012 g. He is to receive ampicillin 100 to 200 mg/kg/24 h divided q 6 h IV per syringe for otitis media. a. Child's weight is ______ kg. b. What is the safe and therapeutic 24-hour dosage range? ______ c. What single-dose range is needed? ______

8. The licensed prescriber orders amoxicillin 180 mg po q 8 h for a 35-lb child. Available is amoxicillin 125 mg/5 mL. Recommended dosage is 25 to 50 mg/kg/24 h divided q 6–8 h. a. Child's weight is ______ kg. b. How many milligrams per kilogram per 24 hours is the child receiving? ______ c. Is the order safe? ______ d. If yes, how many milliliters are needed? ______

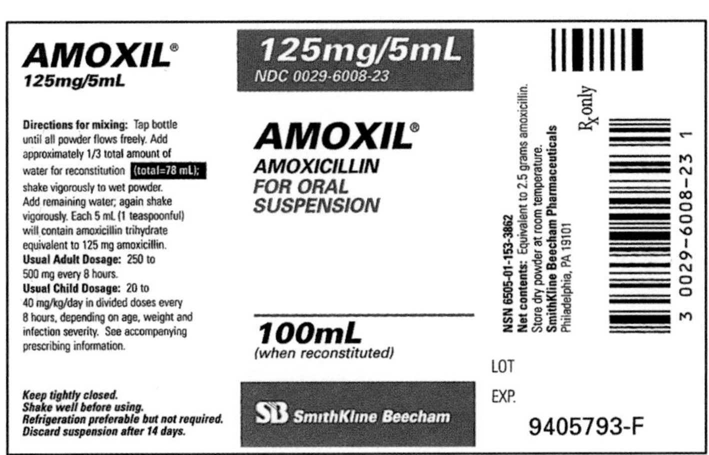

9. The licensed prescriber orders vancomycin 330 mg po q 6 h for a 74-lb child. You have vancomycin 250 mg/5 mL. The recommended daily oral dosage is 40 mg/kg/24 h divided q 6 h. a. Child's weight is ______ kg. b. How many milligrams per kilogram per 24 hours is the child receiving? ______ c. Is the order safe? ______ d. If yes, how many milliliters are needed? ______

10. The licensed prescriber orders morphine sulfate 0.9 mg IV q 4 h for pain. Available is morphine sulfate 0.5 mg/mL. The child weighs 20 lb. The recommended single dose is 0.1 to 0.2 mg/kg q 4 h. a. Child's weight is ______ kg. b. What is the safe and therapeutic dosage range for this child? ______ c. Is the order safe? ______ d. If yes, how many milliliters will you draw up? ______

11. The licensed prescriber orders an infusion of 200 mL of D_5LR over 3 hours to a 6-year-old child. How many milliliters per hour should the IV pump be programmed for? ______

12. A 60-kg child has an order for vancomycin 500 mg IVPB to be delivered over a 1- to 2-hour period. The vial concentration is 50 mg/mL. The recommended infusion concentration is 5 mg/mL. a. How many milliliters of medication will provide 500 mg of vancomycin? ______ b. How many milliliters of IV solution need to be added to the medication to equal the recommended concentration? ______ c. How many drops per minute of vancomycin should be infused? ______

13. The licensed prescriber orders digoxin 0.013 mg po twice a day for an infant weighing 3036 g. The recommended oral dosage for digoxin is 6 to 10 mcg/kg/24 h divided q 12 h. Available is digoxin elixir 50 mcg/mL. a. Child's weight is ______ kg. b. What is a safe and therapeutic 24-hour dosage range for this infant? ______ c. What is a safe single-dose range for this infant? ______ d. Is the order safe? ______ e. If yes, how many milliliters will you give? ______

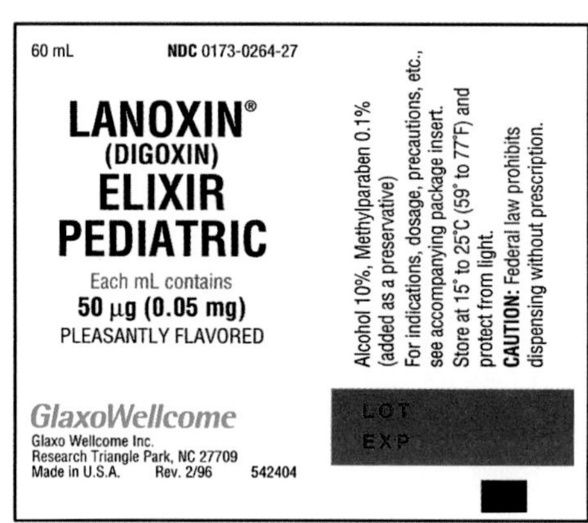

14. Acetaminophen is ordered for an infant who weighs 9 lb. Acetaminophen is available as a 160 mg/5 mL concentration, and the safe and therapeutic dose range is 10 to 15 mg/kg/dose q 6 h. a. Infant's weight is ______ kg. b. What is the single-dose range? ______ c. How many milliliters are needed to deliver the calculated dose range? ______

15. Phenobarbital elixir 72 mg po daily is ordered for a child who weighs 37 lb. Phenobarbital is supplied as 20 mg/5 mL. Recommended dosage is 4 to 6 mg/kg/24 h one or two times per day. a. Child's weight is ______ kg. b. What is the safe and therapeutic 24-hour dosage range needed for this child? ______ c. Is the order safe? ______ d. If yes, how many milliliters will you administer? ______

ANSWERS ON PP. 553–555 AND 560–562.

evolve For additional practice problems, refer to the Pediatric Dosages section of *Elsevier's Interactive Drug Calculation Application*, version 1.

ANSWERS

CHAPTER 18 Dimensional Analysis—Work Sheet, pp. 537–540

1. b. $\frac{x \text{ mg}}{\text{day}} = \frac{25 \text{ mg}}{\text{kg/day}} \times \frac{1 \text{ kg}}{2.2 \text{ lb}} \times \frac{50 \text{ lb}}{1} = 568.18$ or 568.2 mg/day (minimum)

   $\frac{x \text{ mg}}{\text{day}} = \frac{50 \text{ mg}}{\text{kg/day}} \times \frac{1 \text{ kg}}{2.2 \text{ lb}} \times \frac{50 \text{ lb}}{1} = 1136.36$ or 1136.4 mg/day (maximum)

   c. Yes, the order is safe to administer.

   d. $x \text{ cap} = \frac{1 \text{ cap}}{250 \text{ mg}} \times \frac{250 \text{ mg}}{1} = 1$ capsule

2. b. $\frac{x \text{ mg}}{\text{day}} = \frac{0.035 \text{ mg}}{\text{kg/day}} \times \frac{1 \text{ kg}}{2.2 \text{ lb}} \times \frac{6.5 \text{ lb}}{1} = 0.1$ mg/day (minimum)

   $\frac{x \text{ mg}}{\text{day}} = \frac{0.06 \text{ mg}}{\text{kg/day}} \times \frac{1 \text{ kg}}{2.2 \text{ lb}} \times \frac{6.5 \text{ lb}}{1} = 0.18$ mg/day (maximum)

   c. No, the order is not safe.

   d. Question this order.

3. b. $\frac{x \text{ mg}}{\text{dose}} = \frac{5 \text{ mg}}{\text{kg/day}} \times \frac{1 \text{ kg}}{2.2 \text{ lb}} \times \frac{50 \text{ lb}}{1} \times \frac{1 \text{ day}}{4 \text{ doses}} = 28.4$ mg/dose

   c. The order is safe as 25 mg is below 28.4 mg.

   d. $x \text{ mL} = \frac{1 \text{ mL}}{12.5 \text{ mg}} \times \frac{25 \text{ mg}}{1} = 2$ mL

4. a. $x \text{ kg} = \frac{1 \text{ kg}}{2.2 \text{ lb}} \times \frac{28 \text{ lb}}{1} = 12.7$ kg

   First 10 kg: $x \text{ mL} = \frac{100 \text{ mL}}{\text{kg}} \times \frac{10 \text{ kg}}{1} = 1000$ mL/day

   Remaining 2.7 kg: $x \text{ mL} = \frac{50 \text{ mL}}{\text{kg}} \times \frac{2.7 \text{ kg}}{1} = 135$ mL/day

   b. 1000 + 135 = 1135 mL/day

   $\frac{x \text{ mL}}{\text{h}} = \frac{1135 \text{ mL}}{24 \text{ h}} = 47.3$ or 47 mL/h

5. b. $\frac{x \text{ mg}}{\text{dose}} = \frac{14 \text{ mg}}{\text{kg/day}} \times \frac{1 \text{ kg}}{2.2 \text{ lb}} \times \frac{22 \text{ lb}}{1} \times \frac{1 \text{ day}}{2 \text{ doses}} = 70$ mg/dose

   Yes, 70 mg is ordered.

   c. $x \text{ mL} = \frac{5 \text{ mL}}{125 \text{ mg}} \times \frac{70 \text{ mg}}{1} = 2.8$ mL

6. b. $\frac{x \text{ mg}}{\text{day}} = \frac{20 \text{ mg}}{\text{kg/day}} \times \frac{30.3 \text{ kg}}{1} = 606$ mg/day (minimum)

   $\frac{x \text{ mg}}{\text{day}} = \frac{30 \text{ mg}}{\text{kg/day}} \times \frac{30.3 \text{ kg}}{1} = 909$ mg/day (maximum)

   c. $\frac{x \text{ mg}}{\text{dose}} = \frac{606 \text{ mg}}{\text{day}} \times \frac{1 \text{ day}}{2 \text{ doses}} = 303$ mg/dose (minimum)

   $\frac{x \text{ mg}}{\text{dose}} = \frac{909 \text{ mg}}{\text{day}} \times \frac{1 \text{ day}}{2 \text{ doses}} = 454.5$ mg/dose (maximum)

   d. $x \text{ mL} = \frac{5 \text{ mL}}{250 \text{ mg}} \times \frac{300 \text{ mg}}{1} = 6$ mL

7. b. $\frac{x \text{ mg}}{\text{day}} = \frac{0.5 \text{ mg}}{\text{kg/day}} \times \frac{1 \text{ kg}}{2.2 \text{ lb}} \times \frac{94 \text{ lb}}{1} = 21.36 \text{ or } 21.4 \text{ mg/day (minimum)}$

$\frac{x \text{ mg}}{\text{day}} = \frac{2 \text{ mg}}{\text{kg/day}} \times \frac{1 \text{ kg}}{2.2 \text{ lb}} \times \frac{94 \text{ lb}}{1} = 85.45 \text{ or } 85.5 \text{ mg/day (maximum)}$

c. No, 90 mg exceeds the maximum dose of 85.5 mg.

d. No, call the licensed prescriber who wrote the order.

8. b. $\frac{x \text{ mg}}{\text{day}} = \frac{5 \text{ mg}}{\text{kg/day}} \times \frac{1 \text{ kg}}{2.2 \text{ lb}} \times \frac{40 \text{ lb}}{1} = 90.9 \text{ mg/day (minimum)}$

$\frac{x \text{ mg}}{\text{day}} = \frac{7 \text{ mg}}{\text{kg/day}} \times \frac{1 \text{ kg}}{2.2 \text{ lb}} \times \frac{40 \text{ lb}}{1} = 127.27 \text{ or } 127.3 \text{ mg/day (maximum)}$

c. Yes, 60 mg q 12 h = 120 mg/day.

d. $x \text{ tab} = \frac{1 \text{ tab}}{30 \text{ mg}} \times \frac{60 \text{ mg}}{1} = 2 \text{ chewtabs}$

9. b. $\frac{x \text{ mg}}{\text{kg/day}} = \frac{750 \text{ mg}}{\text{dose}} \times \frac{4 \text{ doses}}{1 \text{ day}} \times \frac{2.2 \text{ lb}}{1 \text{ kg}} \times \frac{}{68 \text{ lb}} = 97.05 \text{ or } 97.1 \text{ mg/kg/day}$

c. No, it exceeds the recommended range of 40–60 mg/kg/24h.

10. b. $\frac{x \text{ mg}}{\text{dose}} = \frac{25 \text{ mg}}{\text{kg/day}} \times \frac{1 \text{ kg}}{2.2 \text{ lb}} \times \frac{42 \text{ lb}}{1} \times \frac{1 \text{ day}}{2 \text{ doses}} = 238.63 \text{ mg/dose (minimum)}$

$\frac{x \text{ mg}}{\text{dose}} = \frac{50 \text{ mg}}{\text{kg/day}} \times \frac{1 \text{ kg}}{2.2 \text{ lb}} \times \frac{42 \text{ lb}}{1} \times \frac{1 \text{ day}}{2 \text{ doses}} = 477.27 \text{ mg/dose (maximum)}$

c. $x \text{ mL} = \frac{5 \text{ mL}}{125 \text{ mg}} \times \frac{300 \text{ mg}}{1} = 12 \text{ mL}$

11. $\frac{x \text{ gtt}}{\text{min}} = \frac{60 \text{ gtt}}{1 \text{ mL}} \times \frac{100 \text{ mL}}{30 \text{ min}} = 200 \text{ gtt/min}$

12. b. $\frac{x \text{ mg}}{\text{dose}} = \frac{10 \text{ mg}}{\text{kg/day}} \times \frac{1 \text{ kg}}{2.2 \text{ lb}} \times \frac{58 \text{ lb}}{1} \times \frac{1 \text{ day}}{3 \text{ doses}} = 87.88 \text{ mg/dose (minimum)}$

$\frac{x \text{ mg}}{\text{dose}} = \frac{20 \text{ mg}}{\text{kg/day}} \times \frac{1 \text{ kg}}{2.2 \text{ lb}} \times \frac{58 \text{ lb}}{1} \times \frac{1 \text{ day}}{3 \text{ doses}} = 175.76 \text{ mg/dose (maximum)}$

c. Yes, the order is safe.

d. $x \text{ mL} = \frac{5 \text{ mL}}{100 \text{ mg}} \times \frac{150 \text{ mg}}{1} = 7.5 \text{ mL}$

13. a. $x \text{ kg} = \frac{1 \text{ kg}}{2.2 \text{ lb}} \times \frac{72 \text{ lb}}{1} = 32.7 \text{ kg}$

b. First 20 kg: $x \text{ mL} = \frac{1500 \text{ mL}}{\text{day}} = 1500 \text{ mL/day}$

Remaining 12.7 kg: $x \text{ mL} = \frac{20 \text{ mL}}{\text{kg}} \times \frac{12.7 \text{ kg}}{1} = 254 \text{ mL/day}$

1500 + 254 = 1754 mL/24 h

c. $\frac{x \text{ mL}}{\text{h}} = \frac{1754 \text{ mL}}{24 \text{ h}} = 73.1 \text{ or } 73 \text{ mL/h}$

14. b. $\frac{x \text{ mg}}{\text{dose}} = \frac{5 \text{ mg}}{\text{kg/dose}} \times \frac{1 \text{ kg}}{2.2 \text{ lb}} \times \frac{52 \text{ lb}}{1} = 118.18 \text{ or } 118.2 \text{ mg/dose (minimum)}$

$\frac{x \text{ mg}}{\text{dose}} = \frac{10 \text{ mg}}{\text{kg/dose}} \times \frac{1 \text{ kg}}{2.2 \text{ lb}} \times \frac{52 \text{ lb}}{1} = 236.36 \text{ or } 236.4 \text{ mg/dose (maximum)}$

c. $x \text{ mL} = \frac{5 \text{ mL}}{100 \text{ mg}} \times \frac{100 \text{ mg}}{1} = 5 \text{ mL}$

15. b. $\frac{x \text{ mg}}{\text{dose}} = \frac{25 \text{ mg}}{\text{kg/day}} \times \frac{1 \text{ kg}}{2.2 \text{ lb}} \times \frac{81 \text{ lb}}{1} \times \frac{1 \text{ day}}{4 \text{ doses}} = 230.11$ or 230.1 mg/dose (minimum)

$\frac{x \text{ mg}}{\text{dose}} = \frac{50 \text{ mg}}{\text{kg/day}} \times \frac{1 \text{ kg}}{2.2 \text{ lb}} \times \frac{81 \text{ lb}}{1} \times \frac{1 \text{ day}}{4 \text{ doses}} = 460.22$ or 460.2 mg/dose (maximum)

c. Yes, 350 mg/dose is safe to administer.

d. $x \text{ mL} = \frac{5 \text{ mL}}{500 \text{ mg}} \times \frac{350 \text{ mg}}{1} = 3.5 \text{ mL}$

16. b. $\frac{x \text{ mg}}{\text{dose}} = \frac{15 \text{ mg}}{\text{kg/day}} \times \frac{1 \text{ kg}}{2.2 \text{ lb}} \times \frac{16 \text{ lb}}{1} \times \frac{1 \text{ day}}{3 \text{ doses}} = 36.36$ or 36.4 mg/dose (minimum)

$\frac{x \text{ mg}}{\text{dose}} = \frac{20 \text{ mg}}{\text{kg/day}} \times \frac{1 \text{ kg}}{2.2 \text{ lb}} \times \frac{16 \text{ lb}}{1} \times \frac{1 \text{ day}}{3 \text{ doses}} = 48.48$ or 48.5 mg/dose (maximum)

c. No, the order of 60 mg q 8 h exceeds the safe dose range.

d. $\frac{x \text{ mg}}{\text{kg/day}} = \frac{60 \text{ mg}}{\text{dose}} \times \frac{3 \text{ doses}}{\text{day}} \times \frac{2.2 \text{ lb}}{1 \text{ kg}} \times \frac{}{16 \text{ lb}} = 24.75$ or 24.8 mg/kg/day

e. This is not safe; do not administer. Call the licensed prescriber or pharmacist to check.

17. b. $\frac{x \text{ mg}}{\text{day}} = \frac{0.5 \text{ mg}}{\text{kg/day}} \times \frac{1 \text{ kg}}{2.2 \text{ lb}} \times \frac{19 \text{ lb}}{1} = 4.31$ or 4.3 mg/day (minimum)

$\frac{x \text{ mg}}{\text{day}} = \frac{2 \text{ mg}}{\text{kg/day}} \times \frac{1 \text{ kg}}{2.2 \text{ lb}} \times \frac{19 \text{ lb}}{1} = 17.27$ or 17.3 mg/day (maximum)

c. Yes, it is safe to administer.

d. $x \text{ mL} = \frac{5 \text{ mL}}{5 \text{ mg}} \times \frac{8 \text{ mg}}{1} = 8 \text{ mL}$

18. b. $\frac{x \text{ mg}}{\text{day}} = \frac{100 \text{ mg}}{\text{kg/day}} \times \frac{1 \text{ kg}}{2.2 \text{ lb}} \times \frac{32 \text{ lb}}{1} = 1454.54$ or 1454.5 mg/day

c. $\frac{x \text{ mg}}{\text{day}} = \frac{400 \text{ mg}}{\text{dose}} \times \frac{3 \text{ doses}}{\text{day}} = 1200 \text{ mg/day}$

Yes, this order is safe but may not be therapeutic.

d. $x \text{ mL} = \frac{1 \text{ mL}}{330 \text{ mg}} \times \frac{400 \text{ mg}}{1} = 1.2 \text{ mL}$

19. $\frac{x \text{ mL}}{\text{h}} = \frac{250 \text{ mL}}{3 \text{ h}} = 83.3 \text{ mL/h}$

20. a. $x \text{ mL} = \frac{1 \text{ mL}}{10 \text{ mg}} \times \frac{40 \text{ mg}}{1} = 4 \text{ mL}$

b. $x \text{ mL} = \frac{1 \text{ mL}}{2 \text{ mg}} \times \frac{40 \text{ mg}}{1} = 20 \text{ mL}$

$20 \text{ mL} - 4 \text{ mL} = 16 \text{ mL}$

c. $\frac{x \text{ gtt}}{\text{min}} = \frac{60 \text{ gtt}}{1 \text{ mL}} \times \frac{20 \text{ mL}}{20 \text{ min}} = 60 \text{ gtt/min}$

CHAPTER 18 Dimensional Analysis—Posttest 1, pp. 541–544

1. b. $\frac{x \text{ mg}}{\text{dose}} = \frac{4 \text{ mg}}{\text{kg/day}} \times \frac{1 \text{ kg}}{2.2 \text{ lb}} \times \frac{55 \text{ lb}}{1} \times \frac{1 \text{ day}}{2 \text{ doses}} = 50$ mg/dose (minimum)

$\frac{x \text{ mg}}{\text{dose}} = \frac{6 \text{ mg}}{\text{kg/day}} \times \frac{1 \text{ kg}}{2.2 \text{ lb}} \times \frac{55 \text{ lb}}{1} \times \frac{1 \text{ day}}{2 \text{ doses}} = 75$ mg/dose (maximum)

c. Yes, 60 mg is ordered, and it falls within the 50 to 75 mg/dose range.

d. $x \text{ mL} = \frac{5 \text{ mL}}{20 \text{ mg}} \times \frac{60 \text{ mg}}{1} = 15 \text{ mL}$

2. b. $\frac{x \text{ mg}}{\text{dose}} = \frac{25 \text{ mg}}{\text{kg/day}} \times \frac{1 \text{ kg}}{2.2 \text{ lb}} \times \frac{44 \text{ lb}}{1} \times \frac{1 \text{ day}}{4 \text{ doses}} = 125$ mg/dose (minimum)

$\frac{x \text{ mg}}{\text{dose}} = \frac{50 \text{ mg}}{\text{kg/day}} \times \frac{1 \text{ kg}}{2.2 \text{ lb}} \times \frac{44 \text{ lb}}{1} \times \frac{1 \text{ day}}{4 \text{ doses}} = 250$ mg/dose (maximum)

c. No, 500 mg q 6 h exceeds the recommended dosage for weight.

d. Question this order.

3. b. $\frac{x \text{ mg}}{\text{kg/day}} = \frac{300 \text{ mg}}{\text{dose}} \times \frac{3 \text{ doses}}{1 \text{ day}} \times \frac{2.2 \text{ lb}}{1 \text{ kg}} \times \frac{}{34 \text{ lb}} = 58.23$ or 58.2 mg/kg/day

c. Dosage is safe and therapeutic; it falls in the recommended range.

$x \text{ mL} = \frac{5 \text{ mL}}{125 \text{ mg}} \times \frac{300 \text{ mg}}{1} = 12 \text{ mL}$

4. b. $\frac{x \text{ mg}}{\text{dose}} = \frac{0.1 \text{ mg}}{\text{kg/dose}} \times \frac{1 \text{ kg}}{2.2 \text{ lb}} \times \frac{78 \text{ lb}}{1} = 3.54$ or 3.5 mg/dose (minimum)

$\frac{x \text{ mg}}{\text{dose}} = \frac{0.2 \text{ mg}}{\text{kg/dose}} \times \frac{1 \text{ kg}}{2.2 \text{ lb}} \times \frac{78 \text{ lb}}{1} = 7.09$ or 7.1 mg/dose (maximum)

c. Yes, 4 mg is between 3.54 and 7.09 mg.

d. $x \text{ mL} = \frac{1 \text{ mL}}{15 \text{ mg}} \times \frac{4 \text{ mg}}{1} = 0.27 \text{ mL}$

5. b. $\frac{x \text{ mg}}{\text{dose}} = \frac{10 \text{ mg}}{\text{kg/dose}} \times \frac{1 \text{ kg}}{2.2 \text{ lb}} \times \frac{62 \text{ lb}}{1} = 281.81$ or 281.8 mg/dose (minimum)

$\frac{x \text{ mg}}{\text{dose}} = \frac{15 \text{ mg}}{\text{kg/dose}} \times \frac{1 \text{ kg}}{2.2 \text{ lb}} \times \frac{62 \text{ lb}}{1} = 422.72$ or 422.7 mg/dose (maximum)

c. $x \text{ mL} = \frac{5 \text{ mL}}{160 \text{ mg}} \times \frac{281.82 \text{ mg}}{1} = 8.8 \text{ mL}$ (minimum)

$x \text{ mL} = \frac{5 \text{ mL}}{160 \text{ mg}} \times \frac{422.73 \text{ mg}}{1} = 13.2 \text{ mL}$ (maximum)

6. $\frac{x \text{ mL}}{\text{h}} = \frac{1000 \text{ mL}}{16 \text{ h}} = 62.5 \text{ mL/h}$

7. b. $\frac{x \text{ mg}}{\text{dose}} = \frac{15 \text{ mg}}{\text{kg/day}} \times \frac{1 \text{ kg}}{2.2 \text{ lb}} \times \frac{92 \text{ lb}}{1} \times \frac{1 \text{ day}}{2 \text{ doses}} = 313.64$ or 313.6 mg/dose

c. Yes, 300 mg does not exceed 313.64 mg, so the dose is safe but may not be therapeutic.

d. $x \text{ mL} = \frac{5 \text{ mL}}{125 \text{ mg}} \times \frac{300 \text{ mg}}{1} = 12 \text{ mL}$

8. a. $x \text{ kg} = \frac{1 \text{ kg}}{2.2 \text{ lb}} \times \frac{25 \text{ lb}}{1} = 11.4 \text{ kg}$

b. First 10 kg: $x \text{ mL} = \frac{100 \text{ mL}}{\text{kg}} \times \frac{10 \text{ kg}}{1} = 1000 \text{ mL/24 h}$

Remaining 1.4 kg: $x \text{ mL} = \frac{50 \text{ mL}}{\text{kg}} \times \frac{1.4 \text{ kg}}{1} = 70 \text{ mL/24 h}$

1000 mL/24 h + 70 mL/24 h = 1070 mL/24 h

c. $\frac{x \text{ mL}}{\text{h}} = \frac{1070 \text{ mL}}{24 \text{ h}} = 44.6 \text{ mL/h}$

9. b. $\frac{x \text{ mg}}{\text{kg/day}} = \frac{650 \text{ mg}}{\text{dose}} \times \frac{4 \text{ doses}}{1 \text{ day}} \times \frac{2.2 \text{ lb}}{1 \text{ kg}} \times \frac{}{96 \text{ lb}} = 59.58$ or 59.6 mg/kg/day

c. Yes, it is safe; recommended is 40 to 60 mg/kg/24 h. Child is receiving 59.58 mg/kg/day.

10. b. $\frac{x \text{ mg}}{\text{kg/day}} = \frac{300 \text{ mg}}{\text{dose}} \times \frac{3 \text{ doses}}{1 \text{ day}} \times \frac{2.2 \text{ lb}}{1 \text{ kg}} \times \frac{}{95 \text{ lb}} = 20.84 \text{ mg/kg/day}$

c. The child is receiving 20.84 mg/kg/day. Recommended is 20 to 40 mg/kg/day. The ordered dose is both safe and therapeutic.

11. $\frac{x \text{ mL}}{\text{h}} = \frac{100 \text{ mL}}{6 \text{ h}} = 16.7 \text{ or } 17 \text{ mL/h}$

12. a. $x \text{ mL} = \frac{1 \text{ mL}}{250 \text{ mg}} \times \frac{400 \text{ mg}}{1} = 1.6 \text{ mL}$

b. $x \text{ mL} = \frac{1 \text{ mL}}{50 \text{ mg}} \times \frac{400 \text{ mg}}{1} = 8 \text{ mL}$

$8 \text{ mL} - 1.6 \text{ mL} = 6.4 \text{ mL}$

c. $\frac{x \text{ gtt}}{\text{min}} = \frac{60 \text{ gtt}}{1 \text{ mL}} \times \frac{8 \text{ mL}}{30 \text{ min}} = 16 \text{ gtt/min}$

13. a. $\frac{x \text{ mg}}{\text{kg/day}} = \frac{60 \text{ mg}}{\text{dose}} \times \frac{2 \text{ doses}}{1 \text{ day}} \times \frac{}{30 \text{ kg}} = 4 \text{ mg/kg/day}$

b. No, the ordered dosage is more than the recommended 0.5 to 2 mg/kg/24 h. Also, the maximum dose is 80 mg/25 h, and this is exceeded as well.

c. No, check with the licensed prescriber.

14. b. $\frac{x \text{ mg}}{\text{dose}} = \frac{15 \text{ mg}}{\text{kg/day}} \times \frac{1 \text{ kg}}{2.2 \text{ lb}} \times \frac{89 \text{ lb}}{1} \times \frac{1 \text{ day}}{2 \text{ doses}} = 303.4 \text{ mg/dose (minimum)}$

$\frac{x \text{ mg}}{\text{dose}} = \frac{20 \text{ mg}}{\text{kg/day}} \times \frac{1 \text{ kg}}{2.2 \text{ lb}} \times \frac{89 \text{ lb}}{1} \times \frac{1 \text{ day}}{2 \text{ doses}} = 404.55 \text{ or } 404.6 \text{ mg/dose (maximum)}$

c. Yes, 400 mg/dose is within the recommended single-dose range.

d. $x \text{ mL} = \frac{5 \text{ mL}}{375 \text{ mg}} \times \frac{400 \text{ mg}}{1} = 5.3 \text{ mL}$

15. b. $\frac{x \text{ mg}}{\text{kg/day}} = \frac{90 \text{ mg}}{\text{dose}} \times \frac{4 \text{ doses}}{1 \text{ day}} \times \frac{2.2 \text{ lb}}{1 \text{ kg}} \times \frac{}{11 \text{ lb}} = 72 \text{ mg/kg/24 h}$

c. The order is both safe and therapeutic, between the recommended 50 to 100 mg/kg/24 h.

CHAPTER 18 Dimensional Analysis—Posttest 2, pp. 545–548

1. b. $\frac{x \text{ mg}}{\text{kg/day}} = \frac{450 \text{ mg}}{\text{dose}} \times \frac{4 \text{ doses}}{1 \text{ day}} \times \frac{2.2 \text{ lb}}{1 \text{ kg}} \times \frac{}{70 \text{ lb}} = 56.57 \text{ mg/kg/24 h}$

c. Yes, the child is receiving 56.6 mg/kg/24 h, which is between 40 and 60 mg/kg/24 h.

2. b. $\frac{x \text{ mg}}{\text{day}} = \frac{7 \text{ mg}}{\text{kg/day}} \times \frac{1 \text{ kg}}{2.2 \text{ lb}} \times \frac{62 \text{ lb}}{1} = 197.27 \text{ mg/day (minimum)}$

$\frac{x \text{ mg}}{\text{day}} = \frac{8 \text{ mg}}{\text{kg/day}} \times \frac{1 \text{ kg}}{2.2 \text{ lb}} \times \frac{62 \text{ lb}}{1} = 225.45 \text{ mg/day (maximum)}$

c. $\frac{x \text{ mg}}{\text{dose}} = \frac{197.27 \text{ mg}}{1 \text{ day}} \times \frac{1 \text{ day}}{2 \text{ doses}} = 98.64 \text{ or } 98.6 \text{ mg/dose}$

$\frac{x \text{ mg}}{\text{dose}} = \frac{225.45 \text{ mg}}{1 \text{ day}} \times \frac{1 \text{ day}}{2 \text{ doses}} = 112.73 \text{ or } 112.7 \text{ mg/dose}$

d. Yes, the ordered dose is both safe and therapeutic because it falls within the recommended 24-hour dosage and single-dose ranges.

e. $x \text{ mL} = \frac{5 \text{ mL}}{125 \text{ mg}} \times \frac{100 \text{ mg}}{1} = 4 \text{ mL}$

3. $\frac{x \text{ gtt}}{\text{min}} = \frac{60 \text{ gtt}}{1 \text{ mL}} \times \frac{150 \text{ mL}}{3 \text{ h}} \times \frac{1 \text{ h}}{60 \text{ min}} = 50 \text{ gtt/min}$

4. b. $\frac{x \text{ mg}}{\text{day}} = \frac{25 \text{ mg}}{\text{kg/day}} \times \frac{1 \text{ kg}}{2.2 \text{ lb}} \times \frac{58 \text{ lb}}{1} = 659.09 \text{ or } 659.1 \text{ (minimum)}$

$\frac{x \text{ mg}}{\text{day}} = \frac{50 \text{ mg}}{\text{kg/day}} \times \frac{1 \text{ kg}}{2.2 \text{ lb}} \times \frac{58 \text{ lb}}{1} = 1318.18 \text{ or } 1318.2 \text{ mg/day (maximum)}$

c. $\frac{x \text{ mg}}{\text{dose}} = \frac{659.09 \text{ mg}}{1 \text{ day}} \times \frac{1 \text{ day}}{2 \text{ doses}} = 329.54 \text{ or } 329.5 \text{ mg/dose}$

$\frac{x \text{ mg}}{\text{dose}} = \frac{1318.18 \text{ mg}}{1 \text{ day}} \times \frac{1 \text{ day}}{2 \text{ doses}} = 659.09 \text{ or } 659.1 \text{ mg/dose}$

d. $\frac{x \text{ mg}}{\text{kg/day}} = \frac{400 \text{ mg}}{\text{dose}} \times \frac{2 \text{ doses}}{1 \text{ day}} \times \frac{2.2 \text{ lb}}{1 \text{ kg}} \times \frac{}{58 \text{ lb}} = 30.3 \text{ mg/kg/24 h}$

e. $x \text{ mL} = \frac{5 \text{ mL}}{250 \text{ mg}} \times \frac{400 \text{ mg}}{1} = 8 \text{ mL}$

5. b. $\frac{x \text{ mg}}{\text{kg/day}} = \frac{500 \text{ mg}}{\text{dose}} \times \frac{4 \text{ doses}}{1 \text{ day}} \times \frac{2.2 \text{ lb}}{1 \text{ kg}} \times \frac{}{99 \text{ lb}} = 44.44 \text{ or } 44.4 \text{ mg/kg/24 h}$

c. Yes, the recommended dosage is 50 to 100 mg/kg/24 h.

d. $x \text{ cap} = \frac{1 \text{ cap}}{250 \text{ mg}} \times \frac{500 \text{ mg}}{1} = 2 \text{ capsules}$

6. b. $\frac{x \text{ mg}}{\text{kg/day}} = \frac{200 \text{ mg}}{\text{dose}} \times \frac{2 \text{ doses}}{1 \text{ day}} \times \frac{2.2 \text{ lb}}{1 \text{ kg}} \times \frac{}{66 \text{ lb}} = 13.33 \text{ or } 13.3 \text{ mg/kg/day}$

c. Yes, the dose is safe and therapeutic.

d. $x \text{ mL} = \frac{5 \text{ mL}}{125 \text{ mg}} \times \frac{200 \text{ mg}}{1} = 8 \text{ mL}$

7. b. $\frac{x \text{ mg}}{\text{day}} = \frac{100 \text{ mg}}{\text{kg/day}} \times \frac{1 \text{ kg}}{1000 \text{ g}} \times \frac{2012 \text{ g}}{1} = 201 \text{ mg/day (minimum)}$

$\frac{x \text{ mg}}{\text{day}} = \frac{200 \text{ mg}}{\text{kg/day}} \times \frac{1 \text{ kg}}{1000 \text{ g}} \times \frac{2012 \text{ g}}{1} = 402.4 \text{ mg/day (maximum)}$

c. $\frac{x \text{ mg}}{\text{dose}} = \frac{201 \text{ mg}}{\text{day}} \times \frac{1 \text{ day}}{4 \text{ doses}} = 50.25 \text{ or } 50.3 \text{ mg/dose (minimum)}$

$\frac{x \text{ mg}}{\text{dose}} = \frac{402.4 \text{ mg}}{\text{day}} \times \frac{1 \text{ day}}{4 \text{ doses}} = 100.6 \text{ mg/dose (maximum)}$

8. b. $\frac{x \text{ mg}}{\text{kg/day}} = \frac{180 \text{ mg}}{\text{dose}} \times \frac{3 \text{ doses}}{1 \text{ day}} \times \frac{2.2 \text{ lb}}{1 \text{ kg}} \times \frac{}{35 \text{ lb}} = 33.94 \text{ or } 33.9 \text{ mg/kg/day}$

c. Yes, the ordered dose is within the safe and therapeutic range.

d. $x \text{ mL} = \frac{5 \text{ mL}}{125 \text{ mg}} \times \frac{180 \text{ mg}}{1} = 7.2 \text{ mL}$

9. b. $\frac{x \text{ mg}}{\text{kg/day}} = \frac{330 \text{ mg}}{\text{dose}} \times \frac{4 \text{ doses}}{1 \text{ day}} \times \frac{2.2 \text{ lb}}{1 \text{ kg}} \times \frac{}{74 \text{ lb}} = 39.24 \text{ or } 39.2 \text{ mg/kg/day}$

c. Yes, the dose ordered is safe to administer.

d. $x \text{ mL} = \frac{5 \text{ mL}}{250 \text{ mg}} \times \frac{330 \text{ mg}}{1} = 6.6 \text{ mL}$

10. b. $\frac{x \text{ mg}}{\text{dose}} = \frac{0.1 \text{ mg}}{\text{kg/dose}} \times \frac{1 \text{ kg}}{2.2 \text{ lb}} \times \frac{20 \text{ lb}}{1} = 0.91 \text{ mg/dose (minimum)}$

$\frac{x \text{ mg}}{\text{dose}} = \frac{0.2 \text{ mg}}{\text{kg/dose}} \times \frac{1 \text{ kg}}{2.2 \text{ lb}} \times \frac{20 \text{ lb}}{1} = 1.82 \text{ mg/dose (maximum)}$

c. No, 0.9 mg/dose is not within the safe range to administer. Contact the licensed prescriber.

d. $x \text{ mL} = \frac{1 \text{ mL}}{0.5 \text{ mg}} \times \frac{0.9 \text{ mg}}{1} = 1.8 \text{ mL if dose is approved}$

11. $\frac{x \text{ mL}}{\text{h}} = \frac{200 \text{ mL}}{3 \text{ h}} = 66.7 \text{ or } 67 \text{ mL/h}$

12. a. $x \text{ mL} = \dfrac{1 \text{ mL}}{50 \text{ mg}} \times \dfrac{500 \text{ mg}}{1} = 10 \text{ mL}$

b. $x \text{ mL} = \dfrac{1 \text{ mL}}{5 \text{ mg}} \times \dfrac{500 \text{ mg}}{1} = 100 \text{ mL} - 10 \text{ mL} = 90 \text{ mL}$

c. $\dfrac{x \text{ gtt}}{\text{min}} = \dfrac{60 \text{ gtt}}{1 \text{ mL}} \times \dfrac{100 \text{ mL}}{60 \text{ min}} = 100 \text{ gtt/min}$

13. b. $\dfrac{x \text{ mcg}}{\text{day}} = \dfrac{6 \text{ mcg}}{\text{kg/day}} \times \dfrac{1 \text{ kg}}{1000 \text{ g}} \times \dfrac{3036 \text{ g}}{1} = 18.22 \text{ mcg/day (minimum)}$

$\dfrac{x \text{ mcg}}{\text{day}} = \dfrac{10 \text{ mcg}}{\text{kg/day}} \times \dfrac{1 \text{ kg}}{1000 \text{ g}} \times \dfrac{3036 \text{ g}}{1} = 30.36 \text{ mcg/day (maximum)}$

c. $\dfrac{x \text{ mcg}}{\text{dose}} = \dfrac{18.22 \text{ mcg}}{\text{day}} \times \dfrac{1 \text{ day}}{2 \text{ doses}} \times \dfrac{1 \text{ mg}}{1000 \text{ mcg}} = 0.009 \text{ mg/dose (minimum)}$

$\dfrac{x \text{ mcg}}{\text{dose}} = \dfrac{30.36 \text{ mcg}}{\text{day}} \times \dfrac{1 \text{ day}}{2 \text{ doses}} \times \dfrac{1 \text{ mg}}{1000 \text{ mcg}} = 0.015 \text{ mg/dose (maximum)}$

d. Yes, the ordered dose, 0.013 mg, is between 0.009 and 0.015 mg.

e. $x \text{ mL} = \dfrac{1 \text{ mL}}{50 \text{ mcg}} \times \dfrac{1000 \text{ mcg}}{1 \text{ mg}} \times \dfrac{0.013 \text{ mg}}{1} = 0.26 \text{ mL (a drug rounded to the hundredth)}$

14. b. $\dfrac{x \text{ mg}}{\text{dose}} = \dfrac{10 \text{ mg}}{\text{kg/dose}} \times \dfrac{1 \text{ kg}}{2.2 \text{ lb}} \times \dfrac{9 \text{ lb}}{1} = 40.9 \text{ mg/dose (minimum)}$

$\dfrac{x \text{ mg}}{\text{dose}} = \dfrac{15 \text{ mg}}{\text{kg/dose}} \times \dfrac{1 \text{ kg}}{2.2 \text{ lb}} \times \dfrac{9 \text{ lb}}{1} = 61.36 \text{ or } 61.4 \text{ mg/dose (maximum)}$

c. $x \text{ mL} = \dfrac{5 \text{ mL}}{160 \text{ mg}} \times \dfrac{40.9 \text{ mg}}{1} = 1.28 \text{ or } 1.3 \text{ mL (minimum)}$

$x \text{ mL} = \dfrac{5 \text{ mL}}{160 \text{ mg}} \times \dfrac{61.36 \text{ mg}}{1} = 1.92 \text{ or } 1.9 \text{ mL (maximum)}$

15. b. $\dfrac{x \text{ mg}}{\text{day}} = \dfrac{4 \text{ mg}}{\text{kg/day}} \times \dfrac{1 \text{ kg}}{2.2 \text{ lb}} \times \dfrac{37 \text{ lb}}{1} = 67.27 \text{ or } 67.3 \text{ mg/day (minimum)}$

$\dfrac{x \text{ mg}}{\text{day}} = \dfrac{6 \text{ mg}}{\text{kg/day}} \times \dfrac{1 \text{ kg}}{2.2 \text{ lb}} \times \dfrac{37 \text{ lb}}{1} = 100.9 \text{ mg/day (maximum)}$

Dosage range is 67.27 to 100.9 mg/24 h.

c. Yes, 72 mg/24 h is within the recommended range.

d. $x \text{ mL} = \dfrac{5 \text{ mL}}{20 \text{ mg}} \times \dfrac{72 \text{ mg}}{1} = 18 \text{ mL}$

CHAPTER 18 Proportion Method—Work Sheet, pp. 537–540

Proportion Method:

1. a. 2.2 lb : 1 kg :: 50 lb : x kg

$2.2x = 50$

$x = \dfrac{50}{2.2}$

$x = 22.7$ kg

b. 25 mg/24 h : 1 kg :: x mg/24 h : 22.7 kg

$x = 567.5$ mg/24 h

50 mg/24 h : 1 kg :: x mg/24 h : 22.7 kg

$x = 1135$ mg/24 h

Safe dose range is 567.5 to 1135 mg/24 h.

250 mg : 1 dose :: x mg : 4 doses

$x = 1000$ mg/24 h

c. Yes, the order is safe to administer.

d. 250 mg : 1 cap :: 250 mg : x cap

$250x = 250$

$x = \dfrac{250}{250}$

$x = 1$ capsule

Formula Method:

a. 1 kg = 2.2 lb

$\dfrac{50 \text{ lb}}{2.2 \text{ kg}} = 22.7 \text{ kg}$

b. 25 mg/kg/24 h × 22.7 kg = 567.5 mg/24 h

c. 50 mg/kg/24 h × 22.7 kg = 1135 mg/24 h

d. 250 mg × 4 doses/24 h = 1000 mg/24 h

Proportion Method:

2. a. 2.2 lb : 1 kg :: 6.5 lb : x kg
$2.2x = 6.5$
$x = \frac{6.5}{2.2}$
$x = 2.95$ kg or 3 kg
b. 0.035 mg : 1 kg :: x mg : 3 kg
$x = 0.11$ mg/kg/day
0.06 mg : 1 kg :: x mg : 3 kg
$x = 0.18$ mg
The safe range is 0.11 to 0.18 mg/kg/day.
c. No, the order is not safe.
d. Question this order.
3. a. 2.2 lb : 1 kg :: 50 lb : x kg
$2.2x = 50$
$x = \frac{50}{2.2}$
$x = 22.7$ kg
b. 5 mg/24 h : 1 kg :: x mg/24 h : 22.7 kg
$x = 113.5$ mg/kg/24 h divided by four doses
c. $\frac{113.5 \text{ mg/kg/24 h}}{4 \text{ doses/24 h}} = 28.4$ mg/dose
Safe and therapeutic dose is 28.4 mg/dose, so the 25-mg ordered dose is safe.
d. 12.5 mg : 1 mL :: 25 mg : x mL
$12.5x = 25$
$x = \frac{25}{12.5}$
$x = 2$ mL
4. a. 2.2 lb : 1 kg :: 28 lb : x kg
$2.2x = 28$
$x = \frac{28}{2.2}$
$x = 12.7$ kg
First 0–10 kg = 100 mL/kg/24 h
10 mL/24 h × 10 kg = 1000 mL/24 h
12.7 kg − 10 kg = 2.7 kg
Remaining 2.7 kg × 50 mL/kg = 135 mL/24 h
1000 + 135 = 1135 mL/24 h
b. $\frac{1135 \text{ mL/24 h}}{24 \text{ h}} = 47.3$ or 47 mL/h
5. a. 2.2 lb : 1 kg :: 22 lb : x kg
$2.2x = 22$
$x = \frac{22}{2.2}$
$x = 10$ kg
b. 70 mg : 1 dose :: x mg : 2 doses
$x = 140$ mg/24 h
$\frac{140 \text{ mg/24 h}}{10 \text{ kg}} = 14$ mg/kg/24 h
Child is receiving the recommended dose.
c. 125 mg : 5 mL :: 70 mg : x mL
$125x = 350$
$x = \frac{350}{125}$
$x = 2.8$ mL
6. a. 30.3 kg
b. 20 mg/24 h : 1 kg :: x mg/24 h : 30.3 kg
$x = 606$ mg/24 h
30 mg/24 h : 1 kg :: x mg/24 h : 30.3 kg
$x = 909$ mg/24 h
c. $\frac{606 \text{ mg/24 h}}{2 \text{ doses/24 h}} = 303$ mg/dose
$\frac{909 \text{ mg/24 h}}{2 \text{ doses/24 h}} = 454.5$ mg/dose
303 to 454.5 mg/dose (single dose)
d. 250 mg : 5 mL :: 300 mg : x mL
$250x = 1500$
$x = \frac{1500}{250}$
$x = 6$ mL
7. a. 2.2 lb : 1 kg :: 94 lb : x kg
$2.2x = 94$
$x = \frac{94}{2.2}$
$x = 42.7$ kg
b. 42.7 kg × 0.5 mg/kg/24 h = 21.4 mg/24 h
42.7 kg × 2 mg/kg/24 h = 85.4 mg/24 h
NOTE: 80 mg/24 h is the max dose.
c. No, the child would be receiving 90 mg/24 h.
d. No, call the licensed prescriber who wrote the order.
8. a. 2.2 lb : 1 kg :: 40 lb : x kg
$2.2x = 40$
$x = \frac{40}{2.2}$
$x = 18.2$ kg
b. 18.2 kg × 5 mg/kg/24 h = 91 mg/24 h
18.2 kg × 7 mg/kg/24 h = 127.4 mg/24 h
c. Yes, the order is safe to administer.
d. 30 mg : 1 tab :: 60 mg : x tab
$30x = 60$
$x = \frac{60}{30}$
$x = 2$ chewtabs

9. a. 2.2 lb : 1 kg :: 68 lb : x kg
$2.2x = 68$
$x = \frac{68}{2.2}$
$x = 30.9$ kg
b. $\frac{750 \text{ mg} \times 4 \text{ doses/24 h}}{30.9 \text{ kg}} = \frac{3000}{30.9}$
$= 97.1$ mg/kg/24 h
c. No, it exceeds the recommended 40 to 60 mg/kg/24 h.

10. a. 2.2 lb : 1 kg :: 42 lb : x kg
$2.2x = 42$
$x = \frac{42}{2.2}$
$x = 19.1$ kg
b. $\frac{19.1 \text{ kg} \times 25 \text{ mg/kg/24 h}}{2 \text{ doses/24 h}} = \frac{477.5}{2}$
$= 238.8$ mg/dose
$\frac{19.1 \text{ kg} \times 50 \text{ mg/kg/24 h}}{2 \text{ doses/24 h}} = \frac{955}{2}$
$= 477.5$ mg/dose
Single-dose range is 238.8 to 477.5 mg/dose.
c. 125 mg : 5 mL :: 300 mg : x mL
$125x = 1500$
$x = \frac{1500}{125}$
$x = 12$ mL

11. a. $\frac{100 \text{ mL}}{30 \text{ min}} \times 60$ gtt/mL $= 200$ gtt/min

12. a. 2.2 kg : 1 lb :: 58 lb : x kg
$2.2x = 58$
$x = \frac{58}{2.2}$
$x = 26.4$ kg
b. $\frac{26.4 \text{ kg} \times 10 \text{ mg/kg/24 h}}{3 \text{ doses/24 h}} = \frac{264}{3}$
$= 88$ mg/dose
$\frac{26.4 \text{ kg} \times 20 \text{ mg/kg/24 h}}{3 \text{ doses/24 h}} = \frac{528}{3}$
$= 176$ mg/dose
Single-dose range is 88 to 176 mg/dose.
c. Yes, the dose is safe to administer.
d. 100 mg : 5 mL :: 150 mg : x mL
$100x = 750$
$x = \frac{750}{100}$
$x = 7.5$ mL

13. a. 2.2 lb : 1 kg :: 72 lb : x kg
$2.2x = 72$
$x = \frac{72}{2.2}$
$x = 32.7$ kg
b. First 20 kg — 1500 mL/24 h
Next 12.7 kg × 20 mL — + 254 mL/24 h
1754 mL/24 h
c. $\frac{1754 \text{ mL/24 h}}{24 \text{ h}} = 73.1$ or 73 mL/h

14. a. 2.2 lb : 1 kg :: 52 lb : x kg
$2.2x = 52$
$x = \frac{52}{2.2}$
$x = 23.6$ kg
b. 23.6 kg × 5 mg/kg/dose = 118 mg/dose
23.6 kg × 10 mg/kg/dose = 236 mg/dose
c. 100 mg : 5 mL :: 100 mg : x mL
$100x = 500$
$x = \frac{500}{100}$
$x = 5$ mL

15. a. 2.2 lb : 1 kg :: 81 lb : x kg
$2.2x = 81$
$x = \frac{81}{2.2}$
$x = 36.8$ kg
b. $\frac{36.8 \text{ kg} \times 25 \text{ mg/kg/24 h}}{4 \text{ doses/24 h}} = \frac{920}{4}$
$= 230$ mg/dose
$\frac{36.8 \text{ kg} \times 50 \text{ mg/kg/24 h}}{4 \text{ doses/24 h}} = \frac{1840}{4}$
$= 460$ mg/dose
Single-dose range is 230 to 460 mg/dose.
c. Yes, 350 mg/dose is safe to administer.
d. 500 mg : 5 mL :: 350 mg : x mL
$500x = 1750$
$x = \frac{1750}{500}$
$x = 3.5$ mL

16. a. 2.2 lb : 1 kg :: 16 lb : x kg
$2.2x = 16$
$x = \frac{16}{2.2}$
$x = 7.3$ kg

b. $\frac{7.3 \text{ kg} \times 15 \text{ mg/kg/24 h}}{3 \text{ doses/24 h}} = \frac{109.5}{3}$
$= 36.5$ mg/dose
$\frac{7.3 \text{ kg} \times 20 \text{ mg/kg/24 h}}{3 \text{ doses/24 h}} = \frac{146}{3}$
$= 48.7$ mg/dose

c. No, the order of 60 mg q 8 h exceeds the safe range.

d. $\frac{60 \text{ mg} \times 3 \text{ doses/24 h}}{7.3 \text{ kg}} = 24.7$ mg/kg/24 h
Proof that the ordered dose exceeds the recommended 15 to 20 mg/kg/24 h

e. This is not safe; do not administer. Call the licensed prescriber or pharmacist to check.

17. a. 2.2 lb : 1 kg :: 19 lb : x kg
$2.2x = 19$
$x = \frac{19}{2.2}$
$x = 8.6$ kg

b. 8.6 kg × 0.5 mg/kg/24 h = 4.3 mg/24 h
8.6 kg × 2 mg/kg/24 h = 17.2 mg/24 h

c. Yes, it is safe to administer.

d. 5 mg : 5 mL :: 8 mg : x mL
$5x = 40$
$x = \frac{40}{5}$
$x = 8$ mL

18. a. 2.2 lb : 1 kg :: 32 lb : x kg
$2.2x = 32$
$x = \frac{32}{2.2}$
$x = 14.5$ kg

b. 14.6 kg × 100 mg/kg/24 h = 1460 mg/24 h
The child may receive up to 1460 mg/24 h.

c. 400 mg : 1 dose :: x mg : 3 doses
$x = 1200$ mg/24 h
Yes, this order is safe but may not be therapeutic.

d. 330 mg : 1 mL :: 400 mg : x mL
$330x = 400$
$x = \frac{400}{330}$
$x = 1.2$ mL

19. $\frac{250 \text{ mL}}{3 \text{ h}} = 83.3$ mL/h

20. a. 10 mg : 1 mL :: 40 mg : x mL
$10x = 40$
$x = \frac{40}{10}$
$x = 4$ mL

b. 2 mg : mL :: 40 mg : x mL
$2x = 40$
$x = 40/2 = 20$ mL
20 mL − 4 mL = 16 mL

c. $\frac{20 \text{ mL}}{20 \text{ min}} \times 60$ gtt/mL = 60 gtt/min

CHAPTER 18 Proportion Method—Posttest 1, pp. 541–544

1. a. 2.2 lb : 1 kg :: 55 lb : x kg
$2.2x = 55$
$x = \frac{55}{2.2}$
$x = 25$ kg

b. $\frac{25 \text{ kg} \times 4 \text{ mg/kg/24 h}}{2 \text{ doses/24 h}} = \frac{100}{2}$
$= 50$ mg/dose
$\frac{25 \text{ kg} \times 6 \text{ mg/kg/24 h}}{2 \text{ doses/24 h}} = \frac{150}{2}$
$= 75$ mg/dose
Single-dose range is 50 to 75 mg/dose.

c. Yes, 60 mg is ordered, and it falls within the 50 to 75 mg/dose range.

d. 20 mg : 5 mL :: 60 mg : x mL
$20x = 300$
$x = \frac{300}{20}$
$x = 15$ mL

2. a. 2.2 lb : 1 kg :: 44 lb : x kg
$2.2x = 44$
$x = \frac{44}{2.2}$
$x = 20$ kg

b. $\frac{20 \text{ kg} \times 25 \text{ mg/kg/24 h}}{4 \text{ doses/24 h}} = \frac{500}{4}$
$= 125$ mg/dose
$\frac{20 \text{ kg} \times 50 \text{ mg/kg/24 h}}{4 \text{ doses/24 h}} = \frac{1000}{4}$
$= 250$ mg/dose
Single-dose range is 125 to 250 mg/dose.

c. No, 500 mg q 6 h exceeds the recommended dosage for weight.

d. Question this order.

3. a. 2.2 lb : 1 kg :: 34 lb : x kg
$2.2x = 34$
$x = \frac{34}{2.2}$
$x = 15.5$
b. $\frac{300 \text{ mg} \times 3 \text{ doses/24 h}}{15.5 \text{ kg}} = \frac{900}{15.5}$
$= 58.1$ mg/kg/24 h
c. Dosage is safe and therapeutic; it falls in the recommended range.
125 mg : 5 mL :: 300 mg : x mL
$125x = 1500$
$x = \frac{1500}{125}$
$x = 12$ mL

4. a. 2.2 lb : 1 kg :: 78 lb : x kg
$2.2x = 78$
$x = \frac{78}{2.2}$
$x = 35.5$ kg
b. 35.5 kg × 0.1 mg/kg/dose = 3.55 mg/dose
35.5 kg × 0.2 mg/kg/dose = 7.1 mg/dose
c. Yes, it falls between 3.55 and 7.1 mg/dose.
d. 15 mg : 1 mL :: 4 mg : x mL
$15x = 4$
$x = \frac{4}{15}$
$x = 0.27$ mL

5. a. 2.2 lb : 1 kg :: 62 lb : x kg
$2.2x = 62$
$x = \frac{62}{2.2}$
$x = 28.2$ kg
b. 28.2 kg × 10 mg/kg/dose = 282 mg/dose
28.2 kg × 15 mg/kg/dose = 423 mg/dose
Single-dose range is 282 to 423 mg/dose.
c. 160 mg : 5 mL :: 282 mg : x mL
$160x = 1410$
$x = \frac{1410}{160}$
$x = 8.8$ mL
160 mg : 5 mL :: 423 mg : x mL
$160x = 2115$
$x = \frac{2115}{160}$
$x = 13.2$ mL

6. $\frac{1000 \text{ mL}}{16 \text{ h}} = 62.5$ or 63 mL/h

7. a. 2.2 lb : 1 kg :: 92 lb : x kg
$2.2x = 92$ lb
$x = \frac{92}{2.2}$
$x = 41.8$ kg
b. $\frac{41.8 \text{ kg} \times 15 \text{ mg/kg/24 h}}{2 \text{ doses/24 h}} = \frac{627}{2}$
$= 313.5$ mg/dose
c. Yes, 300 mg is a safe dose to administer but may not be therapeutic; 300 mg does not exceed 313.64 mg.
d. 125 mg : 5 mL :: 300 mg : x mL
$125x = 1500$ mL
$x = \frac{1500}{125}$
$x = 12$ mL

8. a. 2.2 lb : 1 kg :: 25 lb : x kg
$2.2x = 25$
$x = \frac{25}{2.2}$
$x = 11.4$ kg
b. First 10 kg — 1000 mL/24 h
Next 1.4 kg × 50 mL/kg = + 70 mL/24 h
1070 mL/24 h
c. $\frac{1070 \text{ mL/24 h}}{24 \text{ h}} = 44.6$ or 45 mL/h

9. a. 2.2 lb : 1 kg :: 96 lb : x kg
$2.2x = 96$
$x = \frac{96}{2.2}$
$x = 43.6$ kg
b. $\frac{650 \text{ mg} \times 4 \text{ doses/24 h}}{43.6 \text{ kg}} = \frac{2600}{43.6}$
$= 59.6$ mg/kg/24 h
c. Yes, it is safe; recommended is 40 to 60 mg/kg/24 h. Child is receiving 59.6 mg/kg/24 h.

10. a. 2.2 lb : 1 kg :: 95 lb : x kg
$2.2x = 95$
$x = \frac{95}{2.2}$
$x = 43.2$ kg
b. $\frac{300 \text{ mg} \times 3 \text{ doses/24 h}}{43.2 \text{ kg}} = \frac{900}{43.2}$
$= 20.8$ mg/kg/24 h
c. The child is receiving 20.8 mg/kg/24 h; recommended is 20 to 40 mg/kg/24 h. The ordered dose is both safe and therapeutic.

11. $\frac{100 \text{ mL}}{6 \text{ h}} = 16.7$ or 17 mL/h

12. a. 250 mg : 1 mL :: 400 mg : x mL
$250x = 400$
$x = \frac{400}{250}$
$x = 1.6$ mL
b. $400 \text{ mg} \times \frac{1 \text{ mg}}{50 \text{ mL}} = 8 \text{ mL} \rightarrow$
8 mL − 1.6 mL = 6.4 mL
c. $\frac{8 \text{ mL}}{30 \text{ min}} \times 60 \text{ gtt/mL} = x \text{ gtt/min}$
$x = \frac{480}{30}$
$x = 16$ gtt/min

13. a. $\frac{60 \text{ mg} \times 2 \text{ doses/24 h}}{30 \text{ kg}} = \frac{120}{30}$
$= 4$ mg/kg/24 h
b. No, the ordered dosage is more than the recommended 0.5 to 2 mg/kg/24 h. Also, the maximum dose is 80 mg/24 h, and this is exceeded as well.
c. No, check with the licensed prescriber.

14. a. 2.2 lb : 1 kg :: 89 lb : x kg
$2.2x = 89$
$x = \frac{89}{2.2}$
$x = 40.5$ kg
b. $\frac{40.5 \text{ kg} \times 15 \text{ mg/kg/24 h}}{2 \text{ doses/24 h}} = \frac{607.5}{2}$
$= 303.8$ mg/dose
$\frac{40.5 \text{ kg} \times 20 \text{ mg/kg/24 h}}{2 \text{ doses/24 h}} = \frac{810}{2}$
$= 405$ mg/dose
Dosage range is 607.5 to 810 mg/24 h. Single-dose range is 303.8 to 405 mg/dose.
c. Yes, 400 mg/dose is within the recommended single-dose range.
d. 375 mg : 5 mL :: 400 mg : x mL
$375x = 2000$
$x = \frac{2000}{375}$
$x = 5.3$ mL

15. a. 2.2 lb : 1 kg :: 11 lb : x kg
$2.2x = 11$
$x = \frac{11}{2.2}$
$x = 5$ kg
b. $\frac{90 \text{ mg} \times 4 \text{ doses/24 h}}{5 \text{ kg}} = \frac{360}{5}$
$= 72$ mg/kg/24 h
c. The order is both safe and therapeutic, between the recommended 50 to 100 mg/kg/24 h.

CHAPTER 18 Proportion Method—Posttest 2, pp. 545–548

1. a. 2.2 lb : 1 kg :: 70 lb : x kg
$2.2x = 70$
$x = \frac{70}{2.2}$
$x = 31.8$ kg
b. $\frac{450 \text{ mg} \times 4 \text{ doses/24 h}}{31.8 \text{ kg}} = \frac{1800}{31.8}$
$= 56.6$ mg/kg/24 h
c. Yes, the child is receiving 56.6 mg/kg/24 h, which is between 40 and 60 mg/kg/24 h.

2. a. 2.2 lb : 1 kg :: 62 lb : x kg
$2.2x = 62$
$x = \frac{62}{2.2}$
$x = 28.2$ kg
b. 28.2 kg × 7 mg/kg/24 h = 197.4 mg/24 h
28.2 kg × 8 mg/kg/24 h = 225.6 mg/24 h
Dosage range is 197.4 to 225.6 mg/24 h.
c. $\frac{197.4 \text{ mg/24 h}}{2 \text{ doses/24 h}} = 98.7$ mg/dose
$\frac{225.6 \text{ mg/24 h}}{2 \text{ doses/24 h}} = 112.8$ mg/dose
Single-dose range is 98.7 to 112.8 mg/dose.
d. Yes, the ordered dose is both safe and therapeutic because it falls within the recommended 24-hour dosage and single-dose ranges.
e. 125 mg : 5 mL :: 100 mg : x mL
$125x = 500$
$x = \frac{500}{125}$
$x = 4$ mL

3. $\frac{150 \text{ mL}}{180 \text{ min}} \times 60 \text{ gtt/mL} = 50 \text{ gtt/min}$

4. a. 2.2 lb : 1 kg :: 58 lb : x kg
$2.2x = 58$
$x = \frac{58}{2.2}$
$x = 26.4$ kg
b. 26.4 kg × 25 mg/kg/24 h = 660 mg/24 h
26.4 kg × 50 mg/kg/24 h = 1320 mg/24 h
Dosage range is 660 to 1320 mg/24 h.
c. $\frac{660 \text{ mg/24 h}}{2 \text{ doses/24 h}} = 330 \text{ mg/dose}$
$\frac{1320 \text{ mg/24 h}}{2 \text{ doses/24 h}} = 660 \text{ mg/dose}$
Single-dose range is 330 to 660 mg/dose.
d. $\frac{400 \text{ mg} \times 2 \text{ doses/24 h}}{26.4 \text{ kg}} = \frac{800}{26.4}$
$= 30.3$ mg/kg/24 h
e. 250 mg : 5 mL :: 400 mg : x mL
$250x = 2000$
$x = \frac{2000}{250}$
$x = 8$ mL

5. a. 2.2 lb : 1 kg :: 99 lb : x kg
$2.2x = 99$
$x = \frac{99}{2.2}$
$x = 45$ kg
b. $\frac{500 \text{ mg} \times 4 \text{ doses/24 h}}{45 \text{ kg}} = \frac{2000}{45}$
$= 44.4$ mg/kg/24 h
c. Yes, the recommended daily oral dosage is 50 to 100 mg/kg/24 h.
d. 250 mg : 1 cap :: 500 mg : x cap
$250x = 500$
$x = \frac{500}{250}$
$x = 2$ capsules

6. a. 2.2 lb : 1 kg :: 66 lb : x kg
$2.2x = 66$ lb
$x = \frac{66}{2.2}$
$x = 30$ kg
b. $\frac{200 \text{ mg} \times 2 \text{ doses/24 h}}{30 \text{ kg}} = \frac{400}{30}$
$= 13.3$ mg/kg/24 h
c. Yes, the order is safe to administer.
d. 125 mg : 5 mL :: 200 mg : x mL
$125x = 1000$
$x = \frac{1000}{125}$
$x = 8$ mL

7. a. 1000 g : 1 kg :: 2012 g : x kg
$1000x = 2012$
$x = \frac{2012}{1000}$
$x = 2$ kg
b. 2 kg × 100 mg/kg/24 h = 200 mg/24 h
2 kg × 200 mg/kg/24 h = 400 mg/24 h
Dosage range is 200 to 400 mg/24 h.
c. $\frac{200 \text{ mg/24 h}}{4 \text{ doses/24 h}} = 50 \text{ mg/dose}$
$\frac{400 \text{ mg/24 h}}{4 \text{ doses/24 h}} = 100 \text{ mg/dose}$
Single-dose range is 50 to 100 mg/dose.

8. a. 2.2 lb : 1 kg :: 35 lb : x kg
$2.2x = 35$
$x = \frac{35}{2.2}$
$x = 15.9$ kg
b. $\frac{180 \text{ mg} \times 3 \text{ doses/24 h}}{15.9 \text{ kg}} = \frac{540}{15.9}$
$= 33.96$ mg/kg/24 h
c. Yes, the ordered dose is within the safe and therapeutic range.
d. 125 mg : 5 mL :: 180 mg : x mL
$125x = 900$
$x = \frac{900}{125}$
$x = 7.2$ mL

9. a. 2.2 lb : 1 kg :: 74 lb : x kg
$2.2x = 74$
$x = \frac{74}{2.2}$
$x = 33.6$ kg
b. $\frac{330 \text{ mg} \times 4 \text{ doses/24 h}}{33.6 \text{ kg}} = \frac{1320}{33.6}$
$= 39.29$ mg/kg/24 h
c. Yes, the dose ordered is safe to administer.
d. 250 mg : 5 mL :: 330 mg : x mL
$250x = 1650$
$x = \frac{1650}{250}$
$x = 6.6$ mL

10. a. 2.2 lb : 1 kg :: 20 lb : x kg
$2.2x = 20$
$x = \frac{20}{2.2}$
$x = 9.1$ kg
b. 9.1 kg × 0.1 mg/kg/dose = 0.91 mg/dose
9.1 kg × 0.2 mg/kg/dose = 1.82 mg/dose
Safe dose range is 0.91 to 1.82 mg/dose (nearest hundredth with narcotics).
c. No, 0.9 mg is not within the safe range to administer. Contact the licensed prescriber.
d. 0.5 mg : 1 mL :: 0.9 mg : x mL
$0.5x = 0.9$
$x = \frac{0.9}{0.5}$
$x = 1.8$ mL if dose is approved

11. $\frac{200 \text{ mL}}{3 \text{ h}} = 66.7$ or 67 mL/h

12. a. 50 mg : 1 mL :: 500 mg : x mL
$50x = 500$
$x = \frac{500}{50}$
$x = 10$ mL
b. $500 \text{ mg} \times \frac{1 \text{ mL}}{5 \text{ mg}} = 100 \text{ mL} \rightarrow$
100 mL − 10 mL = 90 mL
c. Drop factor = 60 gtt/mL = microgtt
$\frac{100 \text{ mL}}{60 \text{ min}} \times 60 \text{ gtt/min} = x \text{ gtt/min}$
$\frac{6000}{60} = 100 \text{ gtt/min}$

13. a. 1000 g : 1 kg :: 3036 g : x kg
$1000x = 3036$
$x = \frac{3036}{1000}$
$x = 3.0$ kg or 3 kg
b. 3 kg × 6 mcg/kg/24 h = 18 mcg/24 h
3 kg × 10 mcg/kg/24 h = 30 mcg/24 h
Dosage range is 18 to 30 mcg/24 h.
c. $\frac{18 \text{ mcg/24 h}}{2 \text{ doses/24 h}} = 9 \text{ mcg/dose}$
$\frac{30 \text{ mcg/24 h}}{2 \text{ doses/24 h}} = 15 \text{ mcg/dose}$
Single dose is 9 to 15 mcg/dose.
9 mcg = 0.009 mg
15 mcg = 0.015 mg
d. Yes, the ordered dose, 0.013 mg, is between 0.009 mg and 0.015 mg.
e. 50 mcg = 0.05 mg
0.05 mg : 1 mL :: 0.013 mg : x mL
$0.05x = 0.013$
$x = \frac{0.013}{0.05}$
$x = 0.26$ mL (a drug that is measured to the nearest hundredth)

14. a. 2.2 lb : 1 kg :: 9 lb : x kg
$2.2x = 9$
$x = \frac{9}{2.2}$
$x = 4.1$ kg
b. 4.1 kg × 10 mg/kg/dose = 41 mg/dose
4.1 kg × 15 mg/kg/dose = 61.5 mg/dose
Single-dose range is 41 to 61.5 mg/dose.
c. 160 mg : 5 mL :: 41 mg : x mL
$160x = 205$
$x = \frac{205}{160}$
$x = 1.28$ or 1.3 mL
160 mg : 5 mL :: 61.5 mg : x mL
$160x = 61.5$
$x = \frac{307.5}{160}$
$x = 1.92$ or 1.9 mL
Range is 1.28 or 1.3 mL to 1.92 or 1.9 mL/dose.

15. a. 2.2 lb : 1 kg :: 37 lb : x kg
$2.2x = 37$
$x = \frac{37}{2.2}$
$x = 16.8$ kg
b. 16.8 kg × 4 mg/kg/24 h = 67.2 mg/24 h
16.8 kg × 6 mg/kg/24 h = 100.8 mg/24 h
Dosage range is 67.2 to 100.8 mg/24 h.
c. Yes, 72 mg/24 h is within the recommended dosage range.
d. 20 mg : 5 mL :: 72 mg : x mL
$20x = 360$
$x = \frac{360}{20}$
$x = 18$ mL

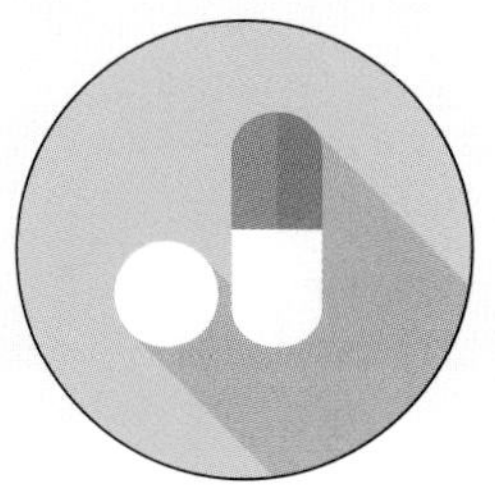

Obstetric Dosages

LEARNING OBJECTIVES

Upon completion of the materials in this chapter, you will be able to perform computations accurately by mastering the following mathematical concepts:

1. Calculating the intravenous (IV) rate of oxytocin (Pitocin) ordered in milliunits per minute
2. Calculating the IV rate of magnesium sulfate ordered in milligrams per minute

In obstetric nursing, oxytocin (Pitocin) and magnesium sulfate are commonly used. Oxytocin is used to either augment or induce labor. Magnesium sulfate is used to prevent seizures in mothers diagnosed with preeclampsia and is also used "off label" to control preterm labor contractions. Both these medications can be titrated, which means that the medication can be adjusted up and down based on patient status.

IV ADMINISTRATION OF MEDICATIONS BY MILLIUNITS/MINUTE

EXAMPLE 1: The licensed prescriber has ordered 1000 mL 5% dextrose in water (D_5W) with 20 units IV oxytocin. Begin at 1 mU/min and then increase by 1 mU/min every 30 minutes until regular contractions occur. Maximum dose is 20 mU/min.

What Is the IV Rate (mL/h) for the Beginning Infusion?

Using the Dimensional Analysis Method

$$\frac{x \text{ mL}}{\text{h}} = \frac{1000 \text{ mL}}{20 \text{ units}} \times \frac{1 \text{ unit}}{1000 \text{ mU}} \times \frac{1 \text{ mU}}{1 \text{ min}} \times \frac{60 \text{ min}}{1 \text{ h}}$$

$$\frac{x \text{ mL}}{\text{h}} = \frac{1000 \times 60}{20 \times 1000}$$

$$x = 3 \text{ mL/h}$$

Using the Ratio-Proportion Method

Step 1. Convert total units in the IV bag to milliunits.

(Formula setup) $1 \text{ unit} : 1000 \text{ mU} :: 20 \text{ units} : x \text{ mU}$

$$x = 1000 \times 20 = 20{,}000 \text{ mU}$$

Step 2. Calculate mL/min.

(Formula setup) $20{,}000\text{ mU} : 1000\text{ mL} :: 1\text{ mU} : x\text{ mL}$

$$20{,}000x = 1000$$

$$x = \frac{1000}{20{,}000}$$

$$x = 0.2\text{ mL/min}$$

Step 3. Calculate mL/h.

(Formula setup) $0.2\text{ mL} : 1\text{ min} :: x\text{ mL} : 60\text{ min (h)}$

$$0.2 : 1 :: x : 60$$

$$x = 3\text{ mL/h}$$

Using the $\frac{D}{A} \times Q$ Method

Step 1. Convert total units in the IV bag to milliunits.

$$20\text{ units} = 20{,}000\text{ mU}$$

Step 2. Calculate mL/min.

(Formula setup) $\frac{D}{A} \times Q = \frac{1\text{ mU/min}}{20{,}000\text{ mU}} \times 1000\text{ mL}$

(Cancel) $\frac{D}{A} \times Q = \frac{1\text{ }\cancel{\text{mU}}\text{/min}}{20{,}000\text{ }\cancel{\text{mU}}} \times 1000\text{ mL} = 0.2\text{ mL/min}$

Therefore 0.2 mL/min of oxytocin is infusing.

Step 3. Calculate mL/h.

(Formula setup) $\frac{\text{Total mL}}{\text{Total min}} \times \frac{60\text{ min}}{1\text{ h}}$

$$\frac{0.2\text{ mL}}{1\text{ min}} \times \frac{60\text{ min}}{1\text{ h}}$$

(Cancel) $\frac{0.2\text{ mL}}{1\text{ }\cancel{\text{min}}} \times \frac{60\text{ }\cancel{\text{min}}}{1\text{ h}} = 3\text{ mL/h}$

The infusion pump should be set at 3 mL/h.

What Is the Maximum IV Rate the Oxytocin Infusion May Be Set for?

Using the Dimensional Analysis Method

$$\frac{x\text{ mL}}{\text{h}} = \frac{1000\text{ mL}}{20\text{ units}} \times \frac{1\text{ unit}}{1000\text{ mU}} \times \frac{20\text{ mU}}{1\text{ min}} \times \frac{60\text{ min}}{1\text{ h}}$$

$$\frac{x\text{ mL}}{\text{h}} = \frac{1000 \times 20 \times 60}{20 \times 1000}$$

$$x = 60\text{ mL/h}$$

Using the Ratio-Proportion Method

Step 1. Convert total units in the IV bag to milliunits.

$$1\text{ unit} : 1000\text{ mU} :: 20\text{ units} : x\text{ mU}$$

$$x = 1000 \times 20 = 20{,}000\text{ mU}$$

Step 2. Calculate mL/min.

$$20{,}000\text{ mU} : 1000\text{ mL} :: 20\text{ mU} : x\text{ mL}$$

$$20{,}000x = 1000 \times 20$$

$$x = \frac{1000 \times 20}{20{,}000} = 1\text{ mL/min}$$

Step 3. Calculate mL/h. $1\text{ mL} : 1\text{ min} :: x\text{ mL} : 60\text{ min (h)}$

$$x = 1 \times 60 = 60\text{ mL/h}$$

Using the $\frac{D}{A} \times Q$ Method

Step 1. Convert units to milliunits.

$$20\text{ units} = 20{,}000\text{ mU}$$

Step 2. Calculate mL/min.

(Formula setup) $\frac{D}{A} \times Q = \frac{20\text{ mU/min}}{20{,}000\text{ mU}} \times 1000\text{ mL}$

(Cancel) $\frac{D}{A} \times Q = \frac{20\ \cancel{\text{mU}}\text{/min}}{20{,}000\ \cancel{\text{mU}}} \times 1000\text{ mL} = 1\text{ mL/min}$

Step 3. Calculate mL/h.

(Formula setup) $\frac{\text{Total mL}}{\text{Total min}} \times \frac{60\text{ min}}{1\text{ h}}$

$$\frac{1\text{ mL}}{1\text{ min}} \times \frac{60\text{ min}}{1\text{ h}}$$

(Cancel) $\frac{1\text{ mL}}{1\ \cancel{\text{min}}} \times \frac{60\ \cancel{\text{min}}}{1\text{ h}} = 60\text{ mL/h}$

Therefore the maximum IV rate is 60 mL/h.

EXAMPLE 2: The licensed prescriber has ordered 500 mL D_5W with 10 units IV oxytocin. Begin at 1 mU/min and then increase by 1 mU/min every 30 minutes until regular contractions occur. Maximum dose is 28 mU/min.

What Is the IV Rate (mL/h) for the Beginning Infusion?

Using the Dimensional Analysis Method

$$\frac{x\text{ mL}}{\text{h}} = \frac{500\text{ mL}}{10\text{ units}} \times \frac{1\text{ unit}}{1000\text{ mU}} \times \frac{1\text{ mU}}{1\text{ min}} \times \frac{60\text{ min}}{1\text{ h}}$$

$$\frac{x\text{ mL}}{\text{h}} = \frac{500 \times 60}{10 \times 1000}$$

$$x = 3\text{ mL/h}$$

Using the Ratio-Proportion Method

Step 1. Convert total units in the IV bag to milliunits.

(Formula setup) $1\text{ unit} : 1000\text{ mU} :: 10\text{ units} : x\text{ mU}$

$$1 : 1000 :: 10 : x$$

$$x = 1000 \times 10$$

$$x = 10{,}000\text{ mU}$$

Step 2. Calculate mL/min.

(Formula setup) $10{,}000 \text{ mU} : 500 \text{ mL} :: 1 \text{ mU} : x \text{ min}$

$$10{,}000x = 500$$

$$x = \frac{500}{10{,}000}$$

$$x = 0.05 \text{ mL/min}$$

Step 3. Calculate mL/h.

(Formula setup) $0.05 \text{ mL} : 1 \text{ min} :: x \text{ mL} : 60 \text{ min/h}$

$$0.05 : 1 :: x : 60$$

$$x = 3 \text{ mL/h}$$

Using the $\frac{D}{A} \times Q$ Method

Step 1. Convert total units in the IV bag to milliunits.

$$10 \text{ units} = 10{,}000 \text{ mU}$$

Step 2. Calculate mL/min.

(Formula setup) $\frac{D}{A} \times Q = \frac{1 \text{ mU/min}}{10{,}000 \text{ mU}} \times 500 \text{ mL}$

(Cancel) $\frac{D}{A} \times Q = \frac{1 \cancel{\text{mU}}\text{/min}}{10{,}000 \cancel{\text{mU}}} \times 500 \text{ mL} = 0.05 \text{ mL/min}$

Therefore 0.05 mL/min of oxytocin is infusing.

Step 3. Calculate mL/h.

(Formula setup) $\frac{\text{Total mL}}{\text{Total min}} \times \frac{60 \text{ min}}{1 \text{ h}}$

$$\frac{0.05 \text{ mL}}{1 \text{ min}} \times \frac{60 \text{ min}}{1 \text{ h}}$$

(Cancel) $\frac{0.05 \text{ mL}}{1 \cancel{\text{min}}} \times \frac{60 \cancel{\text{min}}}{1 \text{ h}} = 3 \text{ mL/h}$

The infusion pump should be set at 3 mL/h.

What Is the Maximum IV Rate the Oxytocin Infusion May Be Set for?

Using the Dimensional Analysis Method

$$\frac{x \text{ mL}}{\text{h}} = \frac{500 \text{ mL}}{10 \text{ units}} \times \frac{1 \text{ unit}}{1000 \text{ mU}} \times \frac{28 \text{ mU}}{1 \text{ min}} \times \frac{60 \text{ min}}{1 \text{ h}}$$

$$\frac{x \text{ mL}}{\text{h}} = \frac{500 \times 28 \times 60}{10 \times 1000}$$

$$x = 84 \text{ mL/h}$$

Using the Ratio-Proportion Method

Step 1. Convert total units in the IV bag to milliunits.

$$1 \text{ unit} : 1000 \text{ mU} :: 10 \text{ units} : x \text{ mU}$$

$$x = 1000 \times 10 = 10{,}000 \text{ mU}$$

Step 2. Calculate mL/min.

$$10{,}000 \text{ mU} : 500 \text{ mL} :: 28 \text{ mU} : x \text{ mL}$$
$$10{,}000x = 500 \times 28$$
$$x = \frac{500 \times 28}{10{,}000} = 1.4 \text{ mL/min}$$

Step 3. Calculate mL/h.

$$1.4 \text{ mL} : 1 \text{ min} :: x \text{ mL} : 60 \text{ min (h)}$$
$$x = 1.4 \times 60 = 84 \text{ mL/h}$$

Using the $\frac{D}{A} \times Q$ Method

Step 1. Convert units to milliunits.

$$10 \text{ units} = 10{,}000 \text{ mU}$$

Step 2. Calculate mL/min.

(Formula setup) $$\frac{D}{A} \times Q = \frac{28 \text{ mU/min}}{10{,}000 \text{ mU}} \times 500 \text{ mL}$$

(Cancel) $$\frac{D}{A} \times Q = \frac{28 \cancel{\text{mU}}\text{/min}}{10{,}000 \cancel{\text{mU}}} \times 500 \text{ mL} = 1.4 \text{ mL/min}$$

Therefore 1.4 mL/min of oxytocin is infusing.

Step 3. Calculate mL/h.

(Formula setup) $$\frac{\text{Total mL}}{\text{Total min}} \times \frac{60 \text{ min}}{1 \text{ h}}$$

$$\frac{1.4 \text{ mL}}{1 \text{ min}} \times \frac{60 \text{ min}}{1 \text{ h}}$$

(Cancel) $$\frac{1.4 \text{ mL}}{1 \cancel{\text{min}}} \times \frac{60 \cancel{\text{min}}}{1 \text{ h}} = 84 \text{ mL/h}$$

Therefore the maximum IV rate is 84 mL/h.

What Is the IV Rate (mL/h) the Oxytocin Infusion May Be Set for at 2 hours?

The licensed prescriber's order is to increase the oxytocin by 1 mU/min every 30 minutes until regular contractions begin. The oxytocin infusion was started at 0900 with 1 mU/min. What is the IV rate (mL/h) 2 hours after the infusion began at 0900?

Step 1. Determine the number of mU/min to be infused at 2 hours.

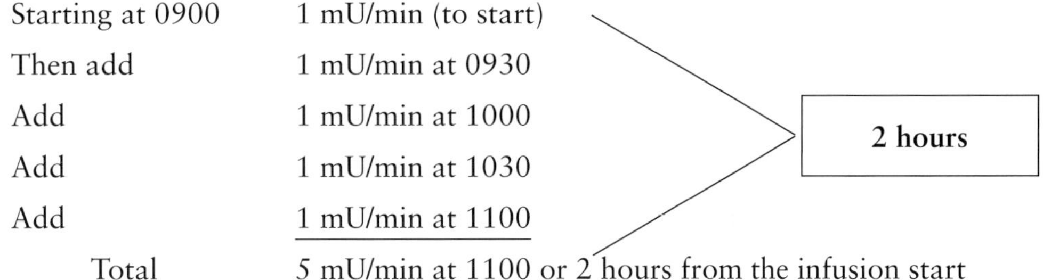

Starting at 0900 — 1 mU/min (to start)
Then add — 1 mU/min at 0930
Add — 1 mU/min at 1000
Add — 1 mU/min at 1030
Add — 1 mU/min at 1100
Total — 5 mU/min at 1100 or 2 hours from the infusion start

Step 2. Calculate the IV flow rate for 5 mU/min.

Using Dimensional Analysis Method

$$\frac{x\text{ mL}}{\text{h}} = \frac{1000\text{ mL}}{10\text{ units}} \times \frac{1\text{ unit}}{1000\text{ mU}} \times \frac{5\text{ mU}}{1\text{ min}} \times \frac{60\text{ min}}{1\text{ h}} = 30\text{ mL/h}$$

$$\frac{x\text{ mL}}{\text{h}} = \frac{1000 \times 5 \times 60}{10 \times 1000}$$

$$\frac{x\text{ mL}}{\text{h}} = 30\text{ mL/h}$$

Using the Ratio-Proportion Method

Step 1. Convert total units in the IV bag to milliunits.

(Formula setup) $1\text{ unit} : 1000\text{ mU} :: 10\text{ units} : x\text{ mU}$

$x = 1000 \times 10 = 10{,}000\text{ mU}$

Step 2. Calculate mL/min.

(Formula setup) $10{,}000\text{ mU} : 1000\text{ mL} :: 5\text{ mU} : x\text{ mL}$

$$10{,}000x = 1000 \times 5$$

$$x = \frac{5000}{10{,}000}$$

$$x = 0.5\text{ mL/min}$$

Step 3. Calculate mL/h.

(Formula setup) $0.5\text{ mL} : \text{min} :: x\text{ mL} : 60\text{ min (h)}$

$$0.5 : 1 :: x : 60$$

$$x = 30\text{ mL/h}$$

Using the $\frac{D}{A} \times Q$ Method

Step 1. Convert total units in the IV bag to milliunits.

$$10\text{ units} = 10{,}000\text{ mU}$$

Step 2. Calculate mL/min.

(Formula setup) $\frac{D}{A} \times Q = \frac{5\text{ mU/min}}{10{,}000\text{ mU}} \times 1000\text{ mL}$

(Cancel) $\frac{D}{A} \times Q = \frac{5\text{ }\cancel{\text{mU}}\text{/min}}{10{,}000\text{ }\cancel{\text{mU}}} \times 1000\text{ mL} = 0.5\text{ mL/min}$

Therefore 0.5 mL/min of oxytocin is infusing.

Step 3. Calculate mL/h.

(Formula setup) $\frac{0.5\text{ mL}}{1\text{ min}} \times \frac{60\text{ min}}{\text{h}} = 30\text{ mL/h}$

Therefore, the IV rate is 30 mL/h 2 hours after the oxytocin was started.

IV ADMINISTRATION OF MEDICATIONS BY MILLIGRAMS/MINUTE

EXAMPLE 1: The licensed prescriber has ordered 1000 mL lactated Ringer's with 20 g magnesium sulfate IV. Bolus with 4 g/30 min and then maintain a continuous infusion at 2 g/h.

What Is the IV Rate (mL/h) for the Bolus Order?

Using the Dimensional Analysis Method

$$\frac{x\text{ mL}}{\text{h}} = \frac{1000\text{ mL}}{20\text{ g}} \times \frac{4\text{ g}}{30\text{ min}} \times \frac{60\text{ min}}{1\text{ h}}$$

$$\frac{x\text{ mL}}{\text{h}} = \frac{1000 \times 4 \times 60}{20 \times 30}$$

$$x = 400\text{ mL/h}$$

Using the Ratio-Proportion Method

Step 1. Calculate the number of milliliters to infuse 4 g.

$$20\text{ g} : 1000\text{ mL} :: 4\text{ g} : x\text{ mL}$$

$$20 : 1000 :: 4 : x$$

$$20x = 4000$$

$$x = 200\text{ mL}$$

Step 2. Calculate mL/h.

(Formula setup) $200\text{ mL} : 30\text{ min} :: x\text{ mL} : 60\text{ min/h}$

$$200 : 30 :: x : 60$$

$$12000 = 30x$$

$$x = 400$$

The IV pump should be set at 400 mL/h.

Using the $\frac{D}{A} \times Q$ Method

Step 1. Calculate the number of milliliters to infuse 4 g.

(Formula setup) $\frac{D}{A} \times Q = \frac{4\text{ g}}{20\text{ g}} \times 1000\text{ mL}$

(Cancel) $\frac{D}{A} \times Q = \frac{4\not{\text{g}}}{20\not{\text{g}}} \times 1000\text{ mL} = 200\text{ mL}$

Step 2. Calculate the bolus rate in mL/h.

(Formula setup) $\frac{\text{Total mL}}{\text{Total min}} \times \frac{60 \text{ min}}{1 \text{ h}}$

$$\frac{200 \text{ mL}}{30 \text{ min}} \times \frac{60 \text{ min}}{1 \text{ h}}$$

(Cancel) $\frac{200 \text{ mL}}{30 \cancel{\text{min}}} \times \frac{60 \cancel{\text{min}}}{1 \text{ h}} = 400 \text{ mL/h}$

The infusion pump should be set at 400 mL/h.

What Is the IV Rate (mL/h) for the Continuous Infusion?

Using the Dimensional Analysis Method

$$\frac{x \text{ mL}}{\text{h}} = \frac{1000 \text{ mL}}{20 \text{ g}} \times \frac{2 \text{ g}}{1 \text{ h}}$$

$$\frac{x \text{ mL}}{\text{h}} = \frac{1000 \times 2}{20}$$

$$x = 100 \text{ mL/h}$$

Using the Ratio-Proportion Method

Calculate the number of milliliters to infuse 2 g/h.

(Formula setup) $20 \text{ g} : 1000 \text{ mL} :: 2 \text{ g} : x \text{ mL}$

$$20 : 1000 :: 2 : x$$

$$20x = 2000$$

$$x = 100 \text{ mL}$$

The IV pump should be set at 100 mL/h.

Using the $\frac{D}{A} \times Q$ Method

Calculate the mL/h to infuse 2 g/h.

(Formula setup) $\frac{D}{A} \times Q = \frac{2 \text{ g/h}}{20 \text{ g}} \times 1000 \text{ mL}$

(Cancel) $\frac{D}{A} \times Q = \frac{2 \cancel{\text{g}}\text{/h}}{20 \cancel{\text{g}}} \times 1000 \text{ mL} = 100 \text{ mL/h}$

The infusion pump should be set at 100 mL/h.

EXAMPLE 2: The licensed prescriber has ordered 500 mL lactated Ringer's with 10 g magnesium sulfate IV. Bolus with 2 g/20 min and then maintain a continuous infusion at 1 g/h.

What Is the IV Rate (mL/h) for the Bolus Order?

Using the Dimensional Analysis Method

$$\frac{x \text{ mL}}{\text{h}} = \frac{500 \text{ mL}}{10 \text{ g}} \times \frac{2 \text{ g}}{20 \text{ min}} \times \frac{60 \text{ min}}{1 \text{ h}}$$

$$\frac{x \text{ mL}}{\text{h}} = \frac{500 \times 2 \times 60}{10 \times 20}$$

$$x = 300 \text{ mL/h}$$

Using the Ratio-Proportion Method

Step 1. Calculate the number of milliliters to infuse 2 g.

$$10 \text{ g} : 500 \text{ mL} :: 2 \text{ g} : x \text{ mL}$$

$$10 : 500 :: 2 : x$$

$$10x = 1000$$

$$x = 100 \text{ mL}$$

Step 2. Calculate mL/h.

(Formula setup) $100 \text{ mL} : 20 \text{ min} :: x \text{ mL} : 60 \text{ min (h)}$

$$100 : 20 :: x : 60$$

$$6000 = 20x$$

$$x = 300 \text{ mL/h}$$

The IV pump will be set at 300 mL/h.

Using the $\frac{D}{A} \times Q$ Method

Step 1. Calculate the milliliters to infuse 2 g.

(Formula setup) $\frac{D}{A} \times Q = \frac{2 \text{ g}}{10 \text{ g}} \times 500 \text{ mL}$

(Cancel) $\frac{D}{A} \times Q = \frac{2 \cancel{\text{g}}}{10 \cancel{\text{g}}} \times 500 \text{ mL} = 100 \text{ mL}$

Step 2. Calculate the bolus rate in mL/h.

(Formula setup) $\frac{\text{Total mL}}{\text{Total min}} \times \frac{60 \text{ min}}{1 \text{ h}}$

$$\frac{100 \text{ mL}}{20 \text{ min}} \times \frac{60 \text{ min}}{1 \text{ h}}$$

(Cancel) $\frac{100 \text{ mL}}{20 \cancel{\text{min}}} \times \frac{60 \cancel{\text{min}}}{1 \text{ h}} = 300 \text{ mL/h}$

The IV pump will be set at 300 mL/h.

What Is the IV Rate (mL/h) for the Continuous Infusion?

Using the Dimensional Analysis Method

$$\frac{x \text{ mL}}{\text{h}} = \frac{500 \text{ mL}}{10 \text{ g}} \times \frac{1 \text{ g}}{1 \text{ h}}$$

$$\frac{x \text{ mL}}{\text{h}} = \frac{500}{10}$$

$$x = 50 \text{ mL/h}$$

Using the Ratio-Proportion Method

Calculate the number of mL/h to infuse 1 g/h.

$$10 \text{ g} : 500 \text{ mL} :: 1 \text{ g} : x \text{ mL}$$

$$10 : 500 :: 1 : x$$

$$10x = 500$$

$$x = 50$$

The IV pump will be set at 50 mL/h.

Using the $\frac{D}{A} \times Q$ Method

Calculate the mL/h to infuse 1 g/h.

(Formula setup) $\frac{D}{A} \times Q = \frac{1 \text{ g/h}}{10 \text{ g}} \times 500 \text{ mL}$

(Cancel) $\frac{D}{A} \times Q = \frac{1 \not{g}\text{/h}}{10 \not{g}} \times 500 \text{ mL} = 50 \text{ mL/h}$

The infusion pump should be set at 50 mL/h.

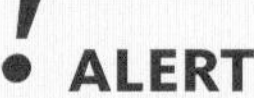

ALERT

Oxytocin and magnesium are high-risk medications. Always use an infusion controller.

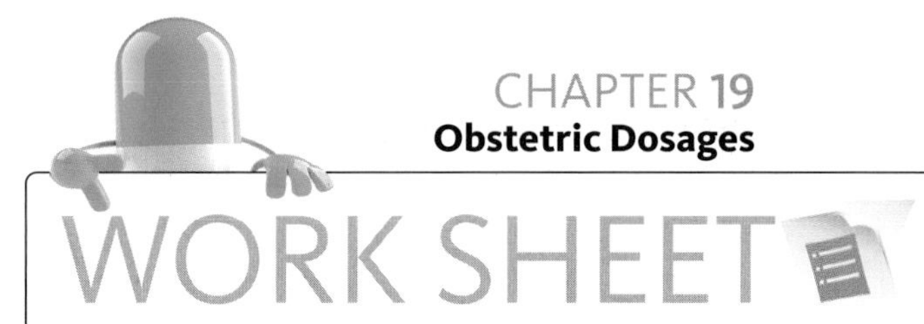

1. The licensed prescriber has ordered 500 mL D_5W with 10 units IV oxytocin. Begin at 2 mU/min and then increase by 1 mU/min every 30 minutes until regular contractions begin. Maximum dose is 30 mU/min.

   a. What is the IV rate for the beginning infusion? ________

   b. What is the IV rate for the maximum infusion? ________

2. The licensed prescriber has ordered 500 mL D_5W with 30 units IV oxytocin. Begin at 2 mU/min at 0900 and then increase by 1 mU/min every 30 minutes until regular contractions begin. Maximum dose is 20 mU/min.

   a. What is the IV rate for the beginning infusion? ________

   b. What is the IV rate for the maximum infusion? ________

   c. What is the IV rate at 2 hours from the start of infusion? ________

3. The licensed prescriber has ordered 500 mL D_5W with 30 units IV oxytocin. Begin at 1 mU/min and then increase by 1 mU/min every 30 minutes until regular contractions occur. Maximum dose is 20 mU/min.

   a. What is the IV rate for the beginning infusion? ________

   b. What is the IV rate for the maximum infusion? ________

   c. What is the IV rate to administer 12 mU/min? ________

4. The licensed prescriber has ordered 1000 mL D_5W with 40 units IV oxytocin. Begin at 2 mU/min and then increase by 1 mU/min every 30 minutes until regular contractions begin. Maximum dose is 20 mU/min.

   a. What is the IV rate for the beginning infusion? ________

   b. What is the IV rate for the maximum infusion? ________

5. The licensed prescriber has ordered 1000 mL lactated Ringer's with 20 g IV magnesium sulfate. Bolus with 2 g/30 min; then maintain a continuous infusion at 2 g/h.

   a. What is the IV rate for the bolus order? ________

   b. What is the IV rate for the continuous infusion? ________

6. The licensed prescriber has ordered 1000 mL lactated Ringer's with 40 g IV magnesium sulfate. Bolus with 1 g/20 min; then maintain a continuous infusion at 1 g/h.

   a. What is the IV rate for the bolus order? ________

   b. What is the IV rate for the continuous infusion? ________

7. The licensed prescriber has ordered 1000 mL lactated Ringer's with 40 g IV magnesium sulfate. Bolus with 6 g/20 min; then maintain a continuous infusion at 4 g/h.

   a. What is the IV rate for the bolus order? ________

   b. What is the IV rate for the continuous infusion? ________

8. The licensed prescriber has ordered 500 mL lactated Ringer's with 10 g IV magnesium sulfate. Bolus with 4 g/30 min; then maintain a continuous infusion at 2 g/h.

   a. What is the IV rate for the bolus order? ________

   b. What is the IV rate for the continuous infusion? ________

ANSWERS ON PP. 579 AND 580–583.

NAME ____________

DATE ____________

ACCEPTABLE SCORE 9

YOUR SCORE ______

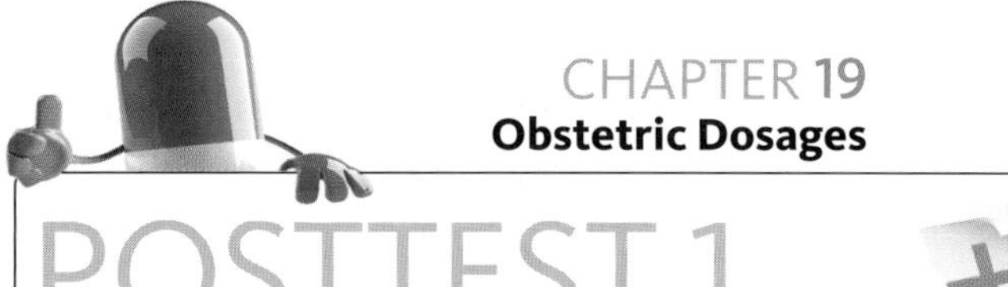

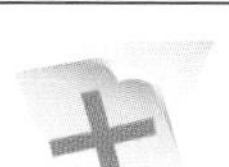

1. The licensed prescriber orders 500 mL of D_5W with 20 units of IV oxytoxin to begin at 2 mU/min at 0900 and then increase by 1 mU/min every 20 minutes until regular contractions begin. Maximum dose is 20 mU/min.

   a. What is the IV rate for the beginning infusion? ______

   b. What is the IV rate for the maximum infusion? ______

   c. What is the IV rate at 2 hours from the start of infusion? ______

2. The licensed prescriber orders 1000 mL of D_5W with 30 units of IV oxytoxin to begin at 2 mU/min and then increase by 1 mU/min every 20 minutes until regular contractions begin. Maximum dose is 30 mU/min.

   a. What is the IV rate for the beginning infusion? ______

   b. What is the IV rate for the maximum infusion? ______

   c. What is the IV rate to administer 7 mU/min? ______

3. The licensed prescriber orders 500 mL lactated Ringer's with 20 g of magnesium sulfate. Bolus with 2 g/30 minutes; then maintain a continuous infusion at 3 g/h.

   a. What is the IV rate for the bolus order? ______

   b. What is the IV rate for the continuous infusion? ______

4. The licensed prescriber orders 500 mL lactated Ringer's with 30 g of magnesium sulfate. Bolus with 2 g/20 minutes; then maintain a continuous infusion at 3 g/h.

a. What is the IV rate for the bolus order? ________

b. What is the IV rate for the continuous infusion? ________

ANSWERS ON PP. 579–580 AND 583–585.

NAME ____________________

DATE ____________________

REQUIRED SCORE **9**

YOUR SCORE ______

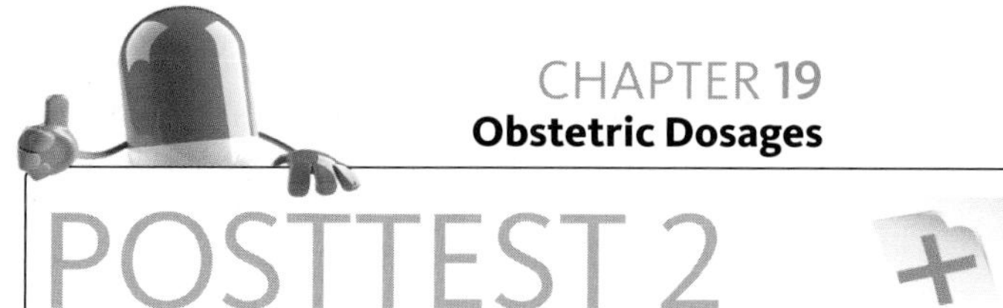

1. The licensed prescriber orders 1000 mL of D_5W with 10 units of IV oxytoxin to begin at 2 mU/min at 0900 and then increase by 2 mU/min every 15 minutes until regular contractions begin. Maximum dose is 30 mU/min.

   a. What is the IV rate for the beginning infusion? ________

   b. What is the IV rate for the maximum infusion? ________

   c. What is the IV rate at 2 hours from the start of infusion? ________

2. The licensed prescriber orders 1000 mL of D_5W with 20 units of IV oxytoxin to begin at 4 mU/min and then increase by 3 mU/min every 20 minutes until regular contractions begin. Maximum dose is 20 mU/min.

   a. What is the IV rate for the beginning infusion? ________

   b. What is the IV rate for the maximum infusion? ________

   c. What is the IV rate to administer 16 mU/min? ________

3. The licensed prescriber orders 1000 mL lactated Ringer's with 20 g of magnesium sulfate. Bolus with 2 g/30 minutes; then maintain a continuous infusion at 2 g/h.

   a. What is the IV rate for the bolus order? ________

   b. What is the IV rate for the continuous infusion? ________

4. The licensed prescriber orders 1000 mL lactated Ringer's with 40 g of magnesium sulfate. Bolus with 2 g/15 minutes; then maintain a continuous infusion at 4 g/h.

a. What is the IV rate for the bolus order? ________

b. What is the IV rate for the continuous infusion? ________

ANSWERS ON PP. 580 AND 585–586.

evolve For additional practice problems, refer to the Obstetric Dosages section of *Elsevier's Interactive Drug Calculation Application*, version 1.

ANSWERS

CHAPTER 19 Dimensional Analysis—Work Sheet, pp. 573–574

1. a. $\frac{x \text{ mL}}{\text{h}} = \frac{500 \text{ mL}}{10 \text{ units}} \times \frac{1 \text{ unit}}{1000 \text{ mU}} \times \frac{2 \text{ mU}}{1 \text{ min}} \times \frac{60 \text{ min}}{1 \text{ h}} = 6 \text{ mL/h}$

   b. $\frac{x \text{ mL}}{\text{h}} = \frac{500 \text{ mL}}{10 \text{ units}} \times \frac{1 \text{ unit}}{1000 \text{ mU}} \times \frac{30 \text{ mU}}{1 \text{ min}} \times \frac{60 \text{ min}}{1 \text{ h}} = 90 \text{ mL/h}$

2. a. $\frac{x \text{ mL}}{\text{h}} = \frac{500 \text{ mL}}{30 \text{ units}} \times \frac{1 \text{ unit}}{1000 \text{ mU}} \times \frac{2 \text{ mU}}{1 \text{ min}} \times \frac{60 \text{ min}}{1 \text{ h}} = 2 \text{ mL/h}$

   b. $\frac{x \text{ mL}}{\text{h}} = \frac{500 \text{ mL}}{30 \text{ units}} \times \frac{1 \text{ unit}}{1000 \text{ mU}} \times \frac{20 \text{ mU}}{1 \text{ min}} \times \frac{60 \text{ min}}{1 \text{ h}} = 20 \text{ mL/h}$

   c. $\frac{x \text{ mL}}{\text{h}} = \frac{500 \text{ mL}}{30 \text{ units}} \times \frac{1 \text{ unit}}{1000 \text{ mU}} \times \frac{6 \text{ mU}}{\text{min}} \times \frac{60 \text{ min}}{\text{h}} = 6 \text{ mL/h}$

3. a. $\frac{x \text{ mL}}{\text{h}} = \frac{500 \text{ mL}}{30 \text{ units}} \times \frac{1 \text{ unit}}{1000 \text{ mU}} \times \frac{1 \text{ mU}}{1 \text{ min}} \times \frac{60 \text{ min}}{1 \text{ h}} = 1 \text{ mL/h}$

   b. $\frac{x \text{ mL}}{\text{h}} = \frac{500 \text{ mL}}{30 \text{ units}} \times \frac{1 \text{ unit}}{1000 \text{ mU}} \times \frac{20 \text{ mU}}{1 \text{ min}} \times \frac{60 \text{ min}}{1 \text{ h}} = 20 \text{ mL/h}$

   c. $\frac{x \text{ mL}}{\text{h}} = \frac{500 \text{ mL}}{30 \text{ units}} \times \frac{1 \text{ unit}}{1000 \text{ mU}} \times \frac{12 \text{ mU}}{\text{min}} \times \frac{60 \text{ min}}{\text{h}} = 12 \text{ mL/h}$

4. a. $\frac{x \text{ mL}}{\text{h}} = \frac{1000 \text{ mL}}{40 \text{ units}} \times \frac{1 \text{ unit}}{1000 \text{ mU}} \times \frac{2 \text{ mU}}{1 \text{ min}} \times \frac{60 \text{ min}}{1 \text{ h}} = 3 \text{ mL/h}$

   b. $\frac{x \text{ mL}}{\text{h}} = \frac{1000 \text{ mL}}{40 \text{ units}} \times \frac{1 \text{ unit}}{1000 \text{ mU}} \times \frac{20 \text{ mU}}{1 \text{ min}} \times \frac{60 \text{ min}}{1 \text{ h}} = 30 \text{ mL/h}$

5. a. $\frac{x \text{ mL}}{\text{h}} = \frac{1000 \text{ mL}}{20 \text{ g}} \times \frac{2 \text{ g}}{30 \text{ min}} \times \frac{60 \text{ min}}{1 \text{ h}} = 200 \text{ mL/h}$

   b. $\frac{x \text{ mL}}{\text{h}} = \frac{1000 \text{ mL}}{20 \text{ g}} \times \frac{2 \text{ g}}{1 \text{ h}} = 100 \text{ mL/h}$

6. a. $\frac{x \text{ mL}}{\text{h}} = \frac{1000 \text{ mL}}{40 \text{ g}} \times \frac{1 \text{ g}}{20 \text{ min}} \times \frac{60 \text{ min}}{1 \text{ h}} = 75 \text{ mL/h}$

   b. $\frac{x \text{ mL}}{\text{h}} = \frac{1000 \text{ mL}}{40 \text{ g}} \times \frac{1 \text{ g}}{1 \text{ h}} = 25 \text{ mL/h}$

7. a. $\frac{x \text{ mL}}{\text{h}} = \frac{1000 \text{ mL}}{40 \text{ g}} \times \frac{6 \text{ g}}{20 \text{ min}} \times \frac{60 \text{ min}}{1 \text{ h}} = 450 \text{ mL/h}$

   b. $\frac{x \text{ mL}}{\text{h}} = \frac{1000 \text{ mL}}{40 \text{ g}} \times \frac{4 \text{ g}}{1 \text{ h}} = 100 \text{ mL/h}$

8. a. $\frac{x \text{ mL}}{\text{h}} = \frac{500 \text{ mL}}{10 \text{ g}} \times \frac{4 \text{ g}}{30 \text{ min}} \times \frac{60 \text{ min}}{1 \text{ h}} = 400 \text{ mL/h}$

   b. $\frac{x \text{ mL}}{\text{h}} = \frac{500 \text{ mL}}{10 \text{ g}} \times \frac{2 \text{ g}}{1 \text{ h}} = 100 \text{ mL/h}$

CHAPTER 19 Dimensional Analysis—Posttest 1, pp. 575–576

1. a. $\frac{x \text{ mL}}{\text{h}} = \frac{500 \text{ mL}}{20 \text{ units}} \times \frac{1 \text{ unit}}{1000 \text{ mU}} \times \frac{2 \text{ mU}}{1 \text{ min}} \times \frac{60 \text{ min}}{1 \text{ h}} = 3 \text{ mL/h}$

   b. $\frac{x \text{ mL}}{\text{h}} = \frac{500 \text{ mL}}{20 \text{ units}} \times \frac{1 \text{ unit}}{1000 \text{ mU}} \times \frac{20 \text{ mU}}{1 \text{ min}} \times \frac{60 \text{ min}}{1 \text{ h}} = 30 \text{ mL/h}$

   c. $\frac{x \text{ mL}}{\text{h}} = \frac{500 \text{ mL}}{20 \text{ units}} \times \frac{1 \text{ unit}}{1000 \text{ mU}} \times \frac{8 \text{ mU}}{\text{min}} \times \frac{60 \text{ min}}{\text{h}} = 12 \text{ mL/h}$

2. a. $\frac{x \text{ mL}}{\text{h}} = \frac{1000 \text{ mL}}{30 \text{ units}} \times \frac{1 \text{ unit}}{1000 \text{ mU}} \times \frac{2 \text{ mU}}{1 \text{ min}} \times \frac{60 \text{ min}}{1 \text{ h}} = 4 \text{ mL/h}$

b. $\frac{x \text{ mL}}{\text{h}} = \frac{1000 \text{ mL}}{30 \text{ units}} \times \frac{1 \text{ unit}}{1000 \text{ mU}} \times \frac{30 \text{ mU}}{1 \text{ min}} \times \frac{60 \text{ min}}{1 \text{ h}} = 60 \text{ mL/h}$

c. $\frac{x \text{ mL}}{\text{h}} = \frac{1000 \text{ mL}}{30 \text{ units}} \times \frac{1 \text{ unit}}{1000 \text{ mU}} \times \frac{7 \text{ mU}}{\text{min}} \times \frac{60 \text{ min}}{\text{h}} = 14 \text{ mL/h}$

3. a. $\frac{x \text{ mL}}{\text{h}} = \frac{500 \text{ mL}}{20 \text{ g}} \times \frac{2 \text{ g}}{30 \text{ min}} \times \frac{60 \text{ min}}{1 \text{ h}} = 100 \text{ mL/h}$

b. $\frac{x \text{ mL}}{\text{h}} = \frac{500 \text{ mL}}{20 \text{ g}} \times \frac{3 \text{ g}}{1 \text{ h}} = 75 \text{ mL/h}$

4. a. $\frac{x \text{ mL}}{\text{h}} = \frac{500 \text{ mL}}{30 \text{ g}} \times \frac{2 \text{ g}}{20 \text{ min}} \times \frac{60 \text{ min}}{1 \text{ h}} = 100 \text{ mL/h}$

b. $\frac{x \text{ mL}}{\text{h}} = \frac{500 \text{ mL}}{30 \text{ g}} \times \frac{3 \text{ g}}{1 \text{ h}} = 50 \text{ mL/h}$

CHAPTER 19 Dimensional Analysis—Posttest 2, pp. 577–578

1. a. $\frac{x \text{ mL}}{\text{h}} = \frac{1000 \text{ mL}}{10 \text{ units}} \times \frac{1 \text{ unit}}{1000 \text{ mU}} \times \frac{2 \text{ mU}}{1 \text{ min}} \times \frac{60 \text{ min}}{1 \text{ h}} = 12 \text{ mL/h}$

b. $\frac{x \text{ mL}}{\text{h}} = \frac{1000 \text{ mL}}{10 \text{ units}} \times \frac{1 \text{ unit}}{1000 \text{ mU}} \times \frac{30 \text{ mU}}{1 \text{ min}} \times \frac{60 \text{ min}}{1 \text{ h}} = 180 \text{ mL/h}$

c. $\frac{x \text{ mL}}{\text{h}} = \frac{1000 \text{ mL}}{10 \text{ units}} \times \frac{1 \text{ unit}}{1000 \text{ mU}} \times \frac{18 \text{ mU}}{\text{min}} \times \frac{60 \text{ min}}{\text{h}} = 108 \text{ mL/h}$

2. a. $\frac{x \text{ mL}}{\text{h}} = \frac{1000 \text{ mL}}{20 \text{ units}} \times \frac{1 \text{ unit}}{1000 \text{ mU}} \times \frac{4 \text{ mU}}{1 \text{ min}} \times \frac{60 \text{ min}}{1 \text{ h}} = 12 \text{ mL/h}$

b. $\frac{x \text{ mL}}{\text{h}} = \frac{1000 \text{ mL}}{20 \text{ units}} \times \frac{1 \text{ unit}}{1000 \text{ mU}} \times \frac{20 \text{ mU}}{1 \text{ min}} \times \frac{60 \text{ min}}{1 \text{ h}} = 60 \text{ mL/h}$

c. $\frac{x \text{ mL}}{\text{h}} = \frac{1000 \text{ mL}}{20 \text{ units}} \times \frac{1 \text{ unit}}{1000 \text{ mU}} \times \frac{16 \text{ mU}}{\text{min}} \times \frac{60 \text{ min}}{\text{h}} = 48 \text{ mL/h}$

3. a. $\frac{x \text{ mL}}{\text{h}} = \frac{1000 \text{ mL}}{20 \text{ g}} \times \frac{2 \text{ g}}{30 \text{ min}} \times \frac{60 \text{ min}}{1 \text{ h}} = 200 \text{ mL/h}$

b. $\frac{x \text{ mL}}{\text{h}} = \frac{1000 \text{ mL}}{20 \text{ g}} \times \frac{2 \text{ g}}{1 \text{ h}} = 100 \text{ mL/h}$

4. a. $\frac{x \text{ mL}}{\text{h}} = \frac{1000 \text{ mL}}{40 \text{ g}} \times \frac{2 \text{ g}}{15 \text{ min}} \times \frac{60 \text{ min}}{1 \text{ h}} = 200 \text{ mL/h}$

b. $\frac{x \text{ mL}}{\text{h}} = \frac{1000 \text{ mL}}{40 \text{ g}} \times \frac{4 \text{ g}}{1 \text{ h}} = 100 \text{ mL/h}$

CHAPTER 19 Ratio-Proportion/Formula Method—Work Sheet, pp. 573–574

Ratio-Proportion

1. a. 1 unit : 1000 mU :: 10 units : x mU
$x = 1000 \times 10 = 10{,}000$ mU
10,000 mU : 500 mL :: 2 mU : x mL/min
$10{,}000x = 500 \times 2$
$x = \frac{1000}{10{,}000} = 0.1$ mL/min
0.1 mL : 1 min :: x mL : 60 min
$x = 60 \times 0.1$ mL/h $= 6$ mL/h

Formula Method

$\frac{2 \cancel{\text{mU}}/\text{min}}{10{,}000 \cancel{\text{mU}}} \times 500 \text{ mL} = 0.1 \text{ mL/min}$

$\frac{0.1 \text{ mL}}{1 \cancel{\text{min}}} \times \frac{60 \cancel{\text{min}}}{1 \text{ h}} = 6 \text{ mL/h}$

Ratio-Proportion	Formula Method
b. 1 unit : 1000 mU :: 10 units : x mU $x = 1000 \times 10 = 10{,}000$ mU 10,000 mU : 500 mL :: 30 mU : x mL/min $10{,}000x = 500 \times 30$ $x = \frac{15{,}000}{10{,}000}$ $x = 1.5$ mL/min 1.5 mL : 1 min :: x mL : 60 min $x = 60 \times 1.5 = 90$ mL/h	$\frac{30 \text{ mU/min}}{10{,}000 \text{ mU}} \times 500 \text{ mL} = 1.5 \text{ mL/min}$ $\frac{1.5 \text{ mL}}{1 \text{ min}} \times \frac{60 \text{ min}}{1 \text{ h}} = 90 \text{ mL/h}$
2. a. 1 unit : 1000 mU :: 30 units : x mU $x = 1000 \times 30 = 30{,}000$ mU 30,000 mU : 500 mL :: 2 mU : x mL/min $30{,}000x = 500 \times 2$ $x = \frac{1000}{30{,}000} = 0.033$ mL/min 0.033 mL : 1 min :: x mL : 60 min $x = 60 \times 0.033 = 2$ mL/h	$\frac{2 \text{ mU/min}}{30{,}000 \text{ mU}} \times 500 \text{ mL} = 0.033 \text{ mL/min}$ $\frac{0.033 \text{ mL}}{1 \text{ min}} \times \frac{60 \text{ min}}{1 \text{ h}} = 2 \text{ mL/h}$
b. 1 unit : 1000 mU :: 30 units : x mU $x = 1000 \times 30 = 30{,}000$ mU 30,000 mU : 500 mL :: 20 mU : x mL/min $30{,}000x = 500 \times 20$ $x = \frac{10{,}000}{30{,}000} = 0.33$ mL/min 0.33 mL : 1 min :: x mL : 60 min $x = 60 \times 0.33 = 19.8$ or 20 mL/h	$\frac{20 \text{ mU/min}}{30{,}000 \text{ mU}} \times 500 \text{ mL} = 0.33 \text{ mL/min}$ $\frac{0.33 \text{ mL}}{1 \text{ min}} \times \frac{60 \text{ min}}{1 \text{ h}} = 19.8 \text{ or } 20 \text{ mL/h}$
c. 1 unit : 10,000 mU :: 30 units : x mU $x = 1000 \times 30 = 30{,}000$ mU 30,000 mU : 500 mL :: 6 mU : x mL $30{,}000x = 500 \times 6$ $x = \frac{3000}{30{,}000} = 0.1$ mL/min 0.1 mL : min :: x mL : 60 min $x = 0.1 \times 60 = 6$ mL/h	$\frac{6 \text{ mU/min}}{30{,}000 \text{ mU}} \times 500 \text{ mL} = 0.1 \text{ mL/min}$ $\frac{0.1 \text{ mL}}{1 \text{ min}} \times \frac{60 \text{ min}}{1 \text{ h}} = 6 \text{ mL/h}$
3. a. 1 unit : 1000 mU :: 30 units : x mU $x = 1000 \times 30 = 30{,}000$ mU 30,000 mU : 500 mL :: 1 mU : x mL/min $30{,}000x = 500$ $x = \frac{500}{30{,}000} = 0.016$ mL/min 0.016 mL : 1 min :: x mL : 60 min $x = 60 \times 0.016 = 1$ mL/h	$\frac{1 \text{ mU/min}}{30{,}000 \text{ mU}} \times 500 \text{ mL} = 0.016 \text{ mL/min}$ $\frac{0.016 \text{ mL}}{1 \text{ min}} \times \frac{60 \text{ min}}{1 \text{ h}} = 1 \text{ mL/h}$
b. 1 unit : 1000 mU :: 30 units : x mU $x = 1000 \times 30 = 30{,}000$ mU 30,000 mU : 500 mL :: 20 mU : x mL/min $30{,}000x = 500 \times 20$ $x = \frac{10{,}000}{30{,}000} = 0.33$ mL/min 0.33 mL : 1 min :: x mL : 60 min $x = 60 \times 0.33 = 19.8$ or 20 mL/h	$\frac{20 \text{ mU/min}}{30{,}000 \text{ mU}} \times 500 \text{ mL} = 0.33 \text{ mL/min}$ $\frac{0.33 \text{ mL}}{1 \text{ min}} \times \frac{60 \text{ min}}{1 \text{ h}} = 19.8 \text{ or } 20 \text{ mL/h}$

Ratio-Proportion	Formula Method
c. 1 unit : 10,000 mU :: 30 units : x mU $x = 1000 \times 30 = 30{,}000$ mU 30,000 mU : 500 mL :: 12 mU : x mL $30{,}000x = 500 \times 12$ $x = \frac{6000}{30{,}000} = 0.2$ mL/min 0.2 mL : min :: x mL : 60 min $x = 0.2 \times 60 = 12$ mL/h	$\frac{12\ \cancel{mU}/min}{30{,}000\ \cancel{mU}} \times 500\ mL = 0.2\ mL/min$ $\frac{0.2\ mL}{1\ \cancel{min}} \times \frac{60\ \cancel{min}}{1\ h} = 12\ mL/h$
4. a. 1 unit : 1000 mU :: 40 units : x mU $x = 1000 \times 40 = 40{,}000$ mU 40,000 mU : 1000 mL :: 2 mU : x mL/min $40{,}000x = 1000 \times 2$ $x = \frac{2000}{40{,}000} = 0.05$ mL/min 0.05 mL : 1 min :: x mL : 60 min $x = 60 \times 0.05$ mL/h $= 3$ mL/h	$\frac{2\ \cancel{mU}/min}{40{,}000\ \cancel{mU}} \times 1000\ mL = 0.05\ mL/min$ $\frac{0.05\ mL}{1\ \cancel{min}} \times \frac{60\ \cancel{min}}{1\ h} = 3\ mL/h$
b. 1 unit : 1000 mU :: 40 units : x mU $x = 1000 \times 40 = 40{,}000$ mU 40,000 mU : 1000 mL :: 20 mU : x mL/min $40{,}000x = 1000 \times 20$ $x = \frac{20{,}000}{40{,}000} = 0.5$ mL/min 0.5 mL : 1 min :: x mL : 60 min $x = 60 \times 0.5 = 30$ mL/h	$\frac{20\ \cancel{mU}/min}{40{,}000\ \cancel{mU}} \times 1000\ mL = 0.5\ mL/min$ $\frac{0.5\ mL}{1\ \cancel{min}} \times \frac{60\ \cancel{min}}{1\ h} = 30\ mL/h$
5. a. 20 g : 1000 mL :: 2 g : x mL $20x = 2000$ $x = 100$ mL 100 mL : 30 min :: x mL : 60 min $30x = 6000$ $x = \frac{6000}{30} = 200$ mL/h	$\frac{100\ mL}{30\ \cancel{min}} \times \frac{60\ \cancel{min}}{1\ h} = 200\ mL/h$
b. 20 g : 1000 mL :: 2 g : x mL $20x = 2000$ $x = 100$ mL 100 mL : 60 min :: x mL : 60 min $60x = 6000$ $x = \frac{6000}{60} = 100$ mL/h	$\frac{2\ \cancel{g}/h}{20\ \cancel{g}} \times 1000\ mL = 100\ mL/h$
6. a. 40 g : 1000 mL :: 1 g : x mL $40x = 1000$ $x = 25$ mL 25 mL : 20 min :: x mL : 60 min $20x = 1500$ $x = \frac{1500}{20} = 75$ mL/h	$\frac{25\ mL}{20\ \cancel{min}} \times \frac{60\ \cancel{min}}{1\ h} = 75\ mL/h$
b. 40 g : 1000 mL :: 1 g : x mL $40x = 1000$ $x = 25$ mL 25 mL : 60 min :: x mL : 60 min $60x = 1500$ $x = \frac{1500}{60} = 25$ mL/h	$\frac{1\ \cancel{g}/h}{40\ \cancel{g}} \times 1000\ mL = 25\ mL/h$

Ratio-Proportion	Formula Method
7. a. $40\text{ g} : 1000\text{ mL} :: 6\text{ g} : x\text{ mL}$ $40x = 6000$ $x = 150\text{ mL}$ $150\text{ mL} : 20\text{ min} :: x\text{ mL} : 60\text{ min}$ $20x = 9000$ $x = \frac{9000}{20} = 450\text{ mL/h}$	$\frac{150\text{ mL}}{20\text{ }\cancel{\text{min}}} \times \frac{60\text{ }\cancel{\text{min}}}{1\text{ h}} = 450\text{ mL/h}$
b. $40\text{ g} : 1000\text{ mL} :: 4\text{ g} : x\text{ mL}$ $40x = 4000$ $x = 100\text{ mL}$ $100\text{ mL} : 60\text{ min} :: x\text{ mL} : 60\text{ min}$ $60x = 6000$ $x = \frac{6000}{60} = 100\text{ mL/h}$	$\frac{4\text{ }\cancel{\text{g}}\text{/h}}{40\text{ }\cancel{\text{g}}} \times 1000\text{ mL} = 100\text{ mL/h}$
8. a. $10\text{ g} : 500\text{ mL} :: 4\text{ g} : x\text{ mL}$ $10x = 2000$ $x = 200\text{ mL}$ $200\text{ mL} : 30\text{ min} :: x\text{ mL} : 60\text{ min}$ $30x = 12{,}000$ $x = \frac{12{,}000}{30} = 400\text{ mL/h}$	$\frac{200\text{ mL}}{30\text{ }\cancel{\text{min}}} \times \frac{60\text{ }\cancel{\text{min}}}{1\text{ h}} = 400\text{ mL/h}$
b. $10\text{ g} : 500\text{ mL} :: 2\text{ g} : x\text{ mL}$ $10x = 1000$ $x = 100\text{ mL}$ $100\text{ mL} : 60\text{ min} :: x\text{ mL} : 60\text{ min}$ $60x = 6000$ $x = \frac{6000}{60} = 100\text{ mL/h}$	$\frac{2\text{ }\cancel{\text{g}}\text{/h}}{10\text{ }\cancel{\text{g}}} \times 500\text{ mL} = 100\text{ mL/h}$

CHAPTER 19 Ratio-Proportion/Formula Method—Posttest 1, pp. 573–574

Ratio-Proportion	Formula
1. a. $1\text{ unit} : 1000\text{ mU} :: 20\text{ units} : x\text{ mU}$ $x = 1000 \times 20 = 20{,}000\text{ mU}$ $20{,}000\text{ mU} : 500\text{ mL} :: 2\text{ mU} : x\text{ mL/min}$ $20{,}000x = 500 \times 2$ $x = \frac{1000}{20{,}000} = 0.05\text{ mL/min}$ $0.05\text{ mL} : 1\text{ min} :: x\text{ mL} : 60\text{ min}$ $x = 60 \times 0.05 = 3\text{ mL/h}$	$\frac{2\text{ }\cancel{\text{mU}}\text{/min}}{20{,}000\text{ }\cancel{\text{mU}}} \times 500\text{ mL} = 0.05\text{ mL/min}$ $\frac{0.05\text{ mL}}{1\text{ }\cancel{\text{min}}} \times \frac{60\text{ }\cancel{\text{min}}}{1\text{ h}} = 3\text{ mL/h}$
b. $1\text{ unit} : 1000\text{ mU} :: 20\text{ units} : x\text{ mU}$ $x = 1000 \times 20 = 20{,}000\text{ mU}$ $20{,}000\text{ mU} : 500\text{ mL} :: 20\text{ mU} : x\text{ mL/min}$ $20{,}000x = 500 \times 20$ $x = \frac{10{,}000}{20{,}000} = 0.5\text{ mL/min}$ $0.5\text{ mL} : 1\text{ min} :: x\text{ mL} : 60\text{ min}$ $x = 60 \times 0.5 = 30\text{ mL/h}$	$\frac{20\text{ }\cancel{\text{mU}}\text{/min}}{20{,}000\text{ }\cancel{\text{mU}}} \times 500\text{ mL} = 0.05\text{ mL/min}$ $\frac{0.5\text{ mL}}{1\text{ }\cancel{\text{min}}} \times \frac{60\text{ }\cancel{\text{min}}}{1\text{ h}} = 30\text{ mL/h}$

Ratio-Proportion | **Formula**

c. 1 unit : 10,000 mU :: 20 units : x mU
$x = 1000 \times 20 = 20{,}000$ mU
20,000 mU : 500 mL :: 8 mU : x mL
$20{,}000x = 500 \times 8$
$$x = \frac{4000}{20{,}000} = 0.2 \text{ mL/min}$$
0.2 mL : 1 min :: x mL : 60 min
$x = 0.2 \times 60 = 12$ mL/h

$$\frac{8 \cancel{\text{mU}}/\text{min}}{20{,}000 \cancel{\text{mU}}} \times 500 \text{ mL} = 0.2 \text{ mL/min}$$
$$\frac{0.2 \text{ mL}}{1 \cancel{\text{min}}} \times \frac{60 \cancel{\text{min}}}{1 \text{ h}} = 12 \text{ mL/h}$$

2. a. 1 unit : 1000 mU :: 30 units : x mU
$x = 1000 \times 30 = 30{,}000$ mU
30,000 mU : 1000 mL :: 2 mU : x mL/min
$30{,}000x = 1000 \times 2$
$$x = \frac{2000}{30{,}000} = 0.066 \text{ mL/min}$$
0.066 mL : 1 min :: x mL : 60 min
$x = 60 \times 0.066 = 4$ mL/h

$$\frac{2 \cancel{\text{mU}}/\text{min}}{30{,}000 \cancel{\text{mU}}} \times 1000 \text{ mL} = 0.066 \text{ mL/min}$$
$$\frac{0.066 \text{ mL}}{1 \cancel{\text{min}}} \times \frac{60 \cancel{\text{min}}}{1 \text{ h}} = 4 \text{ mL/h}$$

b. 1 unit : 1000 mU :: 30 units : x mU
$x = 1000 \times 30 = 30{,}000$ mU
30,000 mU : 1000 mL :: 30 mU : x mL/min
$30{,}000x = 1000 \times 30$
$$x = \frac{30{,}000}{30{,}000} = 1 \text{ mL/min}$$
1 mL : 1 min :: x mL : 60 min
$x = 60 \times 1 = 60$ mL/h

$$\frac{30 \cancel{\text{mU}}/\text{min}}{30{,}000 \cancel{\text{mU}}} \times 1000 \text{ mL} = 1 \text{ mL/min}$$
$$\frac{1 \text{ mL}}{1 \cancel{\text{min}}} \times \frac{60 \cancel{\text{min}}}{1 \text{ h}} = 60 \text{ mL/h}$$

c. 1 unit : 10,000 mU :: 30 units : x mU
$x = 1000 \times 30 = 30{,}000$ mU
30,000 mU : 1000 mL :: 7 mU : x mL
$30{,}000x = 1000 \times 7$
$$x = \frac{7{,}000}{30{,}000} = 0.23 \text{ mL/min}$$
0.4 mL : min :: x mL : 60 min
$x = 0.4 \times 60 = 24$ mL/h

$$\frac{7 \cancel{\text{mU}}/\text{min}}{30{,}000 \cancel{\text{mU}}} \times 1000 \text{ mL} = 0.23 \text{ mL/min}$$
$$\frac{0.23 \text{ mL}}{1 \cancel{\text{min}}} \times \frac{60 \cancel{\text{min}}}{1 \text{ h}} = 13.8 \text{ or } 14 \text{ mL/h}$$

3. a. 20 g : 500 mL :: 2 g : x mL
$20x = 1000$
$x = 50$ mL
50 mL : 30 min :: x mL : 60 min
$30x = 3000$
$$x = \frac{3000}{30} = 100 \text{ mL/h}$$

$$\frac{50 \text{ mL}}{30 \cancel{\text{min}}} \times \frac{60 \cancel{\text{min}}}{1 \text{ h}} = 100 \text{ mL/h}$$

b. 20 g : 500 mL :: 3 g : x mL
$20x = 1{,}500$
$x = 75$ mL
75 mL : 60 min :: x mL : 60 min
$60x = 4500$
$$x = \frac{4500}{60} = 75 \text{ mL/h}$$

$$\frac{3 \cancel{\text{g}}/\text{h}}{20 \cancel{\text{g}}} \times 500 \text{ mL} = 75 \text{ mL/h}$$

Ratio-Proportion	Formula
4. a. 30 g : 500 mL :: 2 g : x mL $30x = 1000$ $x = 33.3$ mL 33.3 mL : 20 min :: x mL : 60 min $20x = 1998$ $x = \frac{1998}{20} = 100$ mL/h	$\frac{33.3 \text{ mL}}{20 \text{ min}} \times \frac{60 \text{ min}}{1 \text{ h}} = 100$ mL/h
b. 30 g : 500 mL :: 3 g : x mL $30x = 1500$ $x = 50$ mL 50 mL : 60 min :: x mL : 60 min $60x = 3000$ $x = \frac{3000}{60} = 50$ mL/h	$\frac{3 \text{ g/h}}{30 \text{ g}} \times 500 \text{ mL} = 50$ mL/h

CHAPTER 19 Ratio-Proportion/Formula Method—Posttest 2, pp. 577–578

Ratio-Proportion	Formula
1. a. 1 unit : 1000 mU :: 10 units : x mU $x = 1000 \times 10 = 10{,}000$ mU 10,000 mU : 1000 mL :: 2 mU : x mL/min $10{,}000x = 1000 \times 2$ $x = \frac{2000}{10{,}000} = 0.2$ mL/min 0.2 mL : 1 min :: x mL : 60 min $x = 60 \times 0.2$ mL/h $= 12$ mL/h	$\frac{2 \text{ mU/min}}{10{,}000 \text{ mU}} \times 1000 \text{ mL} = 0.2$ mL/min $\frac{0.2 \text{ mL}}{1 \text{ min}} \times \frac{60 \text{ min}}{1 \text{ h}} = 12$ mL/h
b. 1 unit : 1000 mU :: 10 units : x mU $x = 1000 \times 10 = 10{,}000$ mU 10,000 mU : 1000 mL :: 30 mU : x mL/min $10{,}000x = 1000 \times 30$ $x = \frac{30{,}000}{10{,}000} = 3$ mL/min 3 mL : 1 min :: x mL : 60 min $x = 60 \times 3 = 180$ mL/h	$\frac{30 \text{ mU/min}}{10{,}000 \text{ mU}} \times 1000 \text{ mL} = 3$ mL/min $\frac{3 \text{ mL}}{1 \text{ min}} \times \frac{60 \text{ min}}{1 \text{ h}} = 180$ mL/h
c. 1 unit : 10,000 mU :: 10 units : x mU $x = 1000 \times 10 = 10{,}000$ mU 10,000 mU : 1000 mL :: 18 mU : x mL $10{,}000x = 1000 \times 18$ $x = \frac{18{,}000}{10{,}000} = 1.8$ mL/min 1.8 mL : min :: x mL : 60 min $x = 1.8 \times 60 = 108$ mL/h	$\frac{18 \text{ mU/min}}{10{,}000 \text{ mU}} \times 1000 \text{ mL} = 1.8$ mL/min $\frac{1.8 \text{ mL}}{1 \text{ min}} \times \frac{60 \text{ min}}{1 \text{ h}} = 108$ mL/h
2. a. 1 unit : 1000 mU :: 20 units : x mU $x = 1000 \times 20 = 20{,}000$ mU 20,000 mU : 1000 mL :: 4 mU : x mL/min $20{,}000x = 1000 \times 4$ $x = \frac{4000}{20{,}000} = 0.2$ mL/min 0.2 mL : 1 min :: x mL : 60 min $x = 60 \times 0.2 = 12$ mL/h	$\frac{4 \text{ mU/min}}{20{,}000 \text{ mU}} \times 1000 \text{ mL} = 0.2$ mL/min $\frac{0.2 \text{ mL}}{1 \text{ min}} \times \frac{60 \text{ min}}{1 \text{ h}} = 12$ mL/h

Ratio-Proportion / **Formula**

b. Ratio-Proportion:

1 unit : 1000 mU :: 20 units : x mU
$x = 1000 \times 20 = 20{,}000$ mU
20,000 mU : 1000 mL :: 20 mU : x mL/min
$20{,}000x = 1000 \times 20$

$$x = \frac{20{,}000}{20{,}000} = 1 \text{ mL/min}$$

1 mL : 1 min :: x mL : 60 min
$x = 60 \times 1 = 60$ mL/h

Formula:

$$\frac{20 \text{ mU/min}}{20{,}000 \text{ mU}} \times 1000 \text{ mL} = 1 \text{ mL/min}$$

$$\frac{1 \text{ mL}}{1 \text{ min}} \times \frac{60 \text{ min}}{1 \text{ h}} = 60 \text{ mL/h}$$

c. Ratio-Proportion:

1 unit : 10,000 mU :: 20 units : x mU
$x = 1000 \times 20 = 20{,}000$ mU
20,000 mU : 1000 mL :: 16 mU : x mL
$20{,}000x = 1000 \times 16$

$$x = \frac{16{,}000}{20{,}000} = 0.8 \text{ mL/min}$$

0.8 mL : min :: x mL : 60 min
$x = 0.8 \times 60 = 48$ mL/h

Formula:

$$\frac{16 \text{ mU/min}}{20{,}000 \text{ mU}} \times 1000 \text{ mL} = 0.8 \text{ mL/min}$$

$$\frac{0.8 \text{ mL}}{1 \text{ min}} \times \frac{60 \text{ min}}{1 \text{ h}} = 48 \text{ mL/h}$$

3. a. Ratio-Proportion:

20 g : 1000 mL :: 2 g : x mL
$20x = 2000$
$x = 100$ mL
100 mL : 30 min :: x mL : 60 min
$30x = 6000$

$$x = \frac{6000}{30} = 200 \text{ mL/h}$$

Formula:

$$\frac{100 \text{ mL}}{30 \text{ min}} \times \frac{60 \text{ min}}{1 \text{ h}} = 200 \text{ mL/h}$$

b. Ratio-Proportion:

20 g : 1000 mL :: 2 g : x mL
$20x = 2000$
$x = 100$ mL
100 mL : 60 min :: x mL : 60 min
$60x = 6000$

$$x = \frac{6000}{60} = 100 \text{ mL/h}$$

Formula:

$$\frac{2 \text{ g/h}}{20 \text{ g}} \times 1000 \text{ mL} = 100 \text{ mL/h}$$

4. a. Ratio-Proportion:

40 g : 1000 mL :: 2 g : x mL
$40x = 2000$
$x = 50$ mL
50 mL : 15 min :: x mL : 60 min
$15x = 3000$

$$x = \frac{3000}{15} = 200 \text{ mL/h}$$

Formula:

$$\frac{50 \text{ mL}}{15 \text{ min}} \times \frac{60 \text{ min}}{1 \text{ h}} = 200 \text{ mL/h}$$

b. Ratio-Proportion:

40 g : 1000 mL :: 4 g : x mL
$40x = 4000$
$x = 100$ mL
100 mL : 60 min :: x mL : 60 min
$60x = 6000$

$$x = \frac{6000}{60} = 100 \text{ mL/h}$$

Formula:

$$\frac{4 \text{ g/h}}{40 \text{ g}} \times 1000 \text{ mL} = 100 \text{ mL/h}$$

NAME ________________

DATE ________________

ACCEPTABLE SCORE **95**

YOUR SCORE ______

COMPREHENSIVE POSTTEST

DIRECTIONS: This test contains 60 questions with a total of 100 points (pts) possible. Each of the 10 separate case sections includes a variety of patient diagnoses. Test items focus on medication dosages, medication calculations, and medication transcription. Use the forms provided, and mark syringes where indicated.

CASE 1—HANDWRITTEN FORMAT *(10 pts)*

Mr. Jones is transferred to your unit from the intensive care unit (ICU). You receive Mr. Jones and look over his orders. It is 1700 on 2/3/24. Refer to the licensed prescriber's order sheet and medication profile sheet on p. 588 for the following questions. Show your work where applicable.

1. Mr. Jones reports pain in his incision. Oxycodone/acetaminophen 5/500 tablets are ordered on the licensed prescriber's order sheet. Oxycodone/acetaminophen is supplied in single tablets issued from the pharmacy. Give ______ *(1 pt)*

2. What regularly scheduled medications would Mr. Jones receive at 0900 each day? Include the amount of medication. a. ______ b. ______ c. ______ d. ______ *(4 pts)*

PHYSICIAN'S ORDERS

1. LABEL BEFORE PLACING IN PATIENT'S CHART 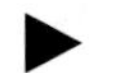
2. INITIAL AND DETACH COPY EACH TIME PHYSICIAN WRITES ORDERS
3. TRANSMIT COPY TO PHARMACY
4. ORDERS MUST BE DATED AND TIMED

Mr. Jones

☐ Inpatient ☐ Outpatient

DATE	TIME	ORDERS	TRANS BY
		Diagnosis: S/P Coronary Art. Bypass Graft Weight: 184.5 lb Height: 5'11"	
		Sensitivities/Drug Allergies: NKDA	
2/3/24	2250	1. Transfer to step-down unit from ICU	
		2. VS q.4. h. × 24 hours then q. 8 hours	
		3. Up in chair 3×day, asst. to walk in hall 2×day	
		4. Intake and output q. 8 hours	
		5. Daily WT.	
		6. Antiembolitic stockings	
		7. Incentive spirometer q.1 h. while awake	
		8. Diet: 3 g Na^+, low cholesterol	
		9. Oxycodone/acetominophen 5/500, 2 tablets by mouth q.4h. p.r.n. pain	
		10. Acetaminophen 650 mg by mouth q.4 h. p.r.n. pain or Temp. $\geq$38 C	
		11. MOM 30 mL by mouth q.day p.r.n. constipation	
		12. Mylanta 30 mL by mouth q.4 h. p.r.n. indigestion	
		13. Zolpidem 10 mg by mouth at bedtime p.r.n. insomnia	
		14. O_2 3 L per nasal cannula	
		15. IVF: D_5 $^1/_2$ NS @ 50 $^{mL}/_h$, maximum 1200 mL IVF/day	
		16. Digoxin 0.25 mg by mouth daily	
		17. E.C. ASA 325 mg by mouth daily	
		18. Omeprazole 20 mg by mouth daily	
		19. Furosemide 20 mg I.V. q.8 h.	
		20. Potassium chloride 10 mEq p.o. twice a day	
		21. Labs A_7, CBC, CXR q. a.m.	
		M. Doctor, M.D.	

Do Not Write Orders If No Copies Remain; Begin New Form **Copies Remaining**

MEDICAL RECORDS COPY				PHYSICIAN'S ORDERS				T-5
B-CLIN. NOTES	E-LAB	G-X-RAY	K-DIAGNOSTIC	M-SURGERY	Q-THERAPY	T-ORDERS	W-NURSING	Y-MISC.

3. Transcribe each as-needed (prn) medication from the licensed prescriber's orders. Include date, medication, dose, route, interval, and time schedule. *(1 pt)*

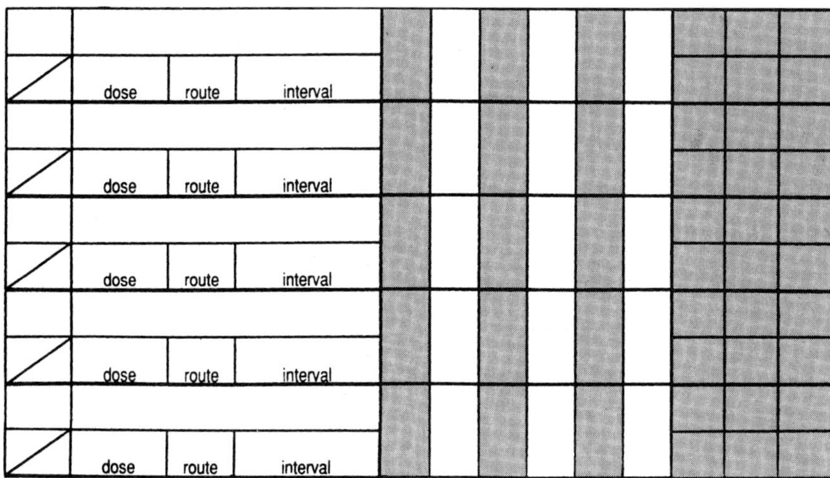
dose route interval
dose route interval
dose route interval
dose route interval
dose route interval

4. Transcribe each regularly scheduled medication from the licensed prescriber's order sheet. Include date, medication, dose, route, interval, and time schedule. *(1 pt)*

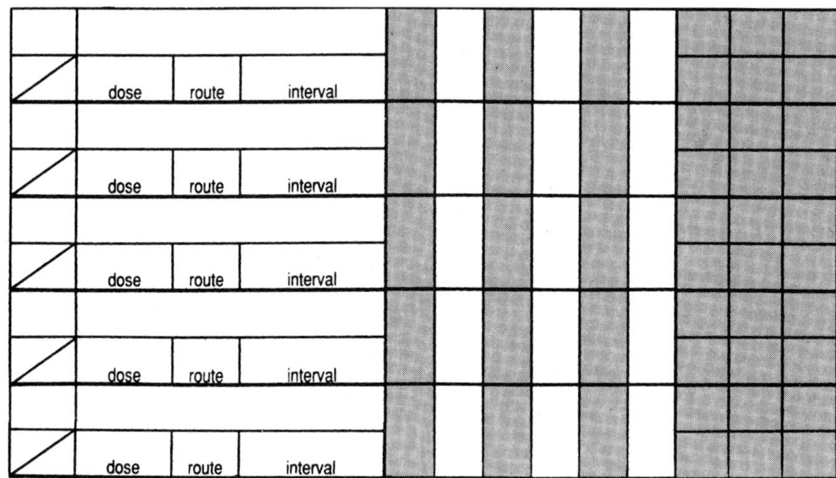
dose route interval
dose route interval
dose route interval
dose route interval
dose route interval

5. Mr. Jones reports insomnia at 2300. What prn medication is available for him? ______ *(1 pt)*

6. It is time to give Mr. Jones his furosemide. You have a premixed intravenous piggyback (IVPB) of furosemide 20 mg in 50 mL of normal saline solution (NS). Infusion time is 30 minutes. Drop factor is 60 gtt/mL. How many drops per minute will be administered? _______ *(1 pt)*

7. Mr. Jones reports constipation. What medication will be given? _______ How much will be administered? _______ *(1 pt)*

CASE 2—HANDWRITTEN FORMAT

(12 pts)

Mrs. Smith is received from the recovery room. You review her orders. It is 1700 on 2/3/24. Refer to the licensed prescriber's order sheet for the following questions. Show your work where applicable.

PHYSICIAN'S ORDERS

1. LABEL BEFORE PLACING IN PATIENT'S CHART ▶
2. INITIAL AND DETACH COPY EACH TIME PHYSICIAN WRITES ORDERS
3. TRANSMIT COPY TO PHARMACY
4. ORDERS MUST BE DATED AND TIMED

Mrs. Smith

☐ Inpatient ☐ Outpatient

DATE	TIME	ORDERS	TRANS BY
2/3/24	1650	Diagnosis: S/P Thyroidectomy Weight: 146.0 lb Height: 5'10"	
		Sensitivities/Drug Allergies: PCN	
		STATUS: ASSIGN TO OBSERVATION ☐ ; ADMIT AS INPATIENT ☐	
		1. Transfer to ward from recovery room.	
		2. VS q.1 hour ×2 hours, then q.4 hours	
		3. HOB ↑45 degrees	
		4. Up in chair 3× day, support head and neck	
		5. Intake and output q. 8 hours	
		6. Incentive spirometer q.1 hour while awake	
		7. Diet: Full liquid	
		8. Hydromorphone 2 mg I.M. q.4 hours p.r.n. pain	
		9. Promethazine 12.5 mg I.M. q.4 hours p.r.n. nausea	
		10. Acetaminophen 650 mg by mouth q.4 hours p.r.n. pain or Temp >38°C	
		11. Zolpidem 5 mg by mouth at bedtime p.r.n. insomnia	
		12. O_2 4 L per nasal cannula	
		13. IVF: NS 75 mL/h	
		14. Levothyroxine 0.15 mg. by mouth daily at 0600	
		15. Omeprazole 40 mg by mouth daily at 0600	
		16. Labs: Ca^+ q. 8 hours × 3 days	
		A_7, CBC q. a.m.	
		17. JP drains × 2 to bulb suction, record output q. 8 hours	
		M. Doctor, M.D.	

Do Not Write Orders If No Copies Remain; Begin New Form Copies Remaining

MEDICAL RECORDS COPY			PHYSICIAN'S ORDERS					T-5
B-CLIN. NOTES	E-LAB	G-X-RAY	K-DIAGNOSTIC	M-SURGERY	Q-THERAPY	T-ORDERS	W-NURSING	Y-MISC.

1. What regularly scheduled medications would Mrs. Smith receive at 0600 each day? Include the amount of each medication. a. _______ b. _______ *(2 pts)*

2. Mrs. Smith reports nausea. Promethazine 25 mg/2 mL is available. How many milliliters will be administered? _______ *(1 pt)*

3. Mrs. Smith reports insomnia at 2200. Zolpidem is supplied in 10-mg tablets. Give _______ tablet(s). *(1 pt)*

4. What prn medications are available for reports of pain? a. _______ b. _______ *(2 pts)*

5. Mrs. Smith reports pain shortly after she is received on the unit from the recovery room. Hydromorphone is available 1 mg/1 mL for injection. How many milliliters will you administer? _______ *(1 pt)*

6. Mrs. Smith has a fever of 38.6° C. Acetaminophen 325-mg tablets is available. How many tablets will be administered? _______ *(1 pt)*

7. Transcribe all regularly scheduled medications from the licensed prescriber's orders. Include date, medication, dose, route, interval, and time schedule. *(2 pts)*

	dose	route	interval									
	dose	route	interval									

CASE 3—ELECTRONIC HEALTH RECORD

(15 pts)

Ms. Davis was admitted with chronic kidney disease (CKD). Admitting serum potassium is 6.2 mEq/dL. Refer to the eMAR for the following questions. Show your work where applicable.

Logout

Pt name: Marie Davis | **Room:** 346 | **Allergies:** Vancomycin
MRN: 3986 | **Admit date:** 12/25/2024 | **Attending:** Dr. Turner
DOB: 10/31/1976

MAR — All | Scheduled | PRN — Close X

Medication	0800	0900	1000	1100	1200	1300
Regular Insulin : Dose 10 units : intravenous : one time dose						
Dextrose 50% : Dose 25 g : intravenous : one time dose						
Erythropoietin (EPOGEN) : Dose 7,500 units : subcutaneous : after dialysis					1200	
Ferrous sulfate (IRON) : Dose 300 mg : by mouth : with meals	0800				1200	
Carvedilol (COREG) : Dose 12.5 mg : by mouth : twice a day	0800					
Sodium bicarbonate : Dose 600 mg : by mouth : 3 times daily	0800				1200	

1. What is Ms. Davis allergic to? _______ *(1 pt)*

2. Before administering medications, the nurse asks the patient to state her name and date of birth. What does the nurse expect to hear? _______ and _______. *(2 pts)*

3. What medication times are shown on the eMAR? _______ *(1 pt)*

4. What medications are due at 0800? _______, _______, _______. *(3 pts)*

5. Draw a line on the syringe to reflect the number of units of regular insulin the patient will receive. *(1 pt)*

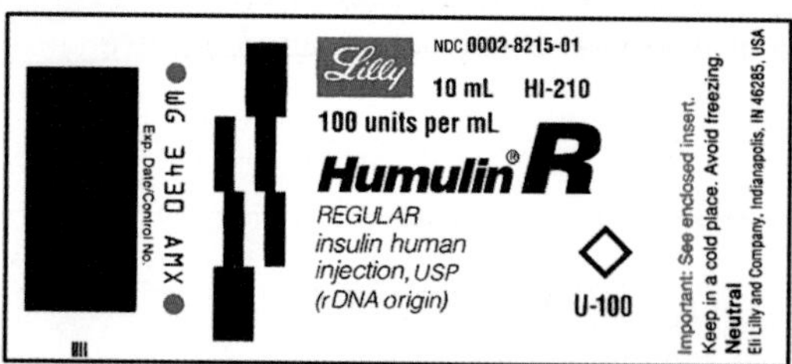

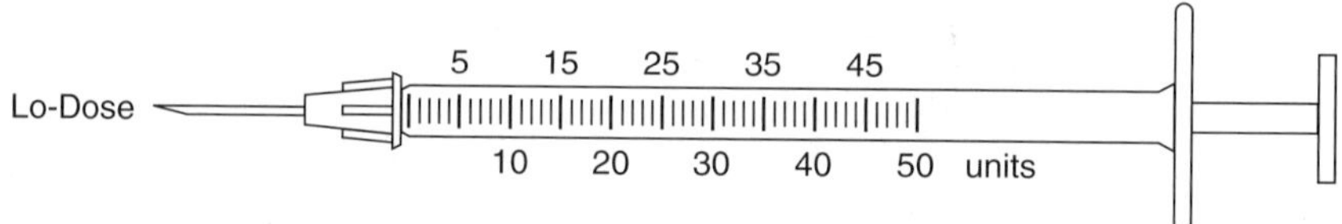

6. How many milliliters of erythropoietin will Ms. Davis receive after her dialysis treatment is complete? Draw a line on the syringe to represent the number of milliliters the patient will receive. *(2 pts)*

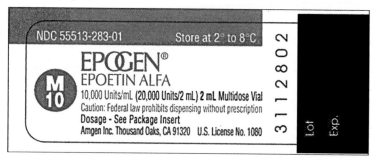

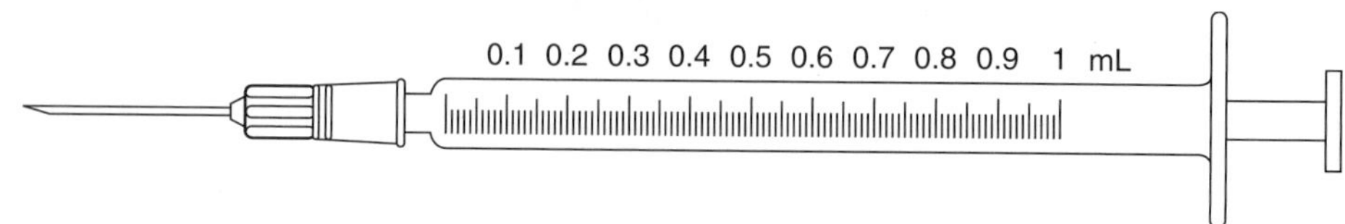

7. The dialysis nurse reports the patient lost 3.5 kg during the dialysis treatment. How many milliliters will the nurse document on the intake and output? _______ *(1 pt)*

8. During the 7 PM to 7 AM shift, Ms. Davis consumed 90 mL of juice and 4 oz of water. The patient voided 2 times during the shift for 100 mL and 80 mL of urine. Calculate the intake and output for this shift. *(2 pts)*

9. The patient is ordered to have 1 unit of blood for anemia. The unit of blood contains 300 mL and is to infuse over 4 hours using a tubing with a 15 drop per milliliter drop factor. How many gtt/min will the nurse infuse the blood? _______ *(2 pts)*

CASE 4—ELECTRONIC HEALTH RECORD

(10 pts)

Mr. Sullivan is a patient admitted with diabetic ketoacidosis (DKA). Admitting serum glucose is 650 mg/dL and potassium is 2.9 mEq/dL. Refer to the eMAR for the following questions. Show your work where applicable.

Logout

Pt name: Bill Sullivan
MRN: 12-856
DOB: 11/10/1969

Room: 346
Admit date: 03/20/2024

Allergies: NKA
Attending: Dr. Spencer

MAR — All | Scheduled | PRN — **Close** X

Medication	0800	0900	1000	1100	1200	1300
Regular insulin 100 units/100 mL : Dose 6 units/h : intravenous : continuous				1100		
1000 mL 0.9% sodium chloride (NS) : Dose over 4 h : intravenous : one time				1100		
Ordansetron (ZOFRAN): Dose 4 mg : intravenous : every 6 h as needed for N&V						
Potassium chloride at 20 mEq/h : Dose 40 mEq/100 mL : intravenous : one time				1100		

1. Calculate the milliliters per hour for the insulin infusion. _______ *(2 pts)*

2. What rate will the nurse infuse the NS infusion? _______ *(1 pt)*

3. When infusing the potassium chloride, how many milliliters per hour will the nurse program for the IV infusion device? _______ *(2 pts)*

4. After 2 hours, the blood glucose level returns 420 mg/dL. The insulin infusion is decreased to 4 mL/h. How many units per hour is the patient receiving? _______ *(2 pts)*

5. Mr. Sullivan reports feeling nauseated. Ondansetron is available in a 2 mg/mL concentration. Draw a line on the syringe to represent the number of milliliters the patient will receive. *(2 pts)*

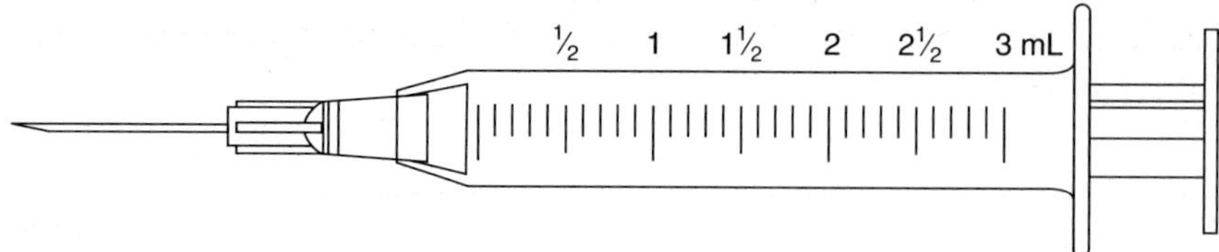

6. Six hours after admission, the patient's blood glucose levels are controlled and the patient is tolerating solid food. The patient's glucose level is 140 mg/dL, and 2 units of Novolog is ordered subcutaneous before eating. Draw a line on the syringe to reflect the number of units the patient will receive. *(1 pt)*

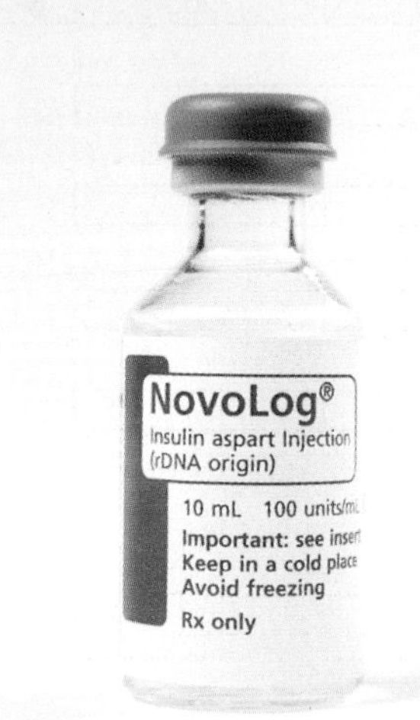

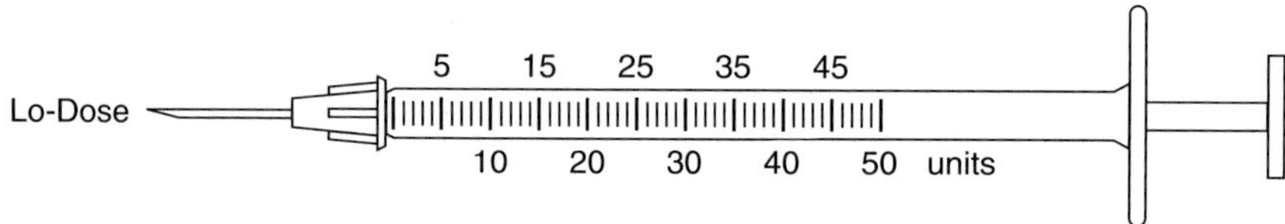

CASE 5—ELECTRONIC HEALTH RECORD

(10 pts)

Mr. Curran was admitted 3 days ago following a cerebral vascular accident (CVA). The patient has a gastrostomy tube (G-tube) for dysphagia. Refer to the eMAR for the following questions. Show your work where applicable.

Logout

Pt name: Tom Curran **Room:** 7834 **Allergies:** NKA
MRN: 87654 **Admit date:** 05/29/2024 **Attending:** Dr. Iyer
DOB: 06/22/1958

MAR Close X

All | Scheduled | PRN

Medication	0800	0900	1000	1100	1200	1300
Phenobarbital : Dose 60 mg : per G-tube : every 12 hours		0900				
Fluoxetine (PROZAC) : Dose 40 mg : per G-tube : daily		0900				
Metoclopramide (REGLAN) : Dose 5 mg : per G-tube : every 6 h before meals				1100		
Dexamethasone (DECADRON) : Dose 0.5 mg : per G-tube : every 12 hours		0900				
Amoxicillin (AMOXIL) : Dose 250 mg : per G-tube : every 6 hours					1200	
Metoprolol (LOPRESSOR) : Dose 100 mg : per G-tube : every 12 hours		0900				

1. How many milliliters of phenobarbital will Mr. Curran receive? Draw a line on the medicine cup to represent the number of milliliters the patient will receive. *(2 pts)*

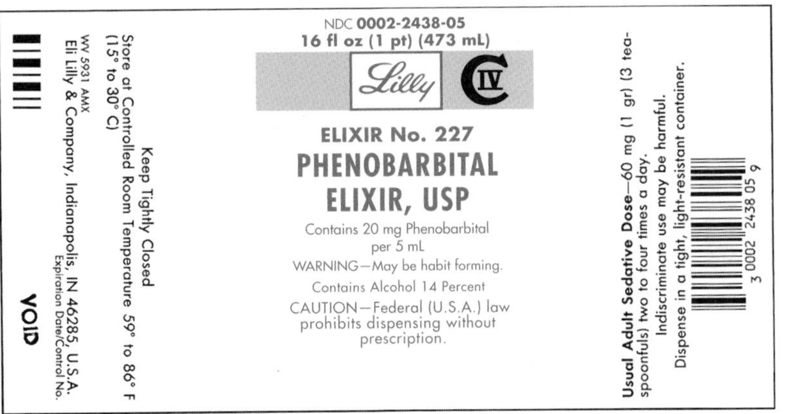

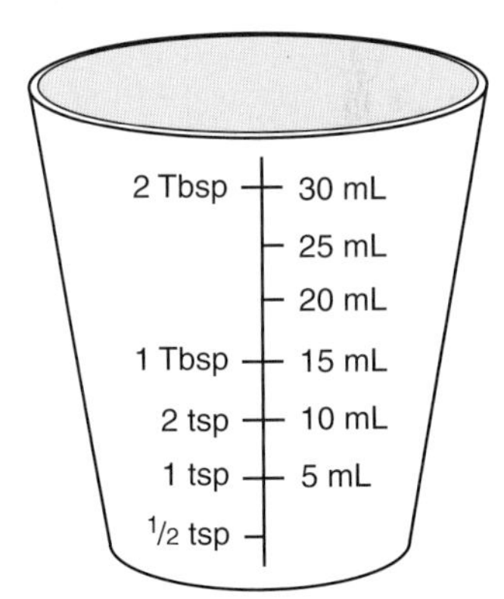

2. How many milliliters of fluoxetine will the patient receive? Draw a line on the medicine cup to represent the number of milliliters the patient will receive. *(1 pt)*

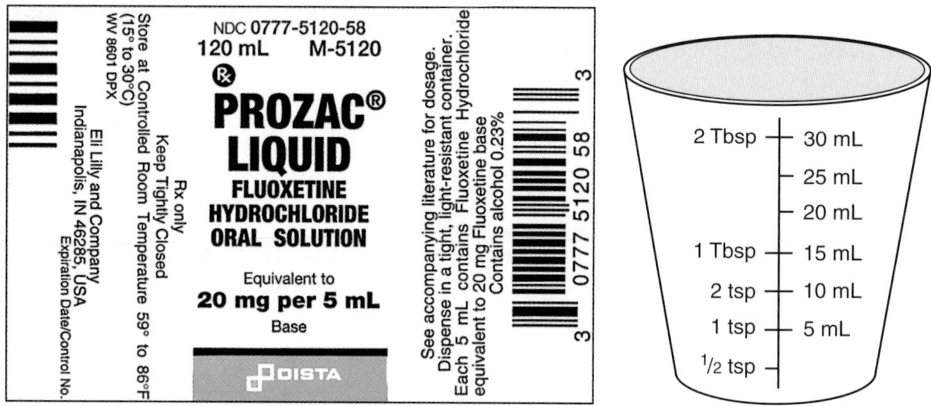

3. What time is the metoclopramide scheduled to be given? _______ *(1 pt)*

4. How many milliliters of metoclopramide will the patient receive when using a concentration of metoclopramide 10 mg/10 mL? Draw a line on the medicine cup to represent the number of milliliters the patient will receive. *(2 pts)*

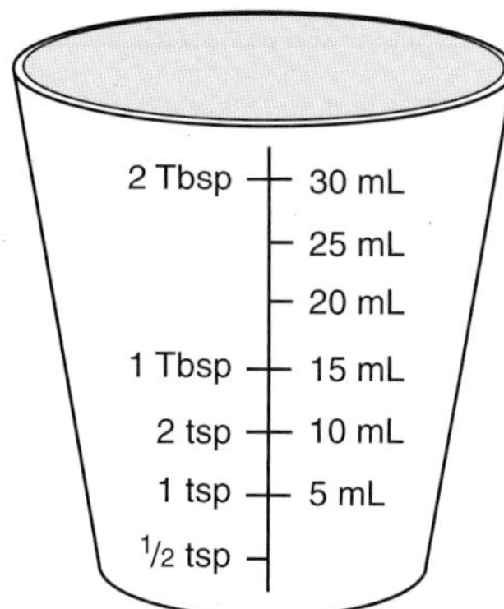

5. It is time to administer dexamethasone to Mr. Curran. How many tablets will the nurse administer? *(1 pt)*

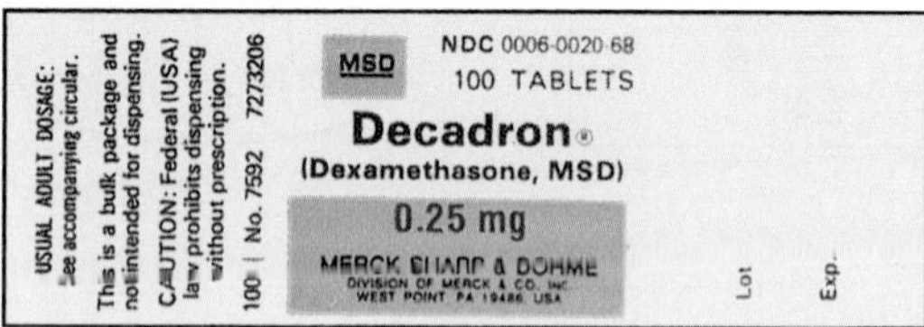

6. It is time to administer the amoxicillin. Calculate the milliliters of amoxicillin Mr. Curran will receive. Draw a line on the medicine cup to represent the number of milliliters the patient will receive. *(2 pts)*

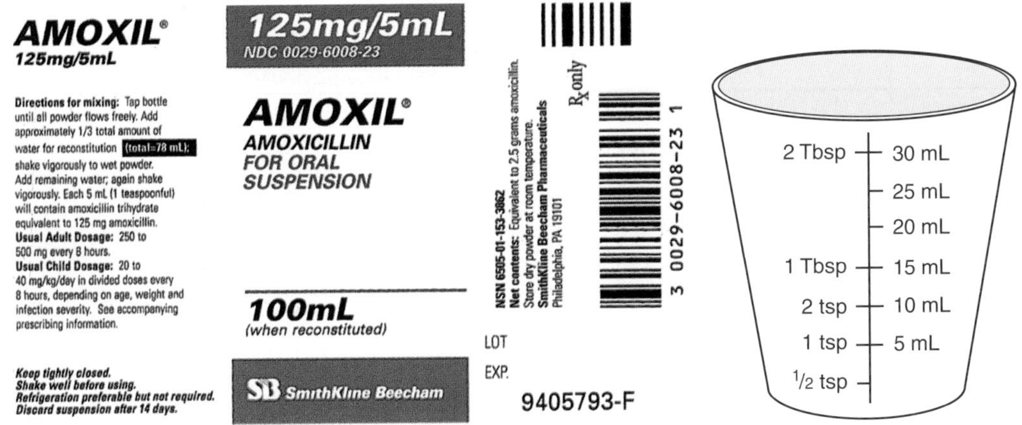

7. It is time to administer the metoprolol to Mr. Curran. How many tablets will be administered? *(1 pt)*

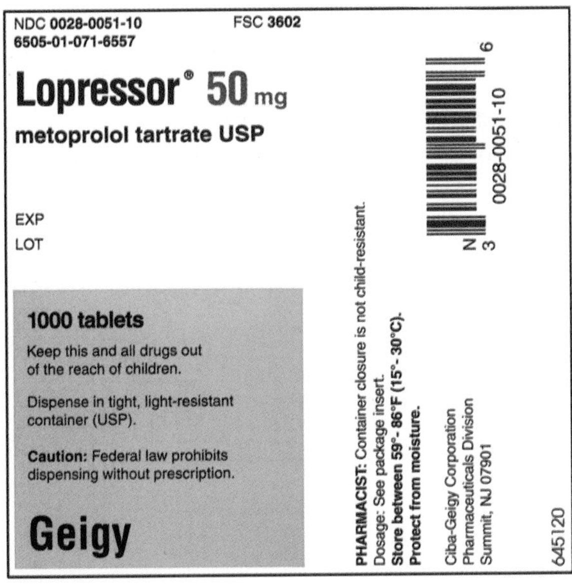

CASE 6—ELECTRONIC HEALTH RECORD

(10 pts)

Mrs. Coleman is a patient admitted from the emergency department with a diagnosis of acute pancreatitis. Refer to the eMAR for the following questions. Show your work where applicable.

Logout

Pt name: Kim Coleman **Room:** 1123 **Allergies:** PCN
MRN: 11-892 **Admit date:** 04/01/2024 **Attending:** Dr. Carl
DOB: 08/01/1951

MAR **Close** X

All | Scheduled | PRN

	1900	2000	2100	2200	2300	2400
Hydromorphone (DILAUDID) : Dose 2 mg : intravenous : every 2h as needed pain						
TPN per fomula : Dose 1800 mL/24 h : intravenous : continuous		2000				
Promethazine (PHENERGAN) : Dose 25 mg : intravenous : every 6 h as needed N&V						
Diphenhydramine (BENADRYL) : Dose 25 mg : intravenous : 2200 as needed for sleep						
Albumin 25% : Dose 100 mL/30 min : intravenous : one time dose			2100			

1. How many milliliters of hydromorphone will Mrs. Coleman receive? Draw a line on the syringe to represent the number of milliliters the patient will receive. *(2 pts)*

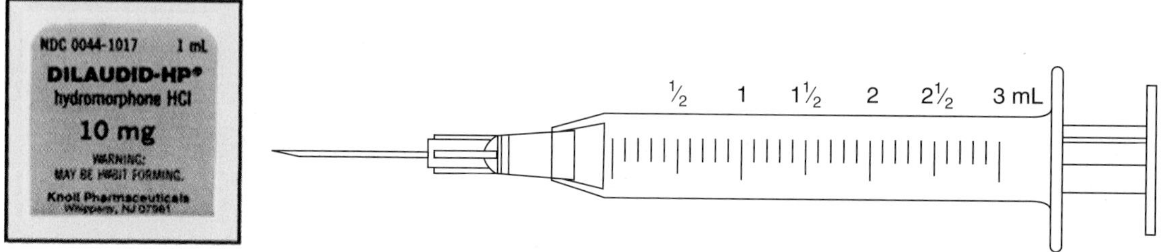

2. How many mL/h will the nurse infuse the TPN? _______ *(1 pt)*

3. Mrs. Coleman is experiencing nausea. How many milliliters of promethazine will the patient receive? Draw a line on the syringe to represent the number of milliliters the patient will receive. *(2 pts)*

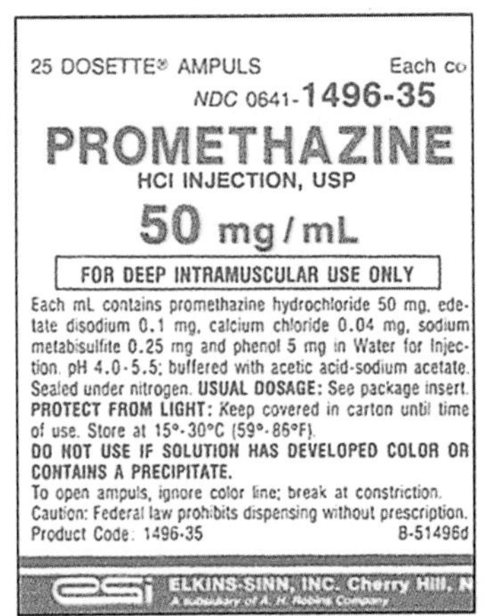

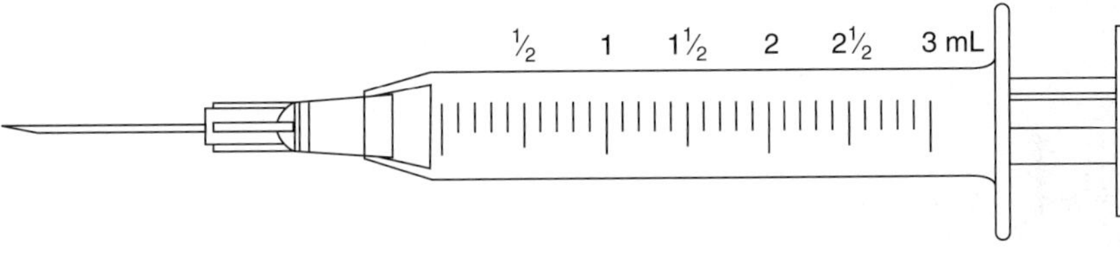

4. Mrs. Coleman reports difficulty sleeping. What medication and dose may the patient receive? _______ *(1 pt)*

5. How many milliliters of diphenhydramine will Mrs. Coleman receive at 2200 if needed for sleep? Draw a line on the syringe to represent the number of milliliters the patient will receive. *(2 pts)*

N 0071-4402-10
Benadryl®
(Diphenhydramine Hydrochloride Injection, USP)
50 mg per mL
HIGH POTENCY
10 mL

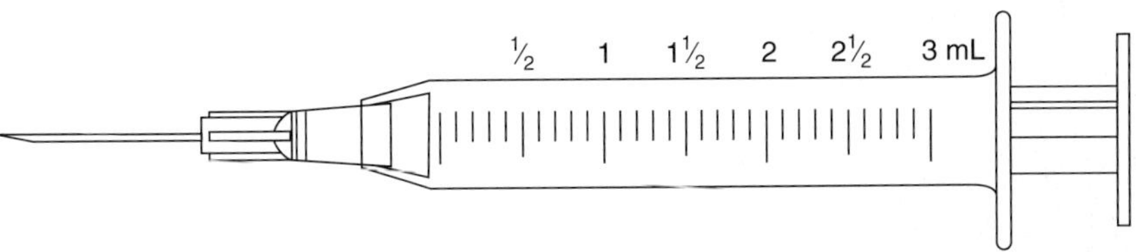

6. The patient's capillary glucose level is 210 mg/dL. The nurse receives a one-time order for Novolog insulin 4 units subcutaneous. Draw a line on the syringe to reflect the number of units the patient will receive. *(1 pt)*

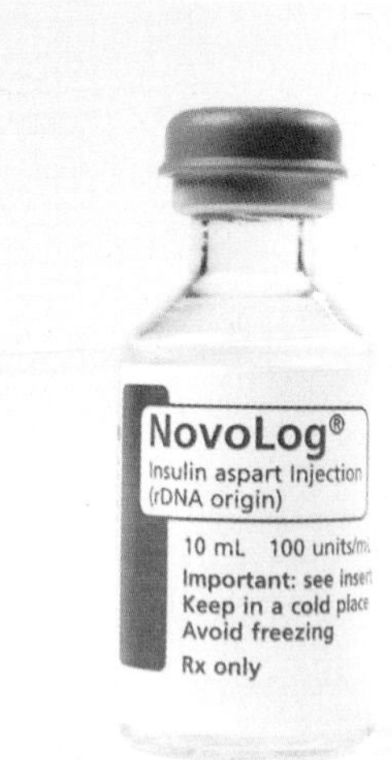

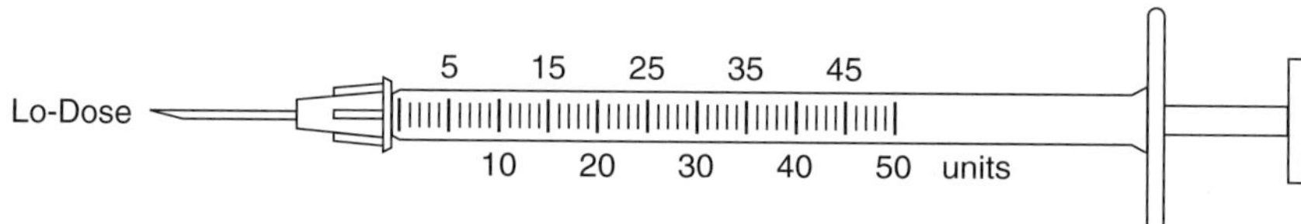

7. It is time for the nurse to administer the scheduled albumin. Using tubing with 10 drops per milliliter, how many drops per minute will the nurse infuse the almumin? _______ *(1 pt)*

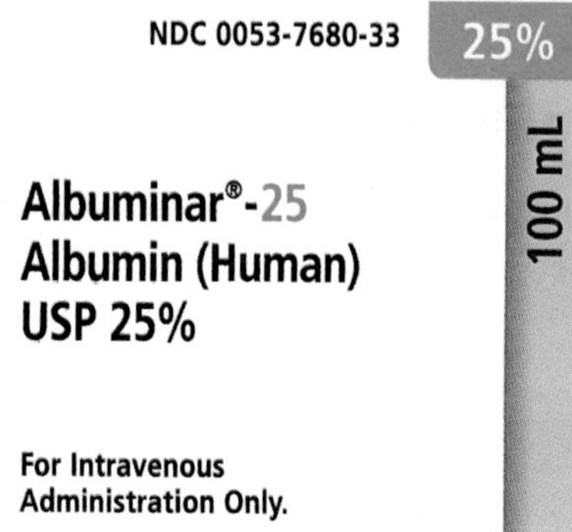

CASE 7—ELECTRONIC HEALTH RECORD

(10 pts)

Ms. Wayne is admitted at 0700 to induce labor. Refer to the eMAR for the following questions. Show your work where applicable.

Logout

Pt name: Linda Wayne **Room:** 3211 **Allergies:** NKA
MRN: 23-458 **Admit date:** 02/14/2024 **Attending:** Dr. Sheets
DOB: 12/07/1998

MAR Close X

All | Scheduled | PRN

0700	0800	0900	1000	1100	1200
Oxytocin (PITOCIN) 10 units/1000mL : Dose 2 mU/min : intravenous : continuous, increase by 2 mU every 20 minutes until active labor occurs					
	800				
Magnesium 10g/500 mL Bolus : Dose 2 g : intravenous : over 30 minutes					
	0830				
Magnesium 10g/500 mL : Dose 1 g/h : intravenous : continuous after bolus					
		0900			
Acetaminophen (TYLENOL) : Dose 650 mg : oral : every 4 h as needed for pain					

1. How many mL/h will the nurse begin the oxytocin infusion at 0800? _______ *(3 pts)*

2. The oxytocin has been increased every 20 minutes. What is the IV rate (mL/h) after 2 hours? _______ *(3 pts)*

3. What is the IV rate (mL/h) for the magnesium bolus? _______ *(2 pts)*

4. What is the IV rate (mL/h) for the magnesium infusion? _______ *(2 pts)*

CASE 8—ELECTRONIC HEALTH RECORD *(10 pts)*

Mr. Keys is admitted with a diagnosis of non-ST elevation myocardial infarction (NSTEMI) and is awaiting a coronary angiogram. Refer to the eMAR for the following questions. Show your work where applicable.

Logout

Pt name: Lee Kays **Room:** 892 **Allergies:** NKA
MRN: 35724 **Admit date:** 03/17/2024 **Attending:** Dr. Nelson
DOB: 03/24/1998

MAR Close X

All | Scheduled | PRN

	0700	0800	0900	1000	1100	1200
Heparin : Dose per weight-based protocol : intravenous : continuous						
Enteric coated aspirin : Dose 81 mg : by mouth : daily		0800				
Clopidogrel (PLAVIX) : Dose 75 mg : by mouth : daily			0900			
Nitroglycerin 50 mg/200mL : Dose 20 mcg/min : intravenous : continuous						
Metoprolol (LOPRESSOR) : Dose 25 mg : by mouth : twice daily			0900			

1. Use the heparin protocol for the following questions. The patient's weight is 77.1 kg.

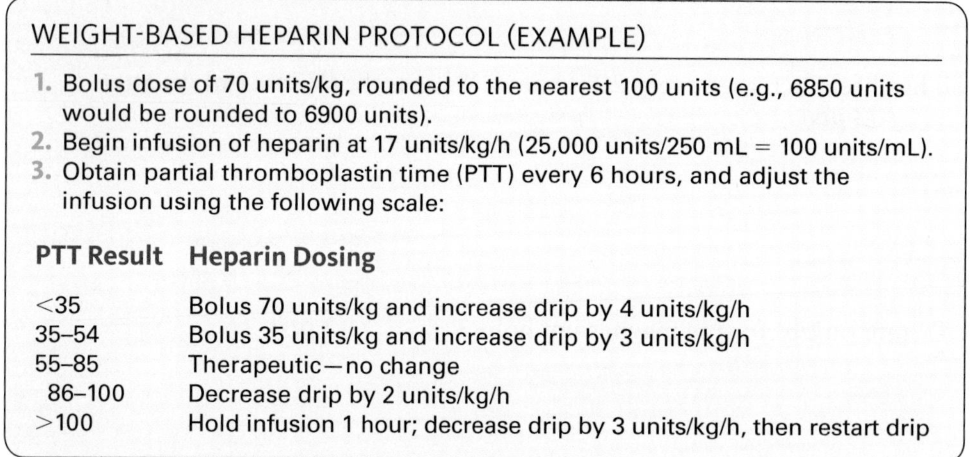

WEIGHT-BASED HEPARIN PROTOCOL (EXAMPLE)

1. Bolus dose of 70 units/kg, rounded to the nearest 100 units (e.g., 6850 units would be rounded to 6900 units).
2. Begin infusion of heparin at 17 units/kg/h (25,000 units/250 mL = 100 units/mL).
3. Obtain partial thromboplastin time (PTT) every 6 hours, and adjust the infusion using the following scale:

PTT Result	Heparin Dosing
<35	Bolus 70 units/kg and increase drip by 4 units/kg/h
35–54	Bolus 35 units/kg and increase drip by 3 units/kg/h
55–85	Therapeutic—no change
86–100	Decrease drip by 2 units/kg/h
>100	Hold infusion 1 hour; decrease drip by 3 units/kg/h, then restart drip

a. How many units of heparin should be administered for the bolus? ______ *(2 pts)*

b. Using the following vial of heparin, draw a line on the syringe to represent the number of milliliters the patient will receive. *(2 pts)*

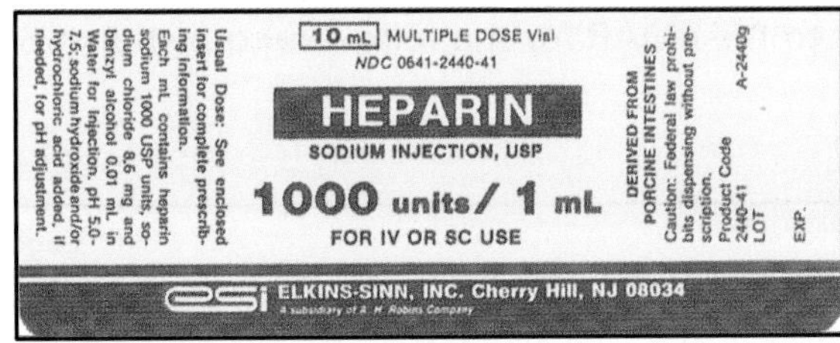

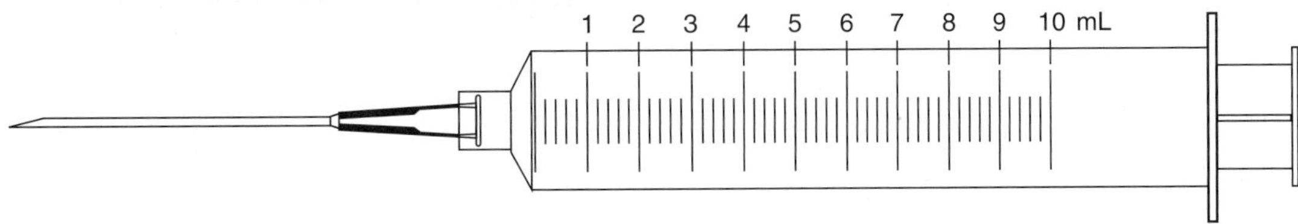

c. How many milliliters per hour would the nurse program the heparin infusion? _______ *(3 pts)*

2. How many milliliters per hour will the nurse program the IV pump when beginning the nitroglycerin infusion? _______ *(3 pts)*

CASE 9—ELECTRONIC HEALTH RECORD

(10 pts)

A 3 year-old child is admitted to the pediatric unit with a diagnosis of acute lymphocytic leukemia (ALL). The child's weight is 40 lb. Refer to the eMAR for the following questions. Show your work where applicable.

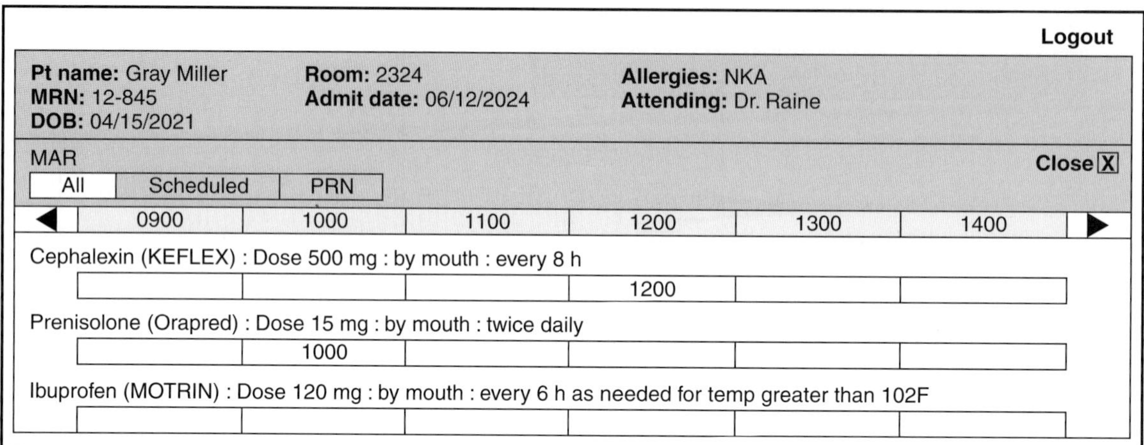

Logout

Pt name: Gray Miller **Room:** 2324 **Allergies:** NKA
MRN: 12-845 **Admit date:** 06/12/2024 **Attending:** Dr. Raine
DOB: 04/15/2021

MAR — All | Scheduled | PRN — Close X

Medication	0900	1000	1100	1200	1300	1400
Cephalexin (KEFLEX) : Dose 500 mg : by mouth : every 8 h				1200		
Prenisolone (Orapred) : Dose 15 mg : by mouth : twice daily		1000				
Ibuprofen (MOTRIN) : Dose 120 mg : by mouth : every 6 h as needed for temp greater than 102F						

1. The recommended dose for cephalexin is 50 to 100 mg/kg/24 h divided in q 8 h schedule.

   a. Is the ordered dose safe and therapeutic (yes or no)? Prove mathematically. _______ *(2 pts)*

   b. Using the following label, how many milliliters would be administered to the patient? _______ *(1 pt)*

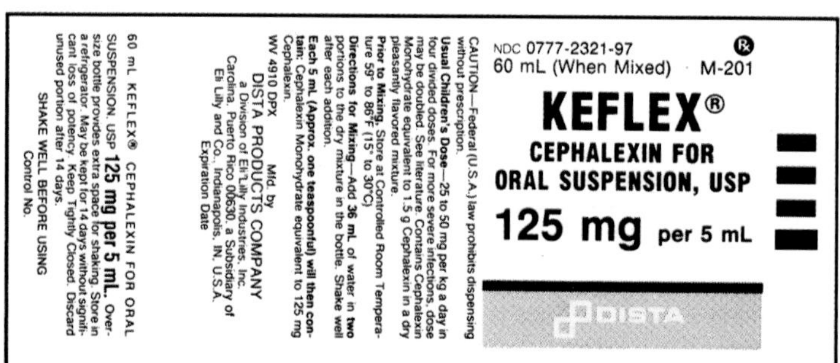

2. The recommended dose for prednisolone is 0.5 to 2 mg/kg/24 h divided twice a day.

   a. Is the dose safe and therapeutic (yes or no)? Prove mathematically. _______ *(2 pts)*

   b. The prednisolone is available in a 15 mg/5 mL concentration. How many milliliters are needed for the dose? _______ *(1 pt)*

3. The recommended dose for ibuprofen is 5 to 10 mg/kg/dose every 6 h.

a. Is the dose safe and therapeutic (yes or no)? Prove mathematically. _______ *(2 pts)*

b. It is available in a 100 mg/5 mL concentration. How many milliliters are needed for the dose? _______ *(1 pt)*

4. Calculate the fluid requirements for this patient. _______ *(1 pt)*

CASE 10–ELECTRONIC HEALTH RECORD *(5 pts)*

Mrs. Taylor, 76, presents to the emergency department with dyspnea and fatigue. The family states that she has a history of heart failure and renal insufficiency and that she is prescribed furosemide 40 mg daily, digoxin 0.25 mg daily, and lisinopril 10 mg daily. Please answer the following questions pertaining to Mrs. Taylor. Show your work where applicable.

1. When assessing Mrs. Taylor's compliance with her prescribed medications, the nurse is aware that the most common medication error for older adults at home is ________. *(1 pt)*

2. Explain how a decrease in cardiac output can affect Mrs. Taylor. _______ *(1 pt)*

3. Mrs. Taylor admits she has been trying to "stretch" her medications, so she has been taking them only every other day. The nurse is aware that the most common reason for patients trying to "stretch" their medications is ________. *(1 pt)*

4. Mrs. Taylor also states that sometimes she can't remember if she has taken her medications. An inexpensive solution to this problem is a ________. *(1 pt)*

5. With discharge teaching, how should the nurse evaluate the effectiveness of the medication teaching? ________. *(1 pt)*

ANSWERS ON PP. 609–612.

ANSWERS

COMPREHENSIVE POSTTEST, pp. 587–608

Case 1, *pp. 587–590*

1. 2 tablets
2. a. Digoxin 0.25 mg
   b. EC ASA 325 mg
   c. Omeprazole 20 mg
   d. Potassium chloride 10 mEq
3.

2/3/24	Oxycodone/acetaminophen 5/500				
	2 dose	p.o. route	q.4 h. interval	prn pain	
2/3/24	Acetaminophen 650 mg				
	650 mg dose	p.o. route	q.4 h. interval	prn pain or Temp >38° C	
2/3/24	MOM				
	30 mL dose	p.o. route	daily interval	prn constipation	
2/3/24	Mylanta				
	30 mL dose	p.o. route	q.4 h. interval	prn indigestion	
2/3/24	Zolpidem				
	10 mg dose	p.o. route	at bedtime interval	prn insomnia	

4.

2/3/24	Digoxin					
	0.25 mg dose	p.o. route	daily interval	09		
2/3/24	E.C. ASA 325 mg					
	325 mg dose	p.o. route	daily interval	09		
2/3/24	Omeprazole					
	20 mg dose	p.o. route	daily interval	09		
2/3/24	Furosemide					
	20 mg dose	I.V. route	q.8 h. interval	08	16	24
2/3/24	Potassium chloride					
	10 mEq dose	p.o. route	twice daily interval	09	17	

5. Zolpidem 10 mg by mouth
6. 100 gtt/min
7. Milk of magnesia 30 mL

Case 2, *pp. 591–592*

1. a. Levothyroxine 0.15 mg
   b. Omeprazole 40 mg
2. 1 mL
3. 0.5 tablet
4. a. Hydromorphone
   b. Acetaminophen
5. 2 mL
6. 2 tablets
7.

2/3/24	Levothyroxine			06
	0.15 mg dose	p.o. route	daily interval	
2/3/24	Tagamet			09
	300 mg dose	p.o. route	daily interval	

Case 3, *pp. 593–594*

1. Vancomycin
2. Marie Davis, October 31, 1976
3. 0800, 0900, 1000, 1100, 1200, and 1300
4. Ferrous sulfate 300 mg, carvedilol 12.5 mg, and sodium bicarbonate 600 mg
5.

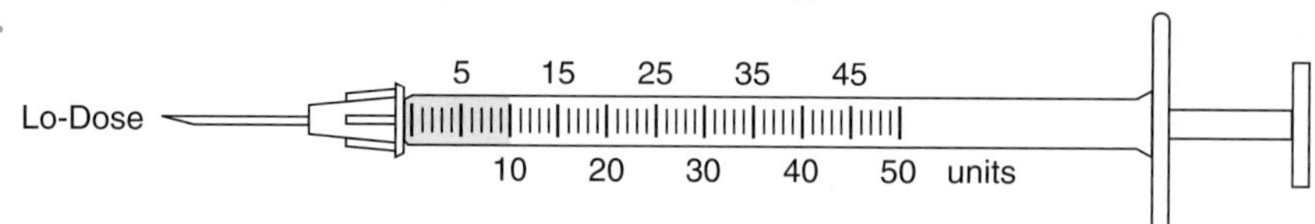

6.

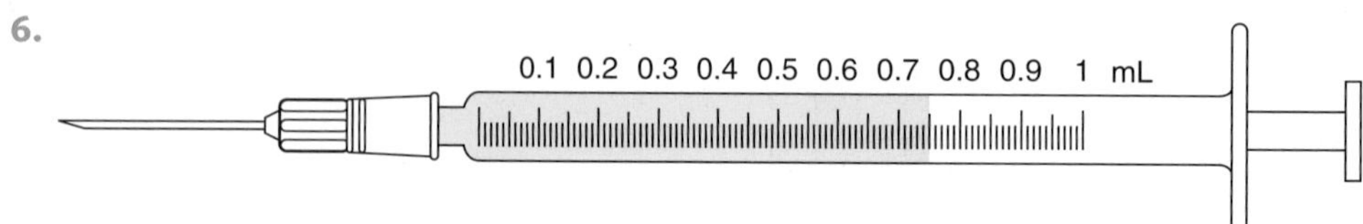

7. 3,500 mL
8. Intake, 210 mL; output, 180 mL
9. 19 gtt/min

Case 4, *pp. 595–596*

1. 6 mL/h
2. 250 mL/h
3. 50 mL/h
4. 4 units/h
5.

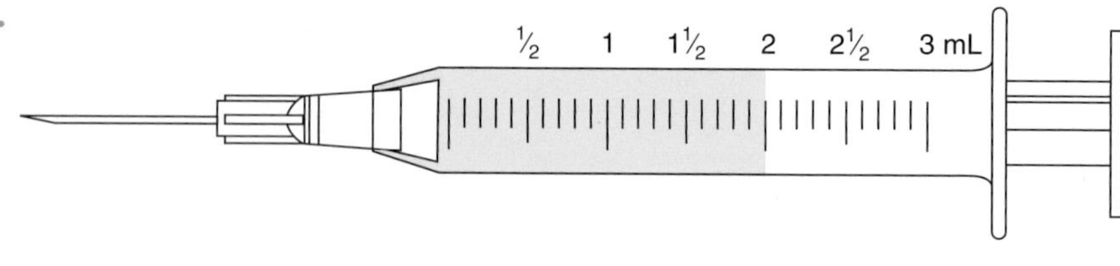

6.

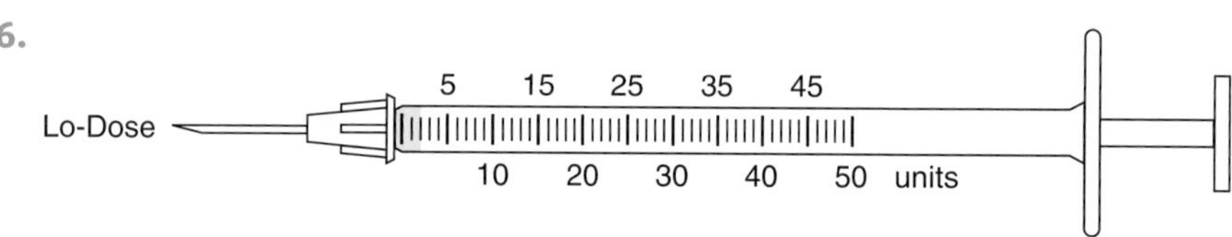

Case 5, *pp. 597–599*

1.

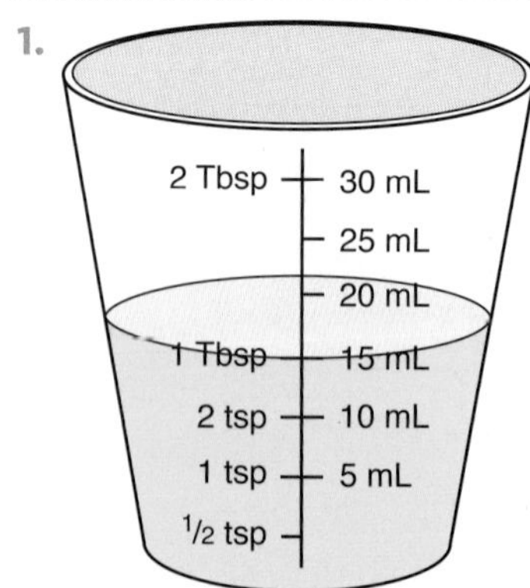

ANSWERS

2.
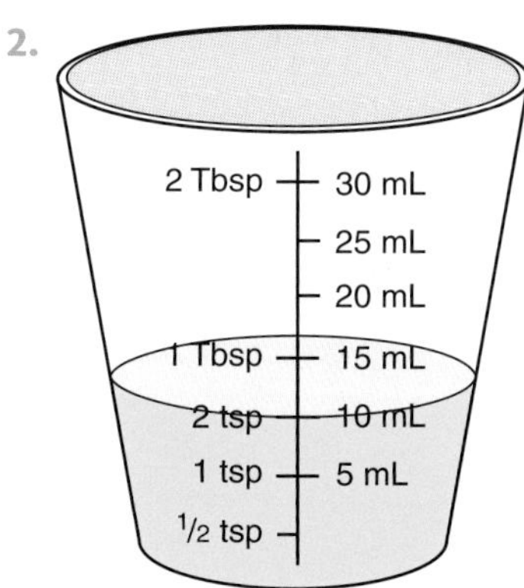

3. 1100

4.
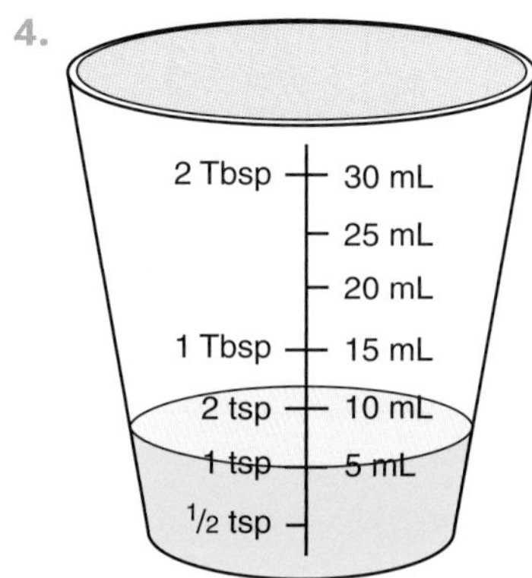

5. 2 tab

6.
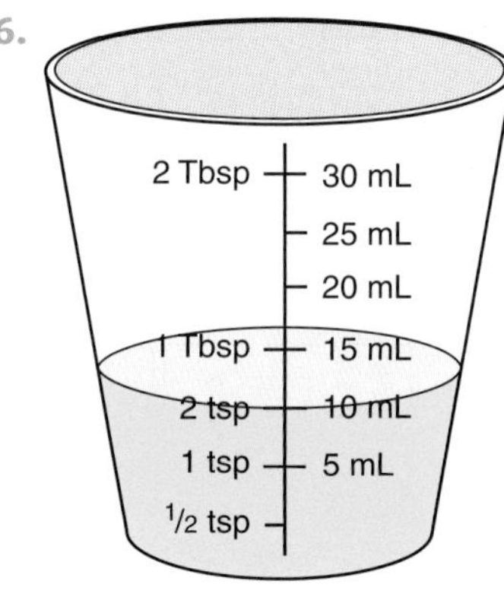

7. 2 tab

Case 6, *pp. 600–602*

1.
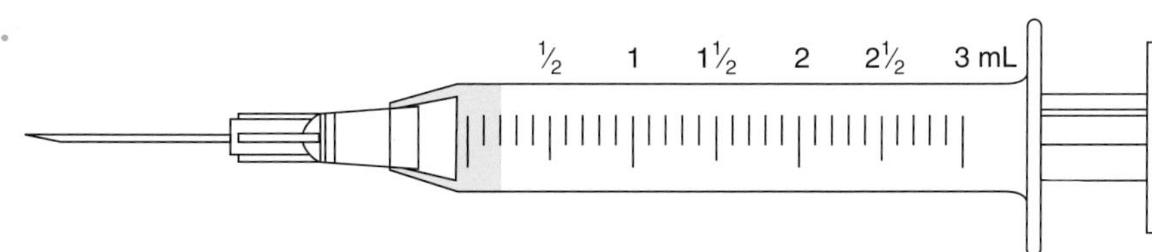

2. 75 mL/h

3.

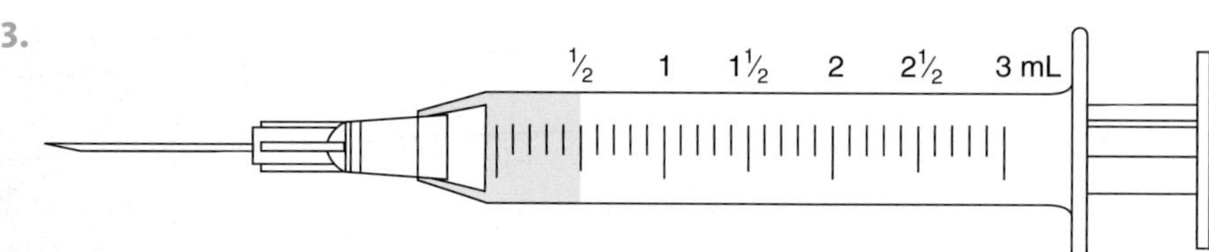

4. Diphenhydramine 25 mg
5.

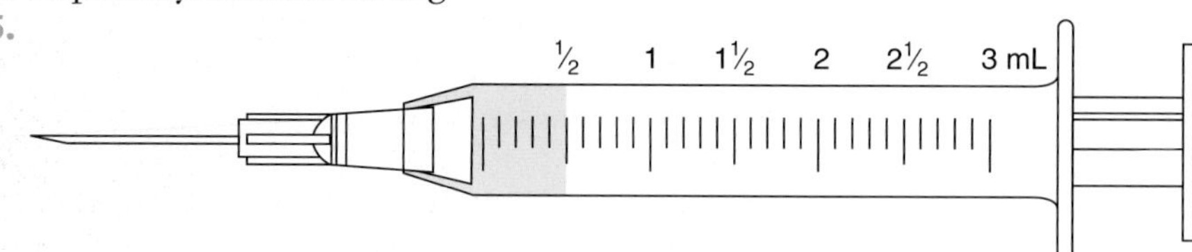

6.

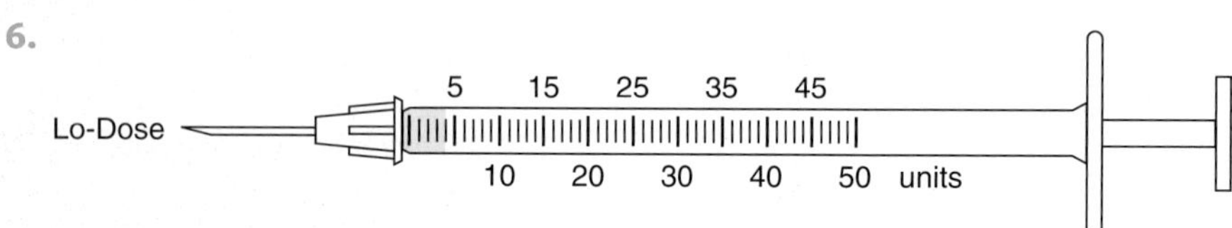

7. 33 gtt/min

Case 7, *p. 603*

1. 12 mL/h
2. 84 mL/h
3. 100 mL/h
4. 50 mL/h

Case 8, *pp. 604–605*

1. a. 5,400 units
   b.

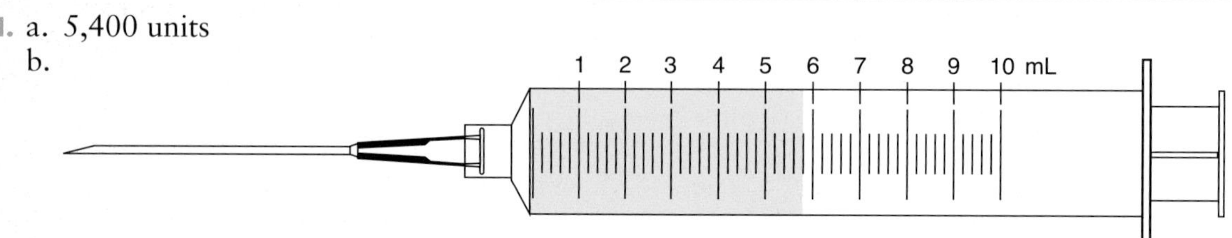

   c. 13.1 mL/h
2. 4.8, 5 mL/h

Case 9, *pp. 606–607*

1. a. Yes, 500 mg is between 303 and 606 mg, b. 20 mL
2. a. Yes, 15 mg is between 4.5 and 18.2 mg, b. 5 mL
3. a. Yes, 100 mg is between 91 and 182 mg, b. 6 mL
4. 18.2 kg; 1000 + 50 mL/kg > 10 kg; 1000 + (50 x 8.2) = 1,410 mL/24 h

Case 10, *p. 608*

1. Omission
2. Decrease the blood flow to the liver and kidneys
3. Inadequate income
4. (2 possible answers) Medication container or a book to record medication administration
5. Have the patient verbally repeat the instructions.

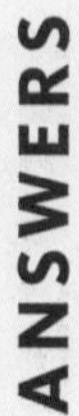

GLOSSARY

Addends the numbers to be added
Ampule a sealed glass container; usually contains one dose of a drug
Buccal between teeth and cheek
Canceling dividing numerator and denominator by a common number
Capsule a small soluble container for enclosing a single dose of medicine
Complex fraction a fraction whose numerator, denominator, or both contain fractions
Decimal fraction a fraction consisting of a numerator that is expressed in numerals, a decimal point that designates the value of the denominator, and the denominator, which is understood to be 10 or some power of 10
Decimal numbers include an integer, a decimal point, and a decimal fraction
Denominator the number of parts into which a whole has been divided
Difference the result of subtracting
Dividend the number being divided
Divisor the number by which another number is divided
Dosage the determination and regulation of the size, frequency, and number of doses
Dose the exact amount of medicine to be administered at one time
Drug a chemical substance used in therapy, diagnosis, and prevention of a disease or condition
Elixir a clear, sweet, hydroalcoholic liquid in which a drug is suspended
Equivalent equal
Extremes the first and fourth terms of a proportion
Fraction indicates the number of equal parts of a whole
Improper fraction a fraction whose numerator is larger than or equal to the denominator
Infusion the therapeutic introduction of a fluid into a vein by the flow of gravity
Injection the therapeutic introduction of a fluid into a part of the body by force
Integer a whole number
Intramuscular within the muscle
Intravenous within the vein
Invert turn upside down
Lowest common denominator the smallest whole number that can be divided evenly by all denominators within the problem
Means the second and third terms of a proportion
Medicine any drug
Milliequivalent the number of grams of a solute contained in 1 mL of a normal solution
Minuend the number from which another number is subtracted
Mixed number a combination of a whole number and a proper fraction
Multiplicand the number that is to be multiplied
Multiplier the number that another number is to be multiplied by
Numerator the number of parts of a divided whole
Oral dosage a medication taken by mouth
Parenteral dosage a dosage administered by routes that bypass the gastrointestinal tract; generally given by injection
Percent indicates the number of hundredths
Product the result of multiplying
Proper fraction a fraction whose numerator is smaller than the denominator
Proportion two ratios that are of equal value and are connected by a double colon, which symbolizes the word *as*
Quotient the answer to a division problem
Ratio the relationship between two numbers that are connected by a colon, which symbolizes the words *is to*
Reconstitution the return of a medication to its previous state by the addition of water or other designated liquid
Subcutaneous beneath the skin
Sublingual under the tongue
Subtrahend the number being subtracted
Sum the result of adding
Suspension a liquid in which a drug is distributed; must be shaken prior to use
Syrup a sweet, thick, aqueous liquid in which a drug is suspended
Tablet a drug compressed into a small disk
Topical on top of the skin or mucous membrane
Unit the amount of a drug needed to produce a given result
Vial a glass container with a rubber stopper; usually contains a number of doses of a drug

APPENDIX **A**

Apothecary System of Measure

The apothecary system of measure is a very old English system and is no longer used for medication ordering and administration. It has been replaced by the metric system.

Physicians occasionally used Roman numerals when writing orders in the apothecary system:

Roman Numeral	Arabic Numeral
i	1
v	5
x	10
l	50
c	100

Addition of Roman numerals is performed when a smaller numeral follows a larger numeral:

xi = 11
xv = 15
li = 51

Addition is performed when a numeral is repeated. However, a numeral is never repeated more than three times:

viii = 8
xii = 12
ccxi = 211

Subtraction is performed when a smaller numeral is placed before a larger numeral:

ix = 9
iv = 4
ic = 99

Subtraction is also performed when a smaller numeral is placed between two larger numerals. The smaller numeral is subtracted from the larger numeral that follows it:

xiv = 14
xxiv = 24
cxc = 190

COMMON APOTHECARY SYSTEM UNITS OF MEASURE

Apothecary Measure of Liquid
16 fluid ounces (fl oz) = 1 pint (pt)
32 fluid ounces (fl oz) = 2 pints (pt) or 1 quart (qt)
4 quarts (qt) = 1 gallon (gal)

APOTHECARY/HOUSEHOLD EQUIVALENTS

Apothecary Measure = Household Measure
8 fluid ounces (fl oz) = 1 standard measuring cup

INDEX